W9-AVJ-751

OCULAR PATHOLOGY

A COLOR ATLAS

Second Edition

OCULAR PATHOLOGY

A COLOR ATLAS

Second Edition

Myron Yanoff MD, FACS
Chairman and Professor, Department of Ophthalmology
Professor, Department of Pathology
Hahnemann University School of Medicine
Adjunct Professor of Pathology
University of Pennsylvania School of Medicine
1988 Distinguished Senior US Scientist Awardee (Humboldt-Awardee)
Former Chairman and William F. Norris and George E. deSchweinitz Professor
Department of Ophthalmology
University of Pennsylvania School of Medicine
Former Director, Scheie Eye Institute and Department of Ophthalmology
Presbyterian-University of Pennsylvania Medical Center
Philadelphia, Pennsylvania

Ben S. Fine MD
Research Associate, Department of Ophthalmic Pathology
Armed Forces Institute of Pathology
Associate Research Professor of Ophthalmology
The George Washington University
Senior Attending Ophthalmologist
The Washington Hospital Center
Washington DC
Clinical Professor of Pathology
Uniformed Services
University of the Health Sciences
Bethesda, Maryland

Gower Medical Publishing New York • London

Distributed in the USA and Canada by:

Raven Press
1185 Avenue of the Americas
New York, NY 10036
USA

Gower Medical Publishing
101 Fifth Avenue
New York, NY 10003
USA

Distributed in Japan by:

Nankodo Company, Ltd.
42-6, Hongo 3-Chome,
Bunkyo-Ku
Tokyo 113
Japan

Distributed in the rest of the world by:

Gower Medical Publishing
Middlesex House
34-42 Cleveland Street
London, W1P 5FB
UK

Library of Congress Cataloging-in-Publication Data

Yanoff, Myron.
Ocular pathology: a color atlas/Myron Yanoff, Ben S. Fine.—2nd ed.
p. cm.
Companion v. to: Ocular pathology: a text and atlas/ Myron Yanoff, Ben S. Fine, 3rd ed. c1989
Includes bibliographical references and index.
ISBN 1-56375-009-0
1. Eye—Diseases and defects—Atlases. 2. Eye—Wounds and injuries—Atlases. I. Fine, Ben S., 1928- . II. Title.
[DNLM: 1. Eye Diseases—pathology—atlases. WW 17 Y24o]
RE50.Y36 1989 Suppl.
617.7'1—dc20
DNLM/DLC
for Library of Congress 91-42755

British Library Cataloguing in Publication Data
Yanoff, Myron
Atlas of ocular pathology. — 2nd ed
I. Title II. Fine, Ben S. (Ben Sion), *1928-*
617.71

ISBN 1-56375-009-0

Editor: Jane Hunter
Art Director: Jill Feltham
Designer: Anne Kenney
Illustrators: Alan Landau, Carol Kalafatic
Editorial Assistant: Alison Marek

10 9 8 7 6 5 4 3 2 1

Printed in Singapore by Imago Productions (FE) PTE Ltd.

PREFACE

In 1988 we published our first edition of *Ocular Pathology: A Color Atlas*. The book, a highly selective color atlas of ocular pathology, was meant to be a companion to the second edition of *Ocular Pathology: A Text and Atlas*, which was published in 1982. Since then, considerable new material has accumulated in such areas as immunohistochemistry, AIDS, and complications of intraocular implant surgery. Much of this new material was incorporated in our third edition of *Ocular Pathology: A Text and Atlas*, published in 1989.

We now have updated the companion Atlas. In addition to revising the accompanying text, we have added 76 new color pictures and have exchanged or updated, or both, numerous other illustrations. Also, in the 10 of the 18 chapters that deal with structures (e.g., conjunctiva, cornea, uvea, retina, etc.) we have added a brief review of normal anatomy at the beginning of each chapter. Finally, in response to an apparent need, we have increased the size of the pages in order to present illustrations that generally are larger than those appearing in the first edition.

Our hope is that this second edition of *Ocular Pathology: A Color Atlas* will give the student (from resident to practicing ophthalmologist and pathologist) a comprehensive overview and understanding of ocular pathology in a concise, interesting format. For a more in-depth review, the reader is referred to the third edition of *Ocular Pathology: A Text and Atlas* and any of the other numerous textbooks of ocular pathology published over the last decade.

It is always with great pleasure that we thank Lorenz E. Zimmerman, MD, who continues to be our teacher in ophthalmic pathology. We also are grateful to Professor G.O.H. Naumann for his superb advice and steadying influence. Abe Krieger, president of Gower Medical Publishing, allowed his enthusiasm and excess energy to flow and energize us. Jane Hunter, our editor at Gower, did a superb job in keeping the project and us on target, and Anne Kenney, who designed this second edition, has produced an elegant book. Most of all we thank Karin L. Yanoff, PhD, and both the Yanoff children (Steven, David, Joanne, and Alexis), and the Fine children (Nina and Sharon) for their loving help and tolerance during our preparation of this book. We deeply miss that wonderful, kind, gentle person whose love, tenderness, and indomitable free spirit are no longer with us. To her, Fruma I. Fine, with much love, we dedicate this book.

Myron Yanoff
Ben S. Fine

Contents

Basic Principles of Pathology

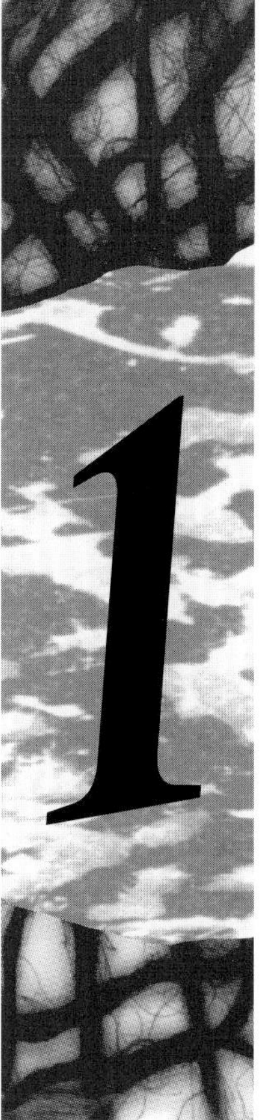

A tissue responds to a noxious stimulus by a process called inflammation. Generally, inflammation may be considered as a nonspecific or specific immune reaction to a foreign agent. The noxious stimulus or foreign agent may be infectious or noninfectious, and any individual tissue or some combination of tissues may be affected.

Both noninfectious agents, such as chemicals or allergens, or infectious agents, such as bacteria and fungi, may induce inflammation. Inflammation may be endogenous or exogenous. Endogenous inflammation is caused by a process occurring in the eye itself, such as phacolytic glaucoma in which leaking denatured lens protein induces a macrophagic inflammatory reaction. Exogenous inflammation is caused by a process occurring at a remote site, an example of which is bacterial endocarditis sending emboli to the retina, resulting in infectious retinitis.

The inflammatory process consists of both cellular components and chemical mediators. The interaction of different factors, including histamine, serotonin, kinins, and others, results in the cardinal signs of inflammation—redness, heat, edema, pain, and loss of function. An inflammatory reaction may be divided into an acute phase, a subacute or intermediate phase, and a chronic phase. The subacute or intermediate phase is most closely related to the immune reaction.

The chronic phase may be divided into nongranulomatous and granulomatous types. The nongranulomatous type is characterized by the presence of lymphocytes and plasma cells. A cause for this type of inflammation usually is not found. The granulomatous type is characterized by the presence of epithelioid cells, and the cause (e.g., tuberculosis and toxoplasmosis) often is found. The granulomatous type commonly shows inflammatory giant cells, such as foreign body, Langhans, and Touton giant cells. The inflammatory pattern may be helpful in identifying a cause. For example, a diffuse granulomatous pattern is seen in sympathetic uveitis, a discrete pattern in sarcoidosis, and a zonal pattern in phacoanaphylactic endophthalmitis.

The entities that cause inflammation will be illustrated in the appropriate chapters. Here, concepts of humoral and cellular immunity are illustrated.

In order to identify causative agents of inflammation, as well as tissue components of many other types of pathological processes, diagnostic immunohistochemistry is an essential component of a modern laboratory of histopathology. A wide spectrum of immunologic reagents now is available, at both the light- and electron-microscopic level, to help identify such diverse things as viral particles, desmin, lambda chains, and S-100 protein. Some examples of tissue immunostaining are given here. Other examples will be found in the appropriate chapters.

TYPES OF INFLAMMATION

Acute (exudative)
Polymorphonuclear leukocytes
Mast cells and eosinophils

Subacute (intermediate)
Healing
Chronicity

Chronic (proliferative)
Nongranulomatous: lymphocytes and plasma cells
Granulomatous: epithelioid cells

FIGURE 1.1

CELLS INVOLVED IN ACUTE INFLAMMATION

Polymorphonuclear leukocyte
Bone-marrow-derived
First line of cellular defense
Drawn to site by chemotaxis
Marginate in venules by adhering to wall junction
Emigrate between endothelial cells into tissue
Remove noxious agents (bacteria) by phagocytosis and lysosomal digestion

Eosinophilic leukocyte
Bone-marrow-derived
Found in allergic and parasitic conditions
Phagocytic
Granules contain proteolytic enzymes

Mast cell (basophilic leukocyte)
Fixed tissue cells
Elaborate heparin and histamine
Basophils can be considered circulating mast cells

FIGURE 1.2

GRANULATION TISSUE INVOLVED IN SUBACUTE INFLAMMATION

Acute and chronic inflammatory cells
Fibroblasts
Vascular endothelial cells

FIGURE 1.3

TYPES OF CHRONIC INFLAMMATION

Granulomatous
Epithelioid cells necessary for diagnosis
Inflammatory giant cells often present
Good chance of finding cause

Nongranulomatous
Lymphocyte (competent immunocyte)
- B-lymphocyte
- T-lymphocyte

Plasma cells
Cause rarely found

FIGURE 1.4

COMPETENT IMMUNOCYTES SEEN IN CHRONIC INFLAMMATION

B-Lymphocyte
Bone-marrow-derived
Active in humoral immunity
Source of immunoglobulin
Plasma cell precursor
Function: immunity to bacteria and neutralization of toxins

T-Lymphocyte
Modified by thymus gland
Active in cell-mediated immunity
Produces a variety of lymphokines
Function: immunity to mycobacteria, viruses, fungi; graft rejection

FIGURE 1.5

MACROPHAGE (HISTIOCYTE) SEEN IN CHRONIC INFLAMMATION

Circulating monocytes and tissue histiocytes
Chief phagocyte
Processes antigen for lymphocytes in immune reaction
Epithelioid cell and giant cell precursor

FIGURE 1.6

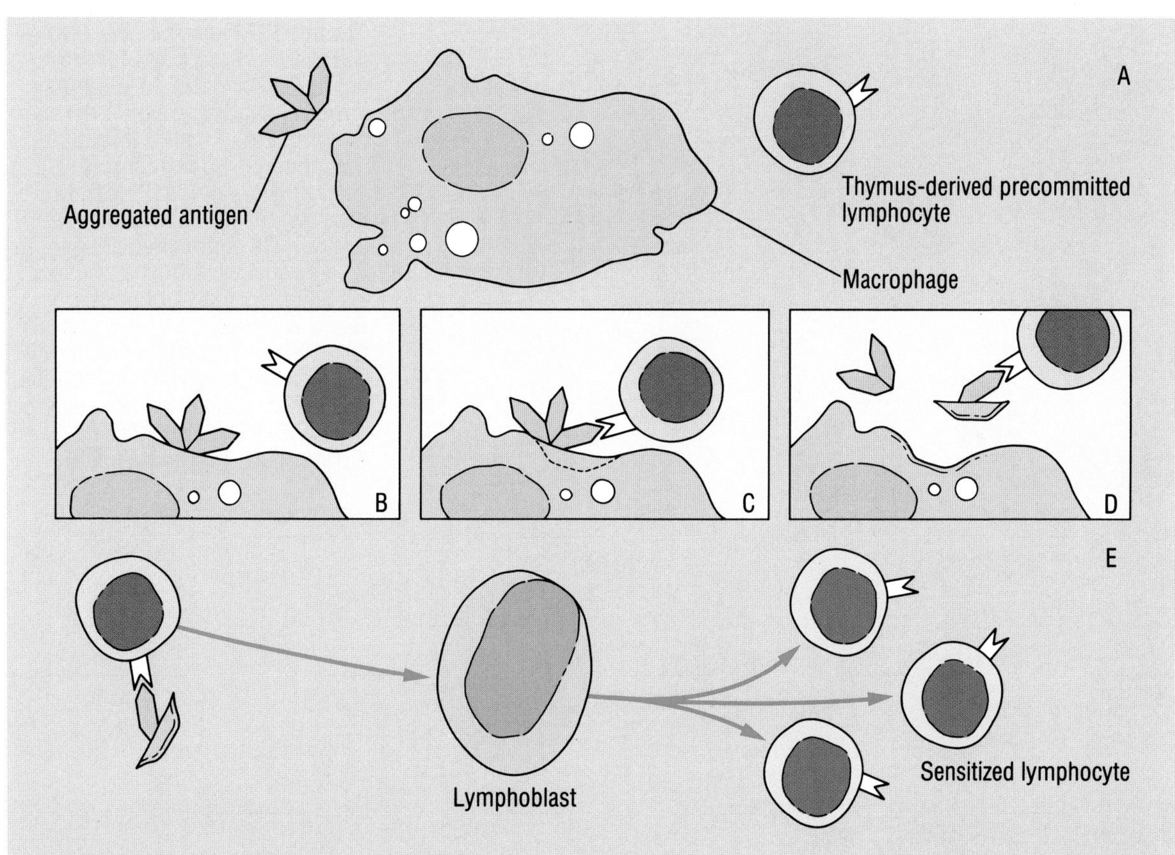

FIGURE 1.7 CELLULAR IMMUNITY. **A** The participants in the cellular immune response include the thymus-derived precommitted lymphocyte (T-cell), bone-marrow- derived monocyte (macrophage), and the aggregated antigens. **B** Aggregated antigen is seen attaching to the surface of the macrophage. **C** The T-cell is shown as it attaches to the aggregated antigen. **D** The substance originating in the macrophage passes into the T-cell, which is attached to the antigen. **E** The combined T-cell, antigen, and macrophagic material causes the T-cell to enlarge into a lymphoblast. Sensitized, or committed, T-lymphocytes arise from lymphoblasts.

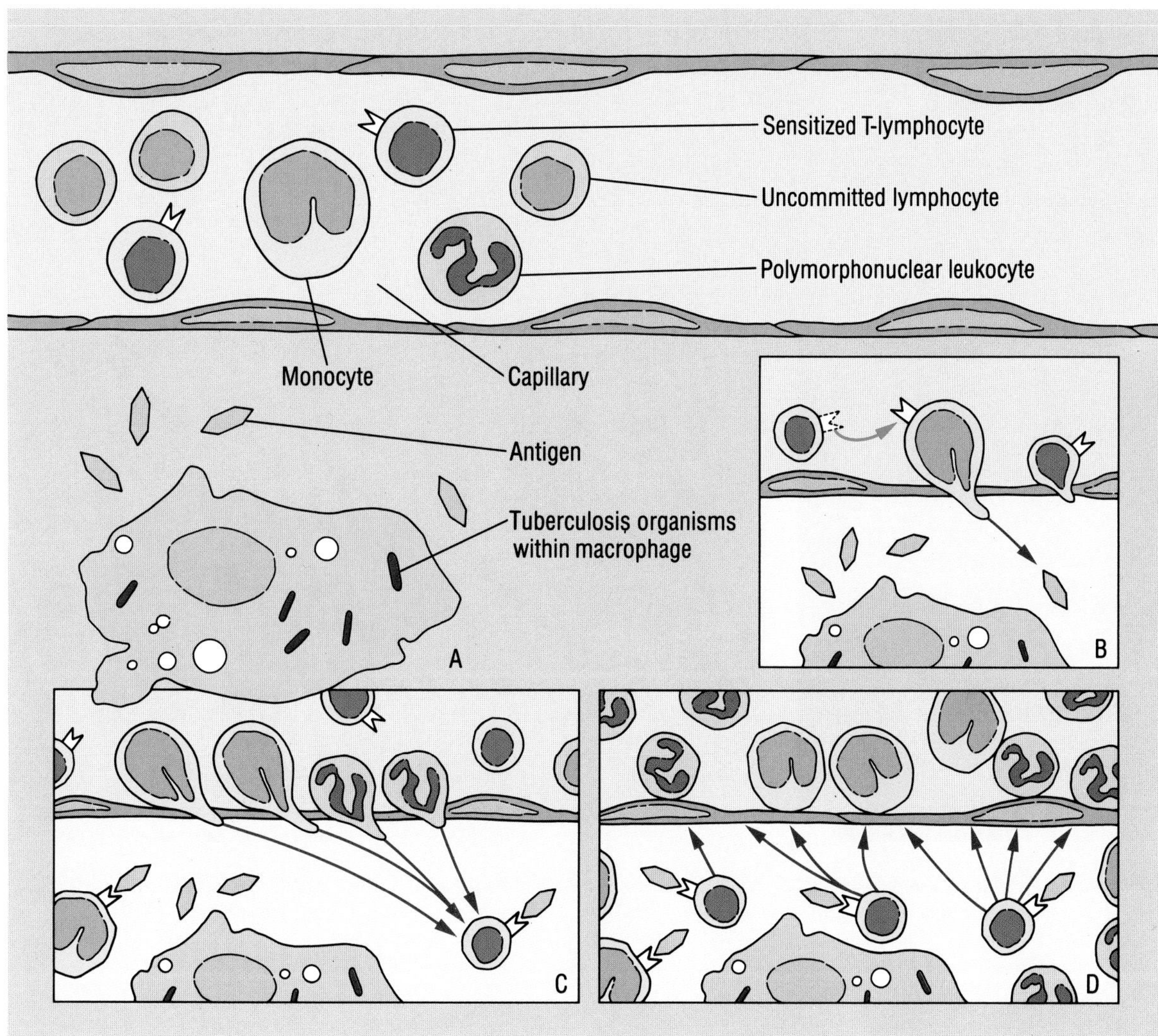

FIGURE 1.8 CELLULAR IMMUNITY. **A** Sensitized T-lymphocytes (SL) are seen in a capillary. Along with the SLs are other leukocytes, including monocytes, at an antigenic site. A macrophage, which contains tubercle bacilli, and antigen may be seen in the surrounding tissue. **B** Monocytes become sensitized when cytophilic antibody from SL is transferred to them. They migrate toward the antigenic stimulus. **C** Biologically active molecules, which cause the monocytes and leukocytes to travel to the area, are released by SL when they have encountered a specific antigen. **D** Monocytes arriving at the site are immobilized by migration-inhibitory factor (MIF), which is released by SL, which also releases cytotoxin and mitogenic factor. Cytotoxin causes tissue necrosis (caseation), and mitogenic factor causes proliferation of cells. Some of these cells undergo transformation, becoming epithelioid cells, causing the formation of a tuberculoma.

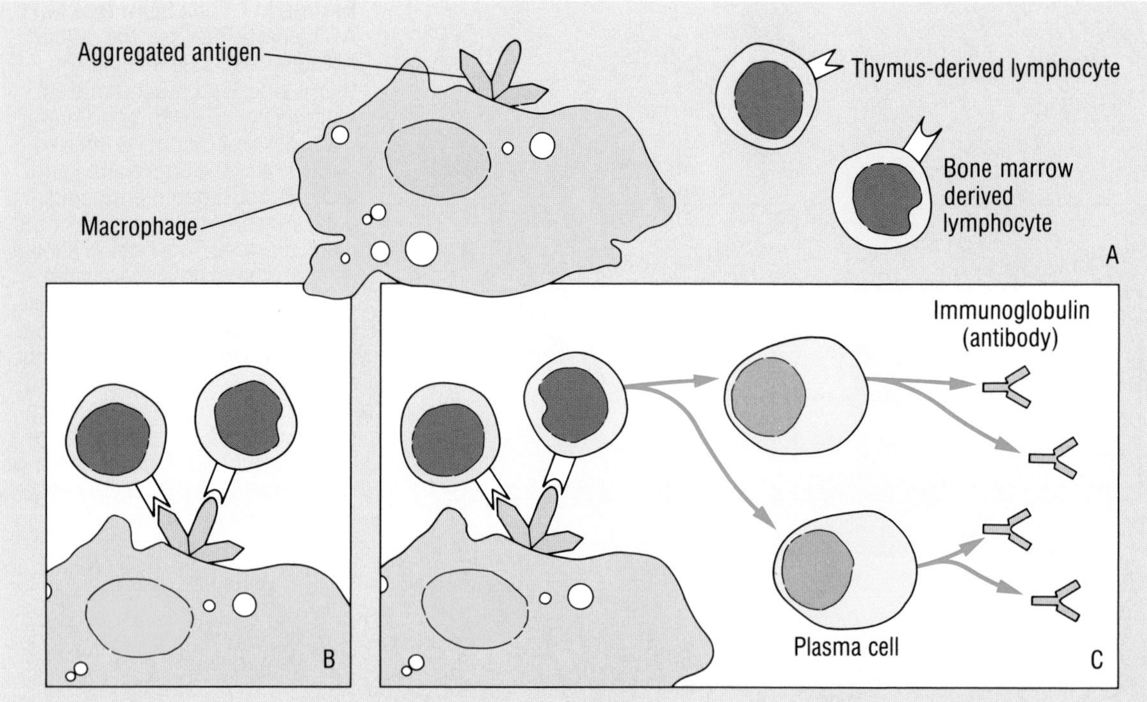

FIGURE 1.9 HUMORAL IMMUNITY. **A, B** Four prerequisites for immunoglobulin formation are demonstrated including thymus-derived lymphocyte (T-cell), thymus-independent bone-marrow-derived lymphocyte (B-cell), bone-marrow-derived monocyte (macrophage), and aggregated antigen. In **A**, aggregated antigens are seen attached to macrophages. In **B**, T- and B-cells are seen attached to different determinants on the aggregated antigen. **C** Cooperative interaction that occurs between the T- and B-cells causes the B-cells to differentiate into plasma cells.

NONINFLAMMATORY CELLULAR AND TISSUE REACTIONS

Hypertrophy—increased size of individual cells
Hyperplasia—increased number of individual cells
Aplasia—lack of embryologic development of a tissue
Hypoplasia—arrest of embryologic development of a tissue
Metaplasia—tranformation of one type of tissue into another
Atrophy—decrease in size of fully developed tissue
Neoplasia—continuous, unregulated increase of cells in a tissue
Degeneration—change in a tissue resulting from previous diseases
Dystrophy—primary inheritable disorder
Necrosis—death of cells
Calcification

FIGURE 1.10

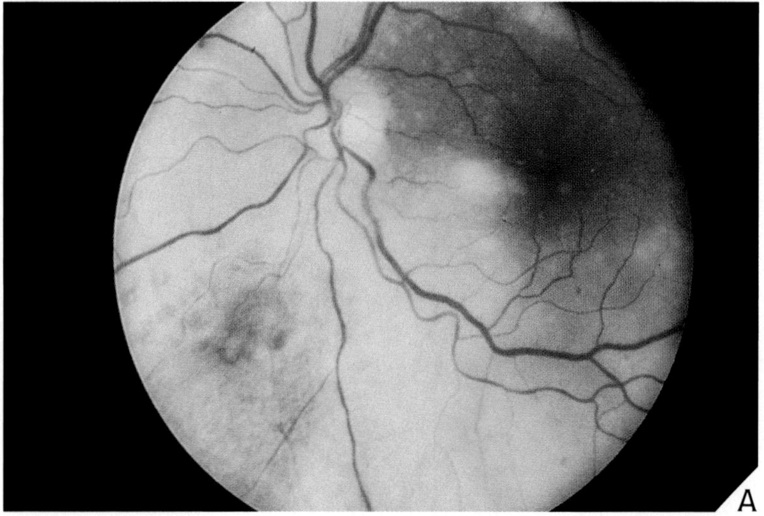

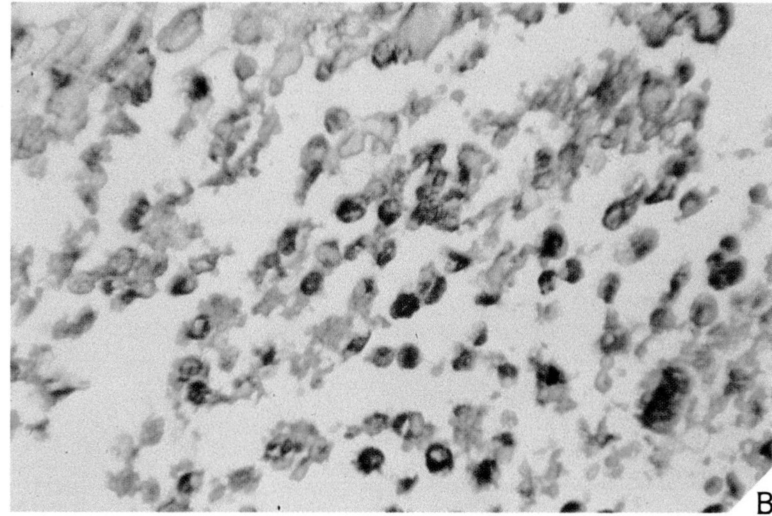

FIGURE 1.11 IMMUNOCYTOCHEMISTRY. **A** Areas of retinal necrosis found in AIDS patient who has HSV retinitis. **B** HS V-1 particles in necrotic retina. Immunoperoxidase stain with anti-HSV-1 antibody. (From Ioachim HL: *Pathology of AIDS*. Gower Medical Publishing, New York, 1989.)

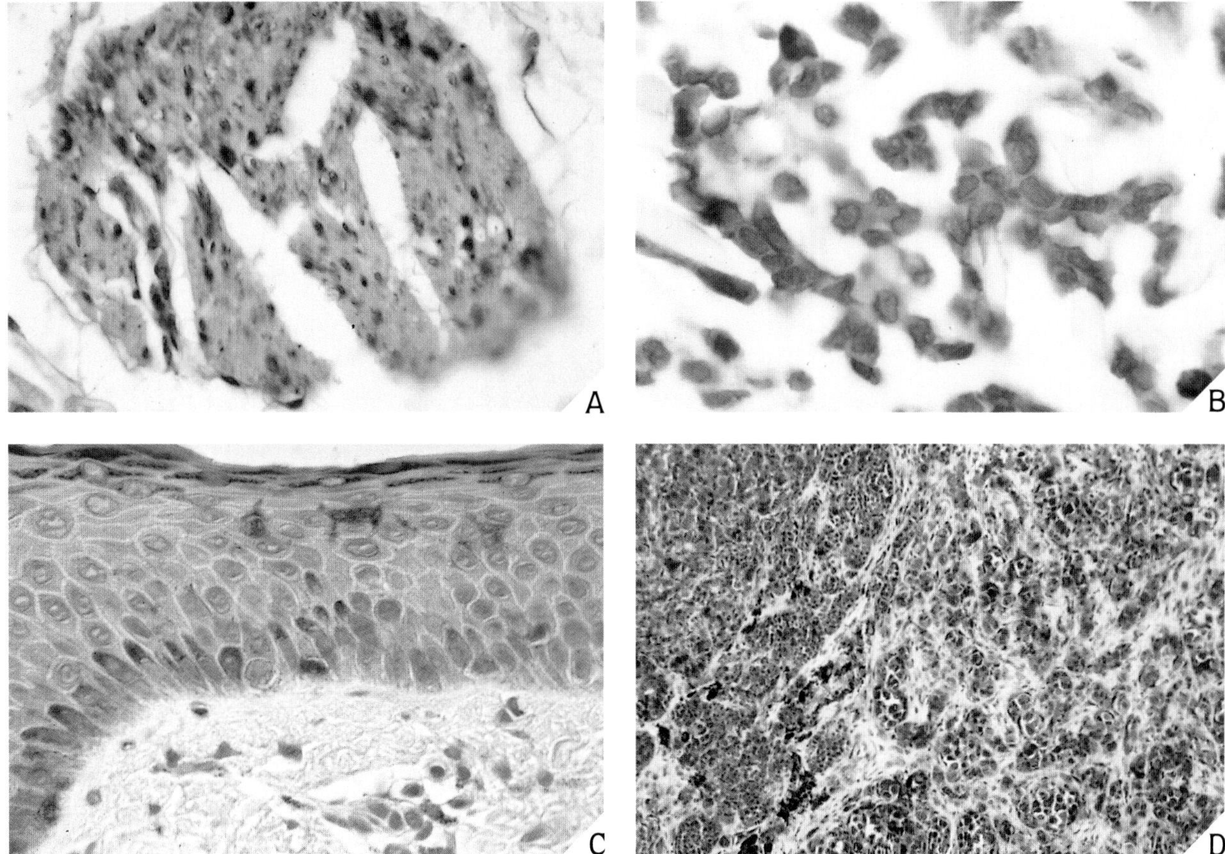

FIGURE 1.12 IMMUNOCYTOCHEMISTRY. A Monoclonal antibody against desmin, one of the cytoskeletal filaments, reacts with both smooth and striated muscles and helps to identify tumors of muscular origin. **B** Monoclonal antibody against lambda chains reacts with lambda chains in plasma cells. **C, D** Polyclonal antibody against S 100 protein identifies melanocytes and Langerhans cells in epidermis **C** and in malignant melanoma cells **D**. (From Shaumburg-Lever G, Lever WF, *Color Atlas of Histopathology of the Skin*. J.B. Lippincott Company, Philadelphia, 1988.)

Bibliography

Blackman M, Kappler J, Marrack P: The role of the T cell receptor in positive and negative selection of developing T cells. Science 248:1335, 1990.

Elias JM, Margiotta M, Gaborc D: Sensitivity and detection efficiency of the peroxidase antiperoxidase (PAP), avidin-biotin peroxidase complex (ABC), and peroxidase-labeled avidinbiotin (LAB) methods. Am J Clin Pathol 92:62, 1989.

Ioachim HL: *Pathology of AIDS*, Philadelphia: JB Lippincott; New York, London: Gower Medical Publishing, 1989, p. 238.

Jakobiec FA, Lefkowitch J, Knowles DM: B- and T-lymphocytes in ocular disease. Ophthalmology 91:635, 1984.

James DG, Graham E, Hamblin A: Review. Immunology of multisystem ocular disease. Surv Ophthalmol 30:155, 1985.

Milanese C, Richardson NE, Reinherz EL: Identification of a T helper cell-derived lymphokine that activates resting T lymphocytes. Science 231:1118, 1986.

Nago K, Yukoro K, Aaronson SA: Continuous lines of basophil/mast cells derived from normal mouse bone marrow. Science 212:333, 1981.

Quigley HA, Kenyon KR: Russell bodies and plasma cells in human conjunctiva. Am J Ophthalmol 76:957, 1973.

Ratech H, Litwin S: Surface immunoglobulin light chain restriction in ß-cell non-Hodgkin's malignant lymphoma. Am J Clin Pathol 91:583, 1989.

Schaumburg-Lever G, Lever WF: *Color Atlas of Histopathology of the Skin*. Philadelphia: JB Lippincott Company, 1988, pp. 10-13.

Truong LD, Rangdaeng S, Cagle P, et al: The diagnostic utility of desmin. A study of 584 cases and review of the literature. Am J Clin Pathol 93:305, 1990.

Turk JL: Immunologic and nonimmunologic activation of macrophages. J Invest Dermatol 74:301, 1980.

Turner RR, Egbert P, Warnke RA: Lymphocytic infiltrates of the conjunctiva and orbit: immunohistochemical staining of 16 cases. Am J Clin Pathol 81:447, 1984.

Weiss SJ, et al: Oxidative autoactivation of latent collagenase by human neutrophils. Science 227:747, 1985.

Williams GT, Williams WJ: Granulomatous inflammation—a review. J Clin Pathol 36:723, 1983.

Zimmerman LE: Ocular lesions of juvenile xanthogranuloma. Nevoxanthoendothelioma. Trans Am Acad Ophthalmol Otolaryngol 69:412, 1965.

Congenital Anomalies

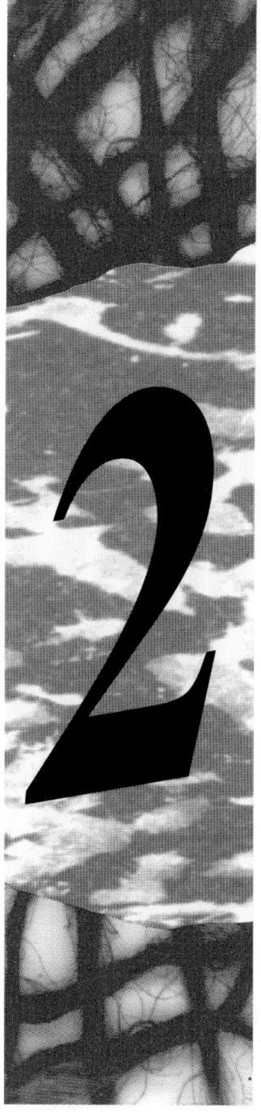

Congenital ocular anomalies that are associated with systemic anomalies may have a variety of causes. Broadly, the causes may be subdivided into:

- chromosomal aberrations;
- infectious embryopathies;
- drug embryopathies;
- phakomatoses;
- other entities.

In chromosomal aberrations, the normal total number of chromosomes (44 autosomes and two sex chromosomes) may be present, but individual chromosomes may have structural alterations, as occurs in the chromosome 18 deletion defect, in which one of the arms of the chromosome is deleted. Alternatively, the total number of chromosomes may be abnormal, either too few (45) as in Turner syndrome or too many (47) as in Down syndrome. Other aberrations, such as mosaicism, also occur.

Infectious embryopathies such as rubella and toxoplasmosis result from infection of the embryo *in utero*, which is especially susceptible during the first trimester of gestation. Similarly, drug embryopathies are caused by substances such as alcohol that cross the blood-placental barrier from mother to fetus, adversely affecting the embryo. Again, the fetus is most susceptible during the first trimester of gestation.

The phakomatoses are a group of congenital tumors of genetic origin that have in common the characteristic of disseminated hamartomas, usually benign. In an individual phakomatosis, the hamartomas tend to affect one type of tissue predominantly; e.g., blood vessels in meningocutaneous angiomatoses (Sturge-Weber syndrome), and peripheral nerves in type 1 neurofibromatosis.

Many other congenital ocular and systemic anomalies, similar to the phakomatoses, have a genetic origin but are not easily classified in groups. Still other anomalies seem to occur by chance, and have no known cause.

CHROMOSOMAL ABERRATIONS SEEN IN CONGENITAL ANOMALIES

Defect in number

Trisomy (47 chromosomes)
- Trisomy 13
- Trisomy 18
- Trisomy 21 (Down syndrome)

Triploidy (69 chromosomes)

Turner syndrome (45 chromosomes)

Deletion defect (46 chromosomes)

Chromosome 5 (*cri-du-chat* syndrome)

Chromosome 11p13 (aniridia-Wilms tumor syndrome)

Chromosome 13 (may be associated with retinoblastoma)

Chromosome 18

Mosaicism

Two or more populations of karyotypically distinct chromosomes

FIGURE 2.1

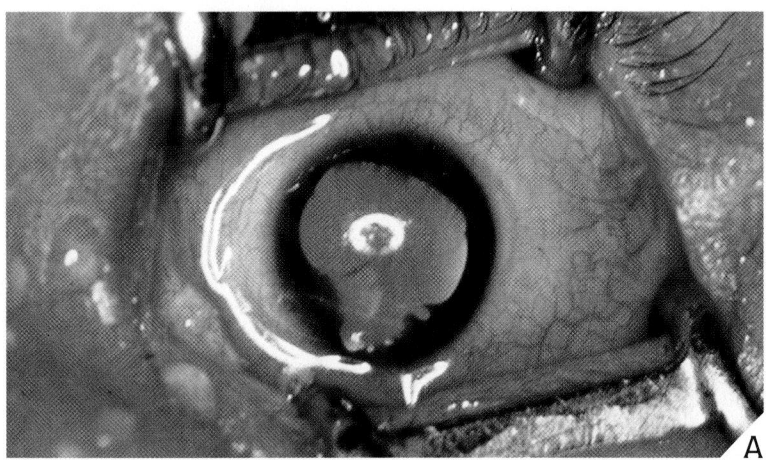

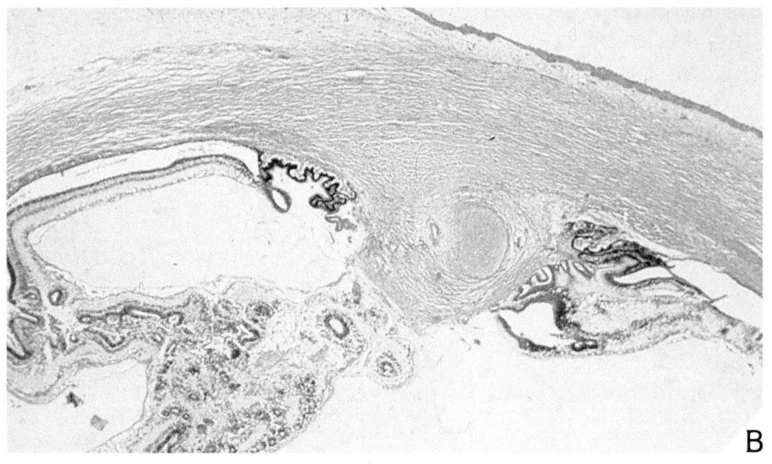

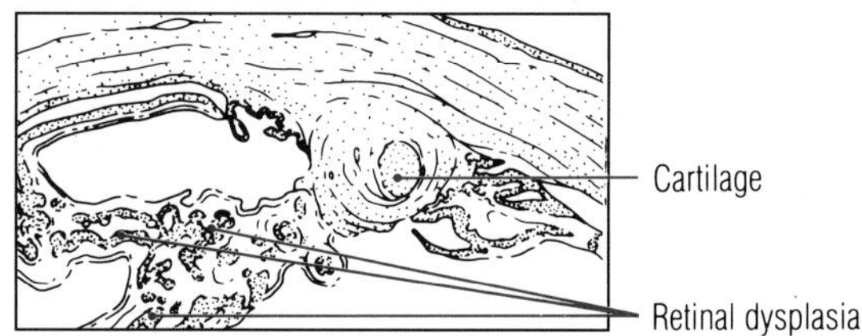

FIGURE 2.2 TRISOMY 13. A An inferior nasal iris coloboma and leukokoria are present. **B** A coloboma of the ciliary body is filled with mesenchymal tissue containing cartilage. Note the retinal dysplasia. Generally, in trisomy 13 cartilage is present in microphthalmic eyes smaller than 10 mm in size. (**A**, courtesy of Dr. DB Schaffer; **B**, reported in Hoepner J, Yanoff M, 1972.)

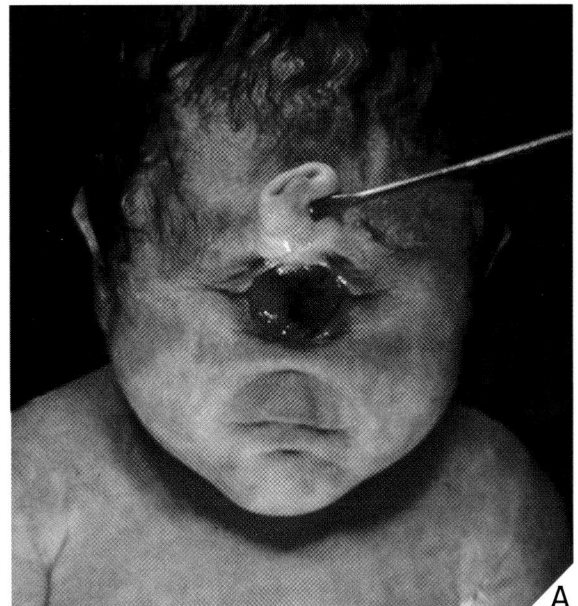

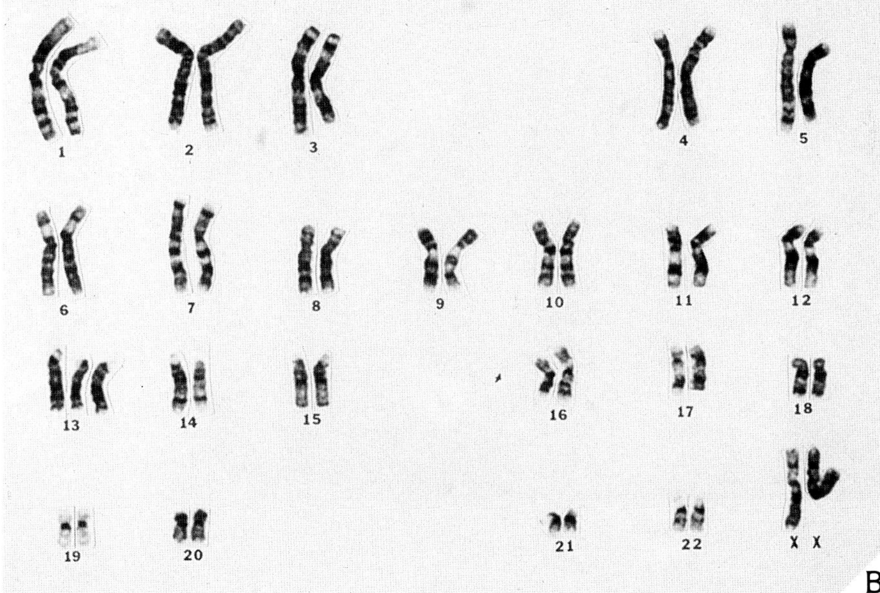

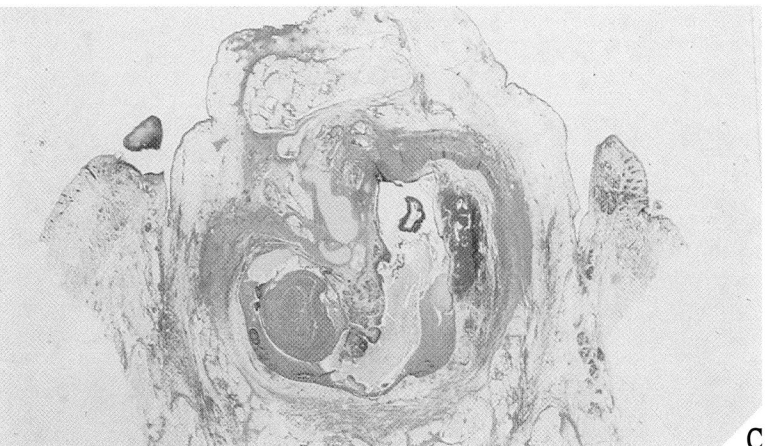

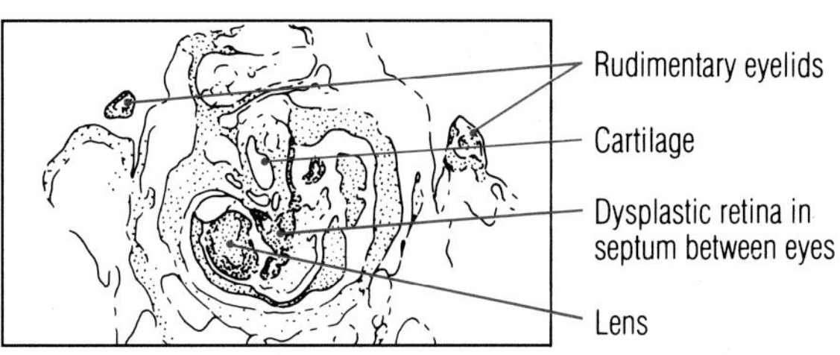

Figure 2.3 Trisomy 13. A The patient was born with clinical cyclops. When the proboscis is lifted, a single pseudo-orbit is seen clinically. Note the fairly well formed eyelids under the proboscis. **B** Karyotype from the same patient shows an extra chromosome (three instead of two) in the 13 group. **C** Histologic section shows that the condition is not true cyclops (a single eye), but the more commonly seen synophthalmos (partial fusion of the two eyes).

Morbid Embryopathies Seen in Congenital Anomalies

Infectious embryopathies
Toxoplasmosis
Cytomegalic inclusion disease
Congenital rubella syndrome
Congenital syphilis

Drug embryopathies
Thalidomide
Lysergic acid diethylamide (LSD)
Fetal alcohol syndrome

Figure 2.4

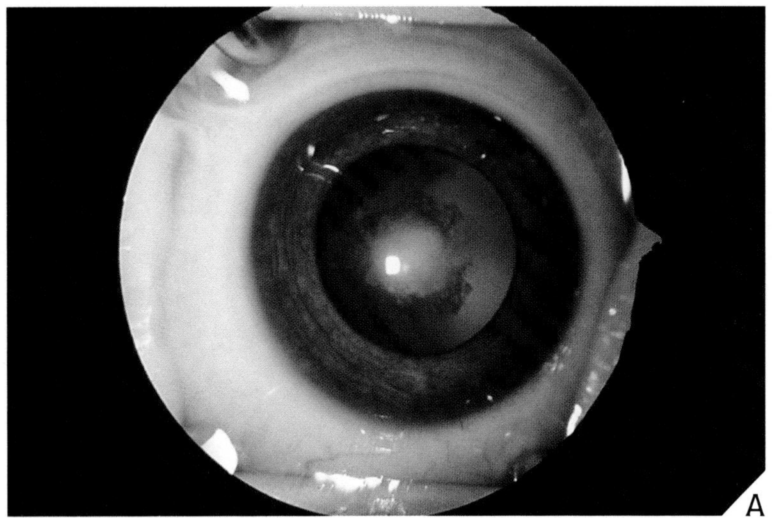

FIGURE 2.5 RUBELLA. A A dense nuclear cataract is seen in the pupillary red reflex, surrounded by a less dense cortical cataract. Congenital infection with rubella is characterized by ocular and cardiovascular abnormalities and deafness. The most common ocular finding is a "salt and pepper" fundus, followed by cataract. **B** Histologic section shows a cataractous lens. **C** High magnification shows retention of lens cell nuclei within the fetal nucleus of the lens. (**A**, courtesy of Dr. DB Schaffer.)

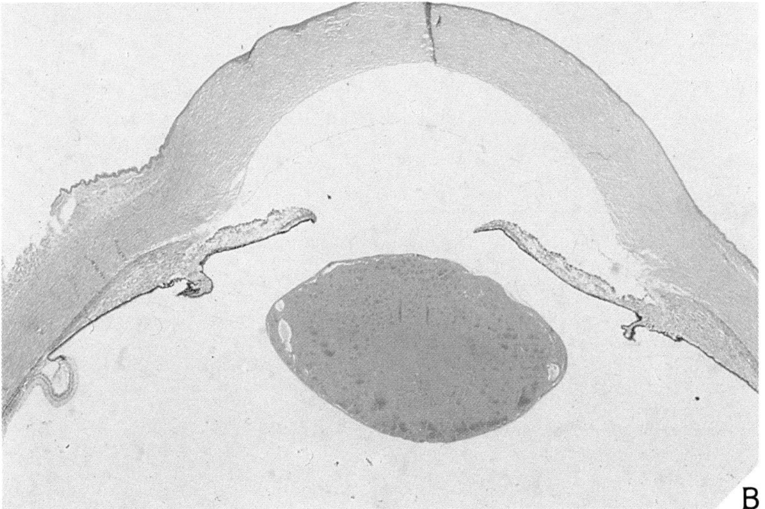

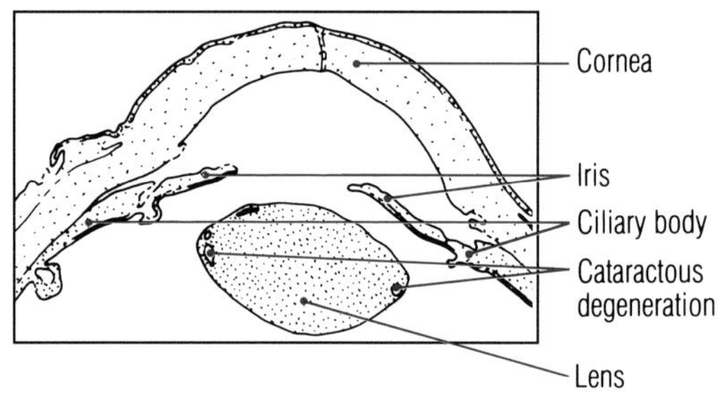

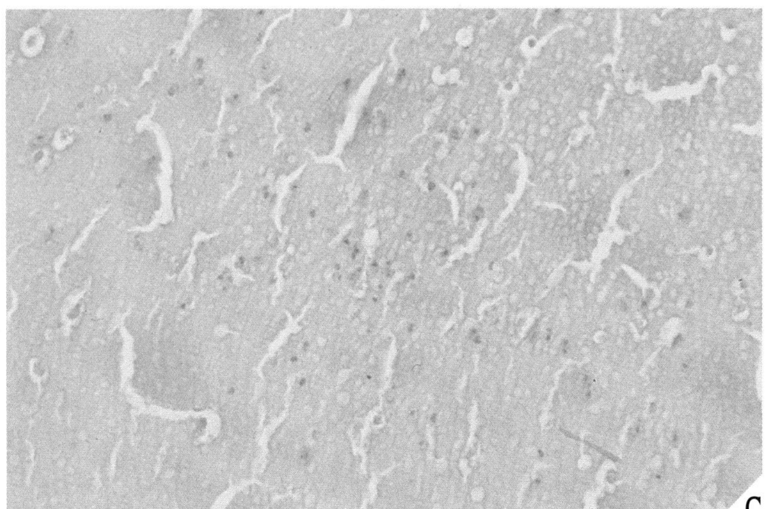

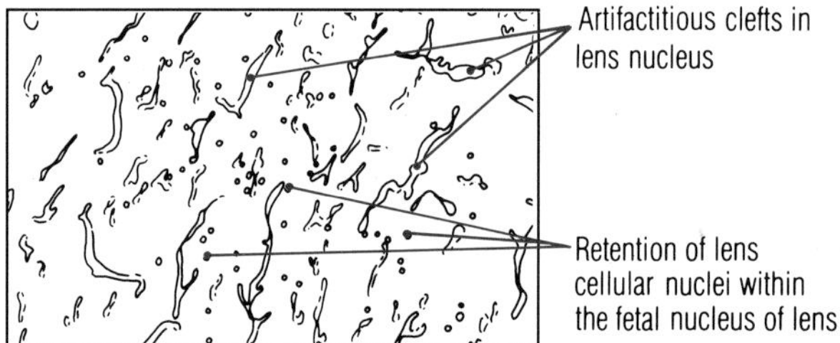

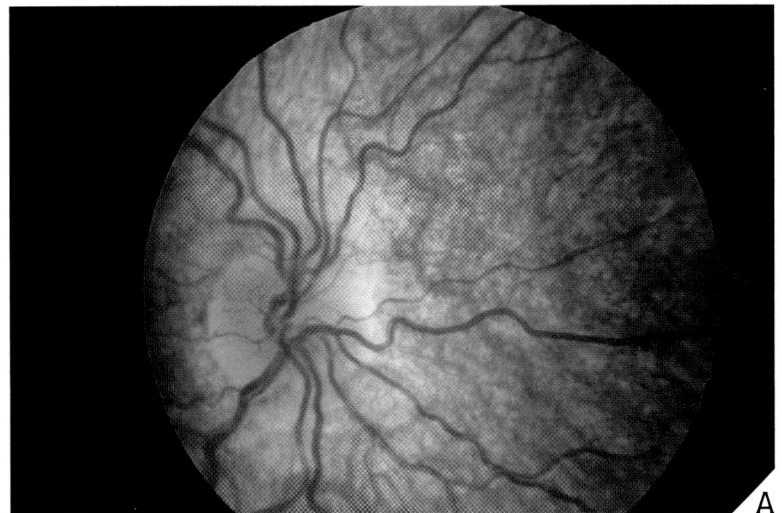

Figure 2.6 Rubella. A Both fine and coarse pigmentation are present in the fundus at the level of the retinal pigment epithelium (RPE). **B** Histologic section shows that the RPE is hypertrophied in this region whereas in other regions, shown in **C**, the pigment epithelium is atrophic and has lost most of its pigment. It is the alternating areas of hypertrophy and atrophy of the RPE that give rise to the clinical picture of "salt and pepper" fundus. (**A**, courtesy of Dr. DB Schaffer.)

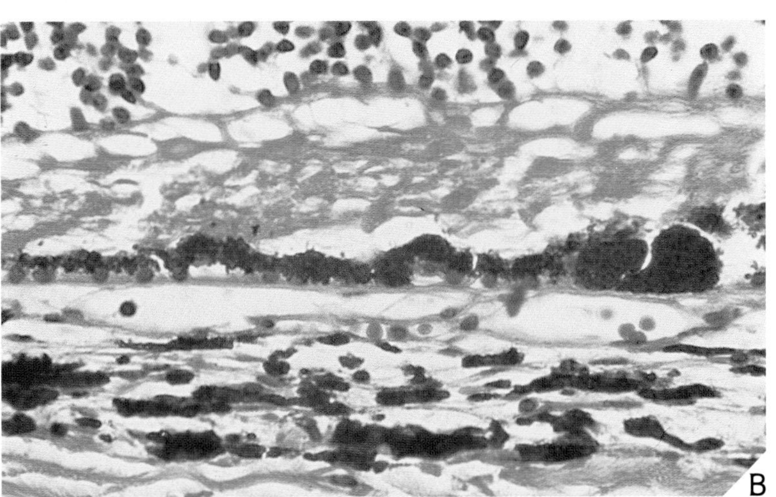

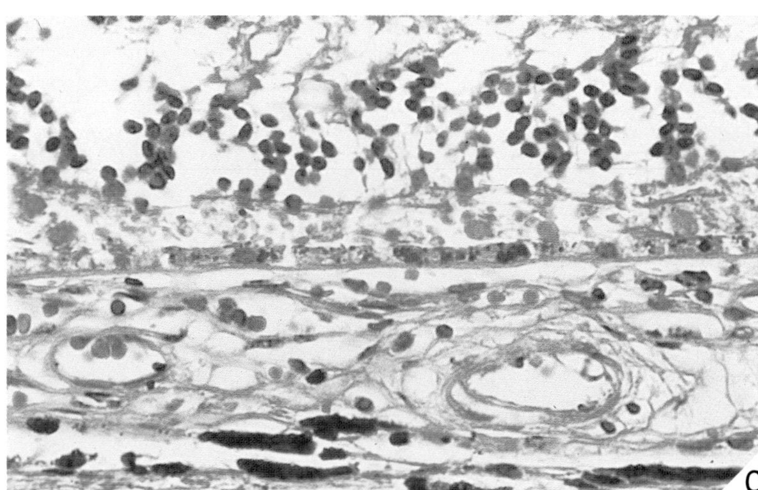

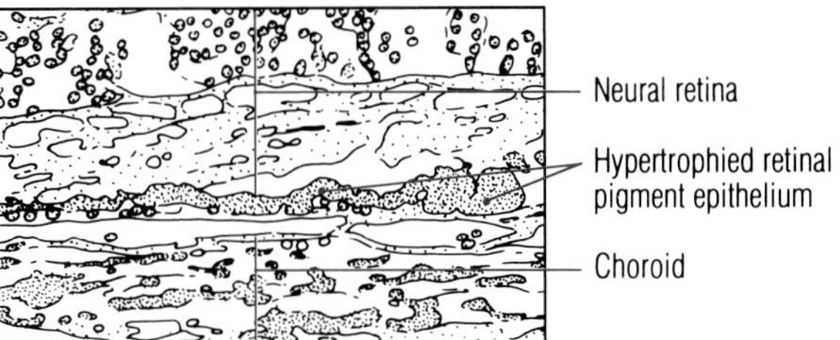

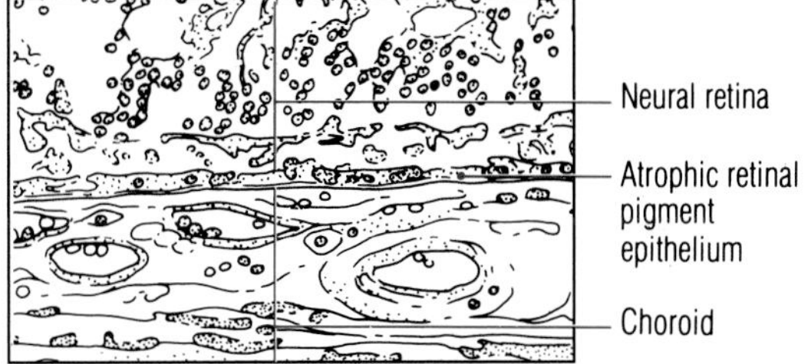

Phakomatoses

Angiomatosis retinae (von Hippel disease)
Meningocutaneous angiomatosis (Sturge-Weber syndrome)
Neurofibromatosis (von Recklinghausen disease)
Tuberous sclerosis (Bourneville disease)
Ataxia telangectasia (Louis-Bar syndrome)
Arteriovenous communication of retina and brain (Wyburn-Mason syndrome)

Figure 2.7

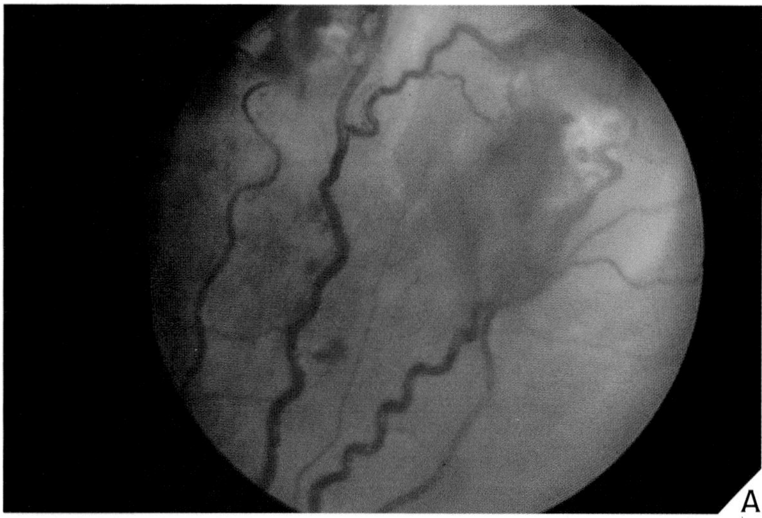

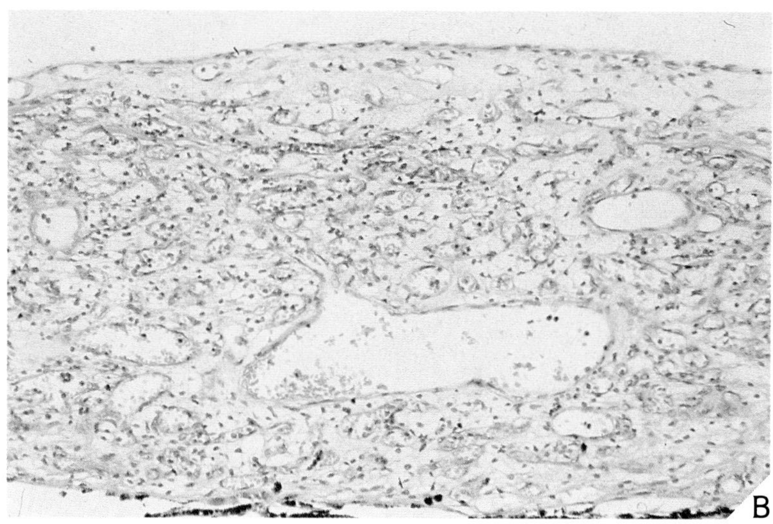

FIGURE 2.8 VON HIPPEL DISEASE. A Superiorly, two round retinal lesions associated with von Hippel disease (angiomatosis retinae) are apparent along with feeder vessels. **B** Histologic section shows two distinct types of cells: endothelial cells lining the numerous capillaries; and, present between the capillaries, stromal cells of unknown origin which appear "foamy." (**B**, courtesy of Dr. DH Nicholson.)

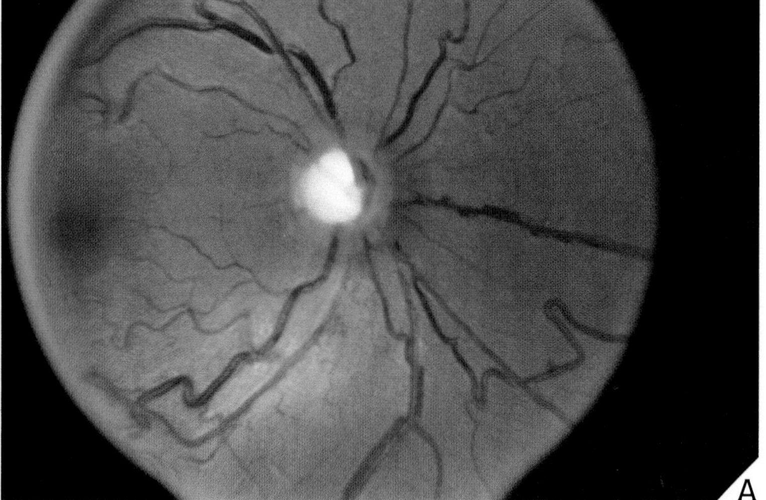

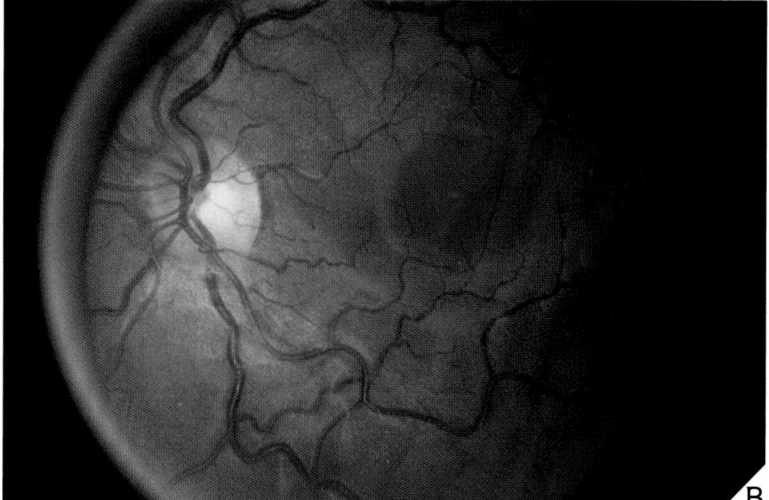

FIGURE 2.9 STURGE-WEBER SYNDROME. A The fundus shows both the characteristic bright red appearance of the involved eye, caused by the choroidal hemangioma, and an enlarged optic nerve cup, secondary to increased intraocular pressure in that eye. **B** The normal fundus of the patient's left eye is shown for comparison. **C** In another case, the choroid is diffusely involved by a cavernous hemangioma. When a choroidal hemangioma occurs in the Sturge-Weber patient, it is diffuse, large, and difficult to distinguish from any normal choroid that might be present. When it occurs in a patient without the syndrome, it is focal, small, and easy to distinguish from the surrounding normal choroid. (**C**, courtesy of Dr. R Cordero-Moreno, from Yanoff M, Fine BS: *Ocular Pathology*, 3rd ed.)

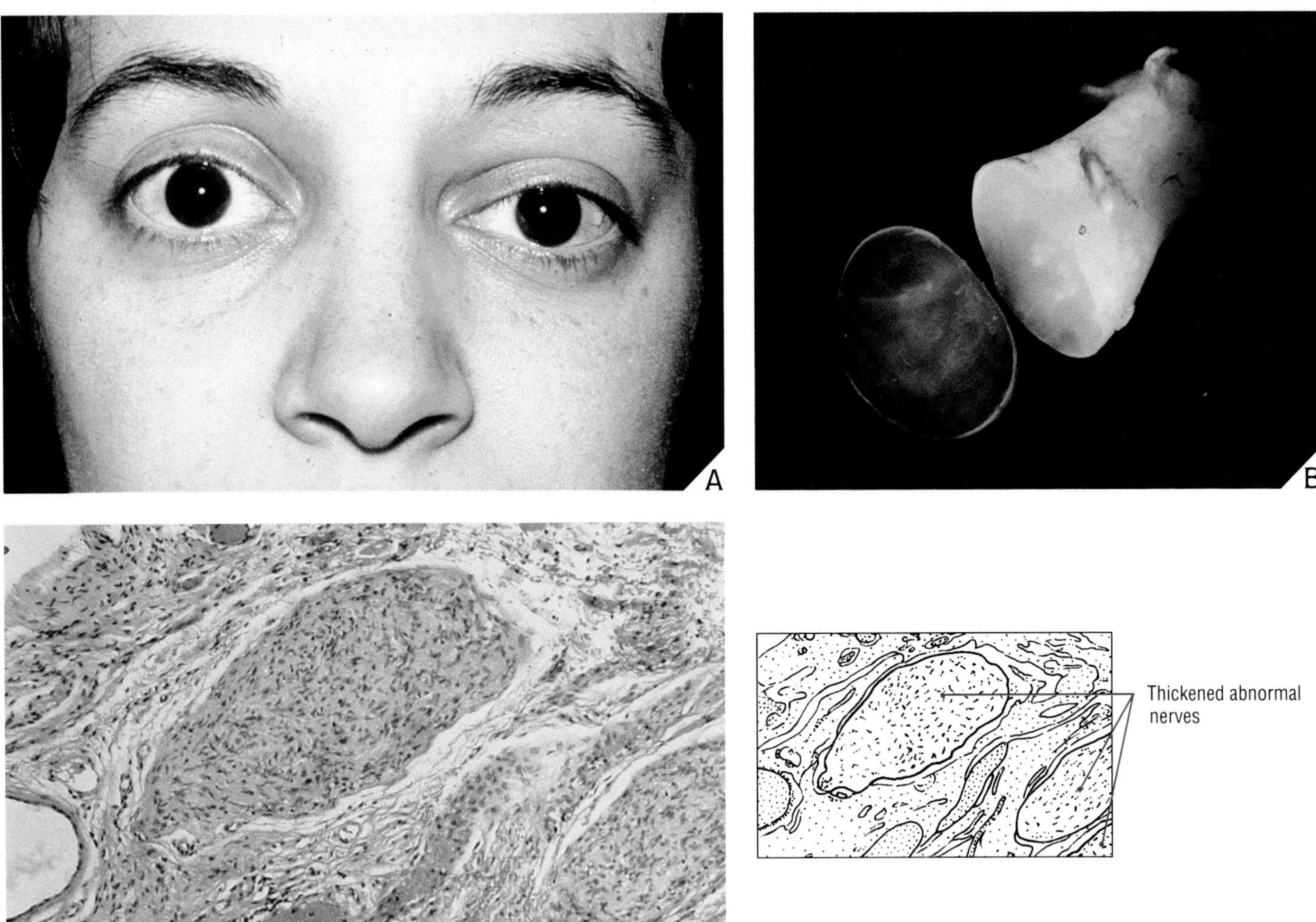

FIGURE 2.10 NEUROFIBROMATOSIS. A A plexiform neurofibroma is enlarging the left upper lid. The neurofibroma was removed. **B** The gross specimen shows a markedly enlarged nerve. A thin slice of the nerve is present at the bottom left. **C** Histologic section from another case shows the markedly enlarged nerves in neurofibromatosis of the orbit. In classic von Recklinghausen disease (type 1 neurofibromatosis or peripheral type) café au lait spots, peripheral neurofibromas, and Lisch nodules predominate. In type 2, or the central type, bilateral acoustic neuromas are characteristic. (**A**, courtesy of Dr. WC Frayer.)

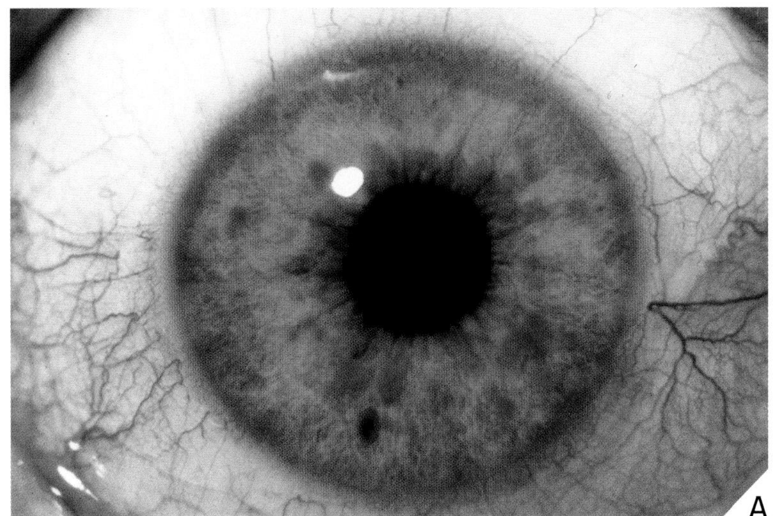

FIGURE 2.11 NEUROFIBROMATOSIS. A Iris shows multiple small spider-like melanocytic nevi, characteristic of neurofibromatosis. **B** The iris nevi, also called Lisch nodules, are caused by collections of nevus cells. **C** The choroid is thickened markedly by the hamartomatous process. Numerous structures such as neural rosettes, tactile nerve endings, and nevi may be found within the thickened choroid. Note the thickened nerves (plexiform neurofibromas) in the sclera.

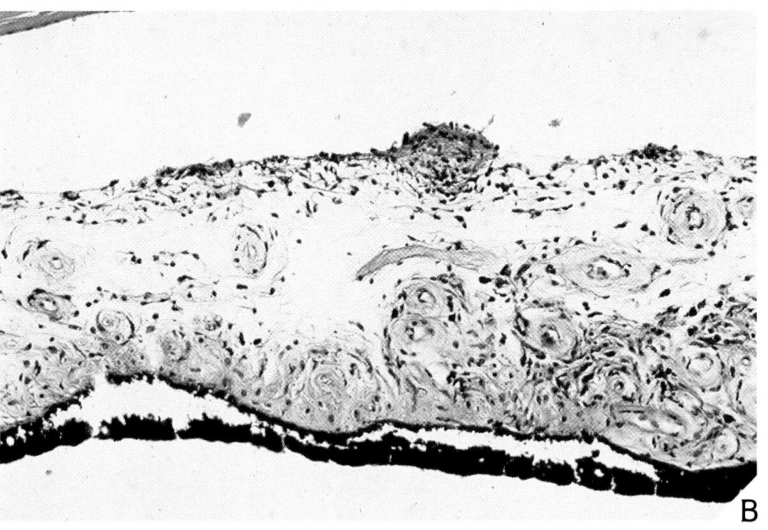

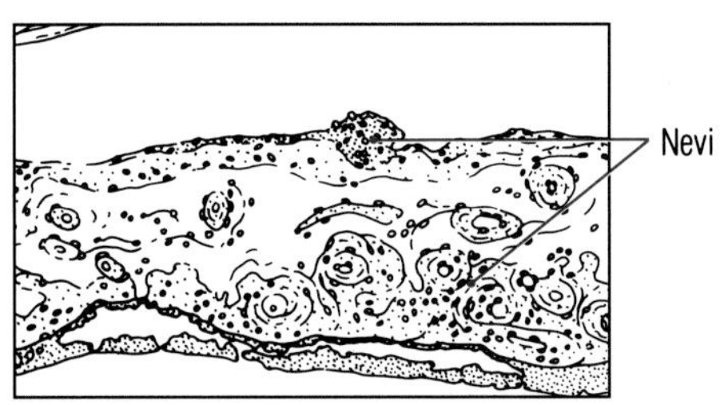

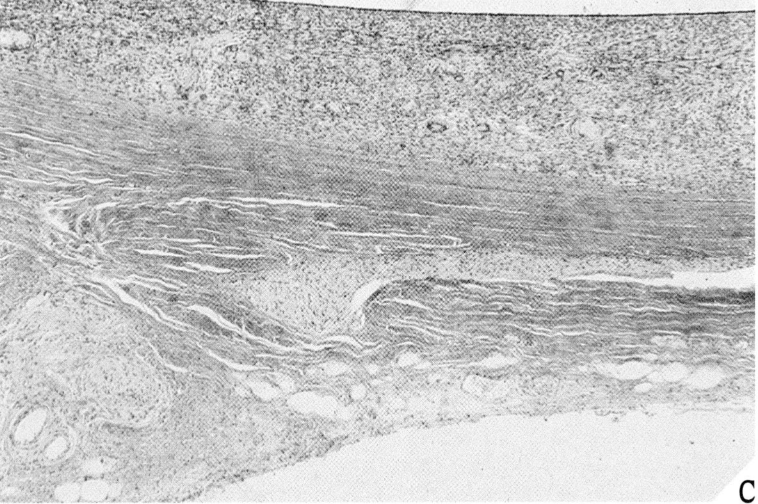

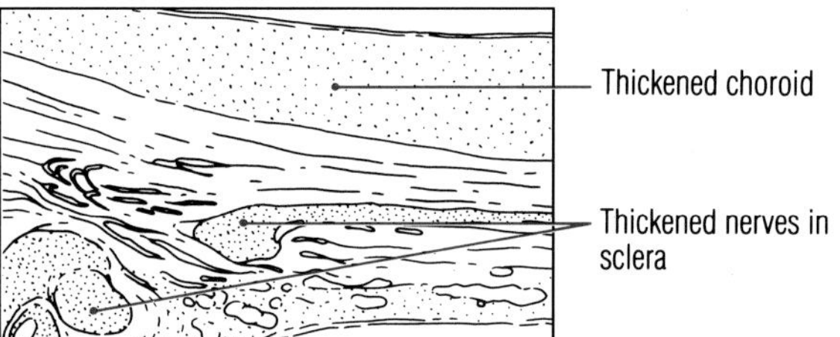

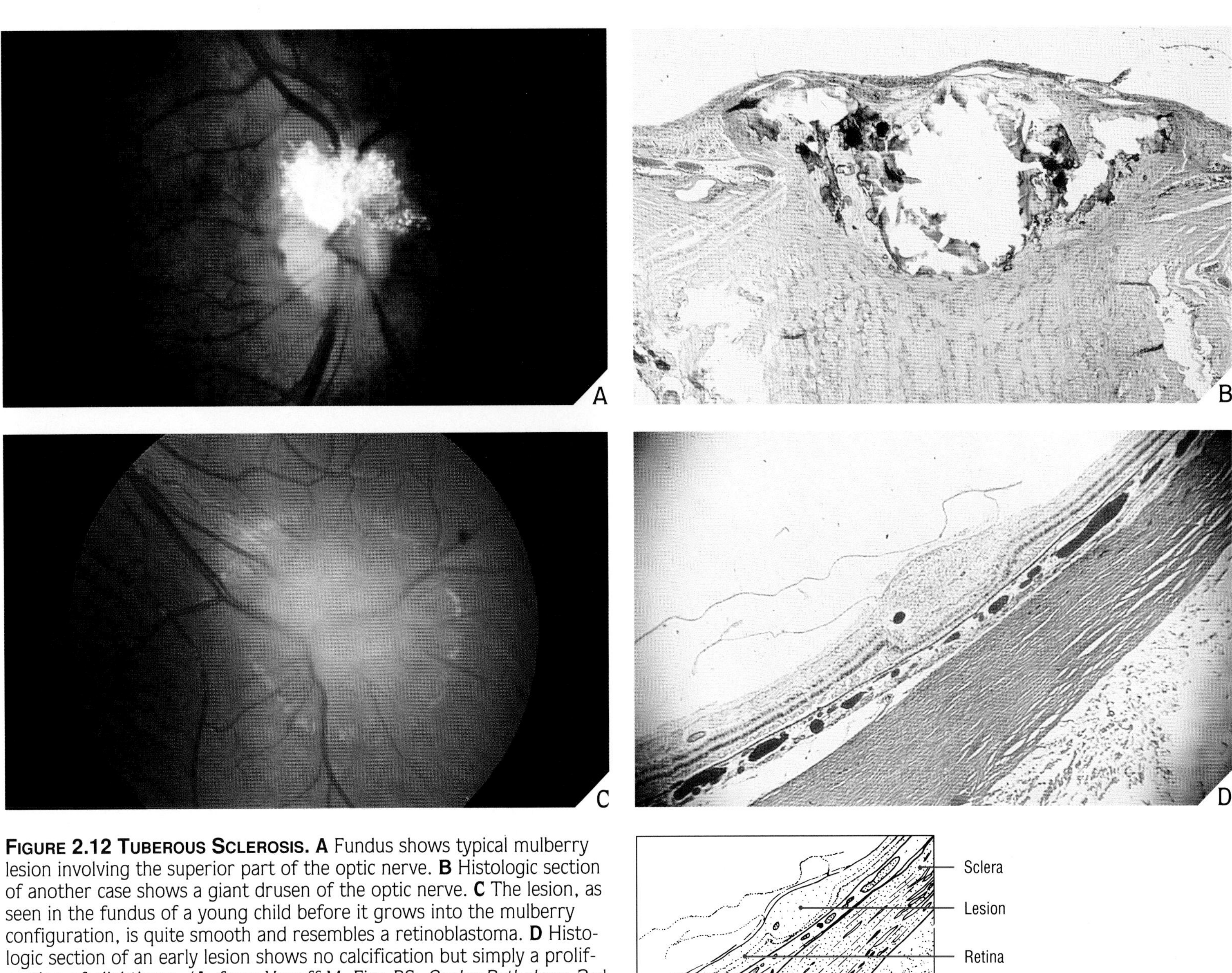

Figure 2.12 Tuberous Sclerosis. A Fundus shows typical mulberry lesion involving the superior part of the optic nerve. **B** Histologic section of another case shows a giant drusen of the optic nerve. **C** The lesion, as seen in the fundus of a young child before it grows into the mulberry configuration, is quite smooth and resembles a retinoblastoma. **D** Histologic section of an early lesion shows no calcification but simply a proliferation of glial tissue. (**A**, from Yanoff M, Fine BS: *Ocular Pathology*, 3rd ed.; **C**, courtesy of Dr. DB Schaffer.)

ASSORTED CONDITIONS SEEN IN CONGENITAL ANOMALIES

Anencephaly (absence of cranial vault)
Anophthalmos (absence of eye)
Microphthalmos (eye diameter less than 15 mm at birth)
Lowe syndrome (oculocerebrorenal syndrome, systemic acidosis, organic aciduria, renal rickets, congenital cataract, glaucoma)
Miller syndrome (oculocerebrorenal syndrome, Wilms tumor, aniridia, genitourinary anomalies)
Leigh syndrome (subacute necrotizing encephalomyelopathy)
de Lange syndrome (mental and growth retardation, characteristic facial appearance, multiple skeletal abnormalities, low-pitched cry)
Meckel syndrome (posterior encephalocele, polydactyly, polycystic kidney)
Menkes disease (defect in copper absorption, cerebral degeneration, arterial changes, sparse and brittle scalp hair)
Dwarfism (many types)

Figure 2.13

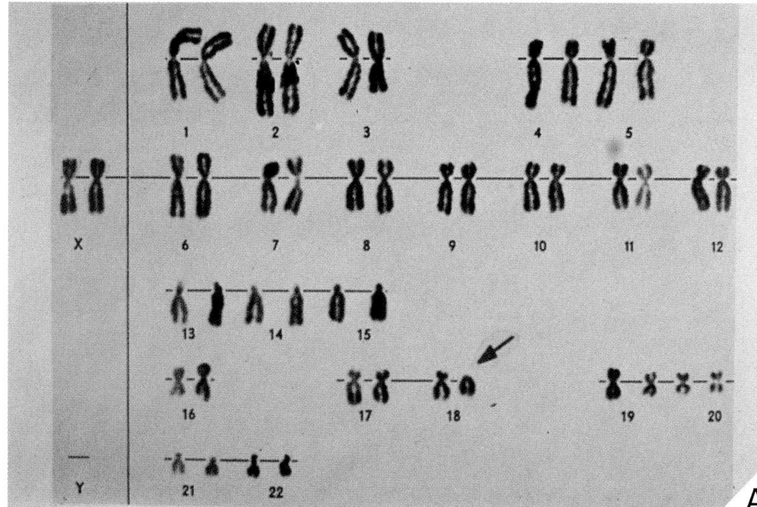

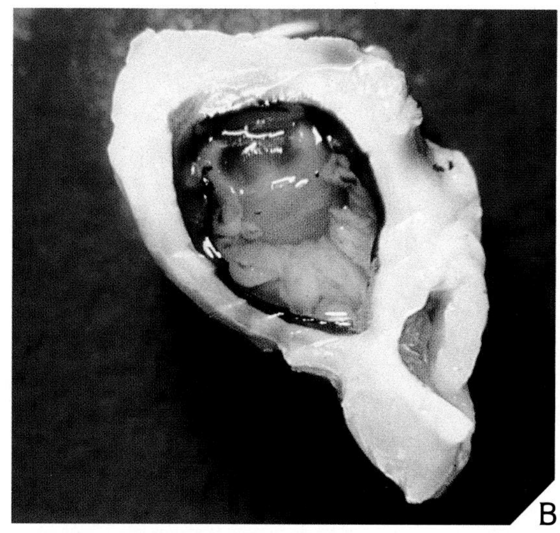

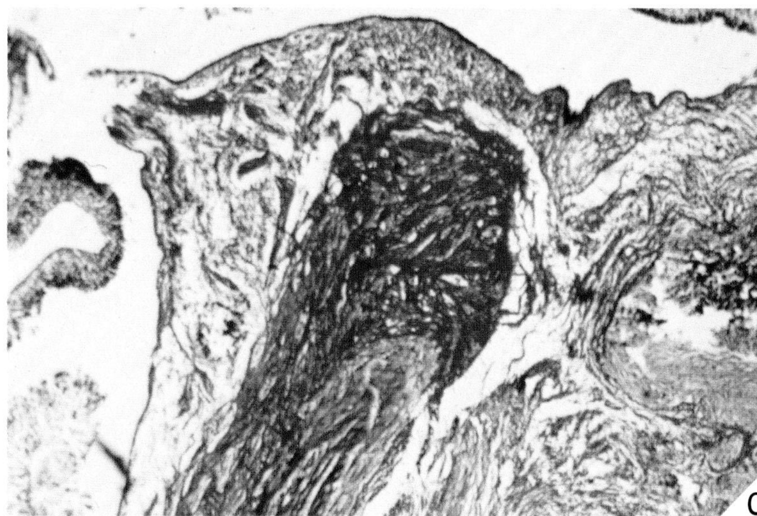

FIGURE 2.14 MICROPHTHALMOS. A Parts of the long and short arms of one of the chromosomes in the 18 group are missing (arrow) in this karyotype. The entity is called chromosome 18 deletion defect. The patient had bilateral microphthalmos with cyst. **B** The opened gross specimen of the patient's left eye shows a small eye and a contiguous cyst (the right eye was similar). **C** Smooth muscle found in the choroid near the optic nerve is bright red when treated with the trichrome stain. (Case reported in Yanoff M, et al., 1970.)

Bibliography

Boetta L, Kuehn SE, Huang A, et al: Wilms tumor locus on 11p13 defined by multiple CpG island-associated transcripts. Science 250:994, 1990.

Cibis GW, Tripathi RC, Tripathi BJ: Glaucoma in Sturge-Weber syndrome. Ophthalmology 91:1061, 1984.

Hardwig P, Robertson DM: von Hippel-Lindau disease: a familial, often lethal, multi-system phakomatosis. Ophthalmology 91:263, 1984.

Hoepner J, Yanoff M: Ocular anomalies in trisomy 13-15: an analysis of 13 eyes with two new findings. Am J Ophthalmol 74:729, 1972.

Krohel GB, et al: Localized orbital neurofibromas. Am J Ophthalmol 100:458, 1985.

Küchle M, Kraus J, Rummelt C: Synophthalmia and holoposencephaly in chromosome 18p deletion defect. Arch Ophthalmol 109:136, 1991.

Mansour AH, Wells CG, Jampol LM, et al: Ocular complications of arteriovenous communications of the retina. Arch Ophthalmol 107:232, 1989.

Mets MB, Maumenee IH: Review. The eye and the chromosome. Surv Ophthalmol 28:20, 1983.

Mulvihill JJ, Parry DM, Sherman JL, et al: Neurofibromatosis 1 (Recklinghausen disease) and neurofibromatosis 2 (bilateral acoustic neurofibromatosis). An update. Ann Intern Med 113:39, 1990.

Streissguth AP, Aase JM, Clarren SK, et al: Fetal alcohol syndrome in adolescents and adults. JAMA 265:1961, 1991.

Wallace MR, Marchuk DA, Andersen LB, et al: Type 1 neurofibromatosis gene: identification of a large transcript disrupted in three NF1 patients. Science 249:181, 1990.

Williams R, Taylor D: Review. Tuberous sclerosis. Surv Ophthalmol 30:143, 1985.

Yanoff M, Rorke LB, Niederer BS: Ocular and cerebral abnormalities in chromosome 18 deletion defect. Am J Ophthalmol 70:391, 1970.

Yanoff M, Schaffer DB, Scheie HG: Rubella ocular syndrome—clinical significance of viral and pathologic studies. Trans Am Acad Ophthalmol Otolaryngol 72:896, 1968.

Nongranulomatous Inflammation

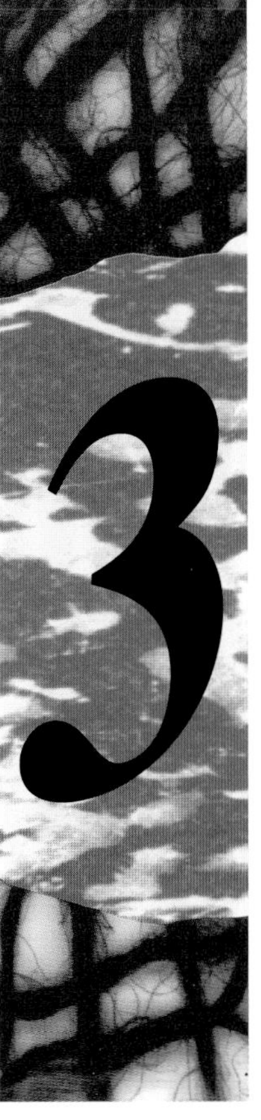

Nongranulomatous inflammation may be designated either suppurative or nonsuppurative. The suppurative form, which has an acute onset and is characterized by the formation of pus, may be manifested in ocular congestion, chemosis, hazy media, hypopyon, pain, and exophthalmos. The polymorphonuclear leukocyte is the predominant inflammatory cell. A reaction in nongranulomatous inflammation may be exogenous (i.e., from outside of the eye), often secondary to the presence of an intraocular foreign body following a penetrating or perforating injury to the eye; or the inflammation may be endogenous (i.e., from within the eye itself), an example of which is necrosis of a uveal melanoma leading to marked endophthalmitis. Nongranulomatous inflammation also may be manifested in the following ways:

- endophthalmitis—inflammation of one or more coats of the eye and adjacent cavities;
- panophthalmitis—inflammation of one or more coats of the eye and adjacent cavities plus scleral involvement and spread to orbital tissue.

Nonsuppurative nongranulomatous inflammation may be acute or chronic. The acute type is characterized by an inflammation in which the polymorphonuclear leukocyte is the predominant cell, as seen in cellulitis secondary to *Streptococcus hemolyticus* infection. The acute type does not lead to suppuration or pus formation. Lymphocytes and plasma cells also may be the predominant cell types, as seen in acute iritis.

In the chronic type of nongranulomatous inflammation, the plasma cell and the lymphocyte usually predominate, as seen in "garden variety" uveitis. Many different entities can cause a nongranulomatous inflammation, including traumatic iridocyclitis, heterochromic iridocyclitis (Fuchs), rheumatoid arthritis, and various idiopathic diseases. Less common causes include Behçet syndrome, Reiter syndrome, and pars planitis. Although the list of possible causes is long, in general, in any given patient a cause rarely is found for chronic nonsuppurative nongranulomatous inflammation.

The sequelae of nongranulomatous inflammation are numerous and range from minor problems to major disorders.

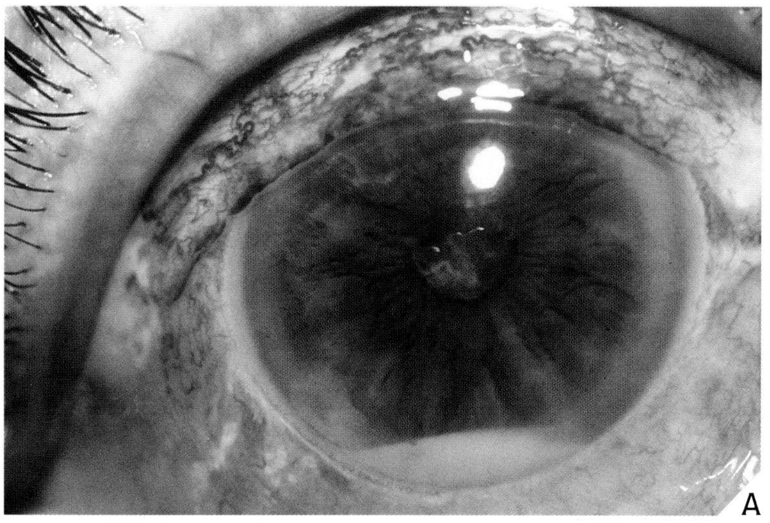

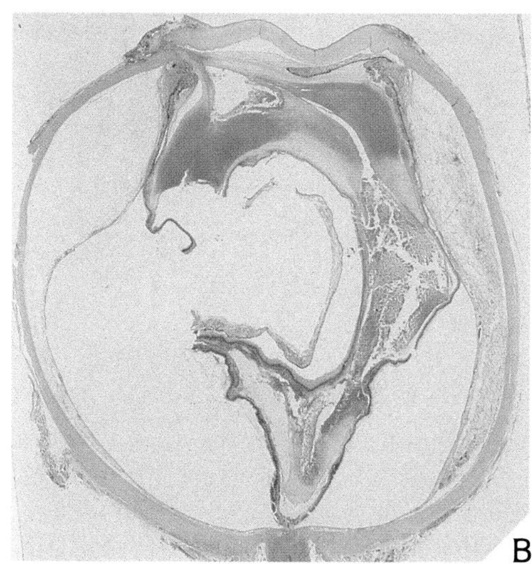

FIGURE 3.1 ENDOPHTHALMITIS. A The patient developed "sterile" endophthalmitis after undergoing extracapsular cataract extraction and a posterior chamber lens implant. Note the hypopyon. **B** Another patient developed bacterial endophthalmitis following intracapsular cataract extraction. The diffuse abscess seen filling the vitreous cavity is characteristic of bacterial infection (fungal infection usually causes multiple tiny abscesses). The retina and its adjacent cavity, the vitreous, are involved but the choroid and sclera are not.

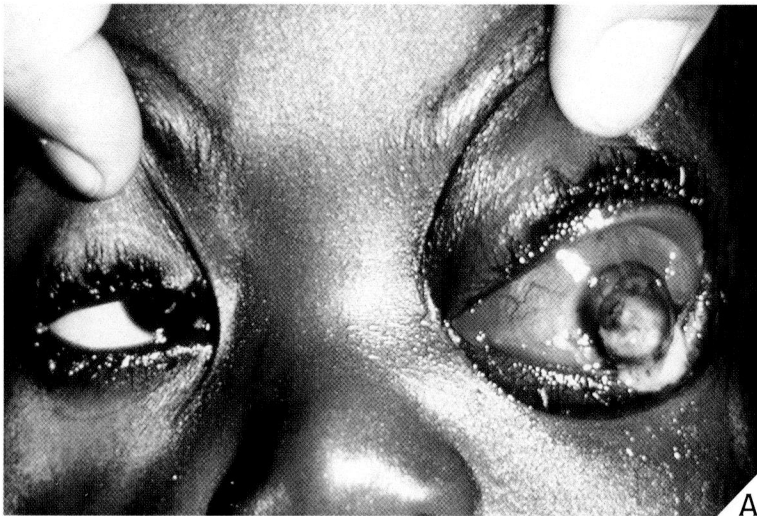

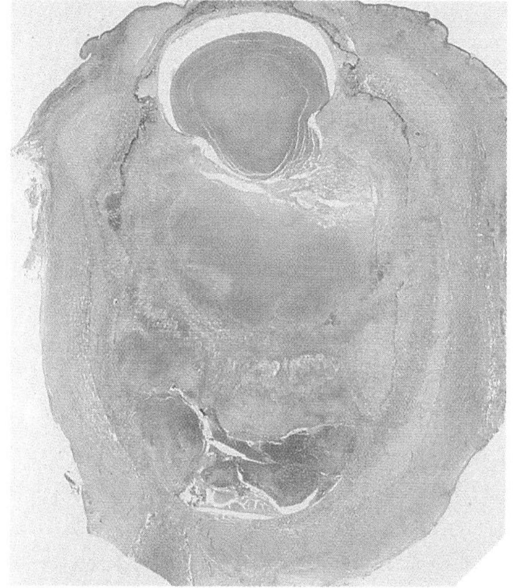

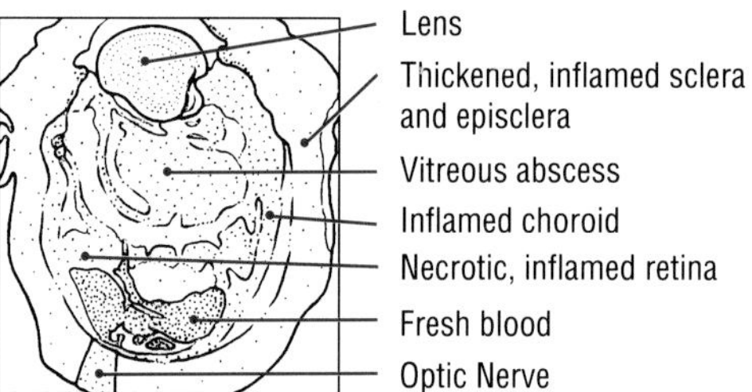

FIGURE 3.2 PANOPHTHALMITIS. A The patient had a regular measles infection and subsequently developed pain and inflammation in the left eye that led to panophthalmitis and corneal perforation. **B** Histologic section shows the corneal perforation. The vitreous body, adjacent retina, choroid, and sclera are all involved, and the inflammation extends through the coats of the eye into the episcleral tissue. (**A**, courtesy of Dr. RE Shannon.)

CAUSES OF SUPPURATIVE INFLAMMATION

Exogenous

Nonsurgical or surgical trauma
Metastatic septic emboli
Spread from sinus inflammation

Endogenous

Iridocyclitis secondary to keratitis or corneal ulcer
Necrosis of uveal melanoma
Behçet syndrome

FIGURE 3.3

MANIFESTATIONS OF BEHÇET SYNDROME

Oral ulceration—aphthous stomatitis
Genital ulceration
Ocular inflammation—recurrent iridocyclitis, hypopyon, and retinal necrosis

FIGURE 3.4

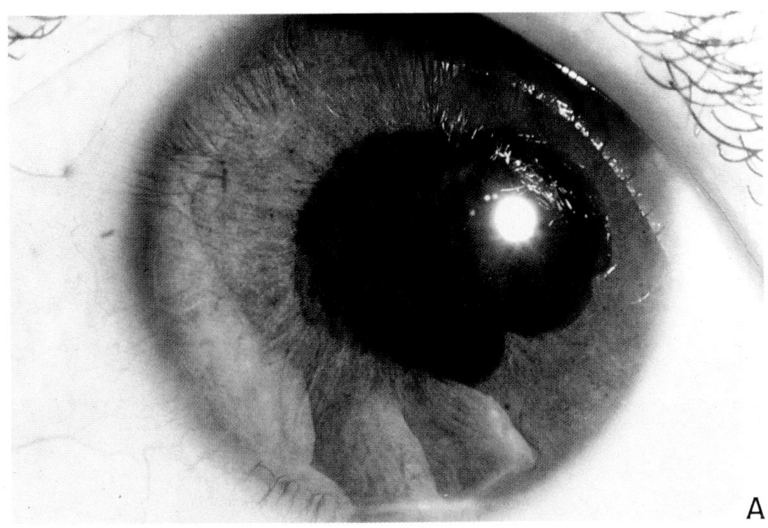

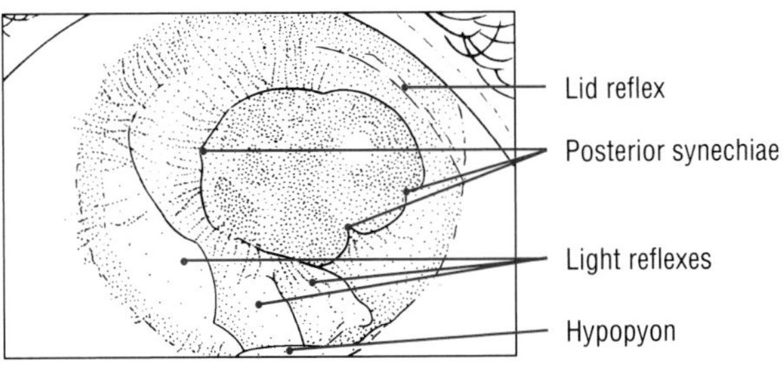

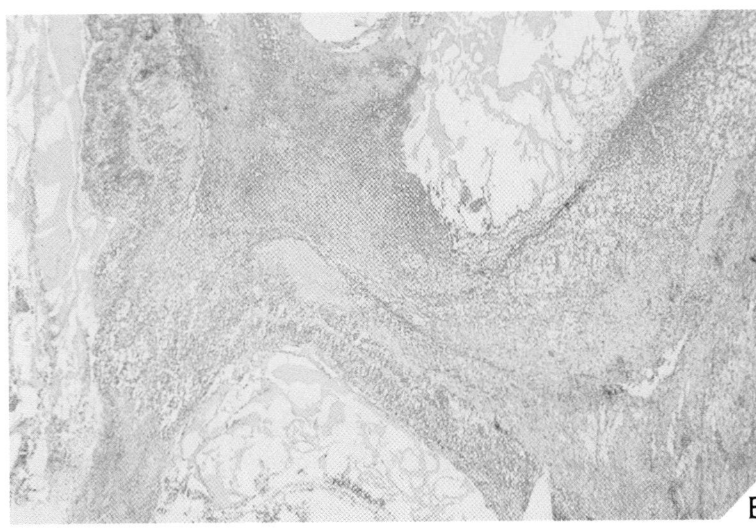

Cyclitic membrane
Detached, necrotic inflamed retina

FIGURE 3.5 BEHÇET SYNDROME. A The patient has a hypopyon. Note the posterior synechiae, a sign of the recurrent iridocyclitis in this patient. **B** A histologic section shows necrosis and perivasculitis of the retina. An organizing cyclitic membrane has caused a detachment of the inflamed retina (**A**, from Yanoff M, Fine BS: *Ocular Pathology*, 3rd ed.; **B**, presented by Dr. TA Makley at the Verhoeff Society, 1976.)

CAUSES OF NONSUPPURATIVE INFLAMMATION

Exogenous
Blunt trauma
Perforating trauma

Endogenous
Idiopathic ("garden variety" uveitis) most common

Associated with systemic diseases
Rheumatoid arthritis
Reiter syndrome (nonbacterial urethritis, conjunctivitis or iridocyclitis, and arthritis)
Crohn disease
Whipple disease

Viral
Rubella
Herpes simplex and *zoster*
Subacute sclerosing panencephalitis (chronic, progressive CNS disease in childhood caused by the measles virus, usually 5 to 7 years after the primary measles infection)

Nonsystemic syndromes
Uveal effusion
Pars planitis
Glaucomatocyclitic crisis (Posner-Schlossman syndrome)
Heterochromic iridocyclitis (Fuchs)

FIGURE 3.6

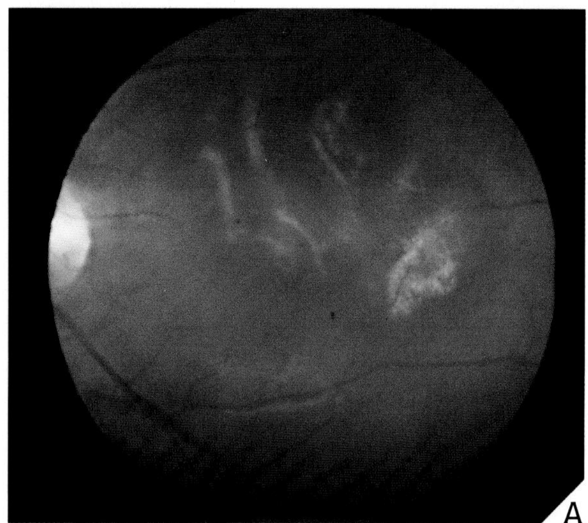

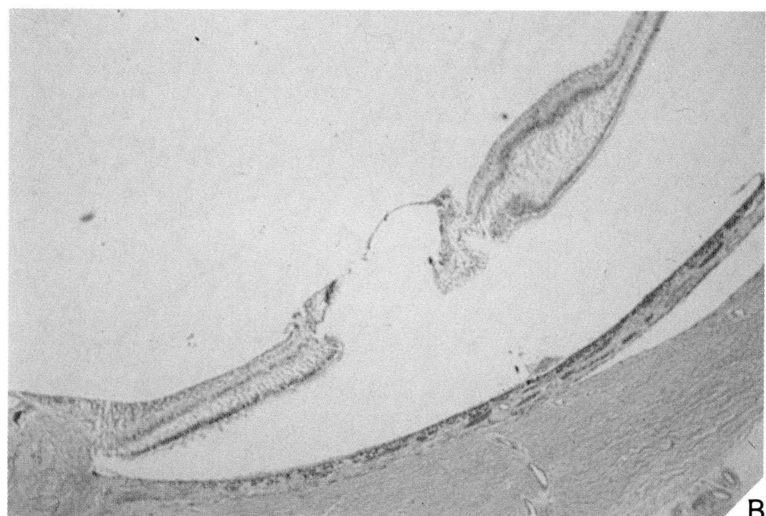

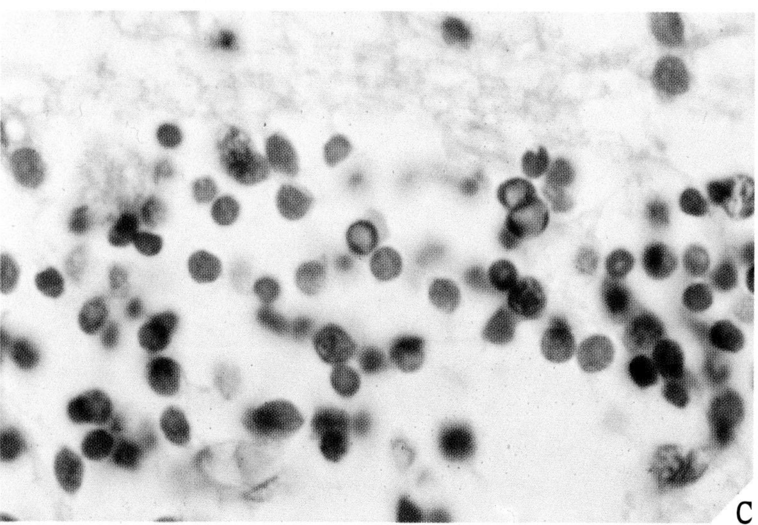

FIGURE 3.7 SUBACUTE SCLEROSING PANENCEPHALITIS (SSPE). A The fundus of a patient who has SSPE shows acute retinitis in the region of the macula. **B** Histologic section shows necrosis of the central macula, resulting in hole formation. **C** Many intranuclear inclusion bodies are present in the inner nuclear layer of the retina. Patients presenting with SSPE frequently have ocular findings, mainly macular lesions and peripheral chorioretinal lesions. (**C**, modified from Nelson DA, et al., 1970.)

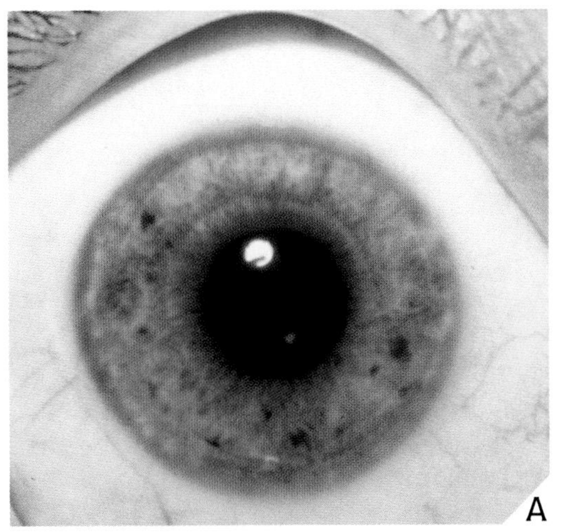

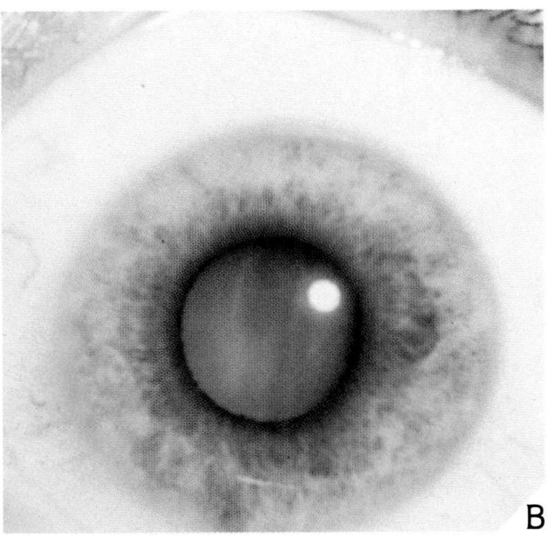

Figure 3.8 Heterochromic Iridocyclitis (Fuchs). A The green iris of the normal uninvolved right eye is darker than in **B**, which shows the light blue iris in the involved left eye. Heterochromia, cataract (present in the left eye), and iris neovascularization are common in this condition. Loss of iris substance may become so severe that paradoxical heterochromia results in which only pigment epithelium remains in the involved eye, which then appears darker than the uninvolved eye. **C** Histologic section shows that diffuse trabeculitis and peripheral iritis are present. The inflammatory cells are mainly lymphocytes and plasma cells. **D** Marked atrophy of the iris and iris neovascularization are present. (**C, D,** reported in Perry H, et al., 1975.)

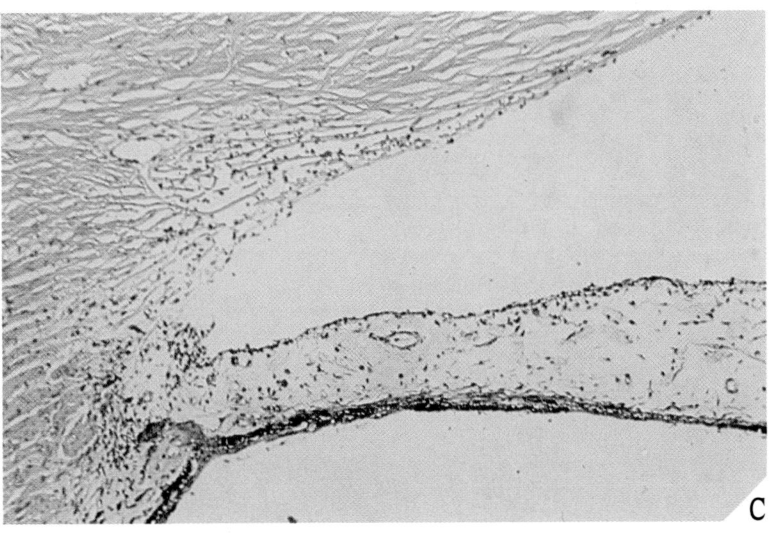

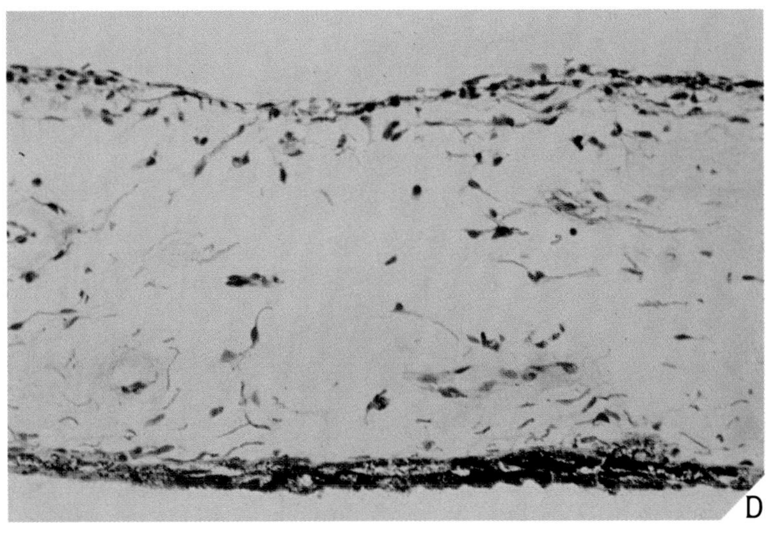

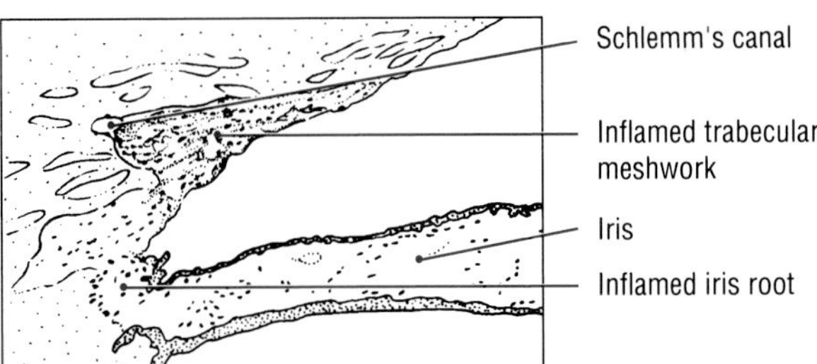

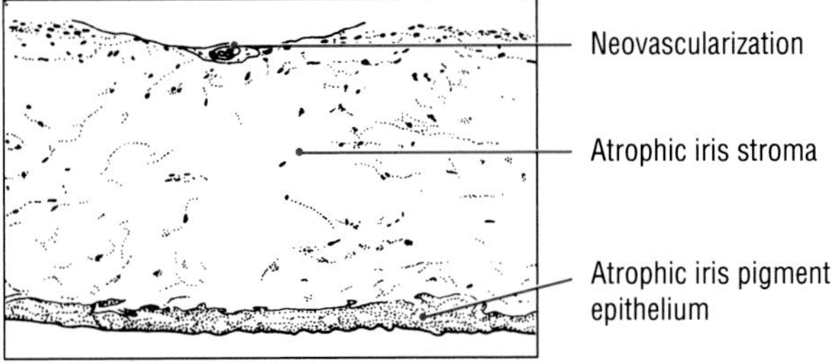

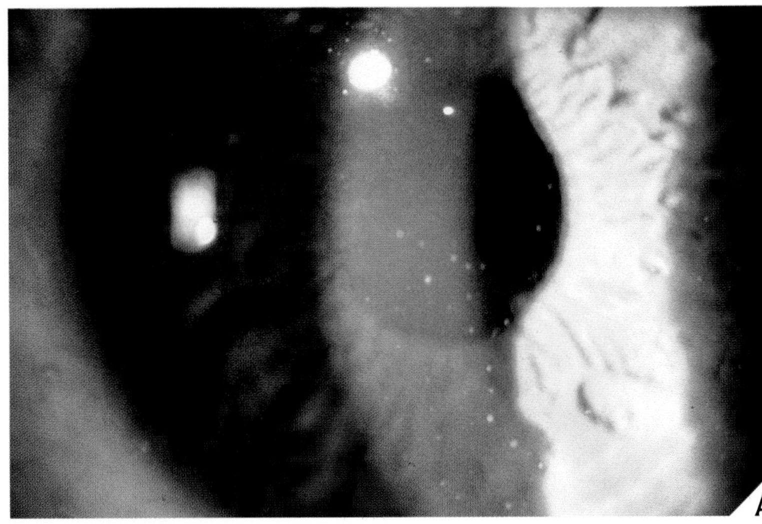

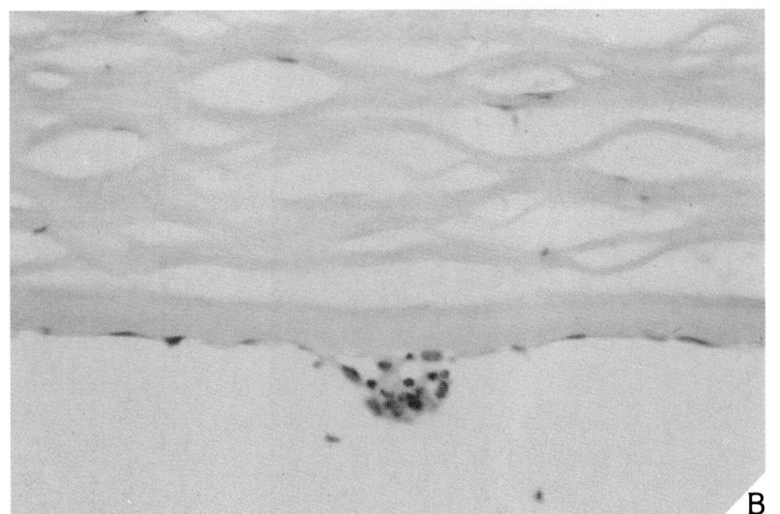

Figure 3.9 Heterochromic Iridocyclitis (Fuchs). A Slit-lamp examination shows typical stellate keratic precipitates (KPs), which tend to change very little over long periods of time. **B** Histologic section shows that the KPs are composed of lymphocytes and histiocytes. (Reported in Perry H, et al., 1975.)

SEQUELAE OF NONGRANULOMATOUS INFLAMMATION

Cornea
Endothelial cell loss
Corneal edema
Scarring
Band keratopathy
Vascularization

Anterior chamber and iris
Scarring
Iris neovascularization
Synechia, peripheral or posterior
Iris necrosis and atrophy

Lens and ciliary body
Cataract
Hyalinization of ciliary processes
Proliferation of ciliary epithelium
Cyclitic membrane

Vitreous and choroid
Posterior vitreous detachment
Cells in vitreous
Vitreous membranes
Atrophy and scarring of choroid

Retina and optic nerve
Perivasculitis of retina
Macular edema
Retinochoroidal scarring
Retinal detachment
Hyperplasia or atrophy of retinal pigment epithelium
Optic atrophy

Glaucoma
Secondary open-angle or closed-angle glaucoma may arise from numerous mechanisms

FIGURE 3.10

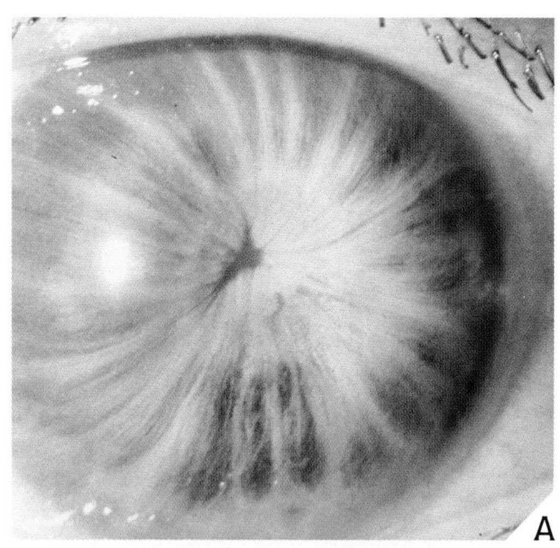

FIGURE 3.11 SEQUELAE OF NONGRANULOMATOUS INFLAMMATION. **A** A membrane has grown across the pupil (occlusion of the pupil) and has adhered to the underlying lens, preventing the pupil from moving (seclusion of the pupil). **B** Aqueous in the posterior chamber has bowed the iris forward (iris bombé), resulting in peripheral anterior synechiae. **C** Histologic section of another case shows iris bombé, posterior synechiae of the iris to the anterior surface of the lens, a cyclitic membrane, and a retinal detachment. All are the result of longstanding chronic uveitis. (**A**, **B**, courtesy of Dr. GOH Naumann.)

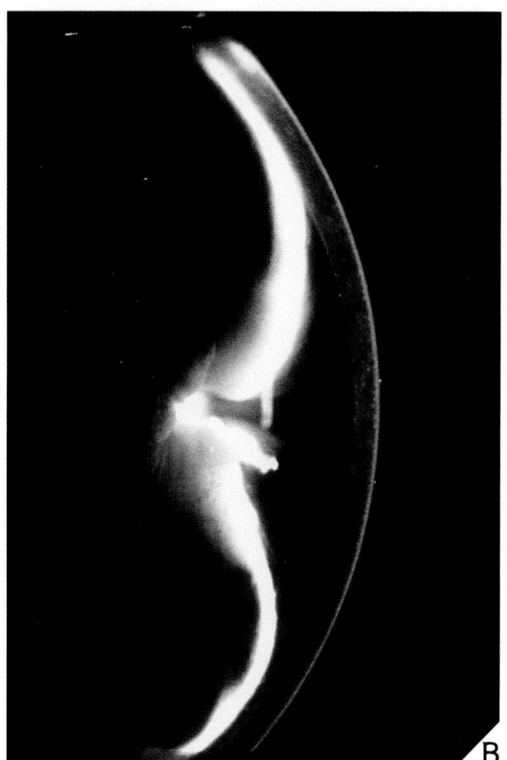

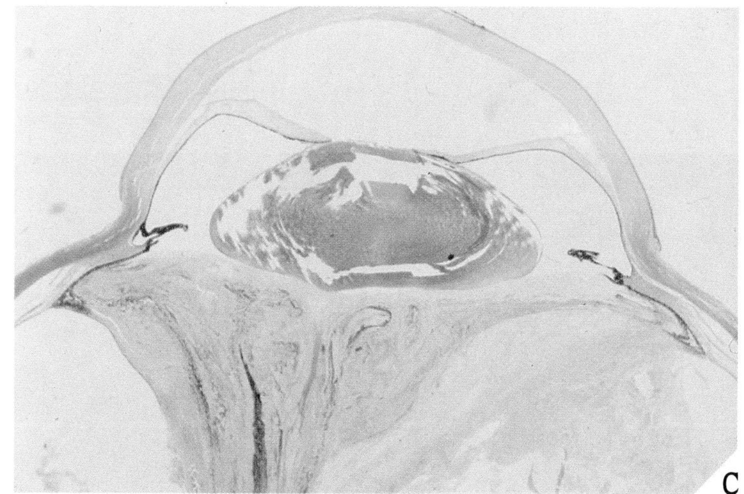

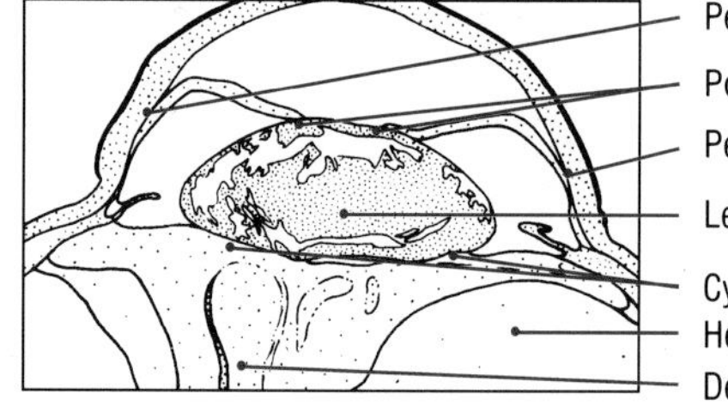

END STAGE OF DIFFUSE OCULAR DISEASE

Atrophy without shrinkage (seen in chronic glaucoma)
Atrophy with shrinkage (atrophia bulbi; seen in chronic uveitis)
Atrophy with shrinkage and disorganization (phthisis bulbi; seen after purulent endophthalmitis)
Intraocular ossification (common with atrophia and phthisis bulbi)
Calcium deposition (may occur in many ocular structures)

FIGURE 3.12

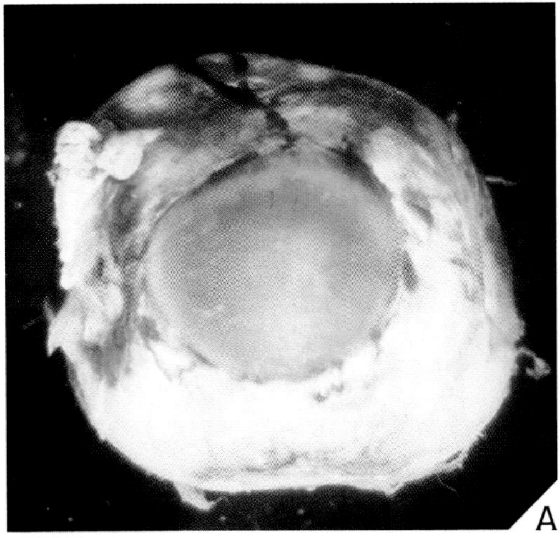

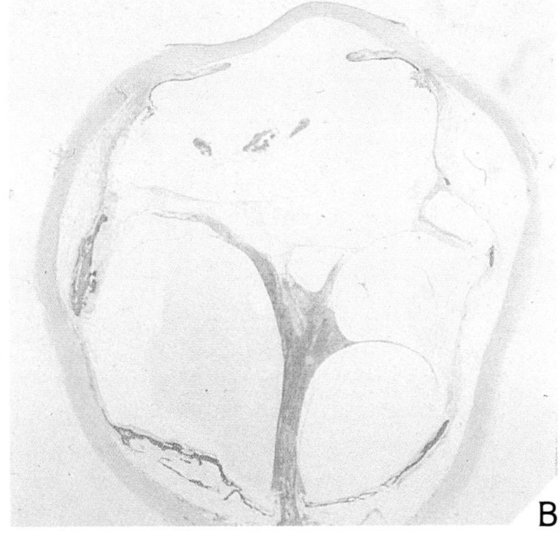

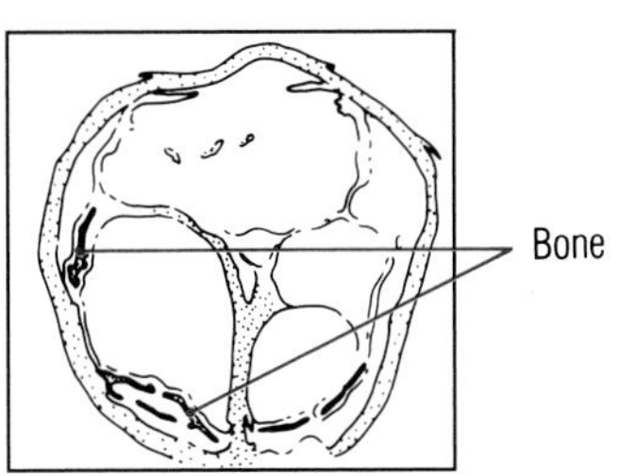

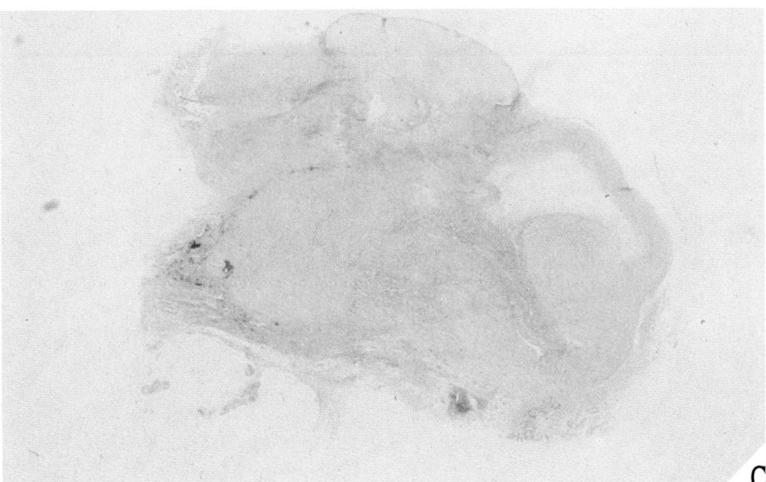

FIGURE 3.13 END STAGE OF DIFFUSE OCULAR DISEASE. A The enucleated eye shows the characteristic squared-off appearance of hypotony. The pull of the horizontal and vertical rectus muscles causes the soft, often shrunken, eye to appear squared-off or cuboidal. Clinically, this type of eye is called a phthisical eye or phthisis bulbi. However, histologically the eye is called atrophia bulbi. **B** Histologic section shows a small atrophic eye that is hypotonus, as evidenced by the ciliary body and choroidal detachments. Extensive formation of a rim of bone in the inner choroid can be seen. **C** In this histologic section, the globe is so disorganized that normal structures are unrecognizable. The condition is called phthisis bulbi. The eye has been completely scarred due to purulent endophthalmitis. (**C**, from Yanoff M, Fine BS: *Ocular Pathology*, 3rd ed.)

Bibliography

de Abreu MT, et al: T-lymphocyte subsets in the aqueous humor and peripheral blood of patients with acute untreated uveitis. Am J Ophthalmol 98:62, 1984.

International study group for Behçet's disease: Criteria for diagnosis of Behçet's disease. Lancet 335:1078, 1990.

Johnson LA, Wirostko E, Wirostko WJ: Crohn's disease uveitis. Parasitization of vitreous by Mollicute-like organisms. Am J Clin Pathol 91:259, 1989.

Kampik A, Patrinely JR, Green WR: Morphologic and clinical features of retrocorneal melanin pigmentation and pigmented pupillary membranes: review of 225 cases. Surv Ophthalmol 27:161, 1982.

Kanski JJ: Juvenile arthritis and uveitis. Surv Ophthalmol 34:253, 1990.

Murray PI, et al: Immunohistochemical analysis of iris biopsy specimens from patients with Fuchs' heterochromic cyclitis. Am J Ophthalmol 109:394, 1990.

Nelson DA, et al: Retinal lesions in subacute sclerosing panencephalitis. Arch Ophthalmol 84:613, 1970.

Pepose JS, et al: Immunocytologic localization of herpes simplex type 1 viral antigens in herpetic retinitis and encephalitis in an adult. Ophthalmology 92:160, 1985.

Perry H, Yanoff M, Scheie HG: Fuchs's heterochromic iridocyclitis. Arch Ophthalmol 93:337, 1975.

Raizman MB, Foster CS: Plasma exhange in the therapy of Behçet's disease. Graefe's Arch Exp Ophthalmol 227:360, 1989.

Sheppard RD, Bornstein MB, Udem SA: Measles virus matrix protein synthesized in a subacute sclerosing panencephalitis cell line. Science 228:1219, 1985.

Wiggins, Jr RE, Steinkuller PG, Hamill MB: Reiter's keratoconjunctivitis. Arch Ophthalmol 108:280, 1990.

Granulomatous Inflammation

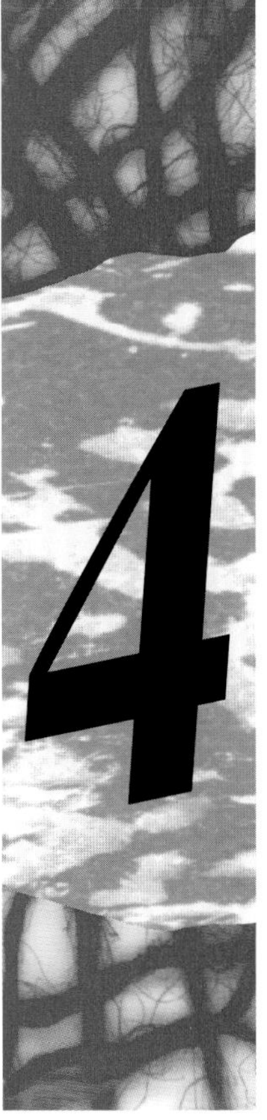

Granulomatous inflammation is a chronic, proliferative reaction characterized by a cellular infiltrate of epithelioid cells. Inflammatory giant cells, lymphocytes, plasma cells, polymorphonuclear leukocytes, and eosinophils also may be present. Granulomatous inflammation is much less common than nongranulomatous inflammation. The identification of an inflammation as granulomatous, however, carries with it a high probability of finding a cause.

Often, clinical information is helpful in determining the cause. For example, juvenile xanthogranuloma (JXG) occurs mainly in infants under six months of age, sarcoid in the third and fourth decades, and rheumatoid scleritis in the fifth and sixth decades. Race may be a factor in diagnosis because sarcoid occurs most commonly in blacks and Vogt-Koyanagi-Harada disease occurs most often in Asians. A history of trauma should be determined. Following trauma, the most frequent complicating granulomatous conditions include sympathetic uveitis, phacoanaphylactic endophthalmitis, and foreign body granulomas.

When nontraumatic granulomatous inflammations are present, it is essential to determine whether the condition is infectious or noninfectious. The major infectious agents are viral entities such as cytomegalovirus and *Herpes zoster*; the main bacterial entities are tuberculosis, leprosy, syphilis, tularemia, and streptothrix or *Actinomyces* (a transitional organism between fungi and bacteria that is classified as a bacterium). A recently recognized entity, Lyme disease, caused by the bacterial spirochete *Borrelia burgdorferi* (similar to the treponeme that causes syphilis), can result in numerous ophthalmic and neuro-ophthalmic findings. Major fungal entities are blastomycosis, cryptococcosis, coccidioidomycosis, aspergillosis, rhinosporidiosis, phycomycosis (mucormycosis or zygomycosis), candidiasis, histoplasmosis, and sporotrichosis. The most common parasitic entities found in granulomatous inflammation include toxoplasmosis, toxocariasis, trichinosis, loa loa, cysticercosis, hydatid cyst, and schistosomiasis.

When it is determined that the inflammation is secondary neither to trauma nor to infection, a number of entities must be considered, such as sarcoidosis, granulomatous scleritis, chalazion, JXG, granulomatous reaction to Descemet membrane, Chediak-Higashi syndrome, allergic granulomatosis, Vogt-Koyanagi-Harada syndrome, and familial chronic granulomatous disease of childhood.

Finally, as mentioned in Chapter 1, the histologic pattern of inflammatory reaction may be quite helpful in diagnosing the particular type of granulomatous disease. If a *diffuse type* of reaction is found, the main causes are sympathetic uveitis, disseminated histoplasmosis and other fungal infections, lepromatous leprosy, JXG, Vogt-Koyanagi-Harada disease, cytomegalic inclusion disease, and toxoplasmosis. The epithelioid cells are distributed randomly against a background of lymphocytes and plasma cells. In the *discrete reaction*, the major causes are sarcoidosis, tuberculoid leprosy, and miliary tuberculosis. An accumulation of epithelioid cells forms nodules surrounded by a narrow rim of lymphocytes and some plasma cells. In the *zonal type* of reaction, the major causes are caseation tuberculosis, some fungal infections, rheumatoid scleritis, chalazion, phacoanaphylactic endophthalmitis, toxocariasis, and cysticercosis. A central nidus is surrounded by pallisaded epithelioid cells that in turn usually are surrounded by lymphocytes and plasma cells.

Another important aspect of the patient's history is the presence of an altered immune system. In 1981 the first case of acquired immune deficiency syndrome (AIDS) was reported in a patient who had pneumonia caused by *Pneumocystis carinii*. AIDS itself is caused by a retrovirus, the human immunodeficiency virus (HIV), usually seen as HIV-1 in this country but as another T-cell lymphotropic retrovirus, HIV-2, in West Africa. Many of the infectious entities described in this chapter can occur as opportunistic ocular infections in patients who have AIDS. Although cytomegalovirus is the most common opportunistic infection, others include *H. simplex* and *zoster*, toxoplasmosis, candidiasis, syphilis, cat-scratch diseases, and *Pneumocystis carinii.* Noninfectious conditions such as Kaposi sarcoma also can occur in patients who have AIDS.

GRANULOMATOUS INFLAMMATION

- Epithelioid cells necessary for diagnosis
- Background of mononuclear cells
- Giant cells often present
- Reaction to persistent antigen

FIGURE 4.1

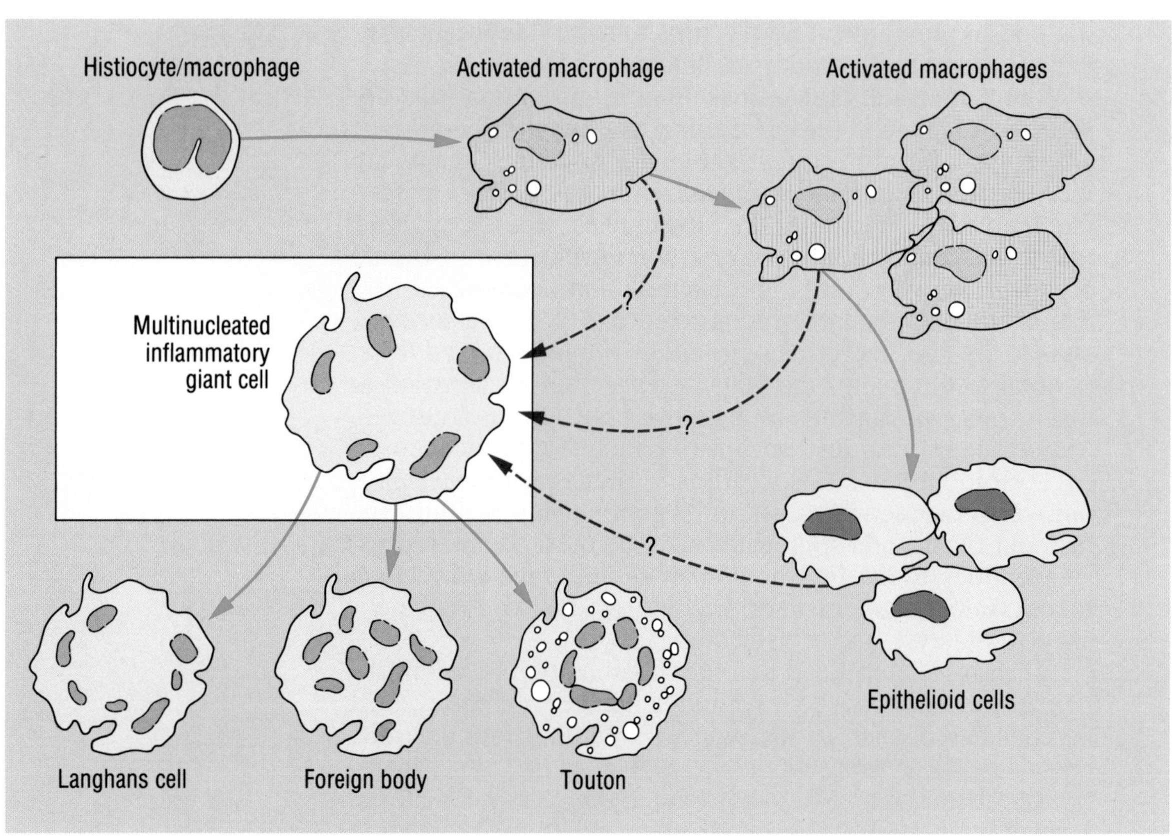

FIGURE 4.2 THEORETICAL ORIGIN OF EPITHELIOID CELLS AND INFLAMMATORY GIANT CELLS.

GRANULOMATOUS INFLAMMATION CAUSED BY TRAUMA

Sympathetic uveitis

Follows penetrating ocular trauma
- May develop 5 days to 20+ years after trauma (2 weeks is "safe period")
- 90% develop 2 weeks to 1 year after trauma (80% 3 weeks to 3 months)

Autoimmune reaction

Diffuse bilateral granulomatous uveitis

Histology
- Diffuse bilateral granulomatous inflammation of uvea
- Sparing of choriocapillaris
- Pigment phagocytosis by epithelioid cells
- Dalen-Fuchs nodules

Phacoanaphylactic endophthalmitis

Follows ocular trauma that results in a ruptured lens

Autoimmune reaction
- Autosensitization to lens protein
- Breakdown or reversal of central tolerance at T-lymphocyte level

Zonal granulomatous reaction

May be found concurrently in eyes that have sympathetic uveitis

FIGURE 4.3

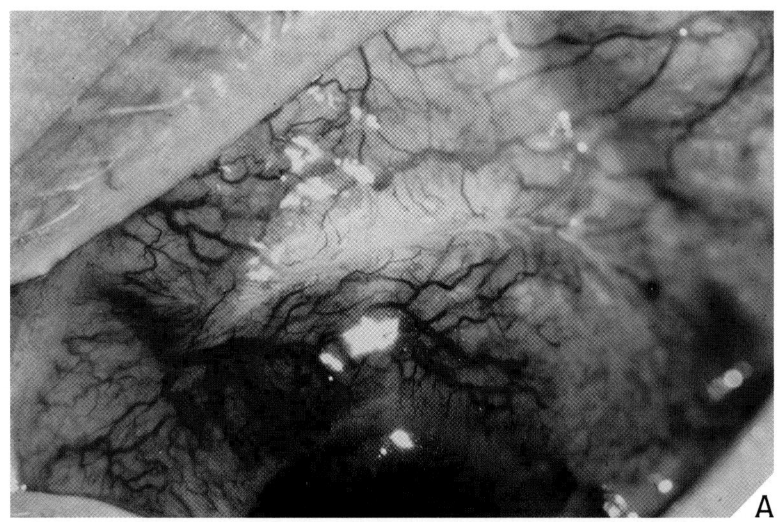

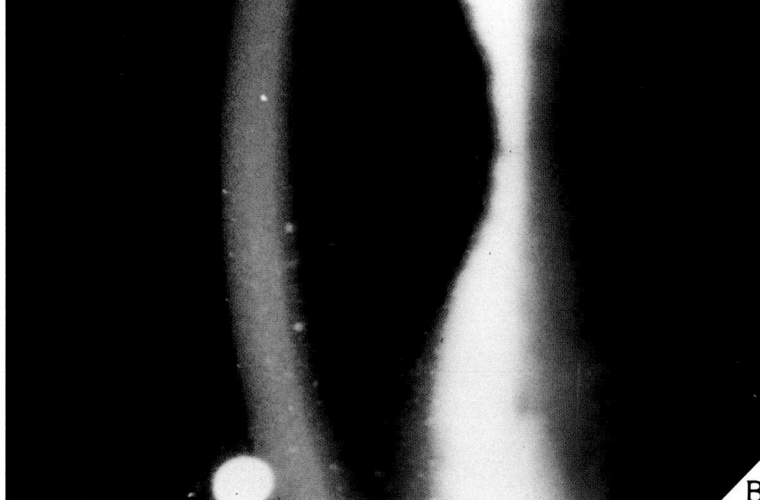

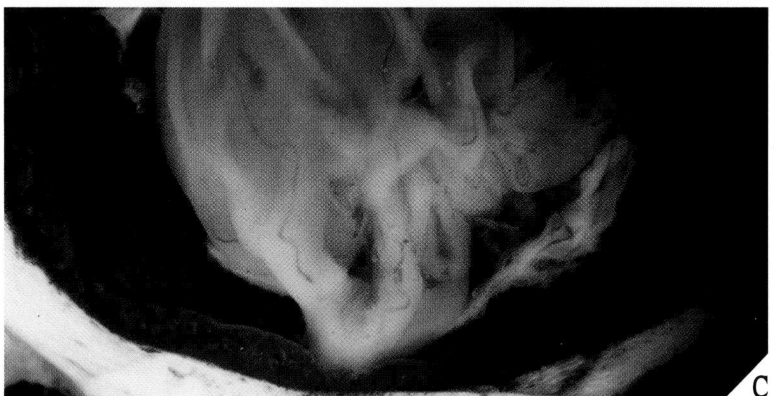

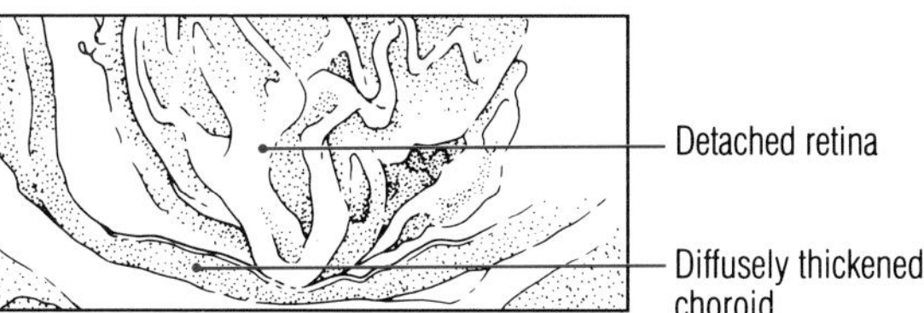

FIGURE 4.4 SYMPATHETIC UVEITIS. A Blunt trauma resulted in rupture of the left globe and a hyphema. The patient developed photophobia in the uninjured right eye seven weeks later. **B** Another patient shows "mutton-fat" keratic precipitates. **C** Enucleated globe shows diffuse thickening of the choroid.

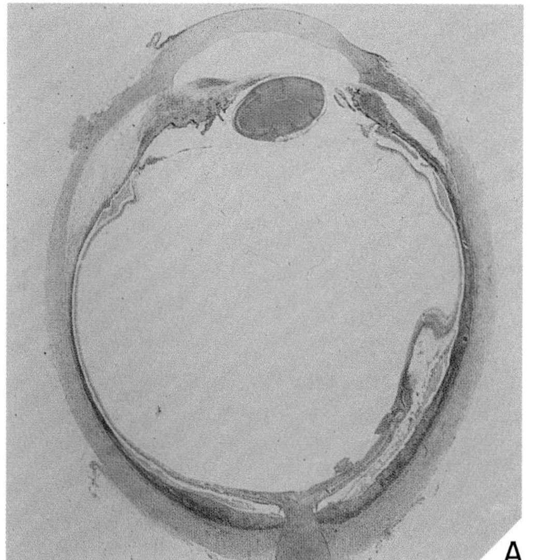

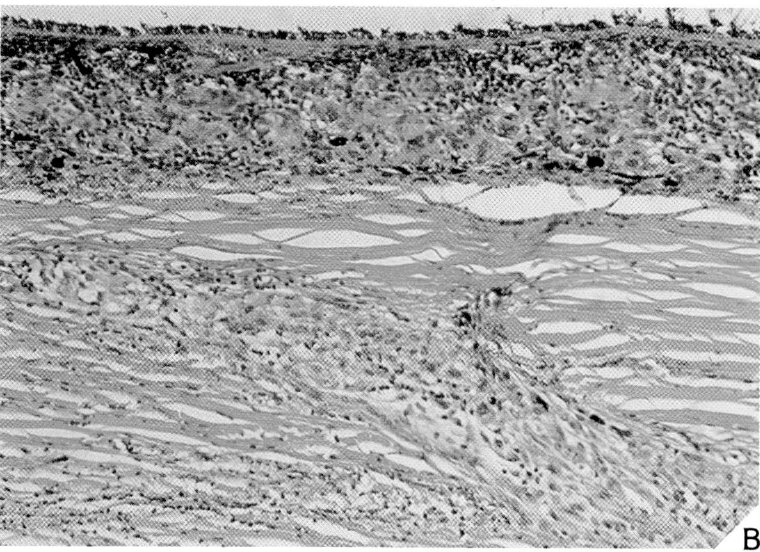

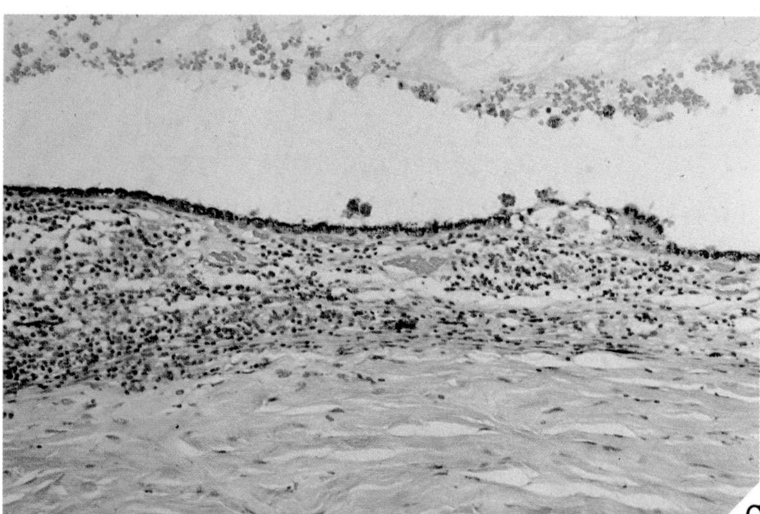

FIGURE 4.5 SYMPATHETIC UVEITIS. A Histologic section shows diffuse thickening of the choroid. **B** The choroid is thickened by a granulomatous inflammatory reaction of the diffuse type. The pale areas represent epithelioid cell formation, and the dark areas consist mainly of lymphocytes. Sparing of the choriocapillaris and pigment phagocytosis by epithelioid cells also are seen. Note the granulomatous inflammatory involvement of a scleral canal in the lower right corner of the picture. **C** A Dalen-Fuchs nodule (i.e., epithelioid cells between the pigment epithelium and the Bruch membrane) is present.

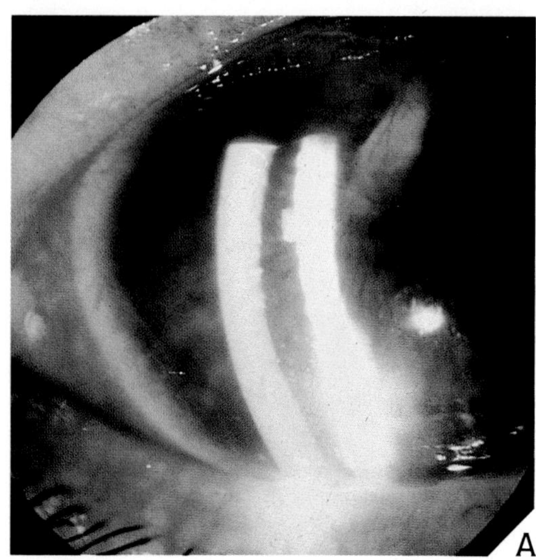

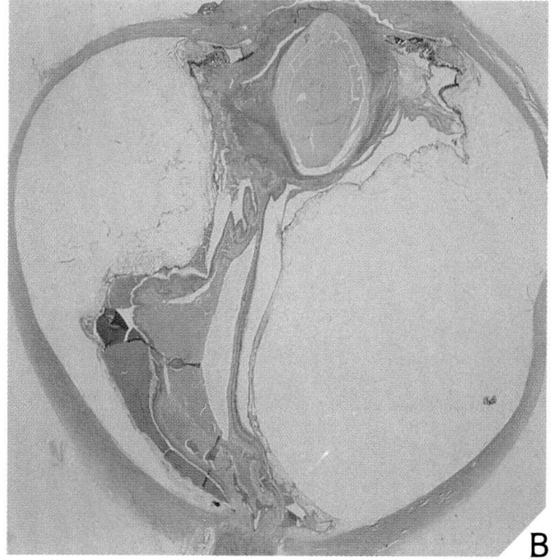

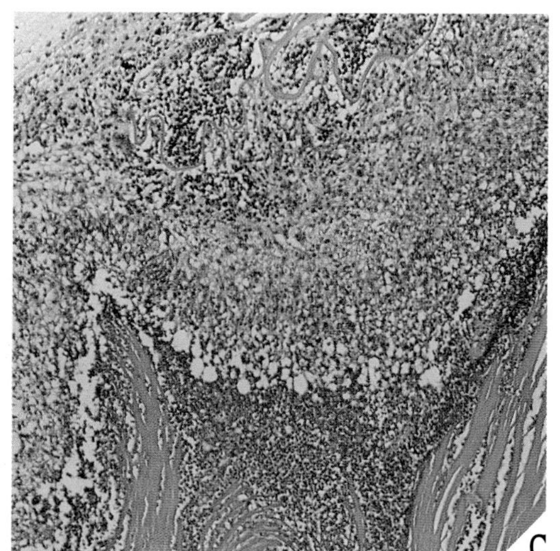

FIGURE 4.6 PHACOANAPHYLACTIC ENDOPHTHALMITIS. A The patient had an iridencleisis in 1971. The eye was injured by blunt trauma in an automobile accident in May 1973. In September 1973, signs of an anterior uveitis developed. Note the small mutton-fat keratic precipitates just to the right of the corneal slit-lamp section in the lower third of the picture. The eye was enucleated in May 1974. **B** The enucleated globe shows iris in the subconjunctival tissue. The lens remnant, mainly nucleus, shows a zonal type of granulomatous reaction, consisting of surrounding epithelioid cells and giant cells, in turn surrounded by lymphocytes and plasma cells, in turn surrounded by granulation tissue. The lens capsule is ruptured posteriorly. **C** Under increased magnification, the typical zonal pattern is seen around the remnant of lens nucleus. (**B**, PAS stain.)

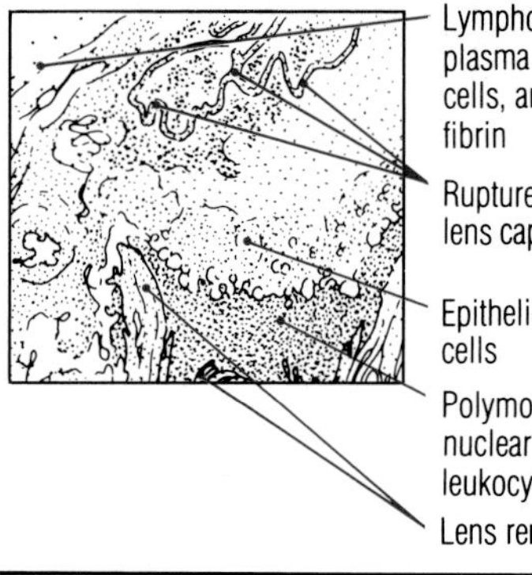

GRANULOMATOUS INFLAMMATION CAUSED BY INFECTIONS

Viral
Cytomegalic inclusion disease
Herpes zoster (shingles)

Bacterial
Tuberculosis
Leprosy
Syphilis
Tularemia
Streptothrix (*Actinomyces*)

Fungal
Blastomycosis
Cryptococcosis
Coccidioidomycosis
Rhinosporidiosis
Phycomycosis (mucormycosis, zygomycosis)
Candidiasis
Histoplasmosis
Sporotrichosis

Parasitic
Toxoplasmosis (protozoa)
Toxocariasis (nematoda)
Trichinosis (nematoda)
Loa loa (nematoda)
Cysticercosis (cestoidea)
Hydatid cyst (cestoidea)
Schistosomiasis (trematoda)

FIGURE 4.7

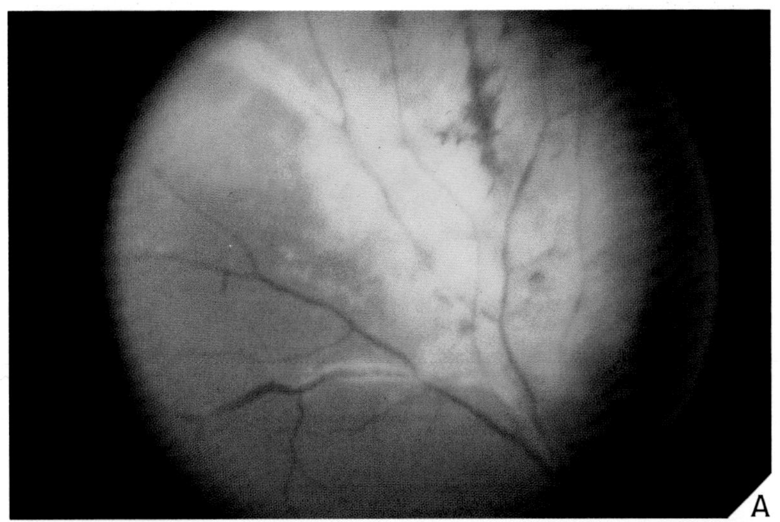

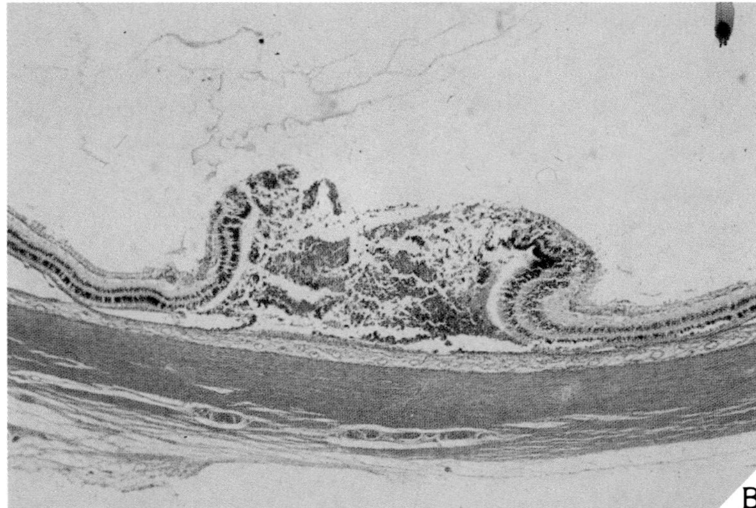

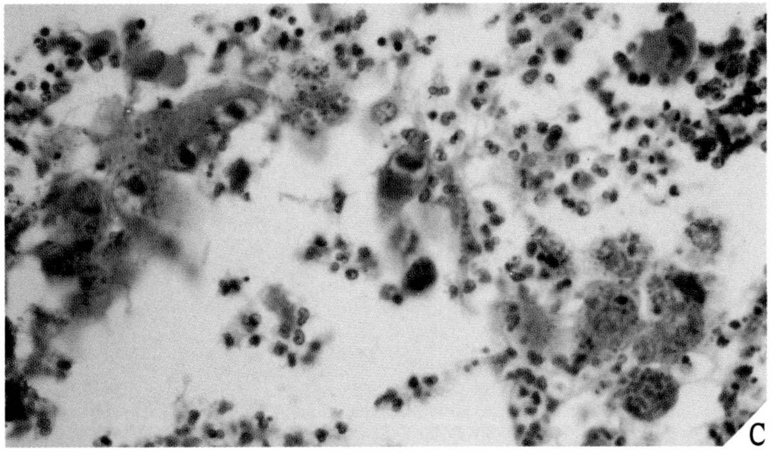

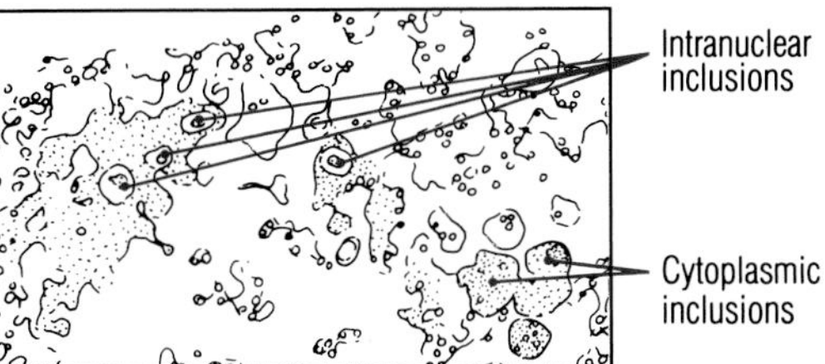

FIGURE 4.8 CYTOMEGALIC INCLUSION DISEASE. A The fundus picture shows the characteristic hemorrhagic exudation ("pizza-pie" appearance) along the retinal vessels. **B** Histologic section shows the relatively normal retina sharply demarcated on each side from the central area of coagulative retinal necrosis, secondary to the infection. The choroid shows a secondary mild and diffuse granulomatous inflammation. **C** Increased magnification shows typical eosinophilic intranuclear inclusion bodies and small round basophilic and cytoplasmic inclusion bodies. (**A**, courtesy Dr. SH Sinclair; **B**, **C**, presented by Dr. Daniel Toussaint at the Verhoeff Society, 1976.)

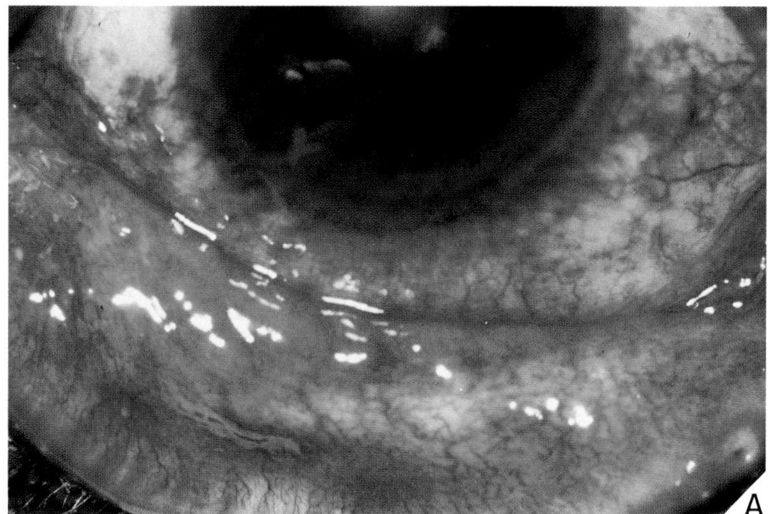

FIGURE 4.9 SYPHILIS. A Small round translucent nodules are seen in the conjunctiva of the inferior fornix. **B** The biopsied nodules show numerous granulomas under the conjunctival epithelium. **C** Increased magnification reveals epithelioid cells within the inflammatory nodules. **D** A special stain demonstrates spirochetes within the inflammatory infiltrate. (**D**, Dieterla; case reported in Spektor FE, et al., 1981.)

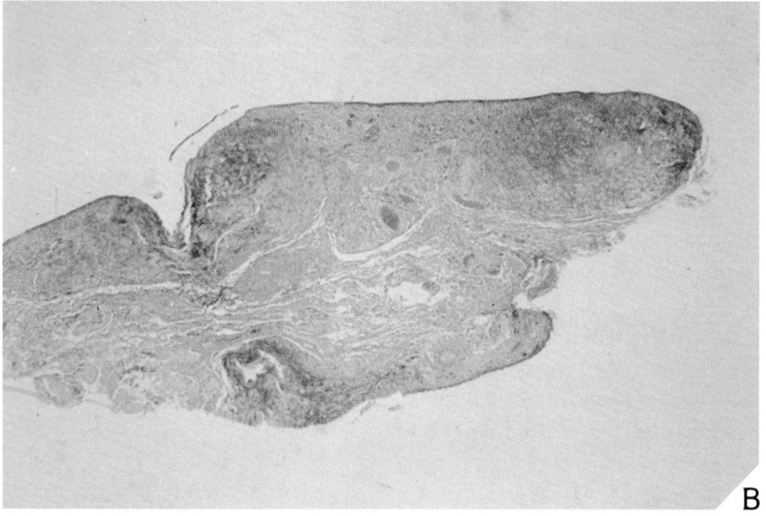

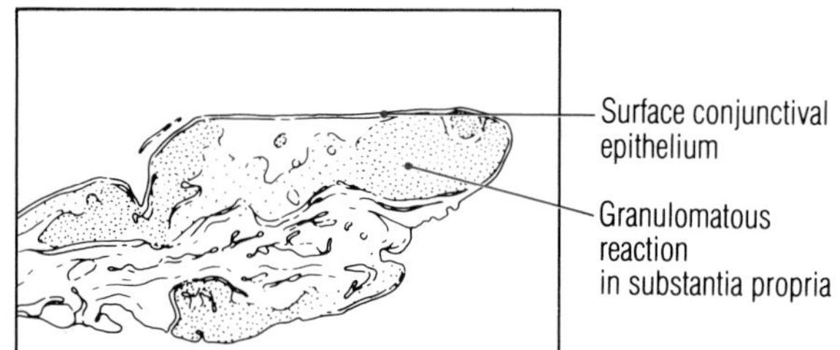

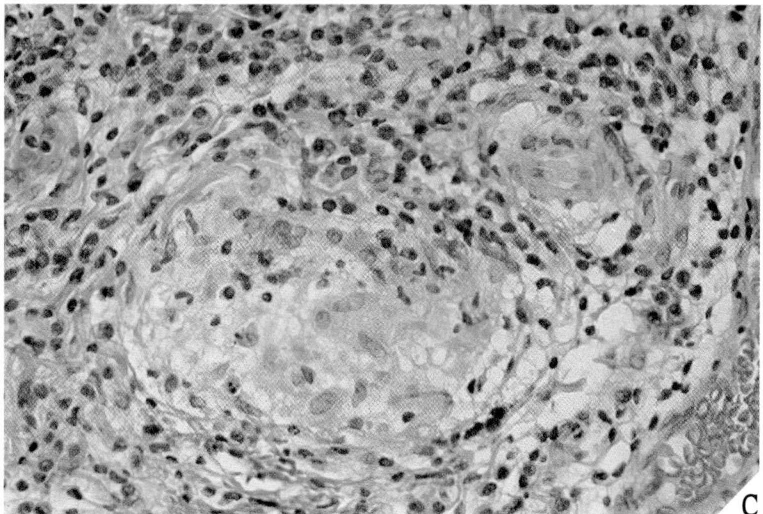

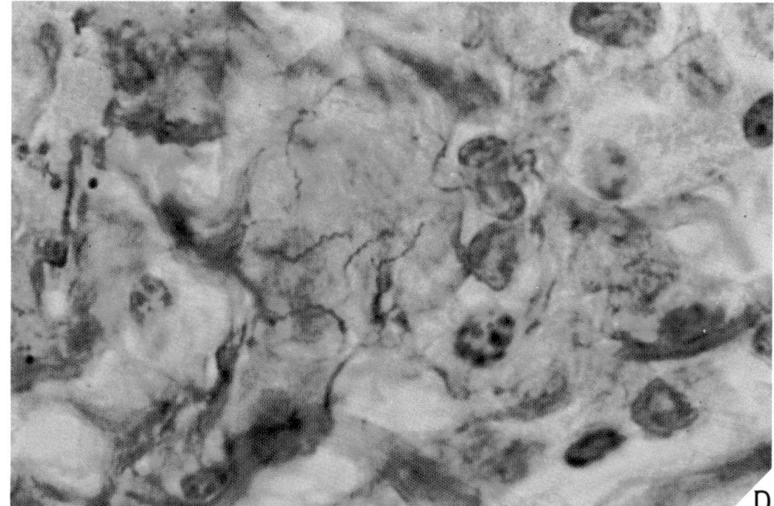

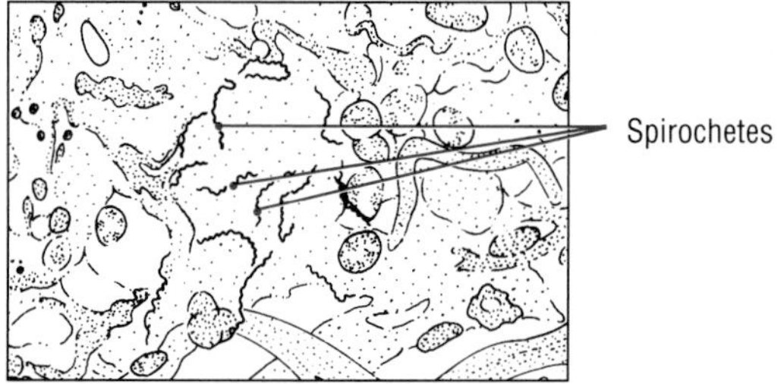

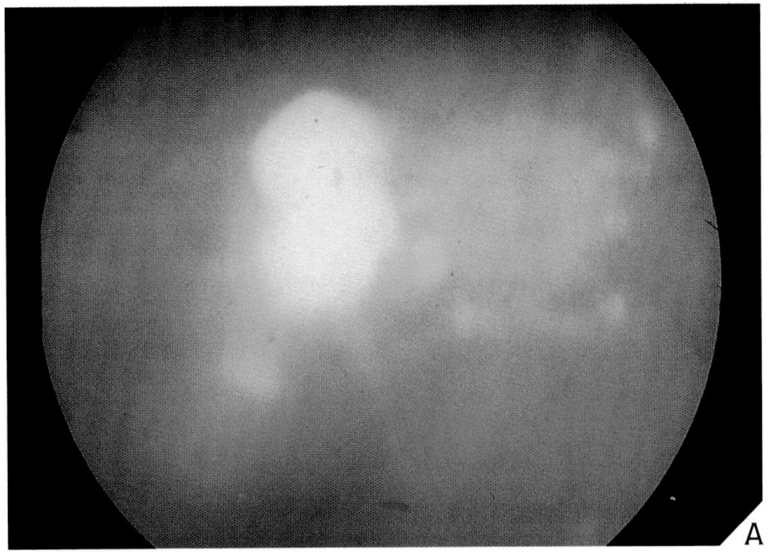

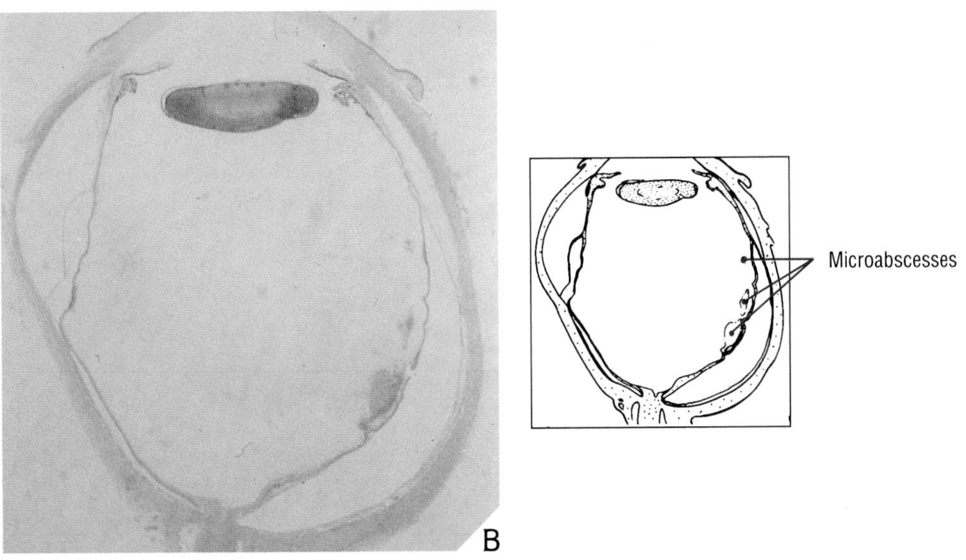

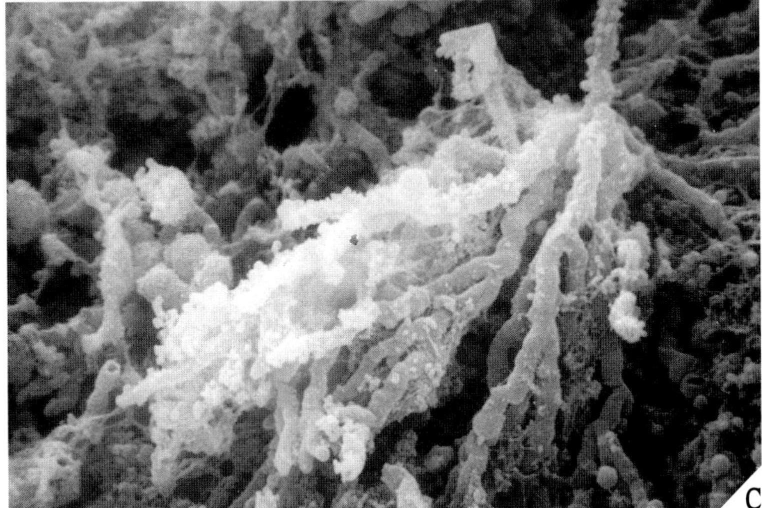

FIGURE 4.10 FUNGAL ENDOPHTHALMITIS. A Immunosuppressed patient developed endophthalmitis. Note the "snowball" opacities in the vitreous just around the optic nerve head. *Candida albicans* was cultured from the blood. **B** Another patient developed decreased vision in his right eye, followed by renal failure two months after a kidney transplant. He died one month later. The histologic section shows microabscesses within the vitreous body characteristic of fungal infection (bacterial infection causes a diffuse vitreous abscess). **C** Scanning electron microscopy demonstrates septate branching *Aspergillus* hyphae. (**C**, courtesy of Dr. RC Eagle Jr, from Yanoff M, Fine BS: *Ocular Pathology*, 2nd ed.)

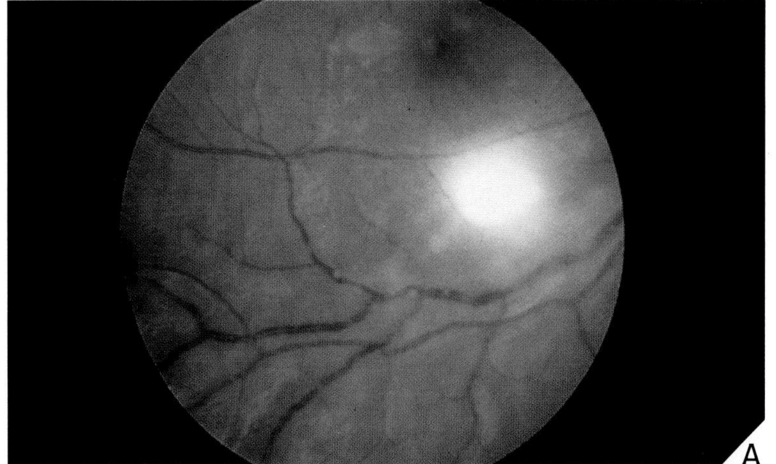

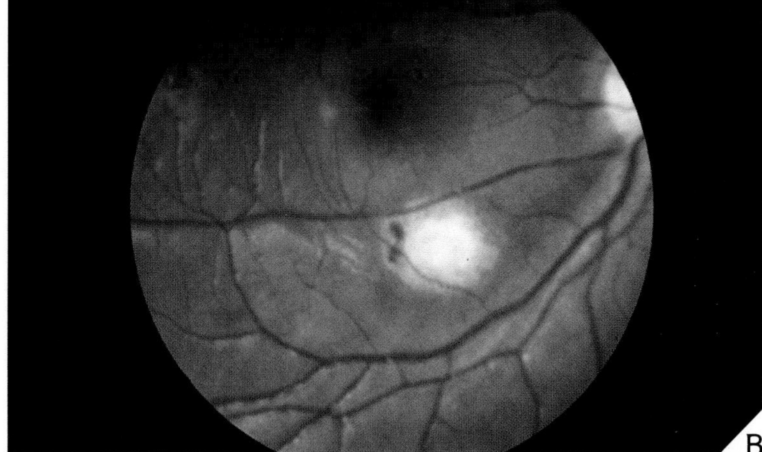

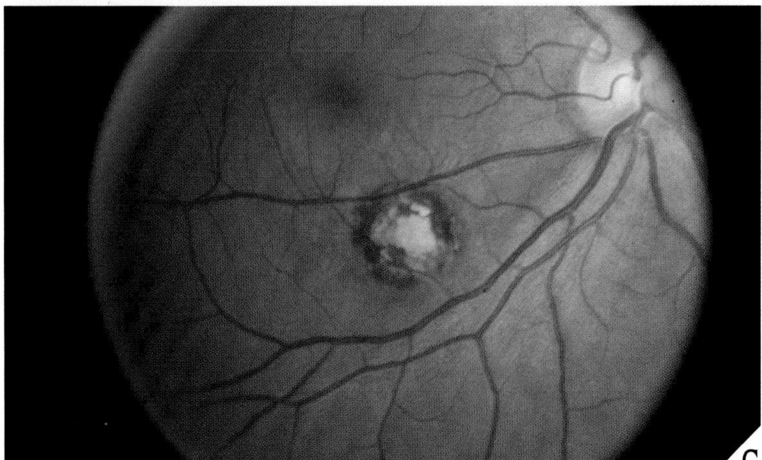

Figure 4.11 Toxoplasmosis. A A 12-year-old girl developed an acute endophthalmitis in her right eye in May 1970. The tiny yellow-white balls on the retinal venules probably represent small granulomas. **B** Early pigmentation is present seven years later. **C** Twelve years later, in 1982, increased pigmentation now makes the lesion appear like a typical toxoplasmosis lesion. (From Yanoff M, Fine BS: *Ocular Pathology*, 3rd ed.)

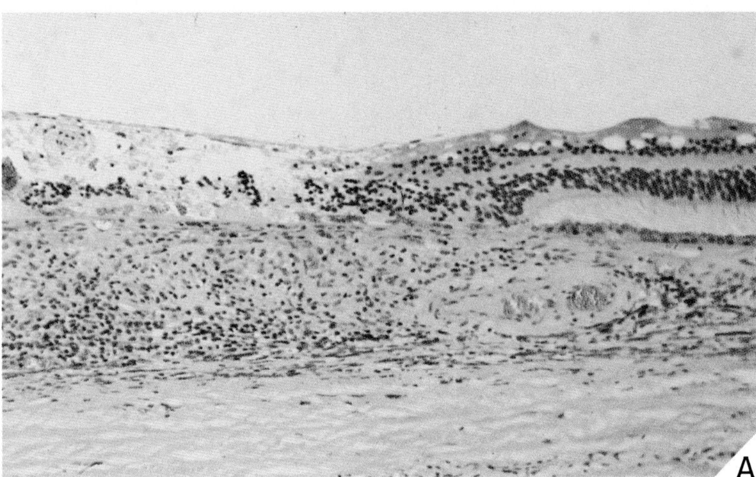

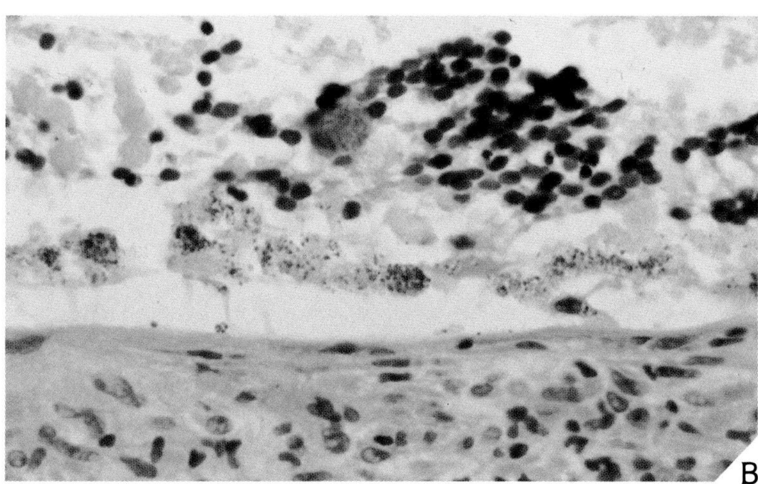

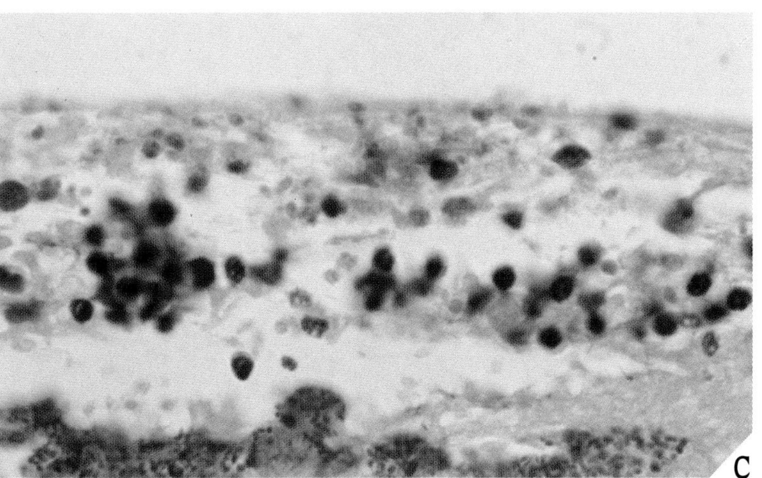

Figure 4.12 Toxoplasmosis. A Histologic section showing an acute coagulative retinal necrosis, whereas the choroid shows a secondary diffuse granulomatous inflammation. **B** A toxoplasmic cyst is present in the retina. Note the tiny nuclei within the cyst. **C** In another section, free forms of the protozoa are present in the necrotic retina. The tiny nuclei are eccentrically placed and the opposite end of the cytoplasm tends to taper.

NONTRAUMATIC, NONINFECTIOUS TYPES OF GRANULOMATOUS INFLAMMATION

- Sarcoidosis
- Granulomatous scleritis
- Chalazion
- Juvenile xanthogranuloma (JXG)
- Granulomatous reaction to Descemet membrane
- Chediak-Higashi syndrome
- Vogt-Koyanagi-Harada syndrome
- Familial chronic granulomatous disease of childhood

FIGURE 4.13

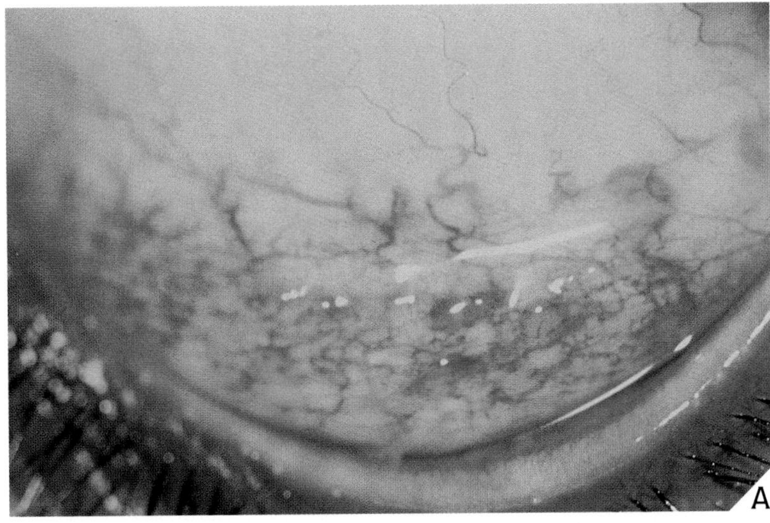

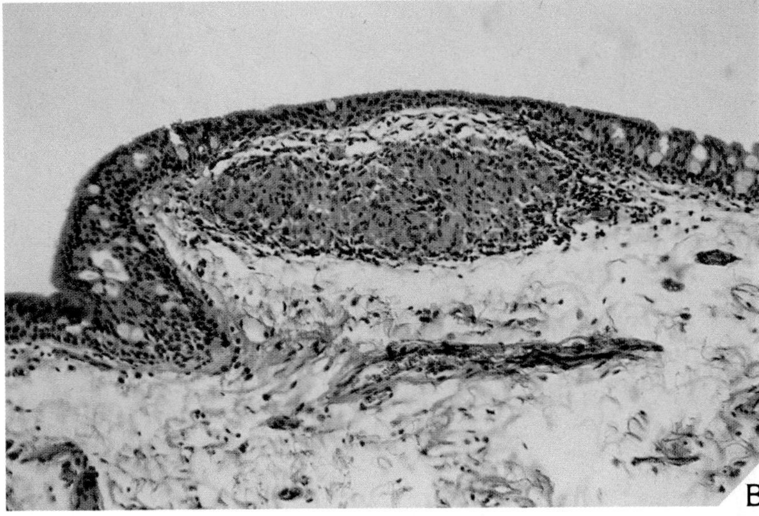

FIGURE 4.14 SARCOIDOSIS. A The patient shows numerous small, round translucent cysts in the conjunctival fornix. **B** A conjunctival biopsy reveals a discrete granuloma, composed of epithelioid cells and surrounded by a rim of lymphocytes and plasma cells. Such granulomas may be found histologically even if no conjunctival nodules are noted clinically.

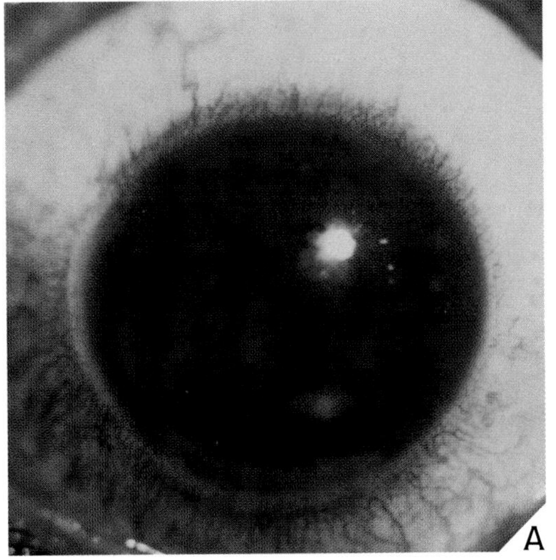

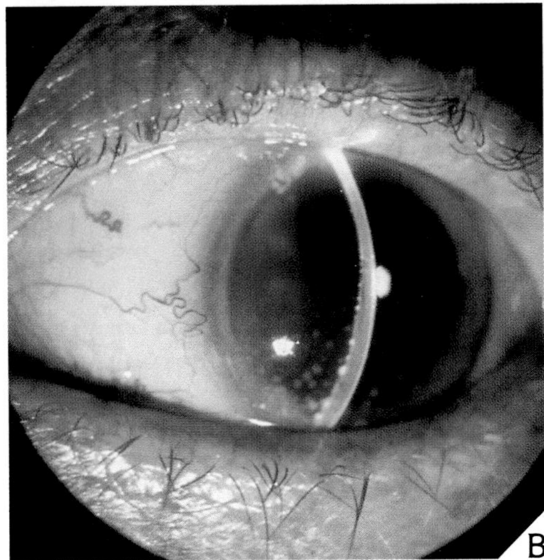

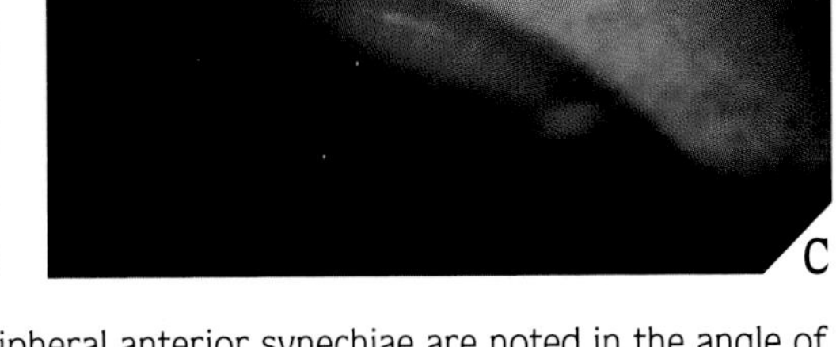

FIGURE 4.15 SARCOIDOSIS. A The iris is involved in the granulomatous process and shows numerous large granulomas. **B** Slit-lamp section shows many mutton-fat keratic precipitates on the posterior corneal surface. **C** Granulomas and peripheral anterior synechiae are noted in the angle of the anterior chamber.

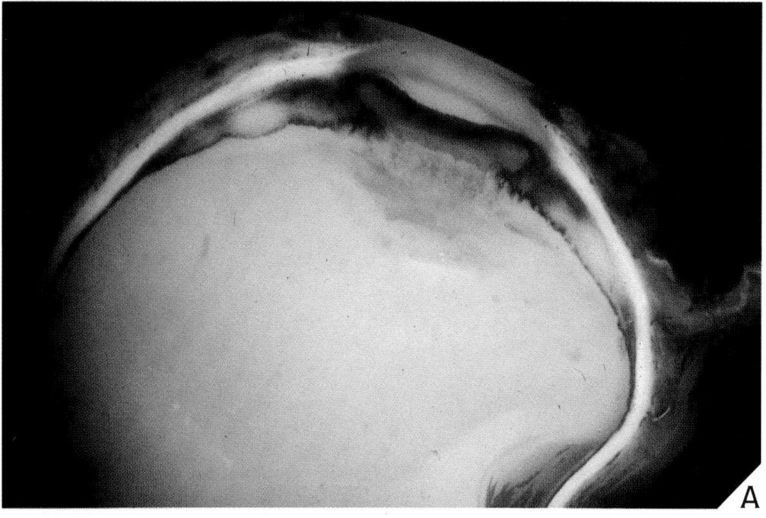

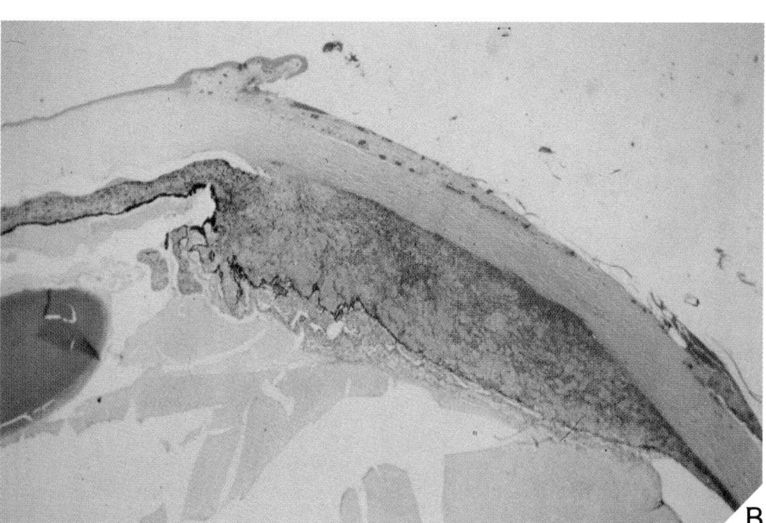

Figure 4.16 Sarcoidosis. A The enucleated globe shows an infiltrate in the ciliary body. **B** The infiltrate consists of a discrete granulomatous inflammation.

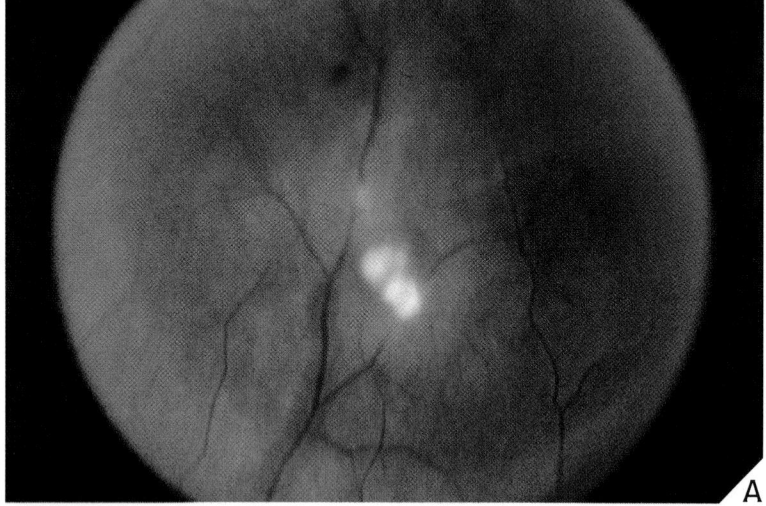

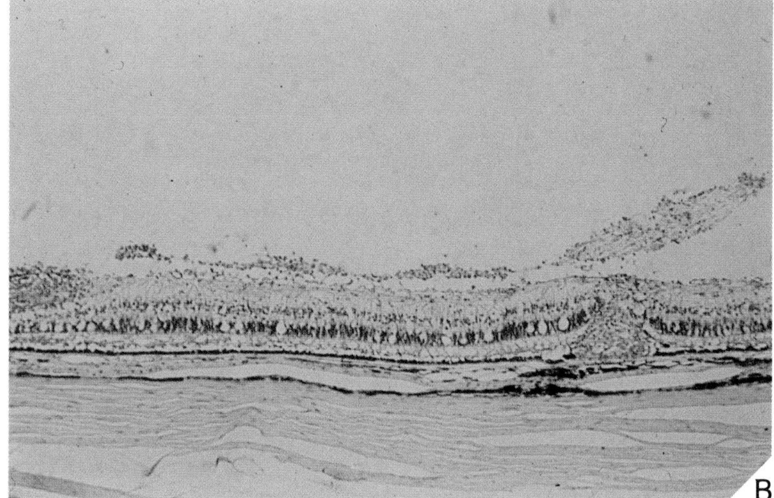

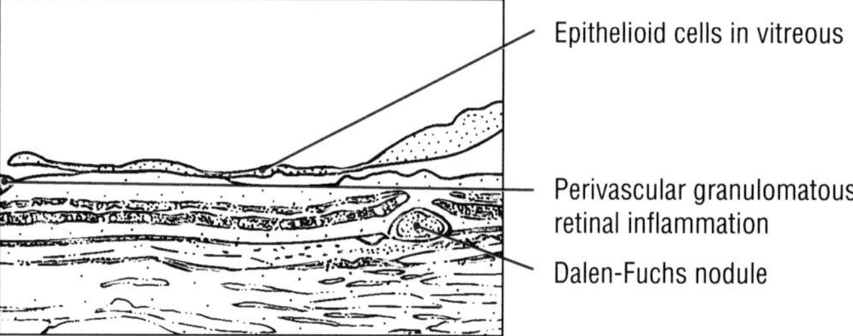

Figure 4.17 Sarcoidosis. A White cellular masses ("balls") are seen in the vitreous compartment on the surface of the retina inferiorly, along with early "candle wax drippings." **B** White balls are caused by accumulations of epithelioid cells in the vitreous, and the candle wax drippings by perivascular granulomatous infiltration in the retina. Candle wax drippings are often an ominous sign, since they may be associated with central nervous system sarcoidosis. Note the Dalen-Fuchs nodule on the right. (**B**, reported in Gass JDM, Olsen CL, 1976.)

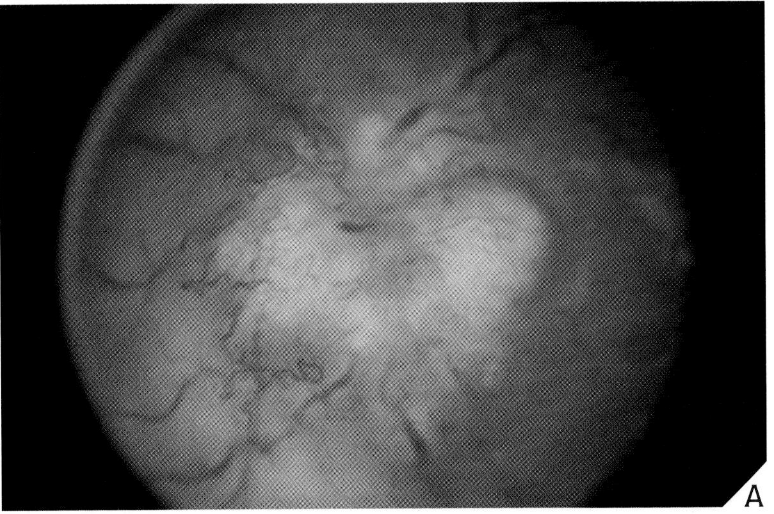

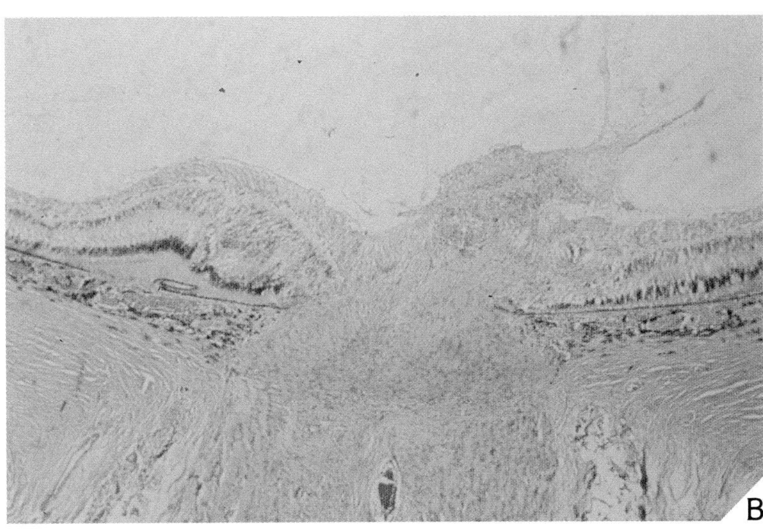

Figure 4.18 Sarcoidosis. A The optic nerve is involved in a mass of granulomas. **B** Histologic section of another patient shows granulomatous inflammation in the anterior portion of the optic nerve. (**A**, courtesy of Dr. AJ Brucker; **B**, reported in Gass JDM, Olsen CL: Trans Am Acad Ophthalmol Otolaryngol 77:739, 1973.)

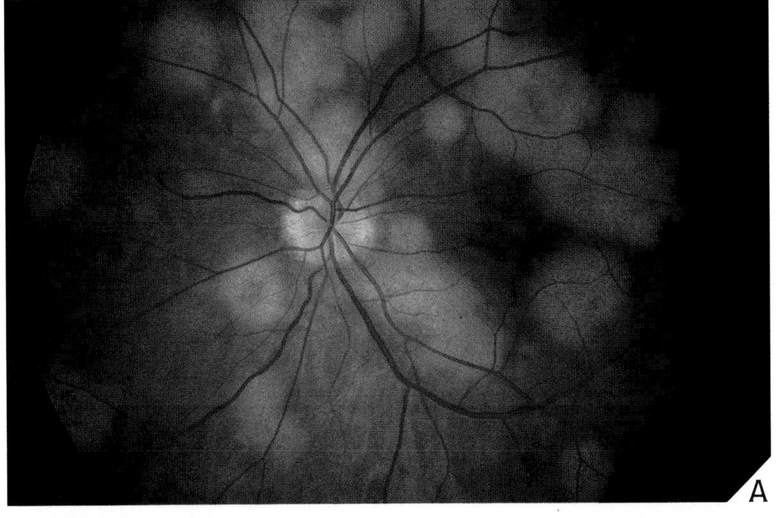

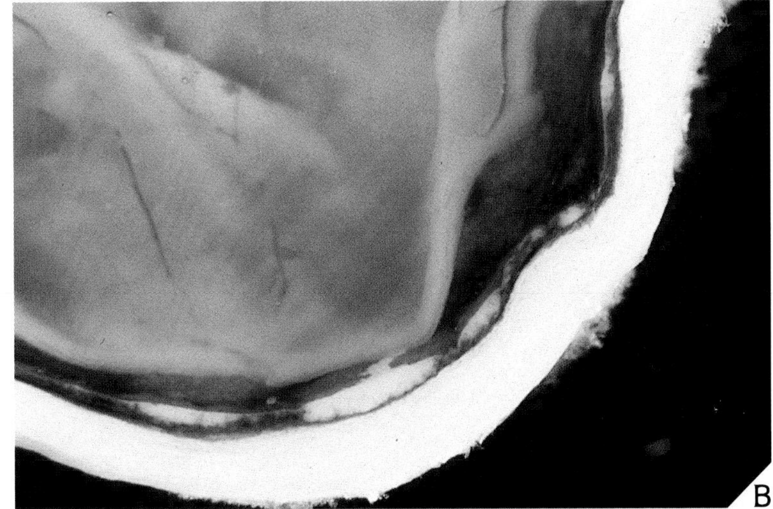

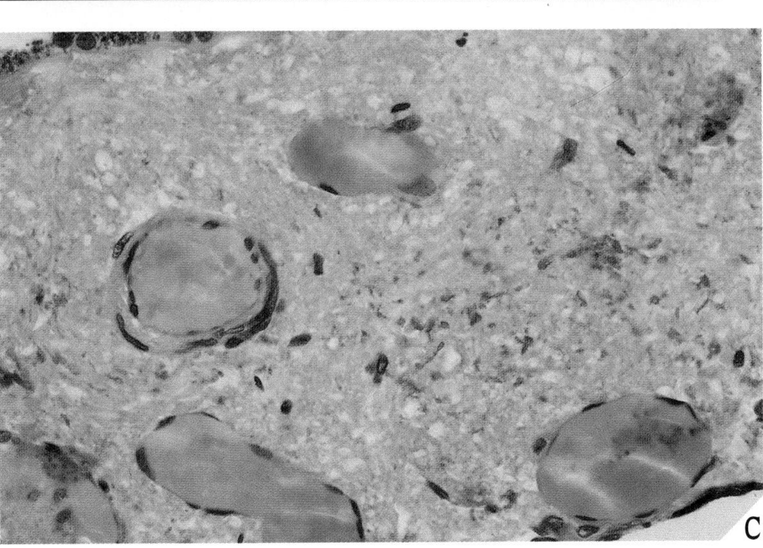

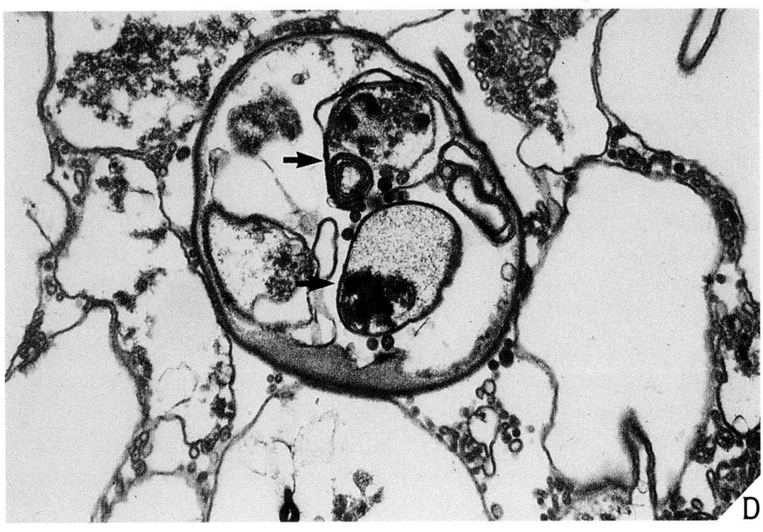

Figure 4.19 Pneumocytis carinii in AIDS. Scattered choroidal infiltrates can be seen in the fundus clinically **A** and in the gross specimen **B** in a patient who had AIDS. **C** The characteristic foamy, eosinophilic, and mostly acellular choroidal infiltrate is shown. **D** An example of the electron-microscopic appearance of *Pneumocystis carinii*, previously thought to be a protozoan parasite of the Sporozoa subphylum, but now believed to be a fungus. (Case presented by Dr. NA Rao at the Verhoeff Society, 1989.)

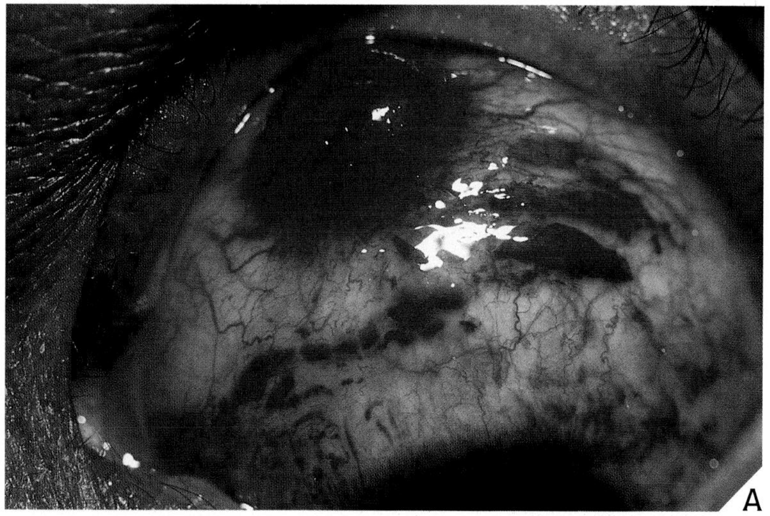

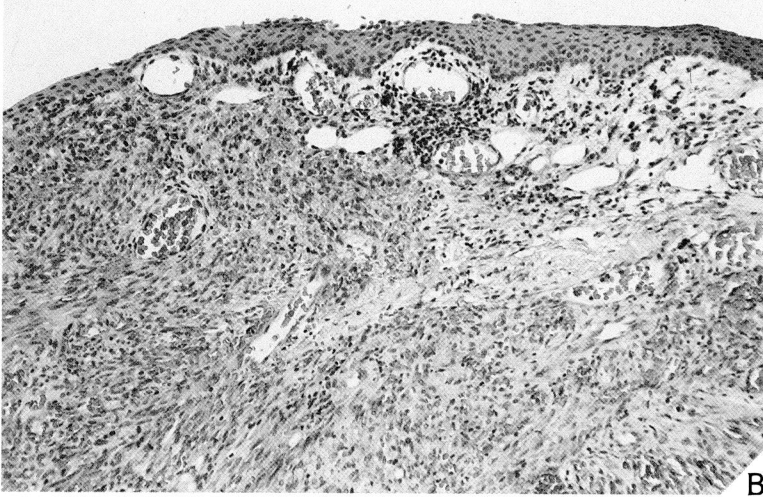

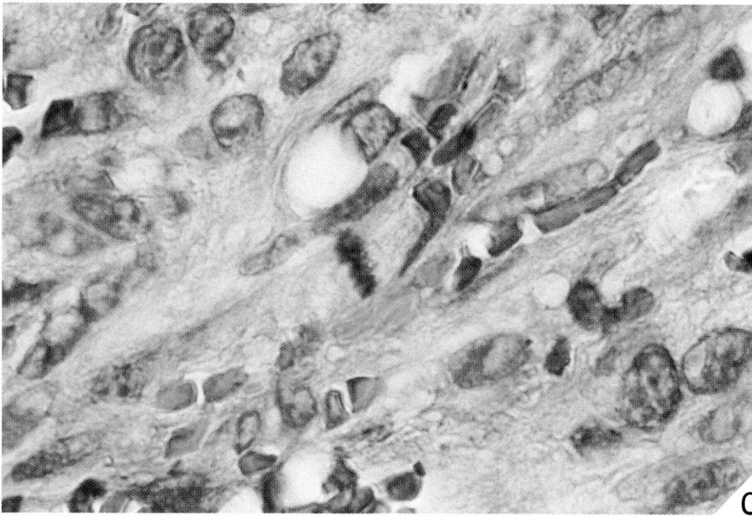

Figure 4.20 Kaposi Sarcoma in AIDS. A A patient who turned out to have AIDS presented with a conjunctival tumor. **B** Biopsy shows neoplastic cells that contain spindle-shaped nuclei and conspicuous nucleoli that are forming bundles or are lining vascular clefts. **C** A mitotic figure is seen. (Case reported by Bedrick JJ, et al., 1981.)

Bibliography

Albert DM, Diaz-Rohena R: A historical review of sympathetic ophthalmia and its epidemiology. Surv Ophthalmol 34:1, 1989.

Bedrick JJ, Schatz NJ, Savino PJ: Conjunctival Kaposi's sarcoma in a patient with myasthenia gravis. Arch Ophthalmol 99:1607, 1981.

Chandler FW, et al: Zygomycosis. Report of four cases with formation of chlamydoconidia in tissue. Am J Clin Pathol 84:99, 1985.

Dugel PU, Gill PS, Frangieh GT, et al: Ocular adnexal Kaposi's sarcoma in acquired immunodeficiency syndrome. Am J Ophthalmol 110:500, 1990.

Forster DJ, Dugel PU, Frangieh GT, et al: Rapidly progressive outer retinal necrosis in the acquired immunodeficiency syndrome. Am J Ophthalmol 110:341, 1990.

Freeman WR, Gross JG, Labelle J, et al: *Pneumocystis carinii* choroidopathy. A new clinical entity. Arch Ophthalmol 107:863, 1989.

Gallin JI, Malech HL: Update on chronic granulomatous diseases of childhood. Immunotherapy and potential for gene therapy. JAMA 263:1533, 1990.

Gass JDM, Olsen CL: Sarcoidosis with optic nerve and retinal involvement. Arch Ophthalmol 94:945, 1976.

Gross JG, Bozzette SA, Mathews WC, et al: Longitudinal study of cytomegalovirus retinitis in acquired immune deficiency syndrome. Ophthalmology 97:681, 1990.

Grossniklaus HE, Specht CS, Allaire G, et al: *Toxoplasma gondii* retinochoroiditis and optic neuritis in acquired immune deficiency syndrome. Ophthalmology 97:1342, 1990.

Jabs DA, Green WR, Fox R, et al: Ocular manifestations of acquired immune deficiency syndrome. Ophthalmol 96:1092, 1989.

Karma A, Huhti E, Poukkula A: Course and outcome of ocular sarcoidosis. Am J Ophthalmol 106:467, 1988.

Khalil M, Lindley S, Matouk E: Tuberculosis of the orbit. Ophthalmology 92:1624, 1985.

Kruger-Lite E, et al: Intraocular cysticercosis. Am J Ophthalmol 99:252, 1985.

Lebowitz MA, Kajobiec FA, Donnenfeld ED, et al: Bilateral epibulbar rheumatoid nodulosis. A new ocular entity. Ophthalmology 95:1256, 1988.

Marak GE, Font RL, Alepa FP: Immunopathogenicity of lens crystallins in the production of experimental lens-induced granulomatous endophthalmitis. Ophthalmic Res 10:33, 1978.

McDonnell PJ, et al: Ocular involvement in patients with fungal infections. Ophthalmology 92:706, 1985.

McLeish WM, Pulido JS, Holland S, et al: The ocular manifestations of syphilis in the human immunodeficiency virus type 1-infected host. Ophthalmology 97:196, 1990.

Nichols CW, et al: Conjunctival biopsy as an aid in evaluation of the patient with suspected sarcoidosis. Ophthalmology 87:287, 1980.

Spaide R, et al: Ocular findings in leprosy in the United States. Am J Ophthalmol 100:411, 1985.

Spektor FE, Eagle RC Jr, Nichols CW: Granulomatous conjunctivitis secondary to *Treponema pallidum.* Ophthalmology 88:863,1981.

Winterkorn JMS: Lyme disease: neurologic and ophthalmic manifestations. Surv Ophthalmol 35:191, 1990.

Zhao M, Jiang Y, Abrahams IW: Association of HLA antigens with Vogt-Koyanagi-Harada syndrome in a Han Chinese population. Arch Ophthalmol 109:368, 1991.

Surgical and Nonsurgical Trauma

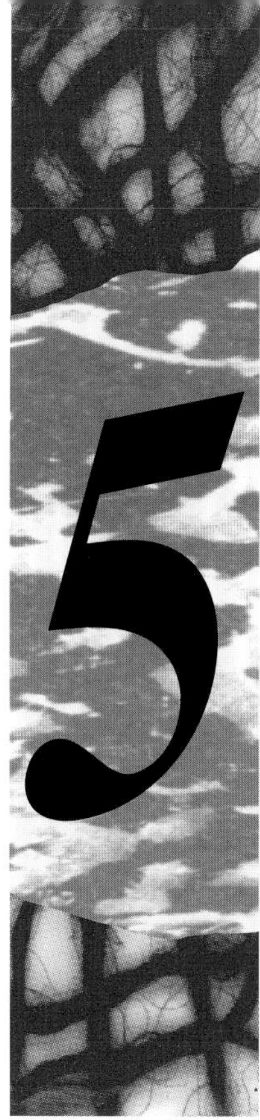

Complications of Intraocular Surgery

Complications of intraocular surgery may occur immediately, during the postoperative period, or may be delayed. The "immediate" period is from the time the decision is made to operate until the patient leaves the operating room. The postoperative period extends from the time the patient leaves the operating room until about three months after surgery. The delayed period occurs after the third month following surgery. Cataract surgery will be used as the prototype for intraocular surgery. Some complications occur that are unpredictable in a specific patient (e.g, intraocular hemorrhage), while others occur because appropriate planning and techniques are not used. It is important to make the correct diagnosis before the surgery is decided upon. There are numerous examples of uveal melanomas and ocular retinoblastomas being discovered after cataracts have been removed, the cataracts having formed secondary to the tumors. Surgical technique must be meticulous. A perfectly performed procedure can end in a disaster simply because of inadequate anesthesia. Even when everything goes well, however, complications may occur. Some of the common and important types of complications will be illustrated.

Aside from complications that occur from the surgery itself, complications also can result from the introduction of a lens implant into the eye. Some examples will be shown.

Complications of Nonsurgical Trauma

Broadly speaking, nonsurgical trauma can be divided into two types: trauma following a contusion and trauma following penetrating and perforating ocular injuries. A contusion results from an external (direct or indirect) force on the eye. The most common contusive injury is one that results from direct, blunt trauma to the eye. The contusion is the injury that results from the force propagated throughout the eye (i.e., the concussive force). Every part of the eye can be affected. An injury may be so severe that a tissue or structure of the eye is partially cut or torn, resulting in a penetrating or perforating injury. When this occurs, the effects of the torn tissue must be considered in addition to the effects of the contusion. Rupture of the globe usually occurs at its thinnest parts: at the limbus, at the sclera just posterior to the insertion of the rectus muscles, or just adjacent to the optic nerve. At the time of perforation, sterile or contaminated objects may be introduced into the interior of the eye, and their added effects also must be considered.

In addition to penetrating and perforating injuries, other types of injuries may involve the eye. Chemicals may be splashed into the eye, or the eyes may be involved in burns or radiation-induced injuries. Injuries to other parts of the body may have ocular effects, e.g., traumatic carotid-carvernous fistula. Examples of some of the most common and important types of nonsurgical trauma will be illustrated.

IMMEDIATE COMPLICATIONS OF INTRAOCULAR SURGERY

Misdiagnosis
Cataract may be secondary to inflammation or neoplasm
Retinal detachment may be secondary to inflammation or neoplasm

Faulty surgical technique
Inadequate facial or ocular anesthesia
Misplacement of incision or sutures
Stripping of Descemet membrane
Iridodialysis

Retrobulbar hemorrhage

Vitreous loss

Expulsive choroidal hemorrhage

FIGURE 5.1

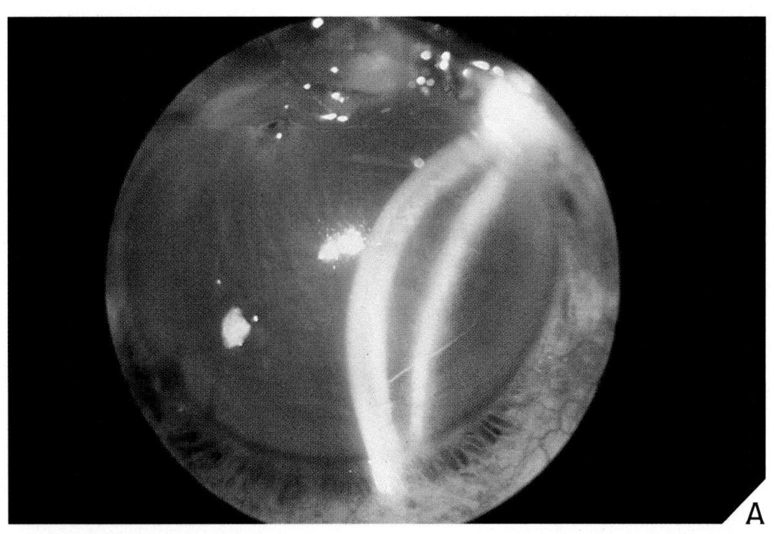

FIGURE 5.2 STRIPPING OF DESCEMET MEMBRANE. A Descemet membrane was stripped over a large area during filtration surgery. The edge of the membrane, free in the anterior chamber, can be seen to the right of the slit-lamp corneal section. **B** The gross specimen shows the stripped membrane between the iris and the cornea. **C** Histology demonstrates the region of filtration. Descemet membrane can be seen in the anterior chamber between the iris and the cornea. (Case reported in Kozart DM, Eagle RC Jr, 1981.)

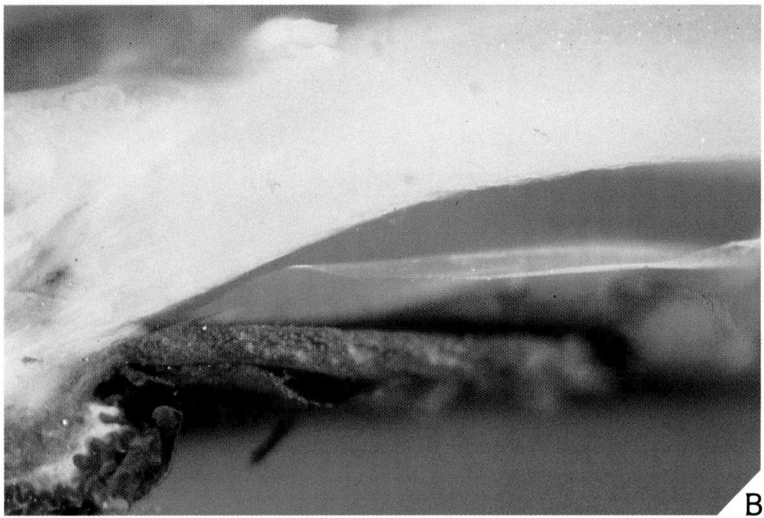

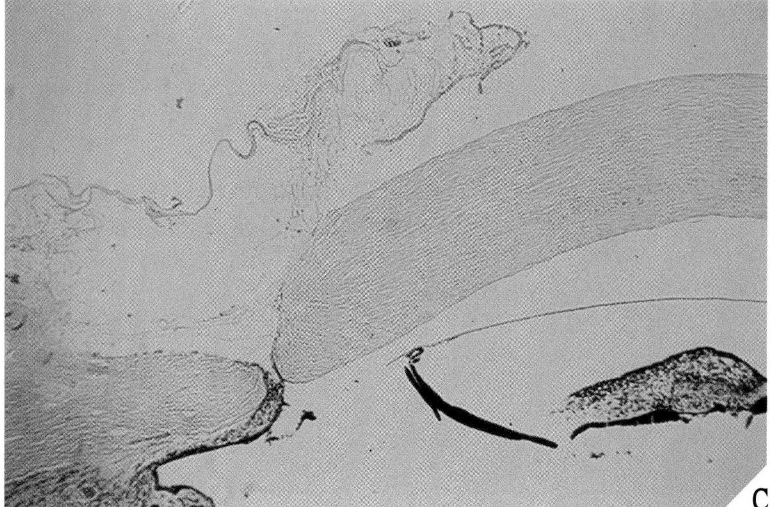

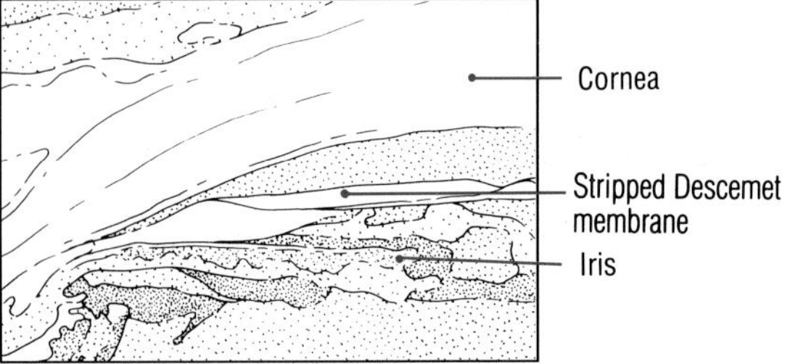

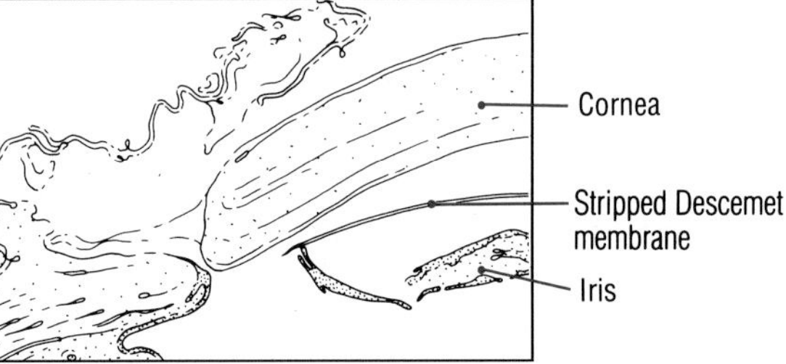

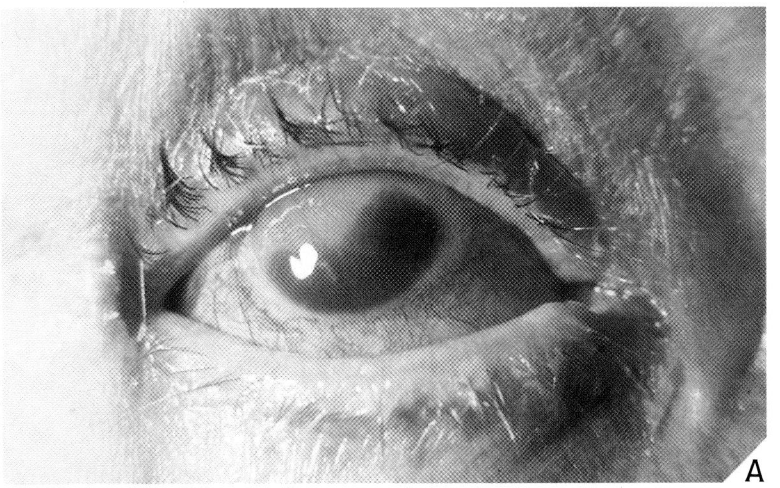

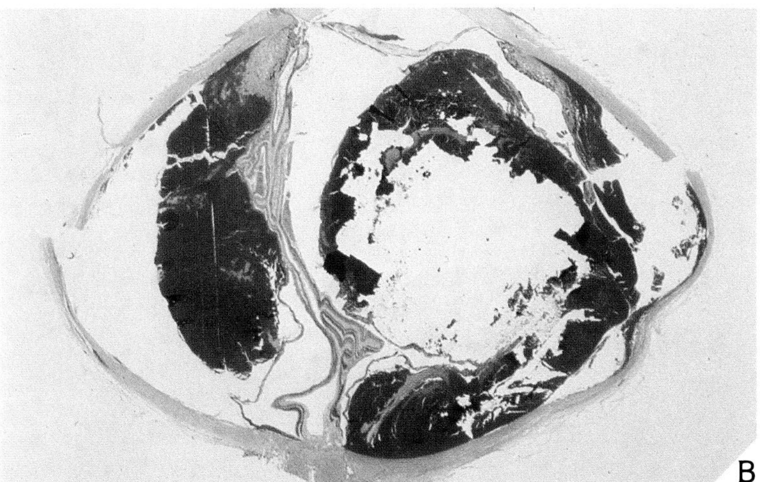

FIGURE 5.3 EXPULSIVE CHOROIDAL HEMORRHAGE. A A large hyphema is present in the anterior chamber. The patient had an expulsive choroidal hemorrhage during surgery. **B** Histologic section shows hemorrhage in the choroid and subretinal space. The retina is in the corneoscleral wound. (**A**, courtesy of Dr. HG Scheie.)

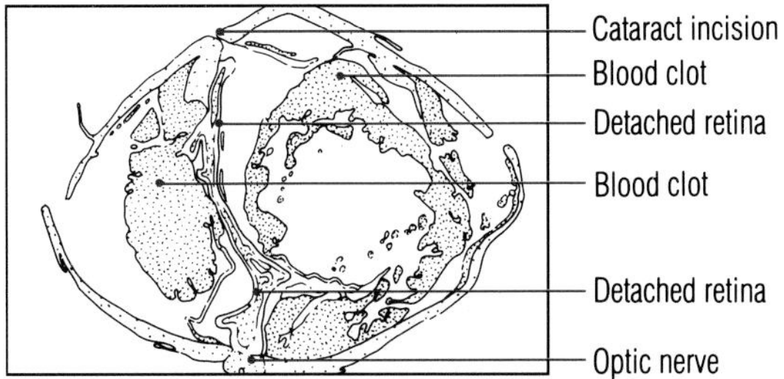

POSTOPERATIVE COMPLICATIONS OF INTRAOCULAR SURGERY

Flat chamber
Faulty wound closure
Choroidal detachment
Aphakic or pseudophakic glaucoma
Choroidal hemorrhage
Iris incarceration or prolapse
Fistulizatlon of cataract wound
Poor wound healing

Striate keratopathy

Hyphema

Corneal edema
Secondary to increased intraocular pressure
Secondary to corneal endothelial damage
Secondary to adherent vitreous or iris
Secondary to splitting off of Descemet membrane
Aggravation of Fuchs combined dystrophy

Subretinal hemorrhage

Retinal detachment

Inflammation—may be infectious (usually bacterial) or noninfectious

FIGURE 5.4

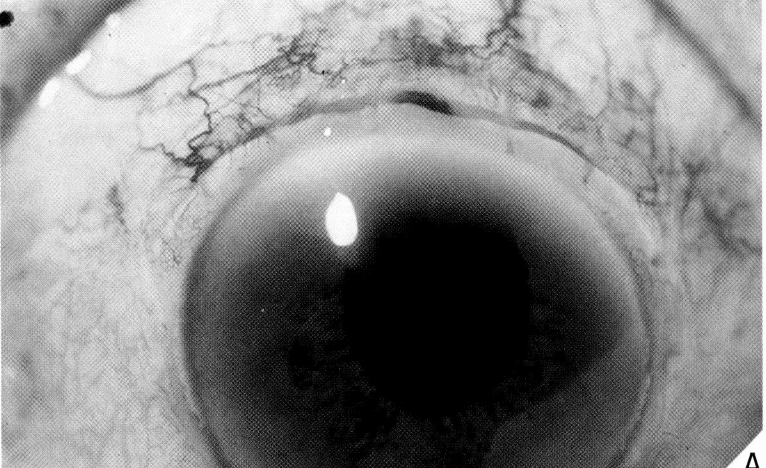

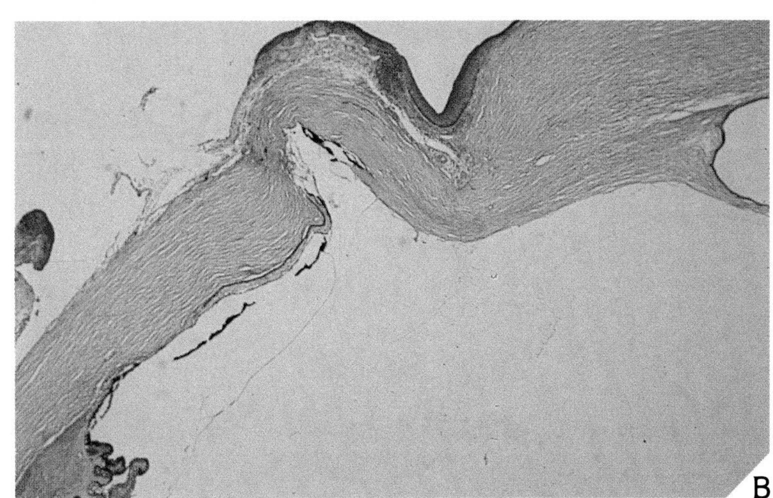

FIGURE 5.5 IRIS IN THE WOUND. A Two weeks postoperatively, the iris has prolapsed through the wound and presents subconjunctivally at the 12-o'clock position. **B** In this case, the iris has become incarcerated within the wound, causing the internal portion of the wound to gape.

DELAYED COMPLICATIONS OF INTRAOCULAR SURGERY

Corneal edema

Elschnig pearls

Soemmerring ring cataract

Retinal detachment

Glaucoma
Peripheral anterior synechiae
Posterior synechiae
Epithelial downgrowth (or cyst)
Stromal overgrowth
Endothelial overgrowth

Inflammation
Infectious—usually fungal or *Staphylococcus epidermidis*
Uveitis
Sympathetic uveitis
Phacoanaphylactic endophthalmitis

Cystoid macular edema

Atrophia or phthisis bulbi

FIGURE 5.6

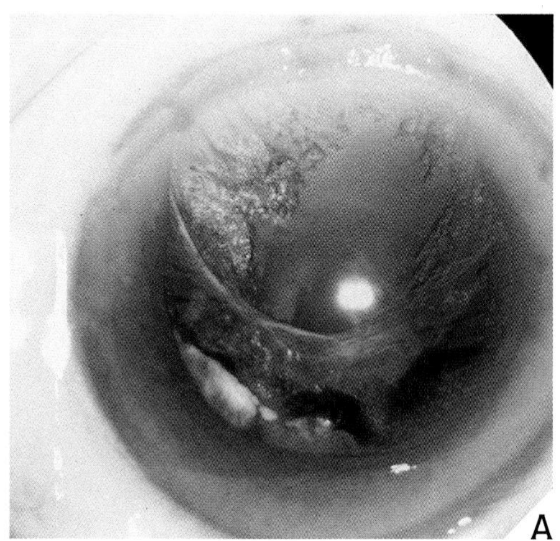

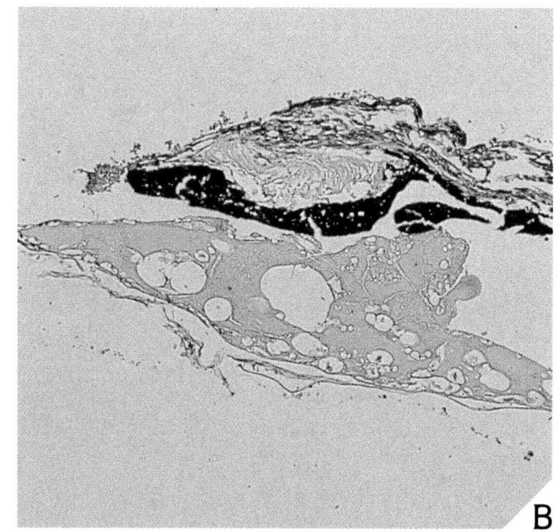

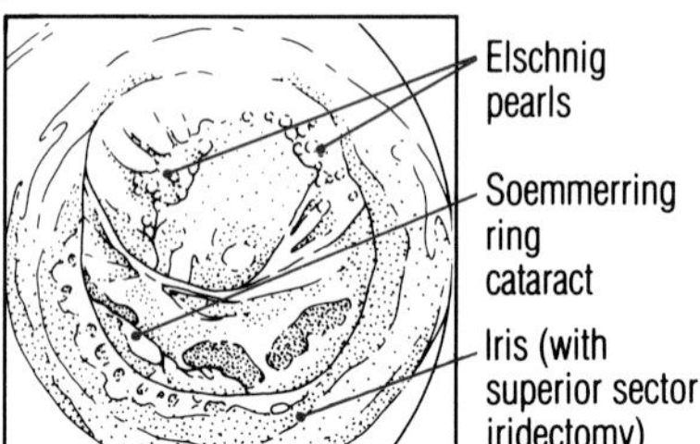

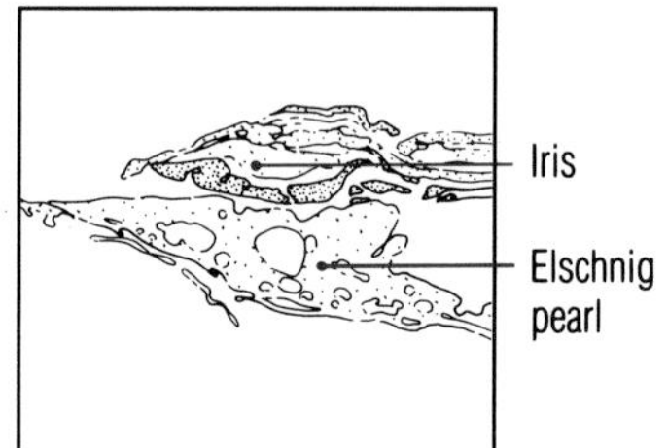

FIGURE 5.7 ELSCHNIG PEARLS AND SOEMMERRING RING CATARACT. A Elschnig pearls are seen as tiny translucent spheres in the superior peripheral pupillary space. Cortical remnants in the form of a Soemmerring ring cataract are noted from six to eight o'clock. **B** Pearls arise from aberrant attempts by the lens cells to form new lens "fibers," often in close association with a Soemmerring ring cataract. A Soemmerring ring cataract is caused by cortical material being trapped in the equatorial portion of the lens in a doughnut configuration. (**A**, from *Ocular Pathology*, 2nd ed, by M Yanoff and BS Fine.)

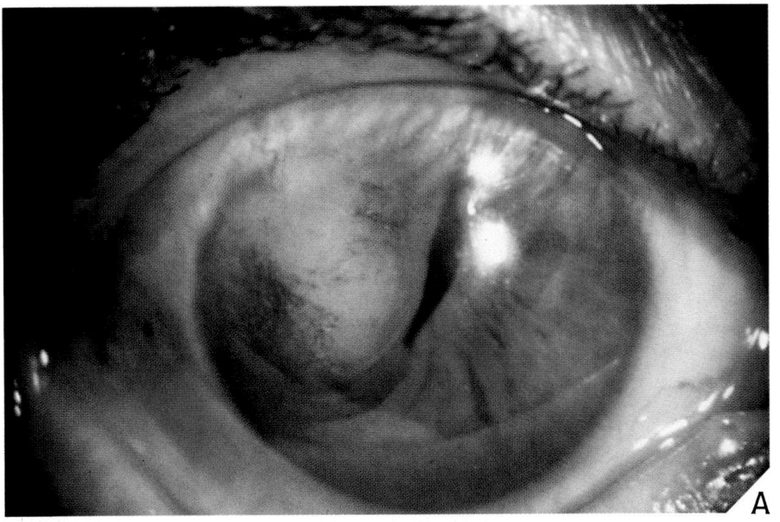

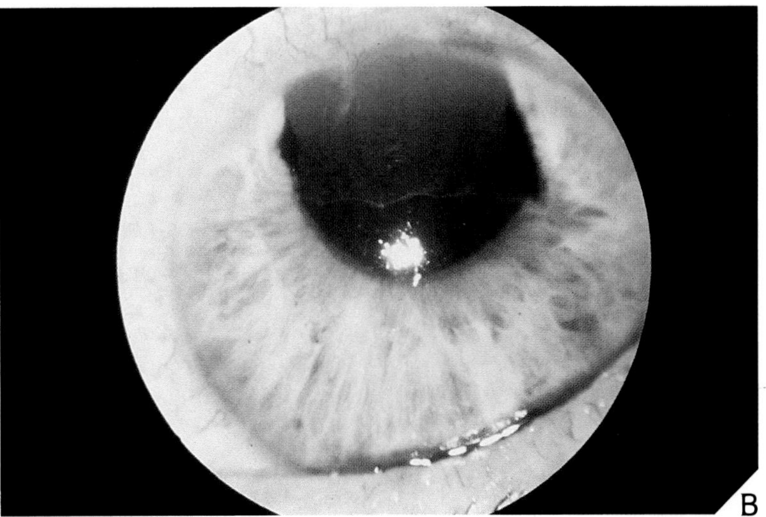

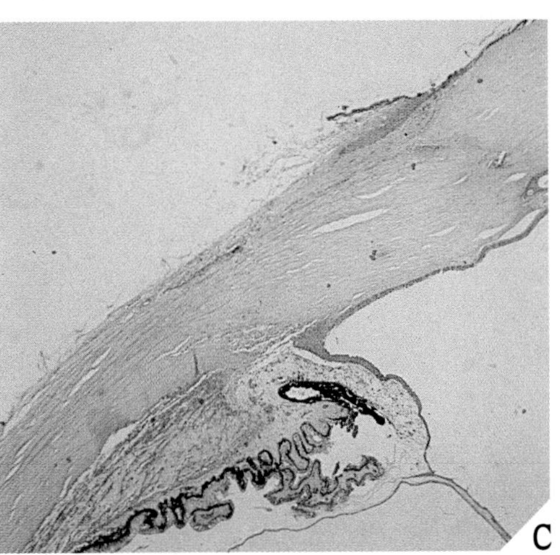

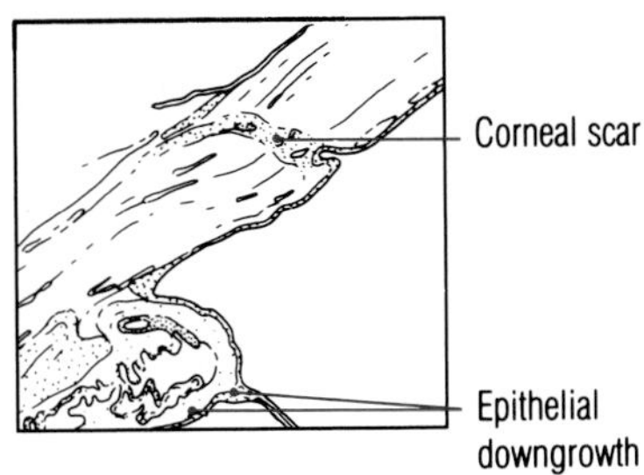

FIGURE 5.8 EPITHELIAL INGROWTH. A Implantation of epithelium on the iris at the time of surgery has resulted in the formation of a large epithelial cyst that obstructs most of the pupil. The milky material within the cyst consists of desquamated epithelial cells. **B** In another case, the epithelium has grown into the eye through the cataract incision and is developing as a downgrowth on the back of the superior one-third of the cornea and onto the superior iris. The line of transition between epithelium and endothelium is seen clearly on the posterior cornea as a horizontal line. **C** Epithelium is present over the posterior surface of the cornea, within the angle, over the iris, and extending posteriorly onto the vitreous. (**B**, case reported in Yanoff M, 1975.)

COMPLICATIONS RELATED TO LENS IMPLANTATION

Stripping of Descemet membrane

Iris atrophy

Lens migration

Subluxation: implant migrates within implanted chamber

Dislocation: implant migrates out of implanted chamber

Glaucoma

Pupillary block

UGH syndrome (uveitis, glaucoma, hyphema)

Corneal edema

Inflammation

Precipitates on implant

Sterile endophthalmitis

Infectious endophthalmitis (incidence 0.07%), e.g., *S. epidermidis* and *P. acnes*, especially after posterior capsulectomy

Secondary membranes

Lens cell proliferation or cicatrization of posterior capsule, or both ("after cataract")

Corneal edema (bullous keratopathy)

Iris-fixated implant

FIGURE 5.9

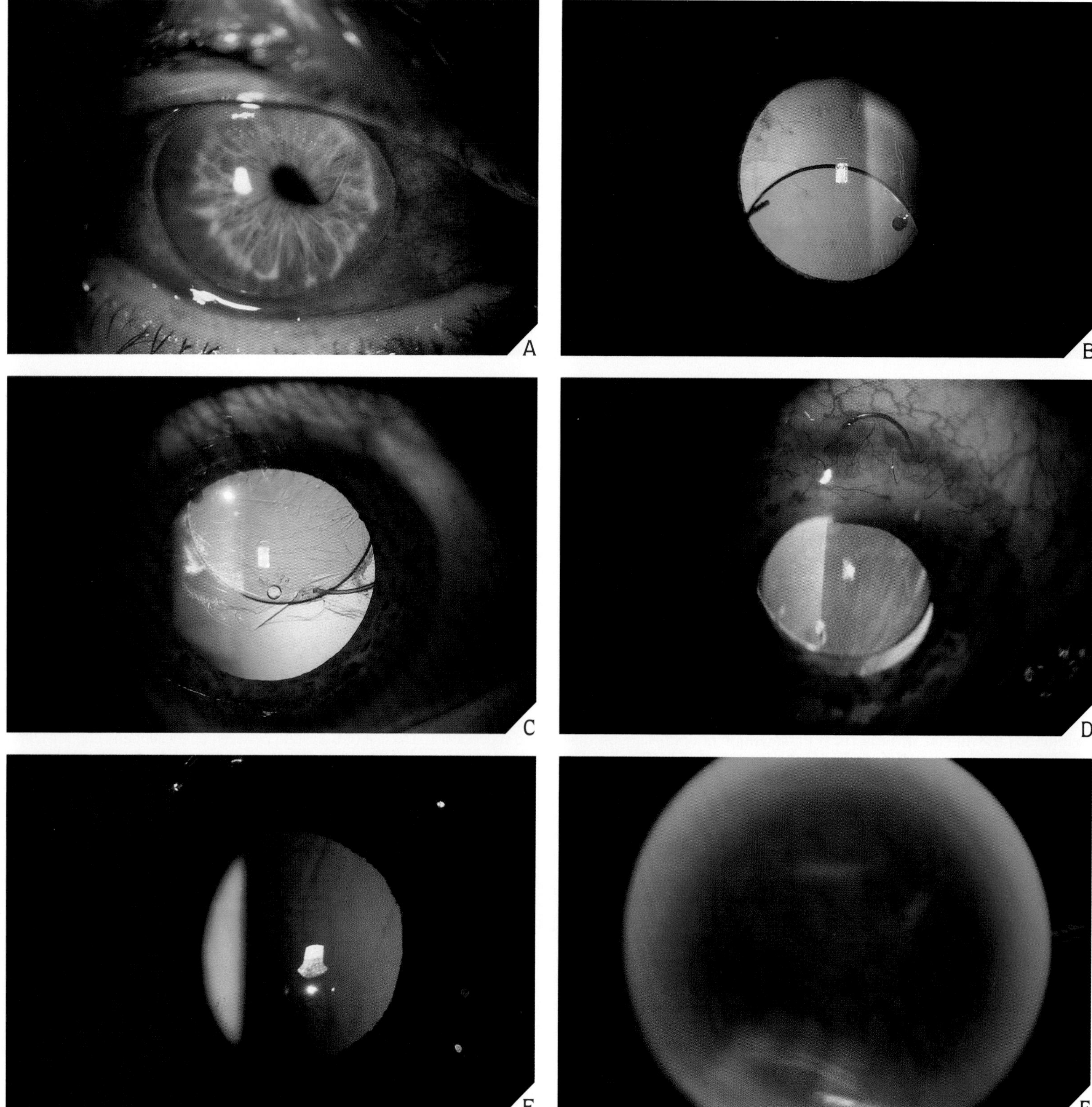

FIGURE 5.10 IMPLANT MIGRATION. A The implant's loop may migrate, as here, into the anterior chamber. The implant's optic also may migrate into the anterior chamber, causing iris capture or entrapment (see Figure 5.13A). The implant may subluxate downward (sunset syndrome, **B**), upward (sunrise syndrome, **C**), out of the eye, as has the superior loop here (**D**), or it may dislocate, as here into the vitreous (**E**, first postoperative day; no implant visible. **F**, implant is in the inferior anterior vitreous compartment).

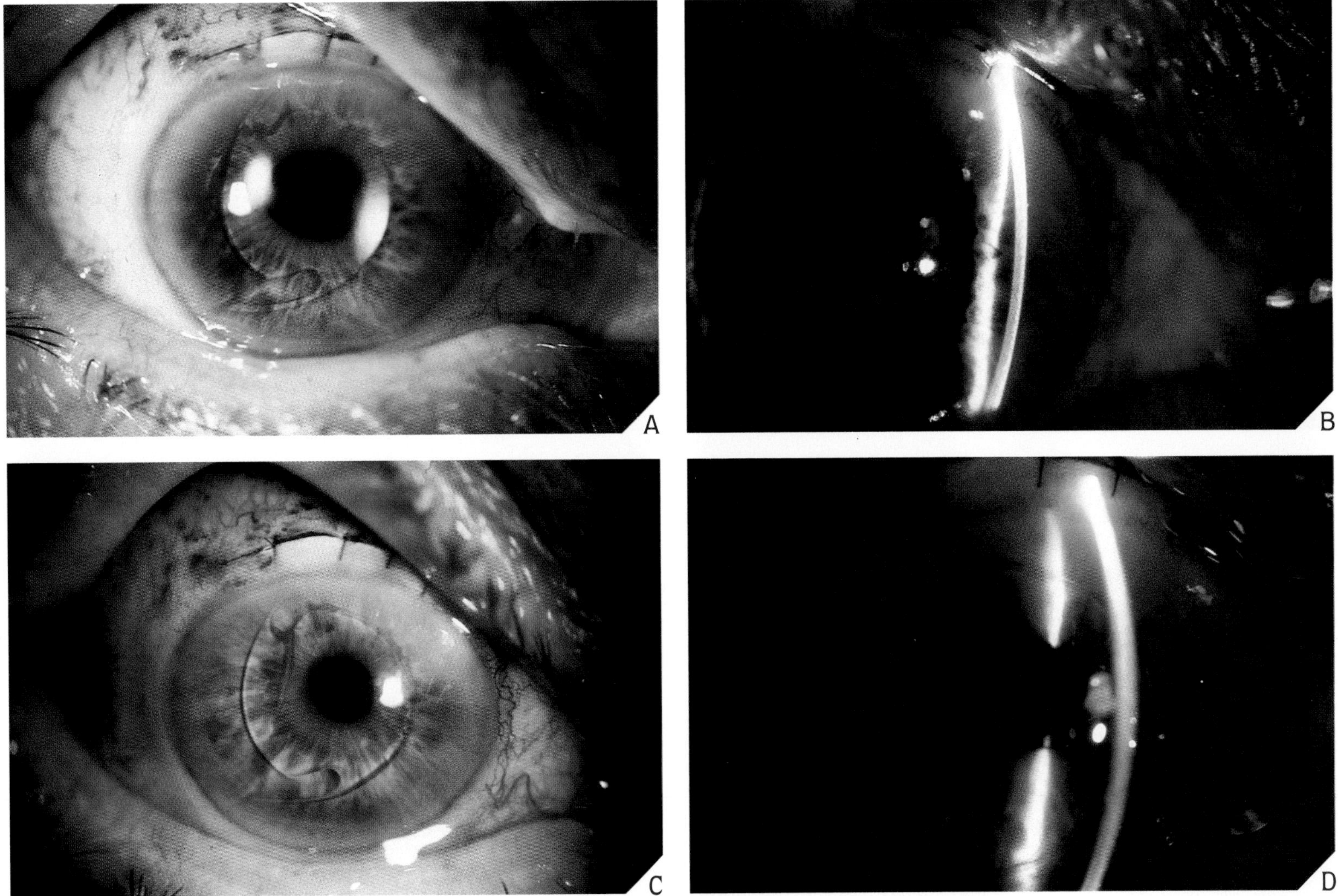

Figure 5.11 Implant-Induced Glaucoma. A, B Pupillary-block glaucoma is noted on the first postoperative day. **C, D** A YAG laser iridectomy "cures" the glaucoma.

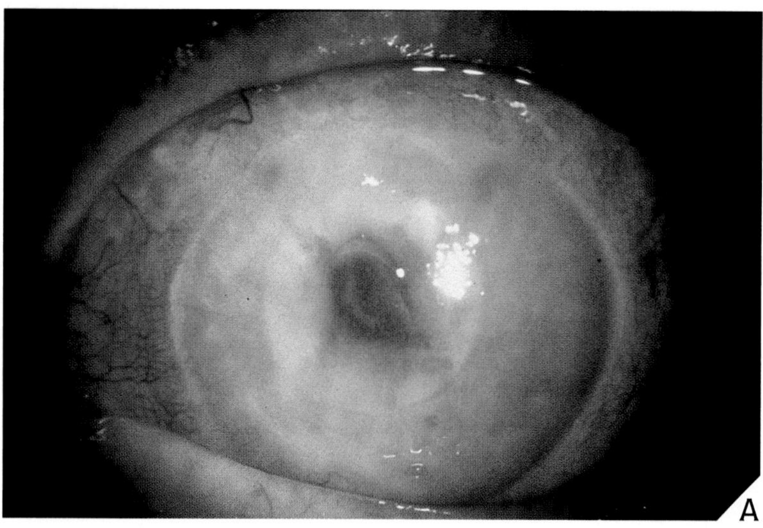

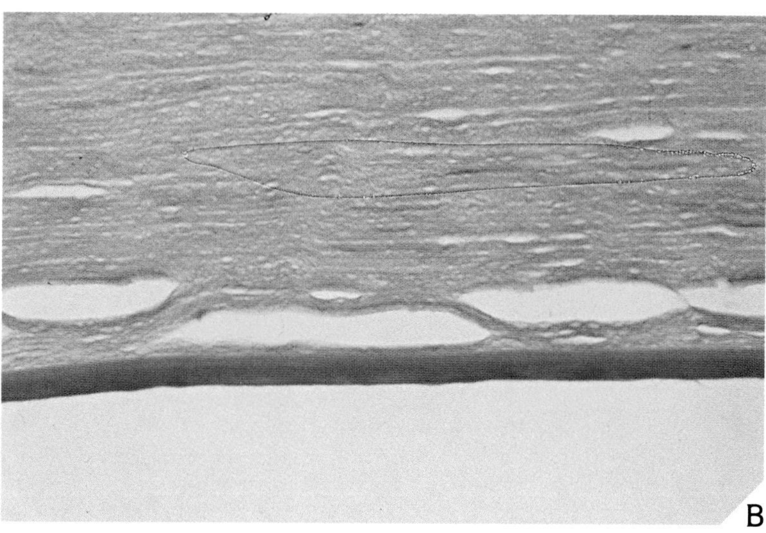

FIGURE 5.12 CORNEAL EDEMA. A Corneal edema has led to bullous keratopathy in this patient with an iris clip intraocular lens. **B** No endothelium is present on the Descemet membrane. The normally seen artifactious clefts in the cornea are largely obliterated by edema fluid in the corneal stroma. (**A**, courtesy of Dr. IM Raber.)

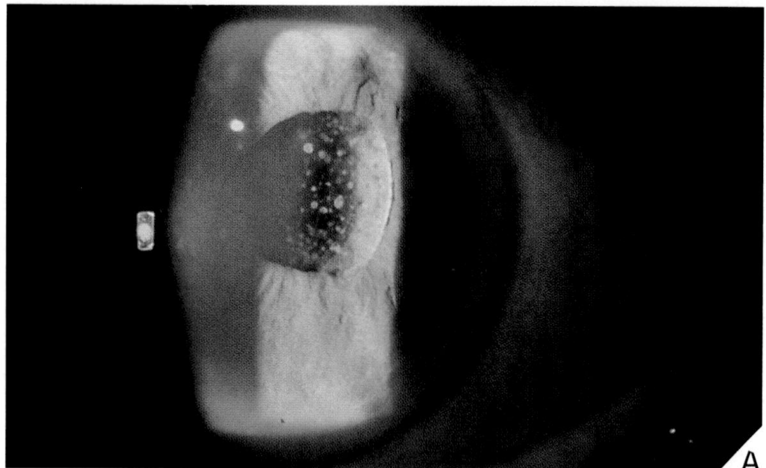

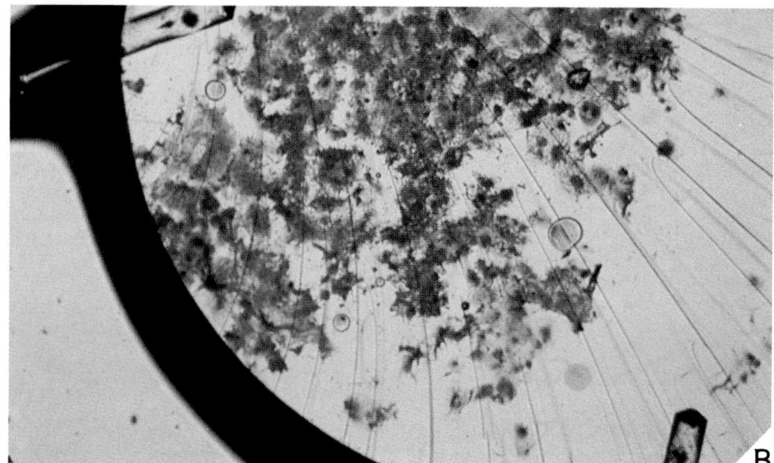

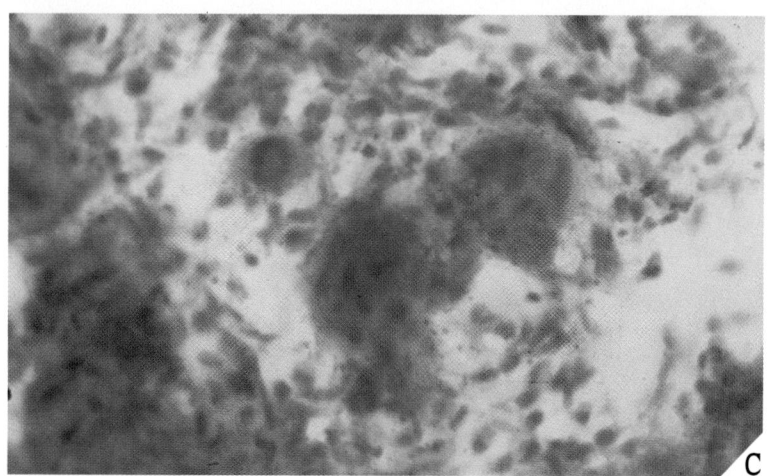

FIGURE 5.13 INFLAMMATION ON IMPLANT. A Large pigmented precipitates are present on the anterior and posterior surface of the lens. Entrapment of the posterior chamber lens has taken place on the right-hand side of the pupil. **B** This anterior chamber lens was removed because of the uveitis, glaucoma, hyphema (UGH) syndrome. The lens is covered with precipitates. **C** Increased magnification shows many histiocytes and multinucleated giant cells on the lens surface. (**B, C**, courtesy of Dr RC Eagle Jr.)

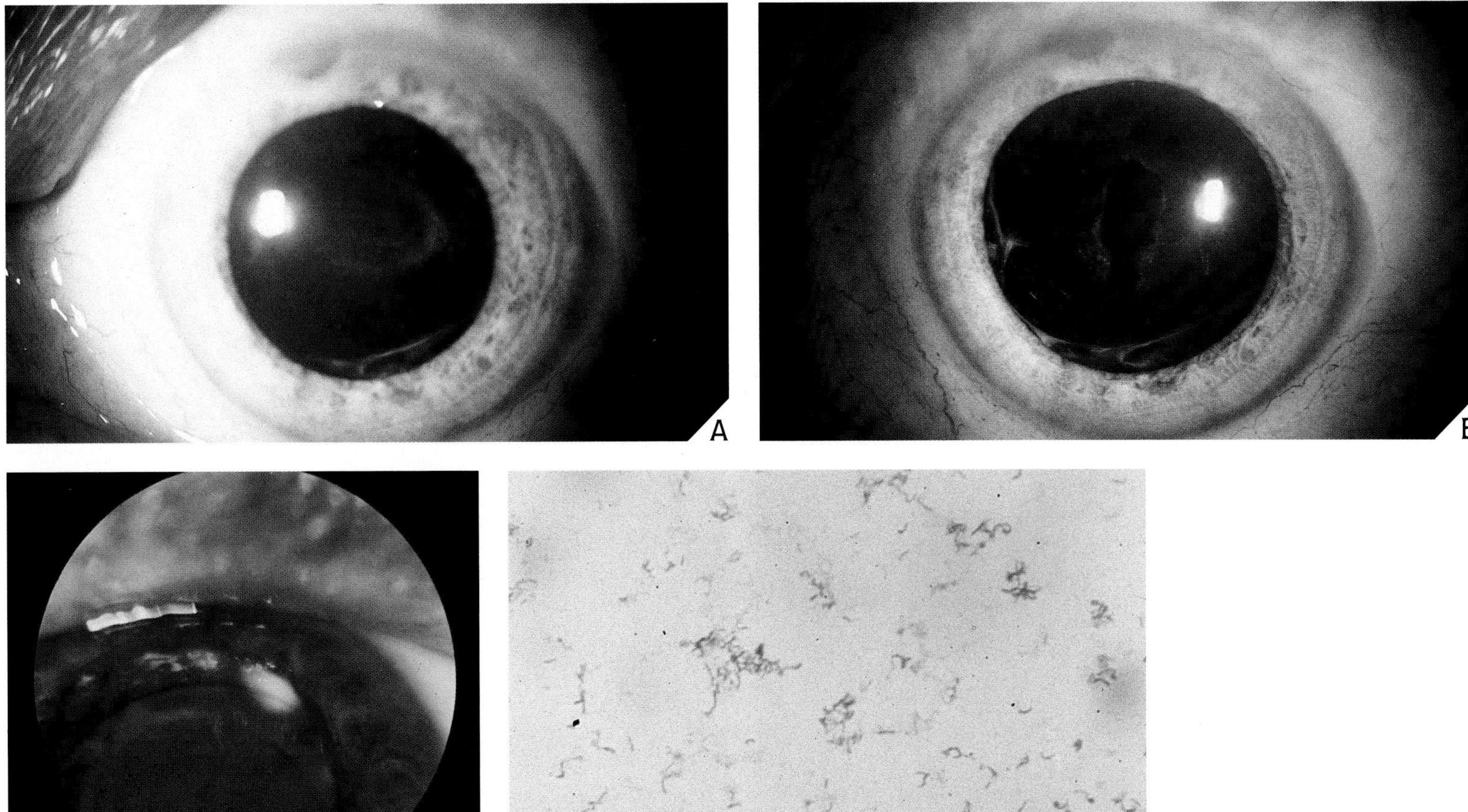

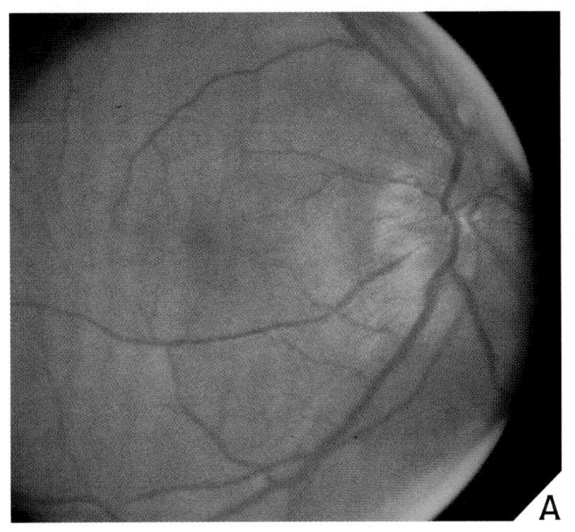

FIGURE 5.14 CICATRIZATION OF POSTERIOR LENS CAPSULE. A thickened, cicatrized posterior lens capsule (**A**) has caused a significant decrease in vision, necessitating a posterior YAG capsulectomy (**B**). In another case, after capsulectomy a thick plaque was noted on the posterior surface of the cornea (**C**). Examination of the surgically removed plaque shows a mass of *P. acnes* (**D**). (**C, D**, courtesy of Dr. AH Friedman.)

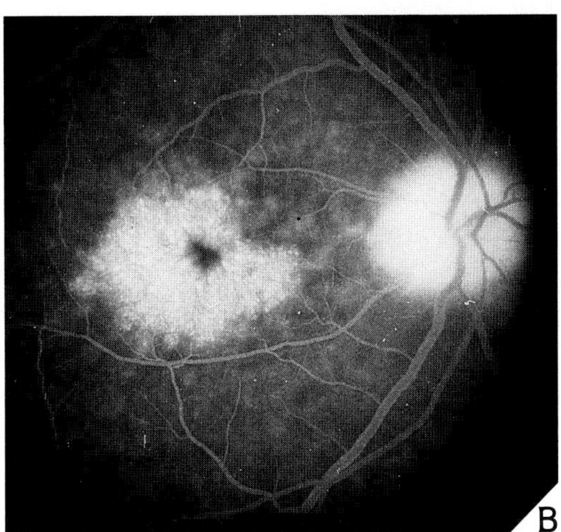

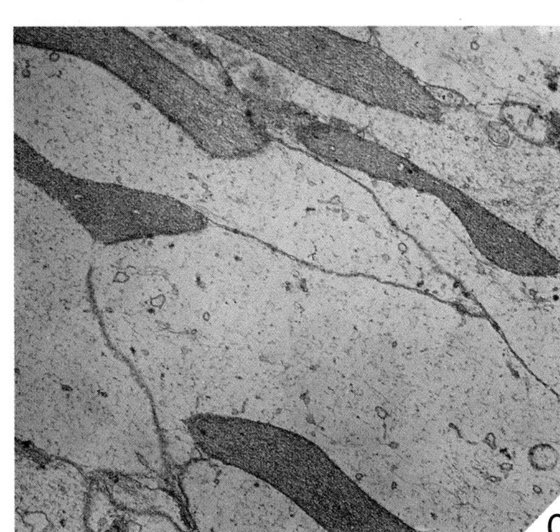

FIGURE 5.15 CYSTOID MACULAR EDEMA. After extracapsular cataract extraction and posterior chamber lens implantation, the patient initially did well. Then however, vision decreased. **A** Examination of the fundus showed cystoid macular edema. **B** The characteristic fluorescein appearance is present. The patient's vision decreased to 20/300. No treatment was given. Nine months later the vision spontaneously returned to 20/20. **C** Electron microscopy of another case shows intracytoplasmic accumulation of fluid within Müller cells. Initially, the fluid in cystoid macular edema is intracytoplasmic and the condition is reversible. Further accumulation of fluid causes the cell membranes to break and fluid to collect extracellularly; presumably, the condition is irreversible. (**C,** modified from Yanoff M, et al., 1984.)

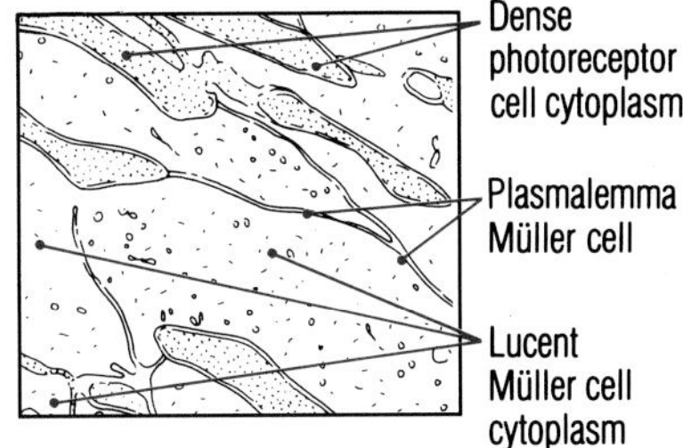

COMPLICATIONS OF NONSURGICAL TRAUMA—CONTUSION

Cornea and conjunctiva	Anterior chamber
Abrasion	Hyphema—may lead to:
Ulceration	•Corneal blood staining
Ruptured Descemet membrane	•Glaucoma
Keloid formation	Angle recession
Blood staining	Iridodialysis
Conjunctival hemorrhage	Cyclodialysis

FIGURE 5.16

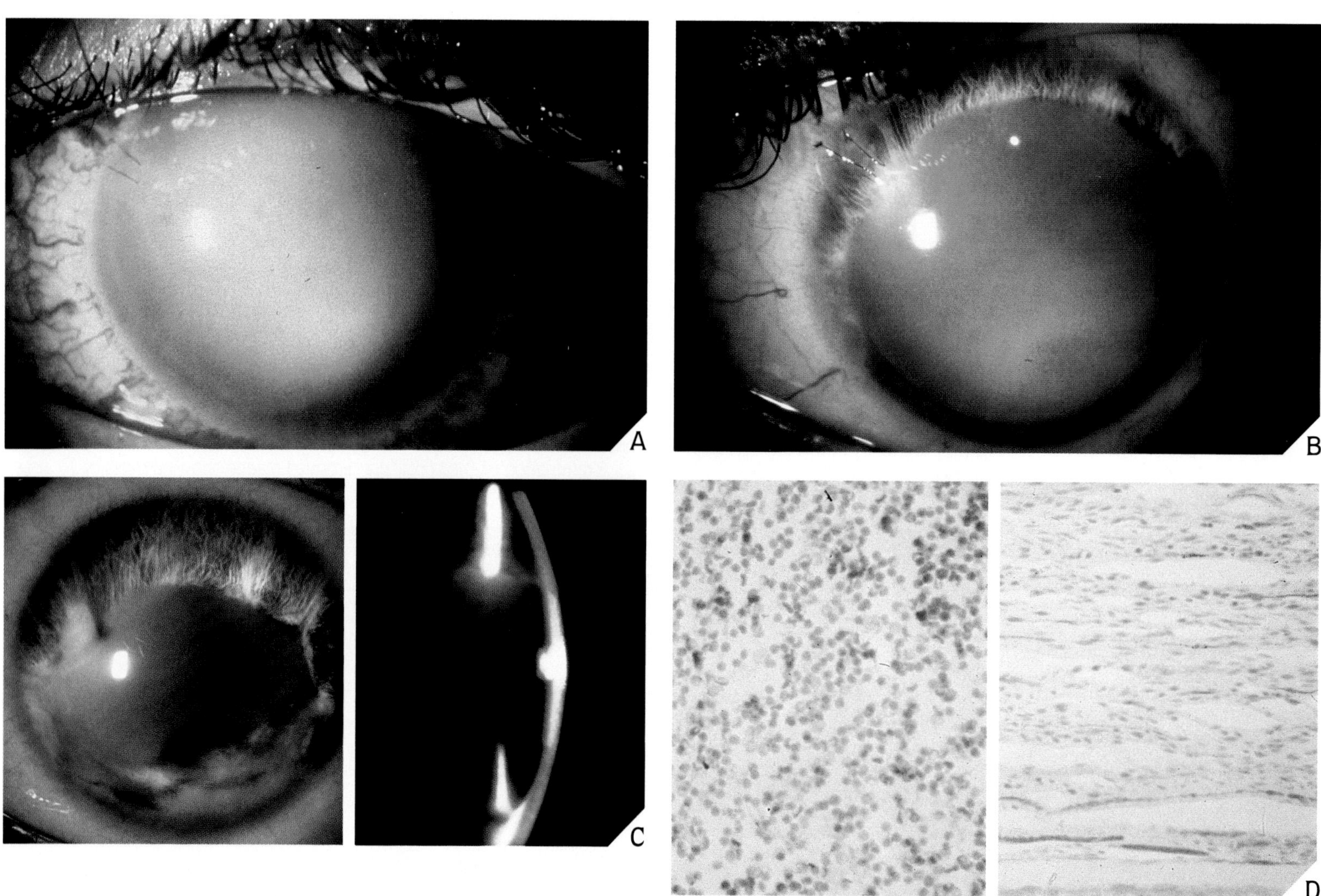

FIGURE 5.17 HYPHEMA. A The patient sustained a blunt trauma that resulted in a total hyphema. One month later, blood staining has occurred. **B** Three months after the initial injury, the hyphema has started to clear peripherally. **C** One year after the trauma, most of the cornea has cleared. **D** Histological sections from a case of corneal blood staining show intact red blood cells in the anterior chamber on the left side. The right side, taken at the same magnification, shows the cornea; both sides are stained for iron. The red blood cells in the cornea have broken up into hemoglobin particles and do not stain for iron. The only positive staining for iron is within the cytoplasm of corneal keratocytes. (**D**, left and right, Perl stain.)

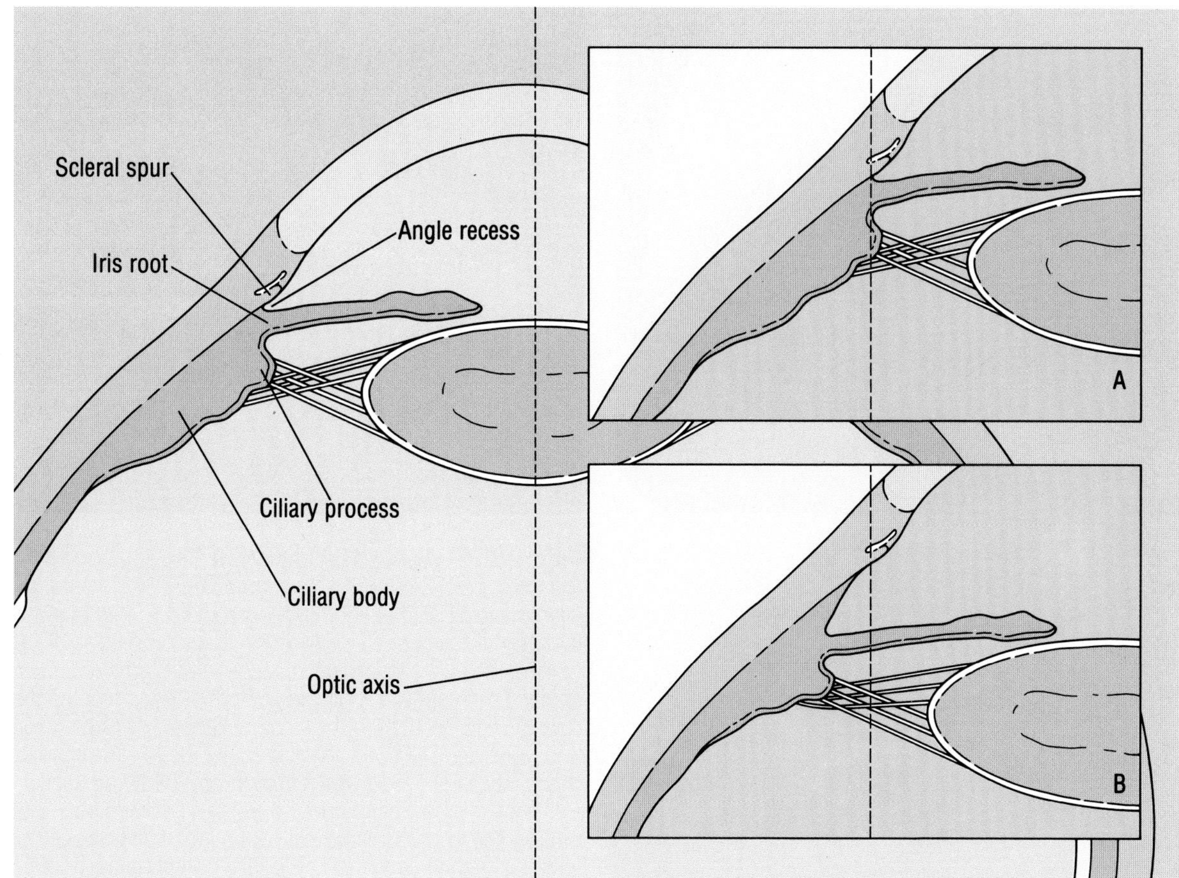

FIGURE 5.18 ANGLE RECESSION. Normal anterior segment. **Inset A** A line drawn parallel to the optic axis in a normal eye passes through the scleral spur, the angle recess, the iris root, and the most anterior portion of the ciliary processes. The ciliary body has a wedge shape, i.e., is pointed at its posterior portion but straight-sided anteriorly. **Inset B** In an eye that has an angle recession (also called postcontusion deformity of the anterior chamber angle), the line parallel to the optic axis that passes through the scleral spur will pass anterior to the angle recess, the iris root, and the most anterior portion of the ciliary body. The ciliary body is fusiform, i.e., pointed posteriorly and anteriorly. (In a fetal or neonatal eye, the line parallel to the optic axis that passes through the scleral spur will pass posterior to the angle recess, the iris root, and the most anterior portion of the ciliary body; the ciliary body also has a normal wedge shape.)

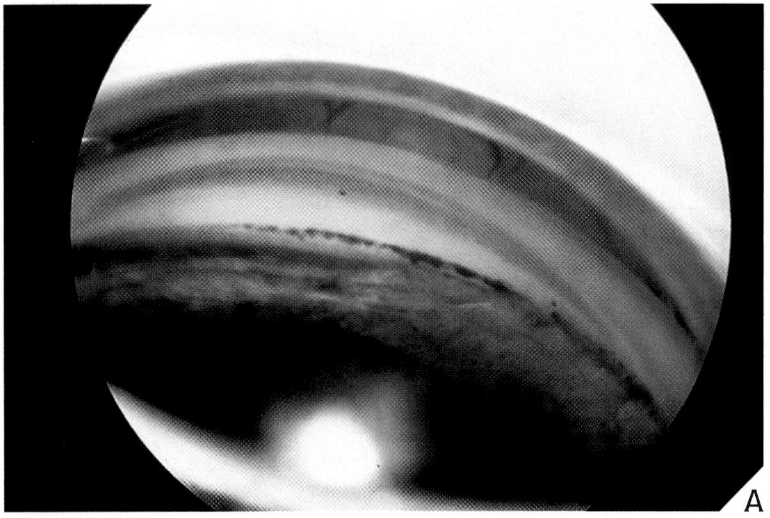

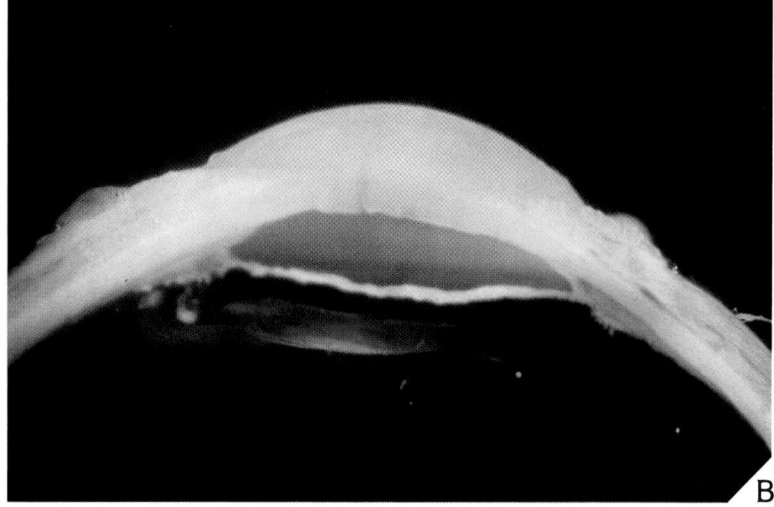

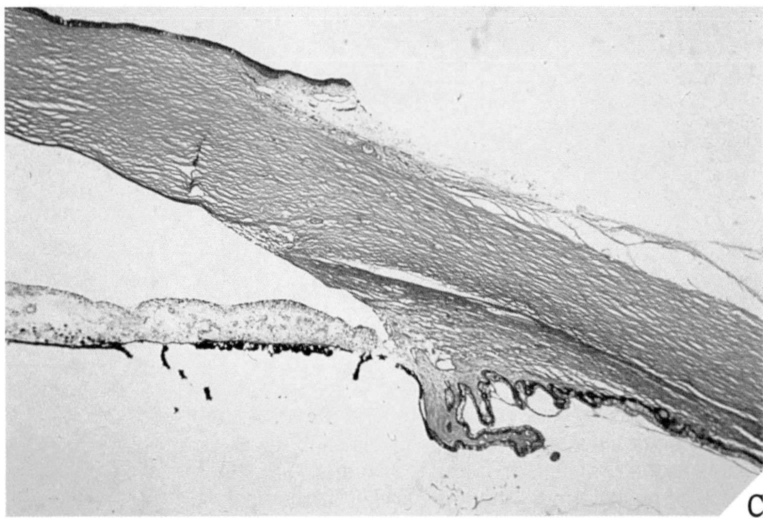

FIGURE 5.19 ANGLE RECESSION. A The angle of the anterior chamber in the eye of a patient who had sustained a blunt trauma is of normal depth over the right side of the figure, except for peripheral anterior synechiae, but is markedly deepened and recessed over the left side. **B** A gross specimen from another case shows the deepened anterior chamber and recessed angle. The fusiform (pointed at both ends) shape of the ciliary body (most clearly seen on the right) is characteristic of angle recession. **C** The ciliary body inserts into the scleral spur normally. The oblique and circular muscles of the ciliary body have atrophied, following a laceration into the anterior face of the ciliary body, and the resulting scar tissue has contracted, pulling the angle recess, iris root, and ciliary processes posteriorly. The anterior wedge shape of the ciliary body has been lost. The entire process results in a fusiform shape of the ciliary body. A number of mechanisms such as trabecular damage and late scarring, peripheral anterior synechiae, and endothelialization of an open angle can lead to secondary glaucoma that would result in optic nerve damage.

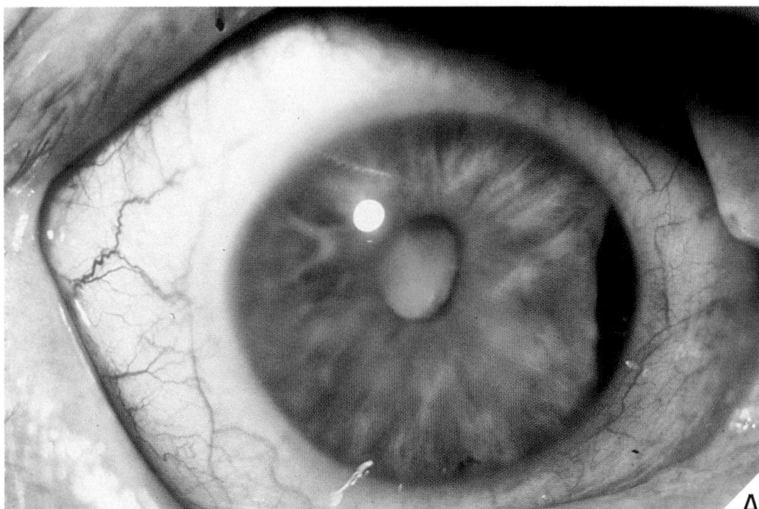

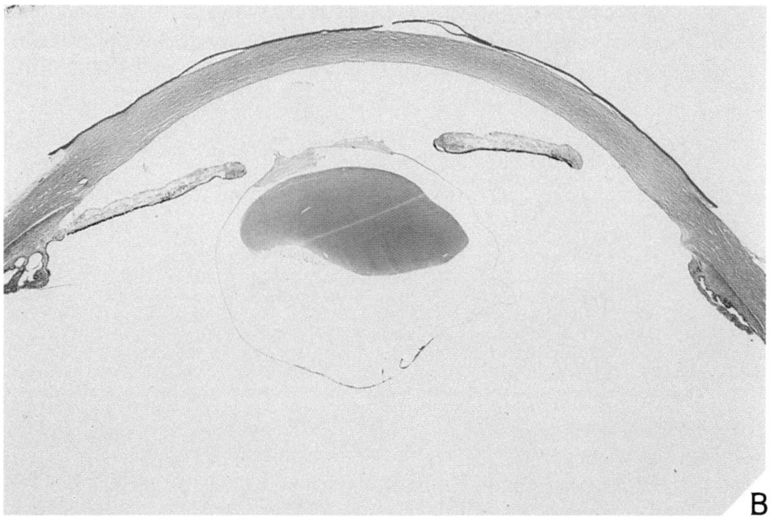

B

FIGURE 5.20 IRIDODIALYSIS. A The patient sustained blunt trauma that resulted in an iridodialysis. Over the next few months he developed a mature cataract. The NLP eye was enucleated. **B** Histological section shows that the liquified cortex has completely leaked out from the lens during tissue processing; all that remains is the nucleus, surrounded by a clear area where the cortex had been, surrounded in turn by the lens capsule. Note the anterior subcapsular cataract. The iridodialysis is seen on the right. In addition, the fusiform shape of the ciliary body, best seen on the left, indicates that an angle recession is present (**A** from *Ocular Pathology*, 3rd ed, by M Yanoff and BS Fine; **B**, PAS stain.)

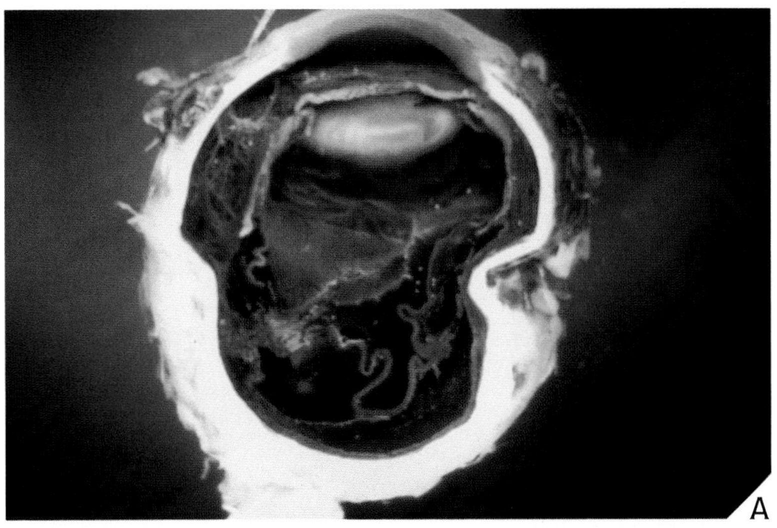

A

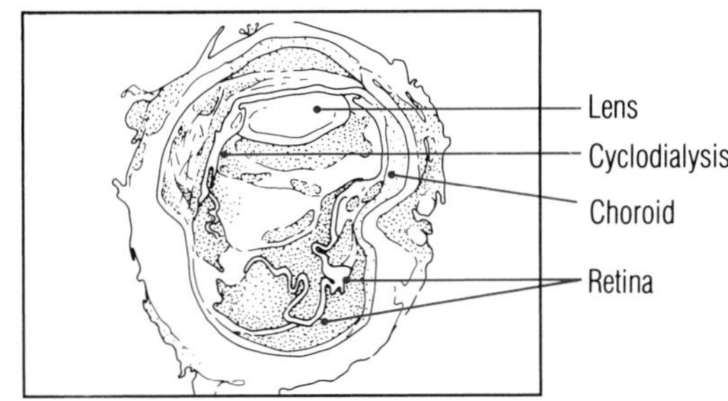

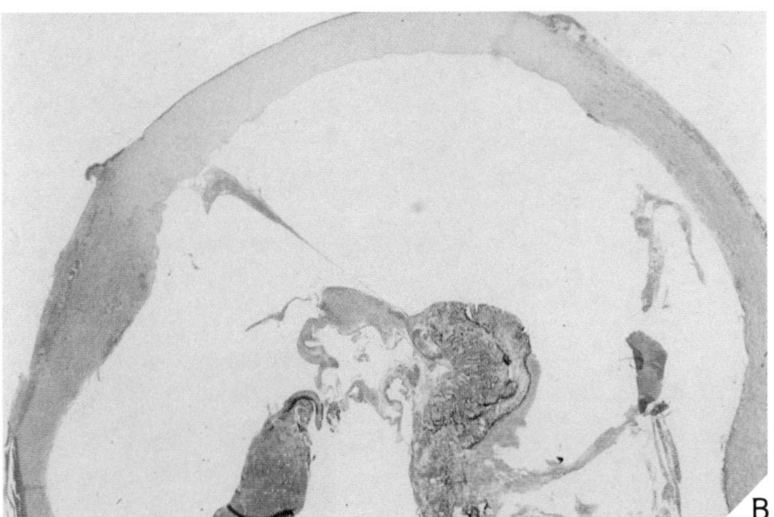

B

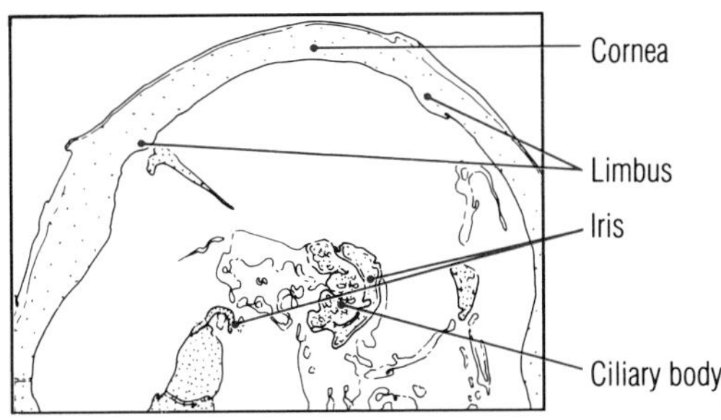

FIGURE 5.21 CYCLODIALYSIS. A The gross eye shows the ciliary body attached to the scleral spur on the right side. The entire ciliary body on the left side, however, is avulsed from the scleral spur, resulting in a cyclodialysis. **B** Histologic section from another case shows the ciliary body and iris in the center of the eye, avulsed from the scleral spur 360°.

COMPLICATIONS OF NONSURGICAL TRAUMA—CONTUSION (CONTINUED)

Lens
Cataract
Rupture
Phacolytic glaucoma
Phacoanaphylactic endophthalmitis
Vossius ring
Subluxation
Dislocation

Ciliary body and choroid
Hemorrhage
Inflammation
Cyclitic membrane
Choroidal rupture
Chorioretinopathy

Vitreous
Inflammation
Hemorrhage
Cholesterolosis

FIGURE 5.22

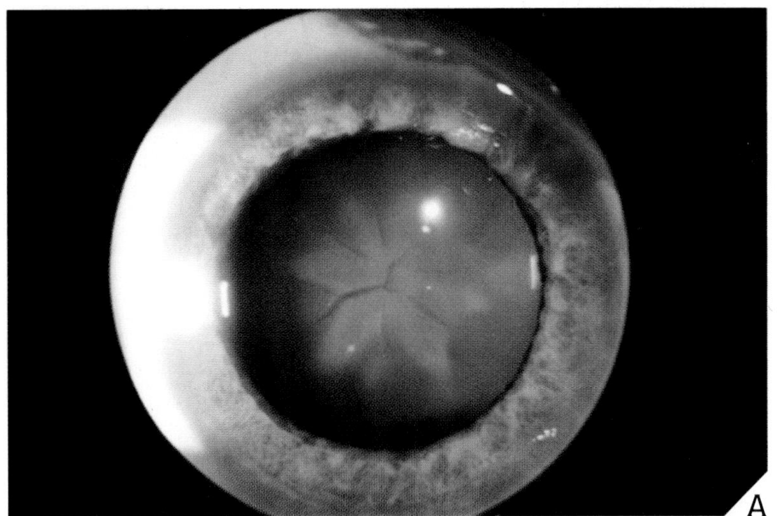

FIGURE 5.23 TRAUMATIC CATARACT. A The patient had blunt trauma from several years earlier. A typical petal-shaped cataract has developed. This may develop in the cortex, under the anterior capsule, or under the posterior capsule. In this case, the cataract is present in both the anterior and posterior cortex. **B** Histologic section of another petal-shaped traumatic cataract shows anterior and posterior cortical degeneration in the form of narrow bands (seen under increased magnification in **C** and **D**). The bands are responsible for the "petals" seen clinically.

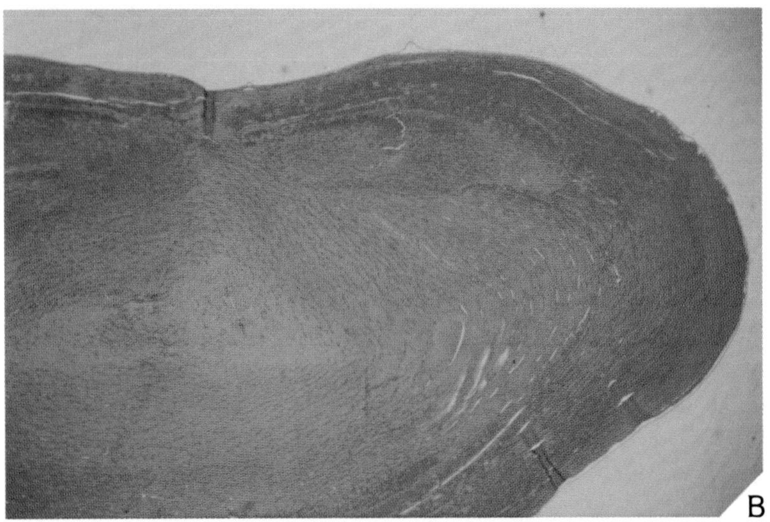

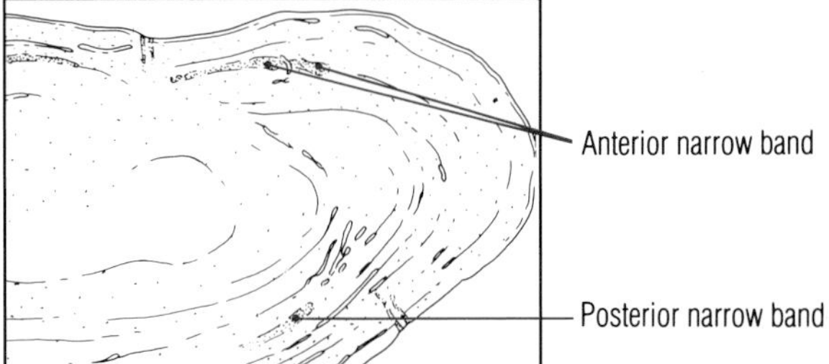

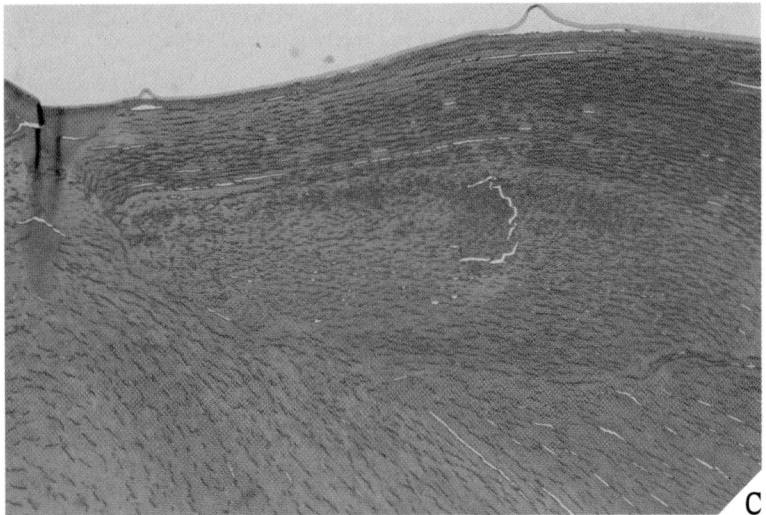

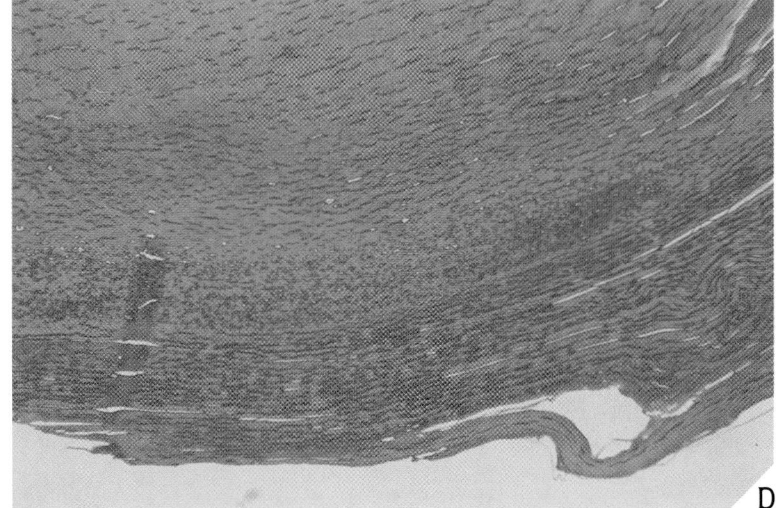

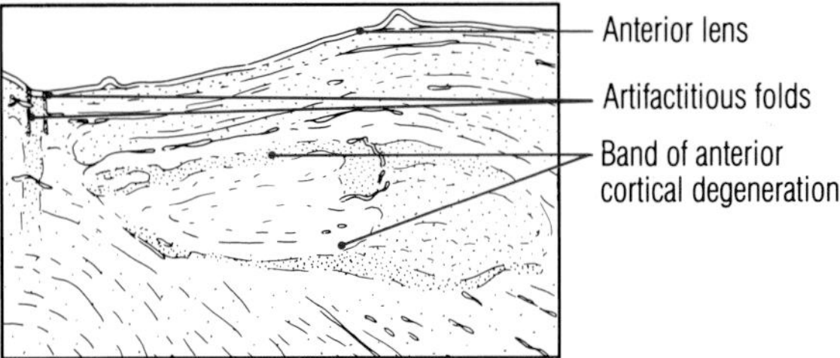

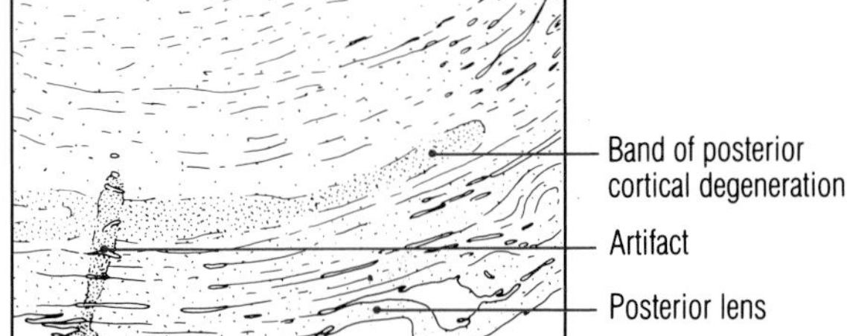

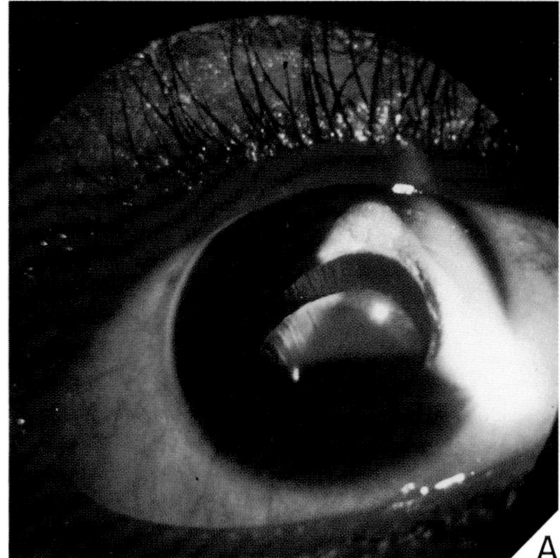

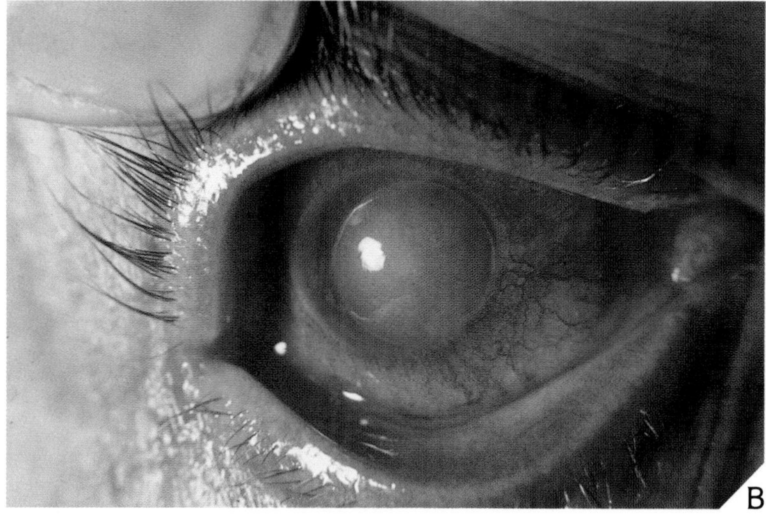

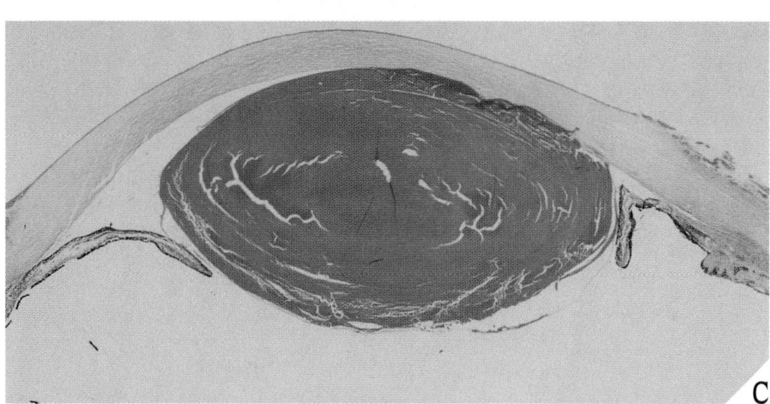

Figure 5.24 Lens Subluxation and Dislocation. A The lens is subluxated inferiorly so that the zonular fibers are easily noted in the superior pupil. When a lens is subluxated, it is still in the posterior chamber but not in its normal position. **B** The lens is dislocated into the anterior chamber. Pupillary block has resulted in peripheral anterior synechiae and closed-angle glaucoma (a similar case is shown histologically in **C**). (**A**, from M Yanoff and BS Fine, *Ocular Pathology*, 2nd ed.)

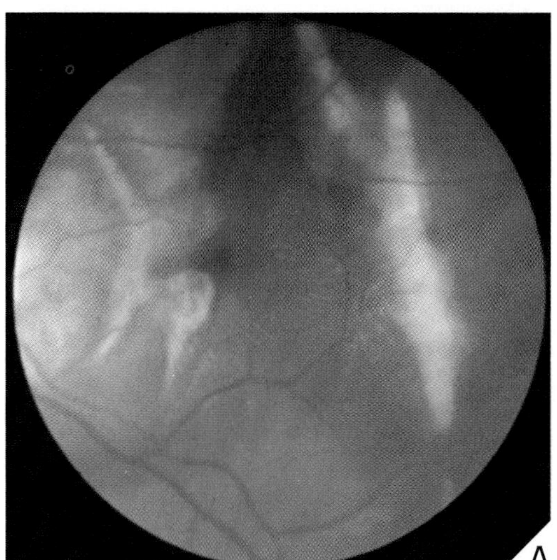

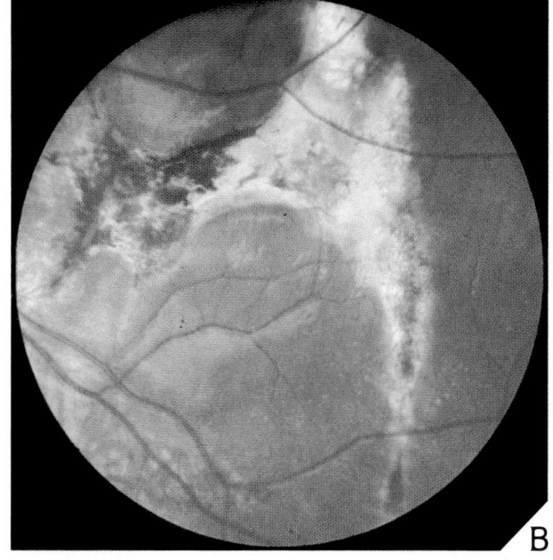

Figure 5.25 Choroidal Rupture. A The patient sustained a blunt trauma that resulted in choroidal ruptures in the posterior pole and in subneural retinal hemorrhages. The optic nerve head is on the left in this eye. **B** One year later, considerable scarring has taken place. These patients must be watched closely for the occurrence of subneural retinal neovascularization that may occur at the edge of the healed rupture. **C** Histologic section of another case shows rupture of the choroid following blunt trauma. (**C**, courtesy of Dr. WR Green, reported in Aguilar JP, Green WR, 1984.)

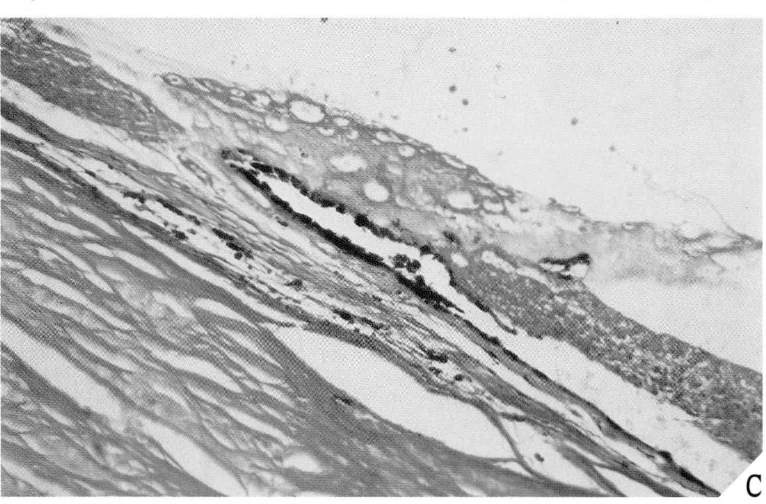

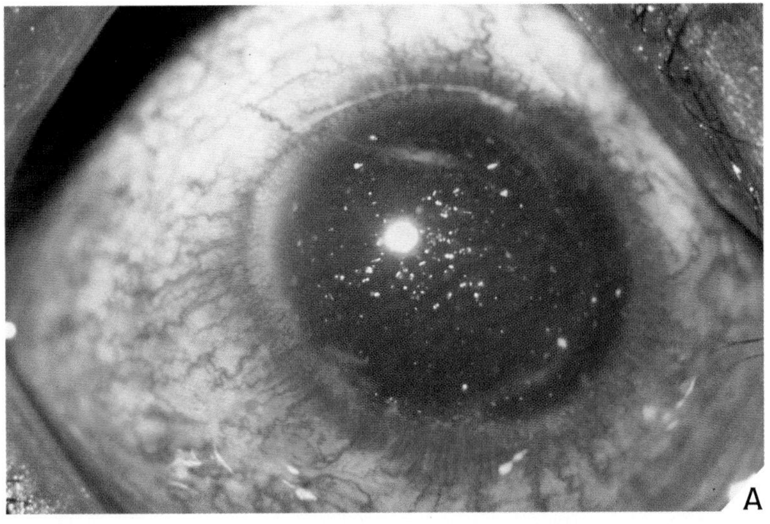

FIGURE 5.26 CHOLESTEROLOSIS. A A traumatic hyphema has been absorbed but cholesterol remains in the anterior chamber. **B** An anterior chamber aspirate of another case shows cholesterol crystals. **C** The cholesterol crystals are birefringent to polarized light. (**B**, unstained; **C**, unstained and polarized.)

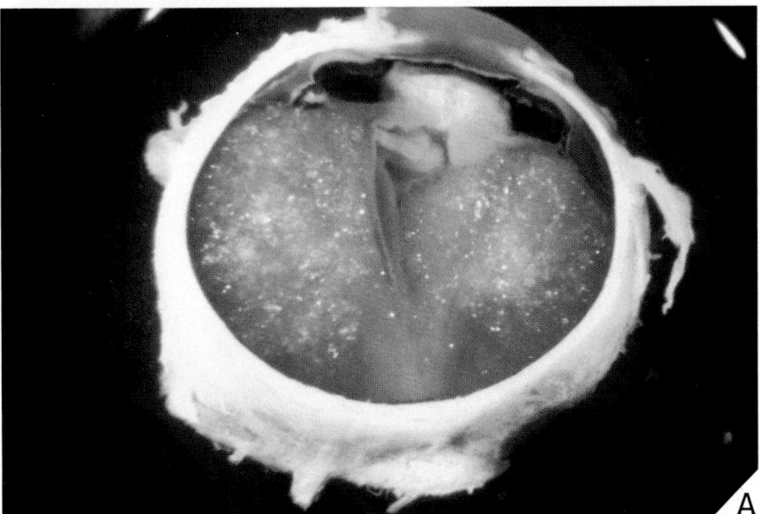

FIGURE 5.27 CHOLESTEROLOSIS. A The subneural retinal space is filled with an exudate containing many cholesterol crystals. Cholesterol often settles out following vitreous or subneural retinal hemorrhages. The cholesterol may be seen free, as in **A** and in Figure 5.26, or the clefts may appear as empty spaces surrounded by foreign body giant cells (**B**). The cholesterol itself is dissolved out by processing of the tissue and only the space remains where the cleft had been. (**B**, from *Ocular Pathology*, 2nd ed, by M Yanoff and BS Fine.)

Retina
Commotio retinae
(Berlin edema)
Hemorrhages
Tears

Optic nerve
Partial or complete avulsion
Hemorrhage
Optic disc edema

Glaucoma
Closed angle
- Secondary to repair
- Organization of hemorrhage and exudate
- Endothelialization
- Iris neovascularization

Open angle
- Cells and debris
- Angle recession
- Trabecular damage

FIGURE 5.28

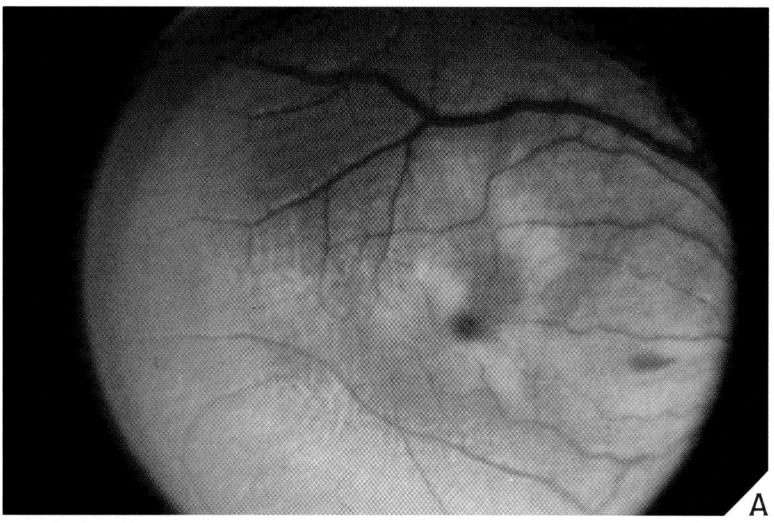

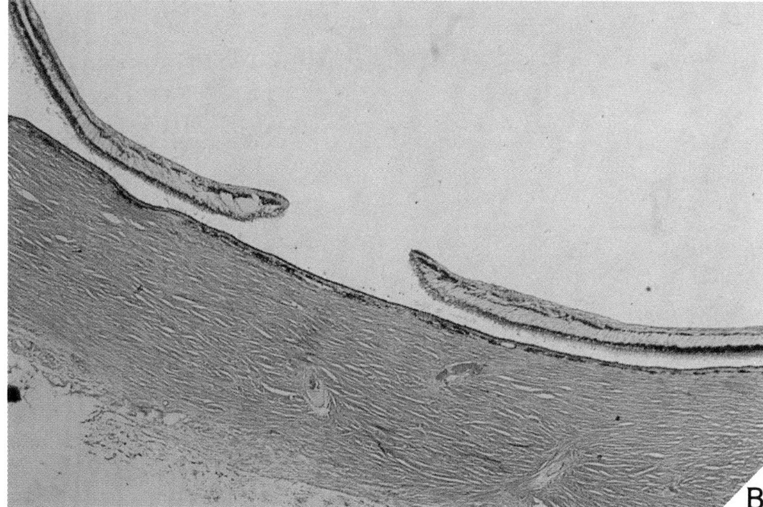

FIGURE 5.29 COMMOTIO RETINAE (BERLIN EDEMA). A The posterior pole is milky and opaque because of damage in the form of vacuolization and degeneration of the inner portion of the photoreceptor and outer nuclear layers. **B** Following commotio retinae, some cases will heal with pigmentation. In other cases, fluid will enter the macular retinal region and cause microcystoid degeneration. Hole formation ultimately may result, as shown here.

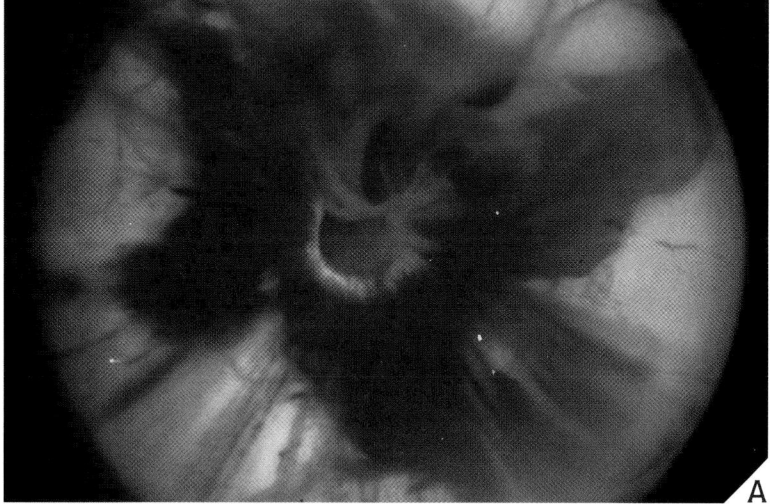

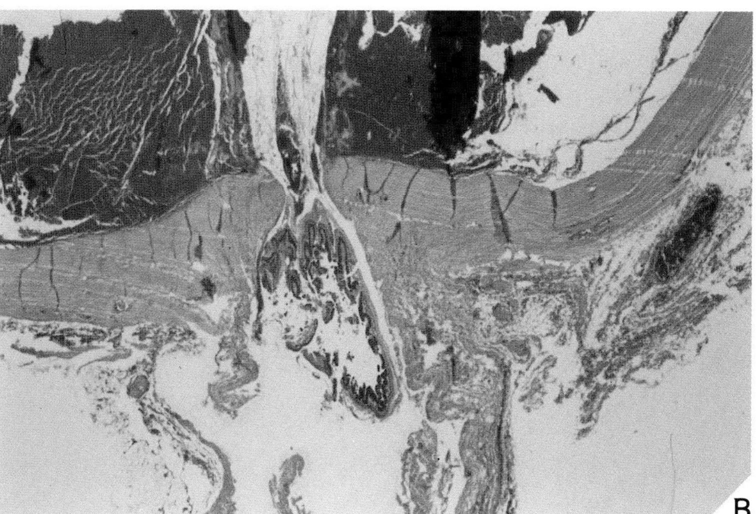

FIGURE 5.30 AVULSION OF THE OPTIC NERVE. A Following trauma, the optic nerve has been avulsed. Note the hole opening into the orbit where the optic nerve had been. **B** The scleral optic nerve canal is not filled with optic nerve but contains retina. (**A**, courtesy of Dr. ME Smith.)

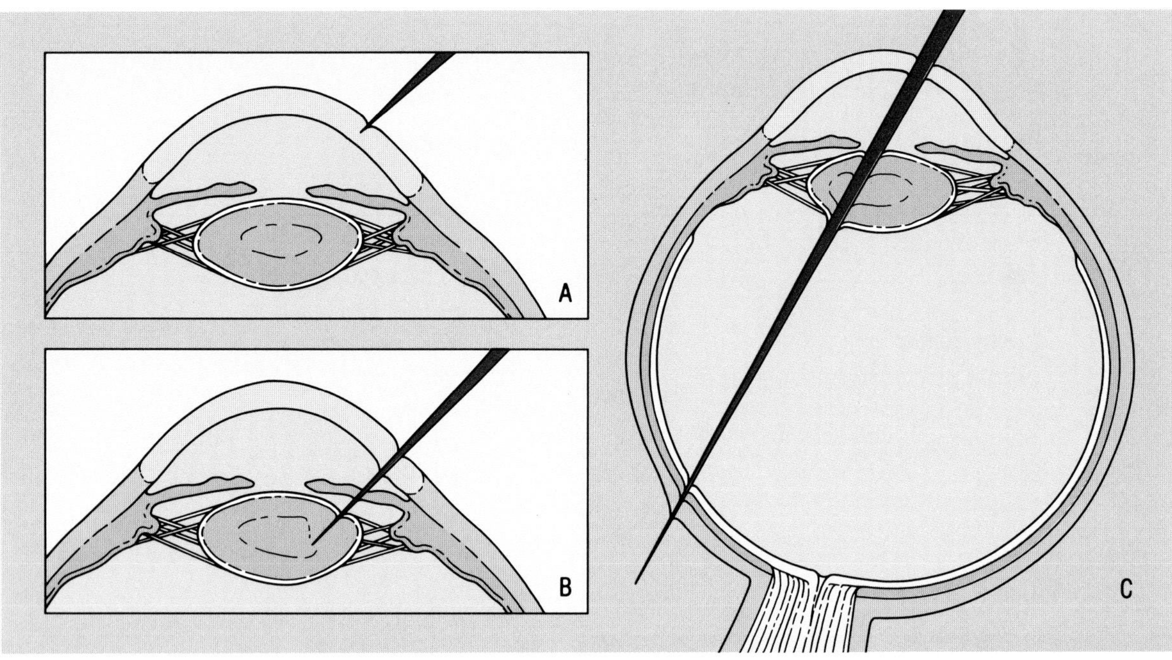

Figure 5.31 Penetration and Perforation of the Globe. **A** The arrow shows a penetrating wound of the cornea. **B** The arrow shows a perforating wound of the cornea and iris and a penetrating wound of the lens and globe. **C** The arrow shows a perforating wound of the cornea, lens, retina, choroid, sclera, and globe.

Penetration and Perforation of the Globe—Definitions

Penetration—into but not through
Perforation—into and through

Figure 5.32

Penetration and Perforation of the Globe—Signs

Decreased visual acuity
Hypotony
Shallow anterior chamber (anterior perforation)
Deep anterior chamber (posterior perforation)
Pupillary alteration
Blood in vitreous
Obvious ocular laceration

Figure 5.33

Penetration and Perforation of the Globe—Effects

Corneal and scleral rupture
Prolapse or loss of intraocular contents
Epithelial downgrowth
Stromal overgrowth
Intraocular infection
Intraocular foreign body
Effects of contusion

Figure 5.34

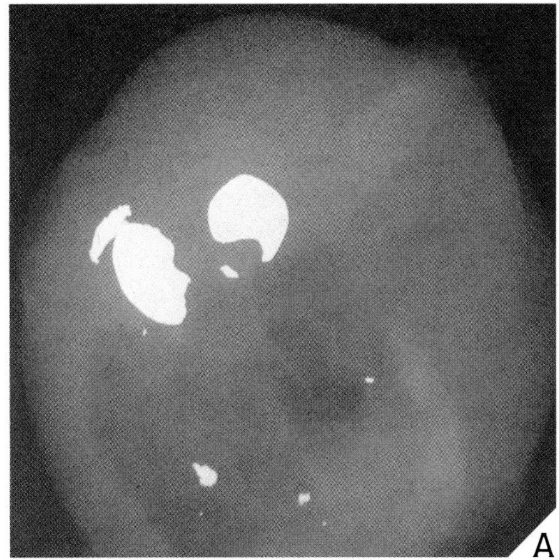

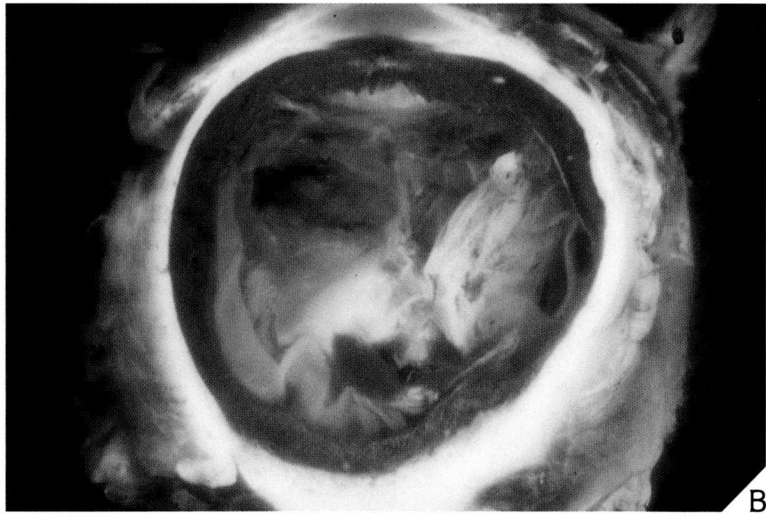

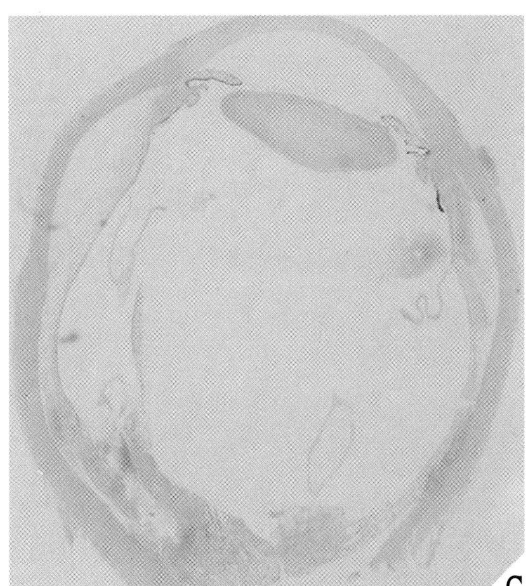

FIGURE 5.35 RUPTURE OF THE GLOBE. A A patient had a gunshot injury to the globe. X-ray examination shows multiple metallic foreign bodies within the globe. The eye was enucleated. **B** The gross specimen shows disorganization, hemorrhage, and retinal detachment. A rupture of the choroid and retina can be seen at the 4-o'clock position at the exit wound site. In enucleating the hypotonus globe, the surgeon cut across the sclera, leaving the optic nerve head with its surrounding sclera, choroid, and retina in the orbit. Obviously, because of uveal tissue left in the orbit, the patient is a candidate for sympathetic uveitis. **C** Histologic section shows the detached retina and the "button-hole" of the posterior segment. Note the opaque black foreign body on the internal surface of the ciliary body on the right side.

INTRAOCULAR FOREIGN BODIES

Inorganic

Relatively inert—gold, silver, platinum, aluminum, and glass

Relatively active—iron and copper

Organic

Vegetable matter—may be contaminated with opportunistic fungi

Cilium

FIGURE 5.36

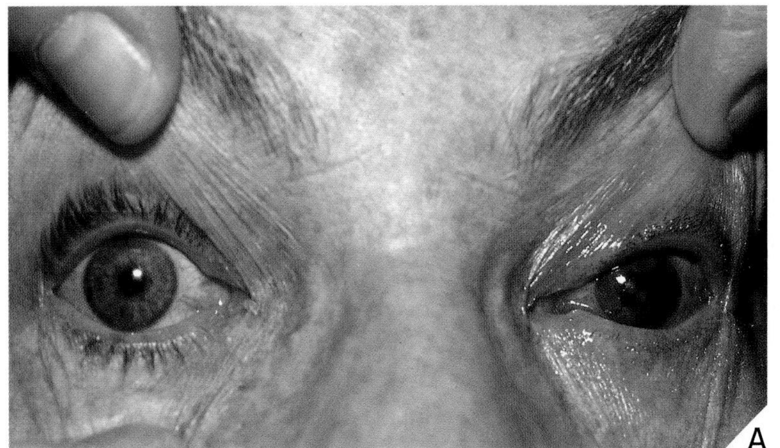

FIGURE 5.37 SIDEROSIS BULBI. A The patient has an intraocular iron foreign body in his left eye. Pigmentation has caused the left iris to become dark. **B** A special stain that shows blue in the presence of iron indicates iron diffusely in the stroma of the iris. Iron also was present in the anterior layer of the iris pigment epithelium. Note the presence of iris neovascularization. **C** The patient had a longstanding hemorrhage in the eye. Iron deposition in the lens has caused hemosiderosis lentis. Hemosiderosis and siderosis are indistinguishable histologically. **D** Iron, as indicated by the blue color, is deposited in the lens epithelium and not in the lens capsule or cortex **B**, Perl stain; **C**, from *Ocular Pathology*, 3rd ed, by M Yanoff and BS Fine; **D**, Perl stain.)

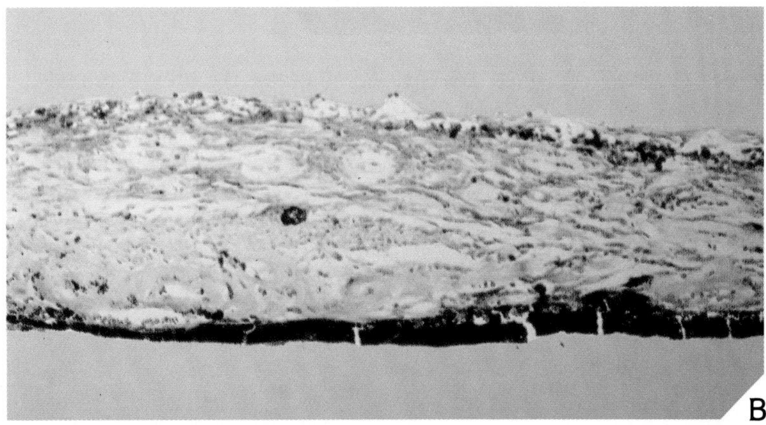

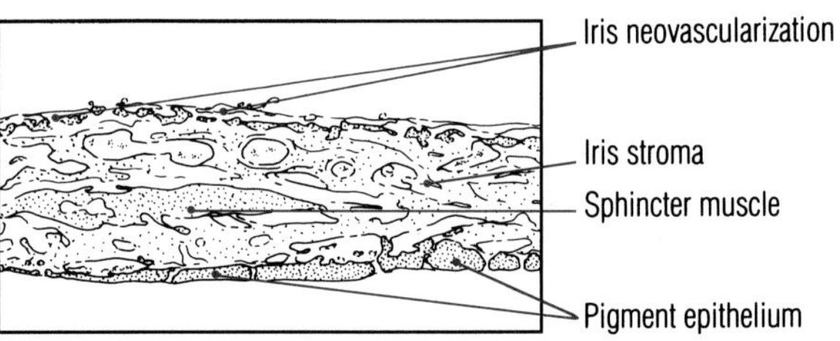

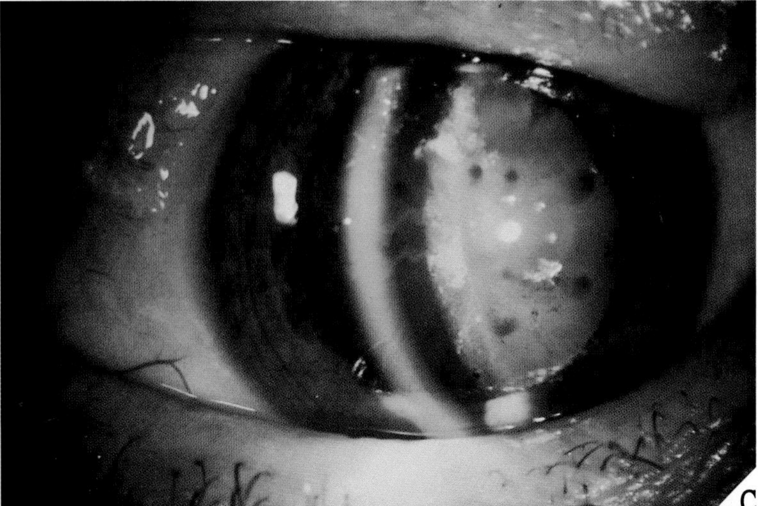

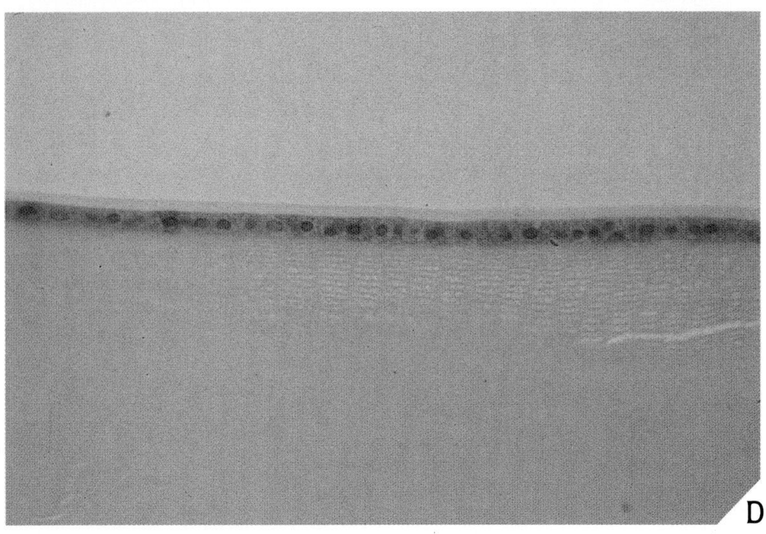

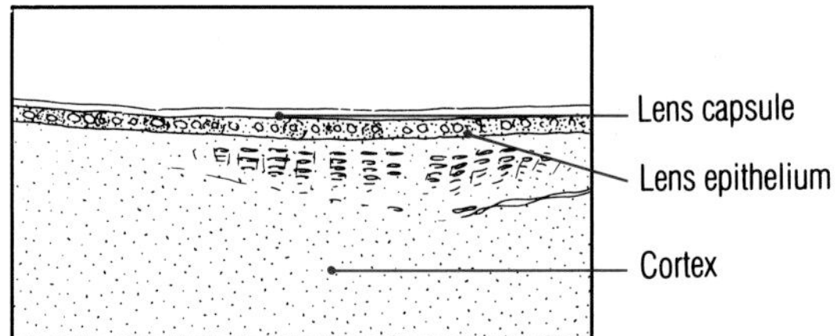

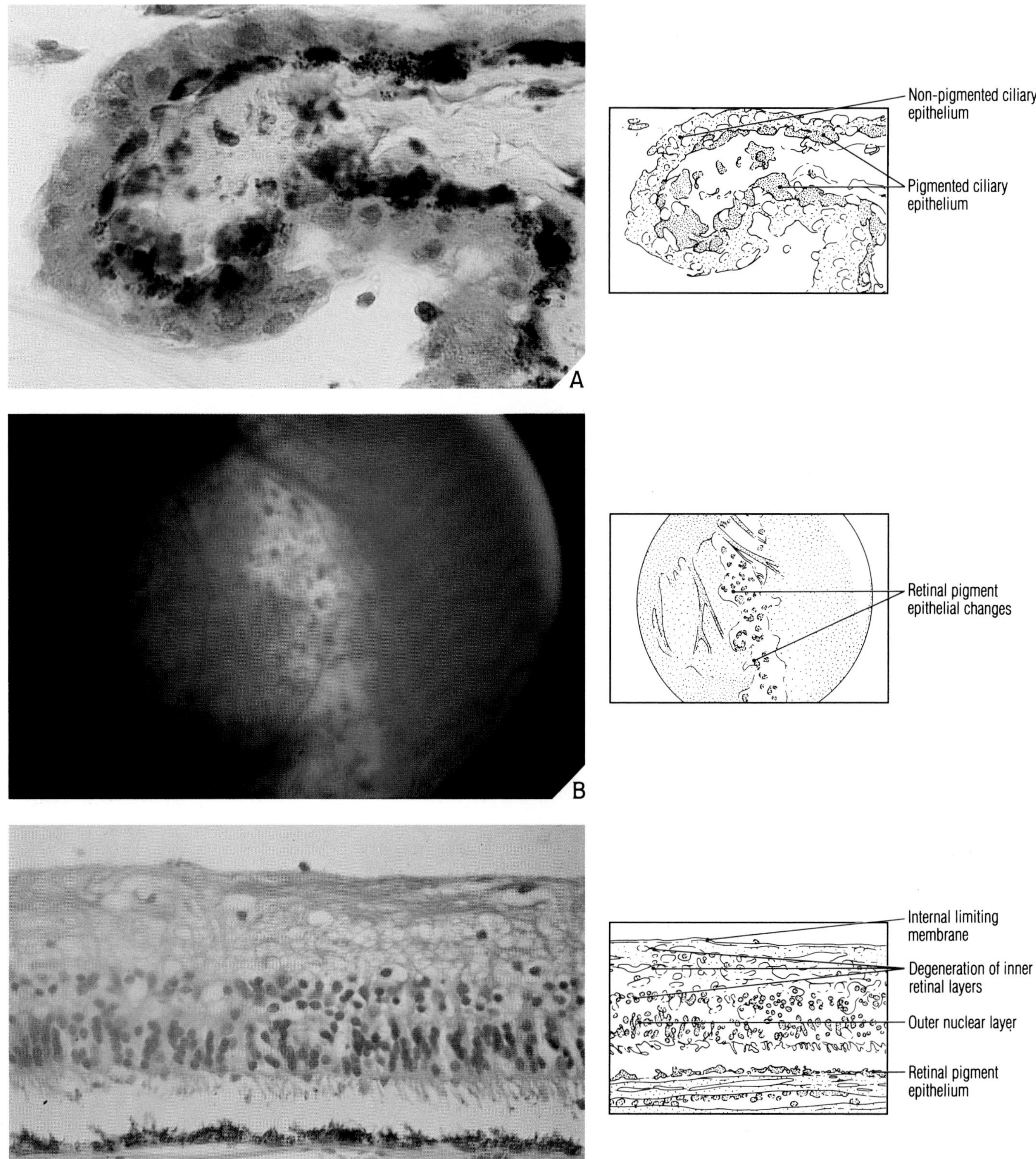

FIGURE 5.38 SIDEROSIS AND HEMOSIDEROSIS BULBI. In both conditions, iron may be deposited in neuroepithelial and lens epithelial structures such as iris pigment epithelium, lens epithelium, and ciliary epithelium (**A**), and in pigment epithelium of the retina (**C**). Iron also may be deposited in the iris stroma, the neural retina, and the trabecular meshwork. The toxic effect of iron may cause retinal damage and scarring in the trabecular meshwork, as well as a secondary chronic open-angle glaucoma. **B** Distinctive changes in the pigment epithelium are caused by an intraocular iron foreign body. **C** In another case, iron is deposited in the neural retina and in the retinal pigment epithelium. (**A**, Perl stain; **B**, courtesy of Dr. AJ Brucker; **C**, Perl stain.)

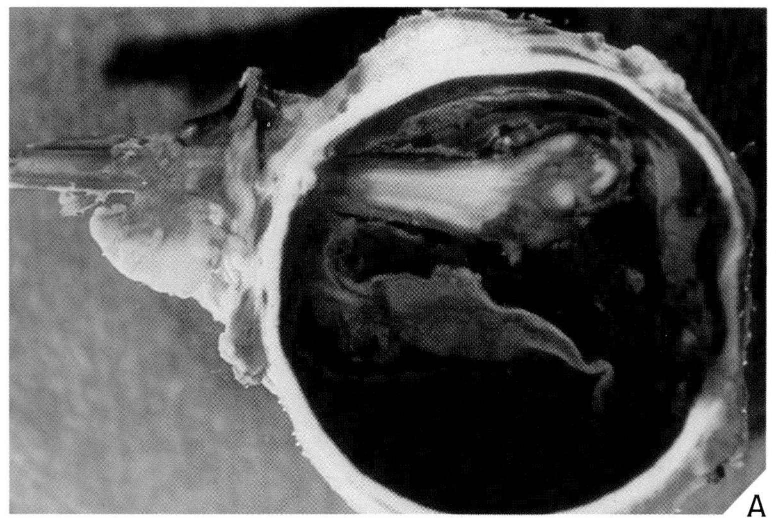

FIGURE 5.39 INTRAOCULAR FOREIGN BODY. A The gross specimen shows a large splinter of wood within the eye. **B** Histology shows a perforation through the limbal cornea. The ciliary body, lower left, is filled with blood. Wood (shown under increased magnification in **C**) is present in the anterior chamber and within the wound. (Case courtesy of Dr. WR Green.)

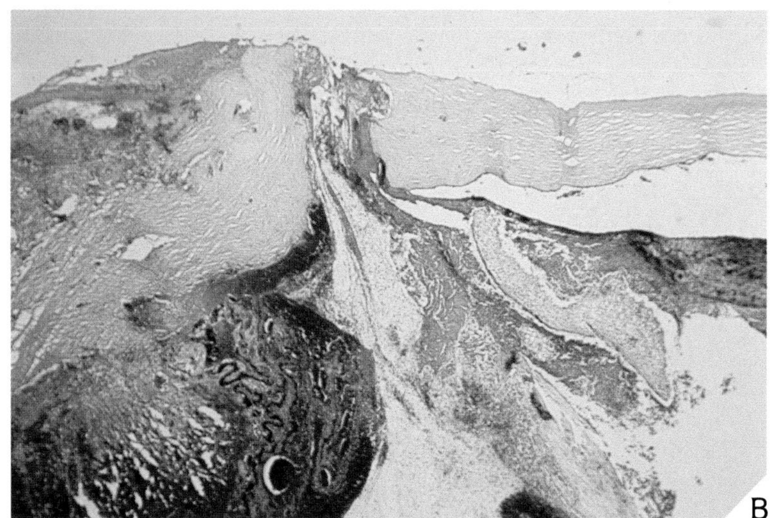

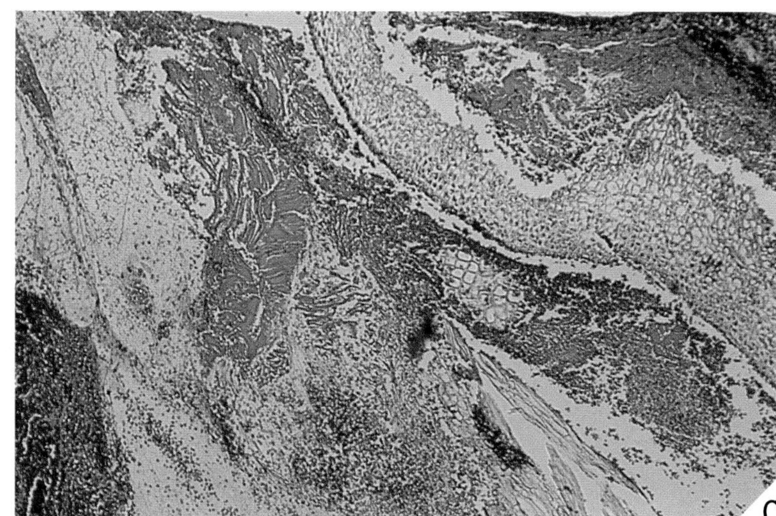

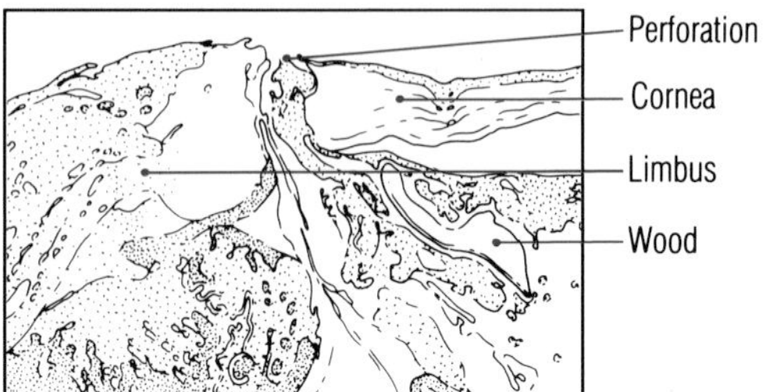

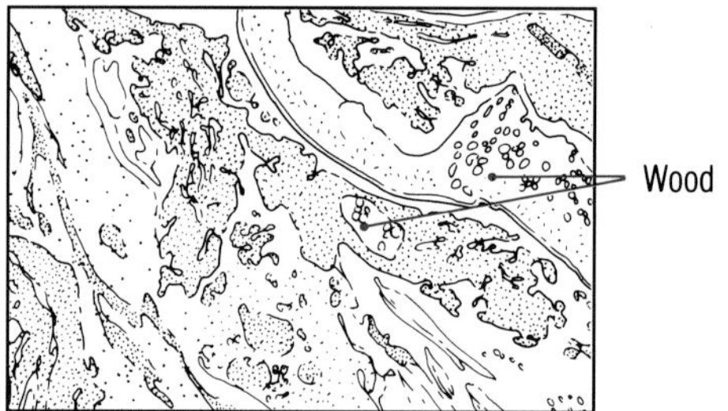

INJURIES

Chemical	Burns	Radiation
Acid	Thermal	
Alkali	Electrical	
Tear gas		
Mustard gas		

FIGURE 5.40

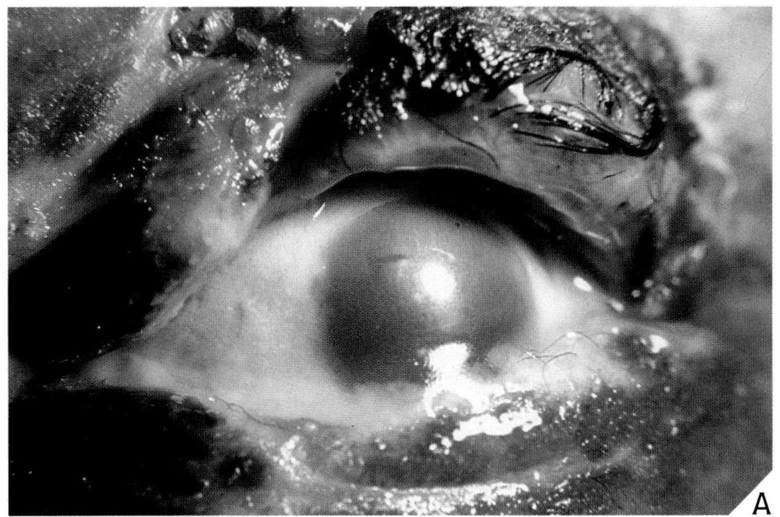

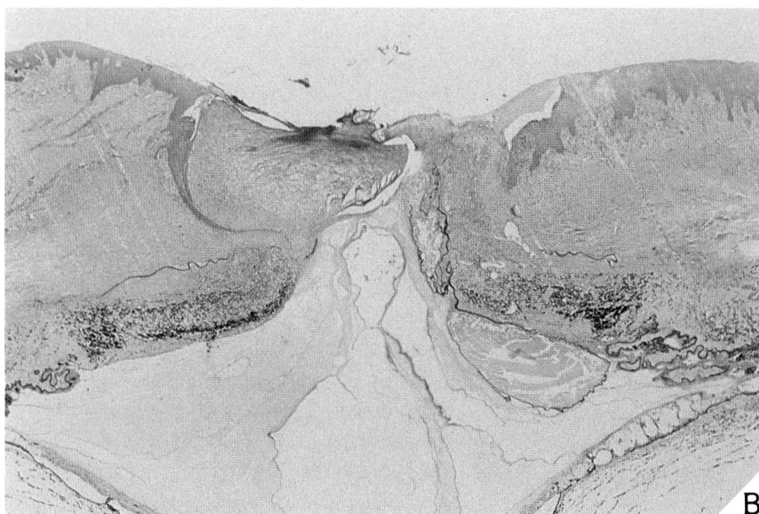

FIGURE 5.41 ALKALI BURN. A Considerable lye has caused a massive burn to the conjunctiva and cornea in this patient's left eye. The "whiteness" of the eye is a measure of the loss of conjunctiva and is always a bad sign in a lye burn. Ultimately, the cornea became necrotic and perforation occurred. **B** Histologic section of another case shows corneal perforation. Lens remnants, including the capsule, are within the corneal wound. Note the thickened cornea and proliferation of corneal epithelium into the stroma. The proliferating epithelium, along with keratocytes and polymorphonuclear leukocytes, secretes collagenase that causes a "melting" of the corneal stroma. The eye is hypotonus, as evidenced by the massive choroidal detachment. (**B**, PAS stain.)

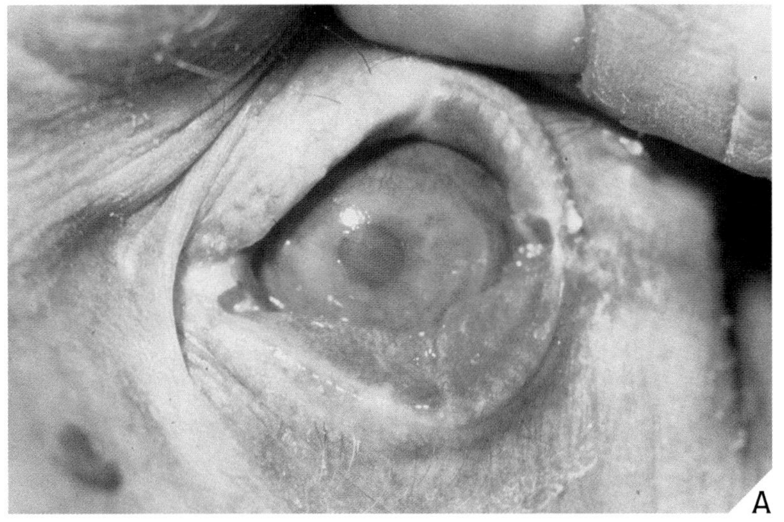

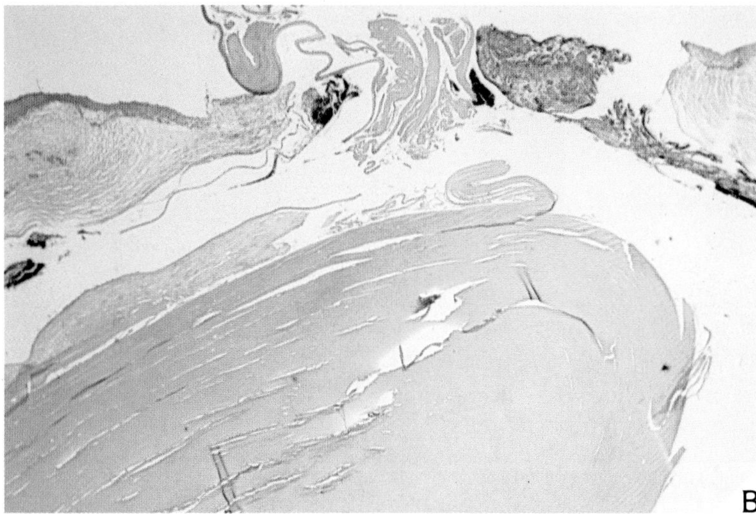

FIGURE 5.42 RADIATION INJURY. A The patient had radiation therapy for sebaceous carcinoma of the eyelid. Note the scarring of the cornea and ciliary injection. **B** Another patient who received radiation therapy for basal cell carcinoma of the eyelid shows corneal perforation. Note the vascularized cornea. Lens remnants and iris are present within the corneal perforation.

Bibliography

Aguilar JP, Green WR: Choroidal rupture. A histopathologic study of 47 cases. Retina 4:269, 1984.

Champion R, Green WE: Intraocular lenses: a histopathologic study of eyes, ocular tissues, and intraocular lenses obtained surgically. Ophthalmology 92:1628, 1985.

Eagle RC, Yanoff M: Cholesterolosis of the anterior chamber. Albrecht v Graefes Arch klin exp Ophthal 193:121, 1975.

Fox GM, Joondeph BC, Flynn HW Jr, et al: Delayed-onset pseudophakic endophthalmitis. Am J Ophthalmol 111:163, 1991.

Harris M, et al: Corneal endothelial overgrowth of angle and iris. Evidence of myoblastic differentiation in three cases. Ophthalmology 91:1154, 1984.

Kappelhof JP, et al: An ultrastructural study of Elschnig's pearls in the pseudophakic eye. Am J Ophthalmol 101:58, 1986.

Kattan HM, Flynn HW Jr, Pflugelder SC, et al: Nosocomial endophthalmitis survey. Current incidence of infection after intraocular surgery. Ophthalmol 98:227, 1991.

Katz LJ, Cantor LB, Spaeth GL: Complications of surgery in glaucoma. Early and late bacterial endophthalmitis following glaucoma filtration surgery. Ophthalmology 92:959, 1985.

Kozart DM, Eagle RC Jr: Stripping of Descemet's membrane after glaucoma surgery. Ophthalmic Surgery 12:420, 1981.

Kozart DM, Yanoff M, Katowitz JA: Tolerated eyelash embedded in the retina. Arch Ophthalmol 91:235, 1974.

Lahav M: The decreased incidence of retinal detachment after cataract surgery. Trans Am Ophthalmol Soc 86:321, 1988.

Liesegang TL, Bourne WM, Ilstrup DM: Prospective 5-year postoperative study of cataract extraction and lens implantation. Trans Am Ophthalmol Soc 87:57, 1989.

Maumenee AE, Schwartz MF: Acute intraoperative choroidal effusion. Am J Ophthalmol 100:147, 1985.

Pearson PA, Owen DG, van Meter WS, et al: Vitreous loss rates in extracapsular cataract surgery by residents. Ophthalmology 96:1225, 1989.

Potts AM, Distler JA: Shape factor in the penetration of intraocular foreign bodies. Am J Ophthalmol 100:183, 1985.

Rao GN, Aquavella JV, Goldberg SH, Berk SL: Pseudophakic bullous keratopathy. Relationships to preoperative corneal endothelial status. Ophthalmology 91:1135, 1984.

Rummelt V, et al: A 32-year follow-up of the rigid Schreck anterior chamber lens. A clinicopathological correlation. Arch Ophthalmol 108:401, 1990.

Sipperly JO, Quigley HA, Gass JDM: Traumatic retinopathy in primates. The explanation of commotio retinae. Arch Ophthalmology 96:2267, 1978.

Speaker MG, Guerriero PN, Met JA, et al: A case-control study of risk factors for intraoperative suprachoroidal expulsive hemorrhage. Ophthalmology 98:202, 1991.

Tawara A: Transformation and cytotoxicity of iron in siderosis bulbi. Invest Ophthalmol Vis Sci 27:226, 1986.

Tesluk GC, Spaeth GL: The occurrence of primary open-angle glaucoma in the fellow eye of patient with unilateral angle-cleavage glaucoma. Ophthalmology 92:904, 1985.

Yanoff M: In vitro biology of corneal epithelium and endothelium. Trans Am Ophthalmol Soc 73:571, 1975.

Yanoff M, et al: Pathology of human cystoid macular edema. Surv Ophthalmol 28 (Suppl):505, 1984.

Lid and Lacrimal Drainage System

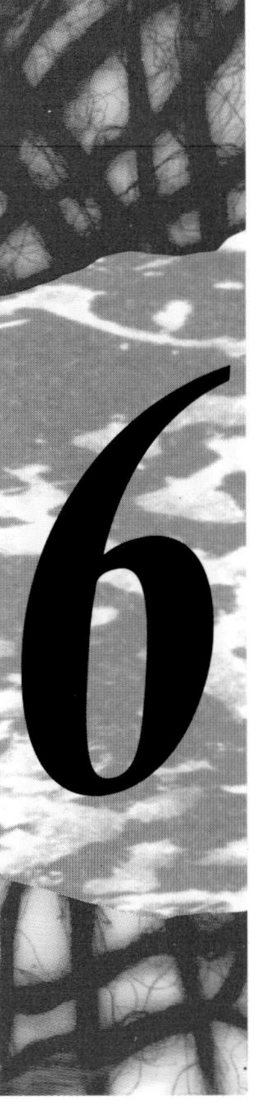

The skin of the eyelids is representative of skin elsewhere in the body. Some conditions, however, either affect the eyelids uniquely or are more common in eyelid structures. The terminology used in dermatopathology will be reviewed where applicable to lid pathology.

Congenital abnormalities may affect the lids alone, or may affect the eyes, or may be part of a generalized systemic defect. At the other end of the spectrum, aging changes often involve the eyelids and lead to characteristic and easily defined clinical entities, such as dermatochalasis.

Inflammation commonly involves the eyelids. Although infectious inflammation may occur, allergic conditions are the most common. Many of the inflammatory conditions that involve the eyelids have the same histological characteristics as those previously described in Chapters 3 and 4.

Many systemic dermatoses may have lid involvement. The spectrum spans congenital lesions such as ichthyosis congenita, inflammatory conditions such as contact dermatitis, systemic syndromes such as collagen diseases, and so forth. The eyelids may be involved alone or may participate in the systemic involvement.

Cysts, pseudoneoplasms, and neoplasms frequently involve the eyelids. Lesions may arise from the surface epithelium, the epidermal appendages, or the dermis. Pigmented tumors of the eyelids are considered in Chapter 17 (on ocular melanotic tumors); soft tissue tumors are described mainly in Chapter 14 (on the orbit).

The lacrimal drainage system may be involved with congenital abnormalities, inflammation, and tumors. Some of the common entities are discussed below.

NORMAL ANATOMY OF THE LIDS

Skin
Epidermis
Dermis

Subcutaneous tissue

FIGURE 6.1

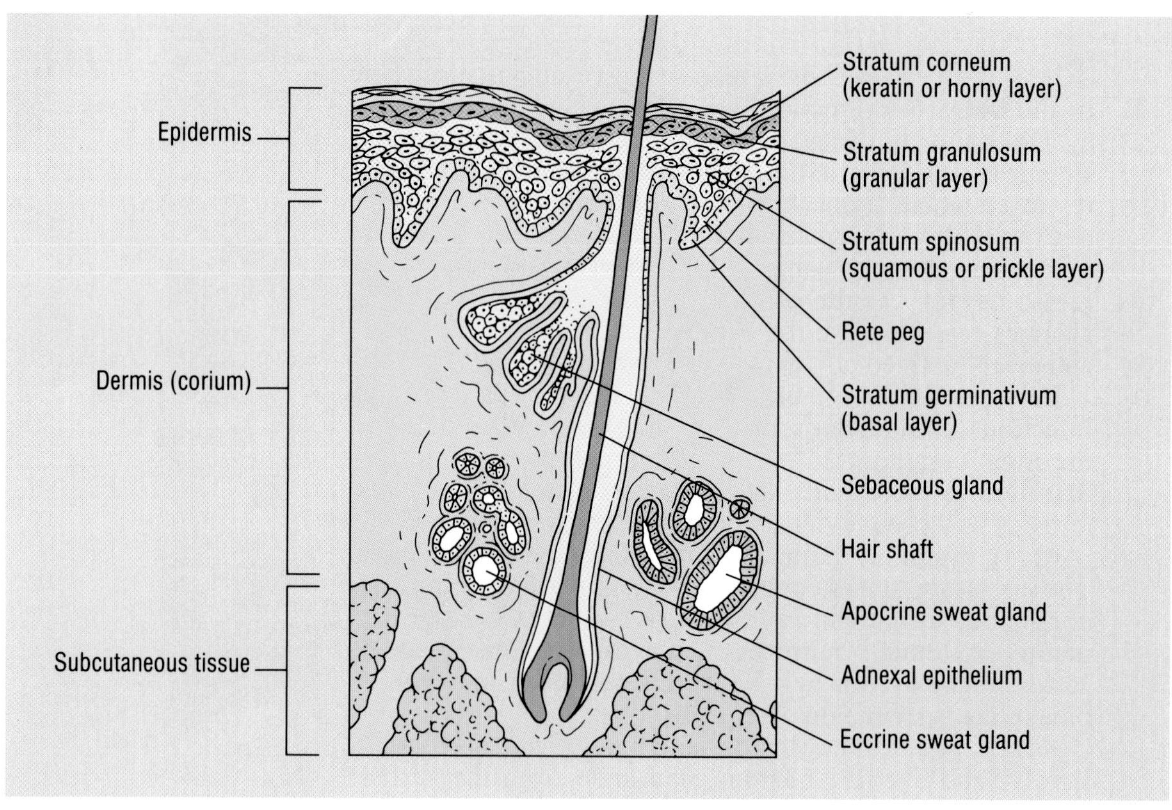

FIGURE 6.2

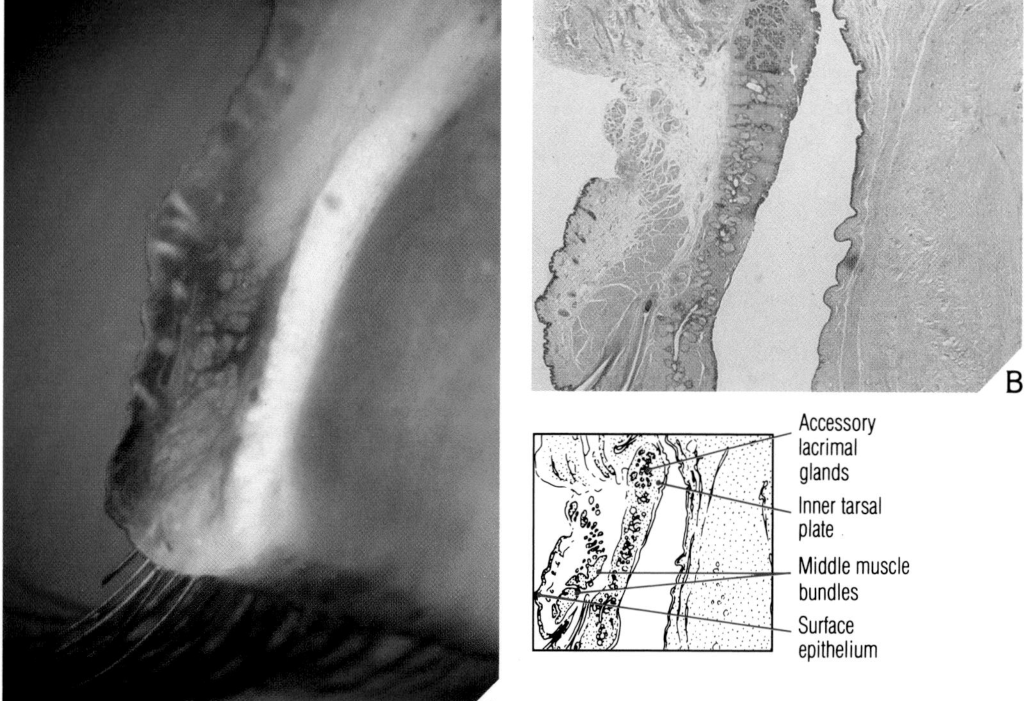

FIGURE 6.3 NORMAL ANATOMY. A Cross section of the eyelid shows the inner white tarsal plate, the middle layers of muscle fibers, and the surface epithelium. Note the cilia coming out of the lid margin inferiorly. **B** Histologic section shows the inner tarsal plate containing the meibomian glands, the middle muscular bundles, and the surface epithelium. The cilia exit from the middle portion of the lid margin inferiorly. Apocrine sweat glands, eccrine sweat glands, sebaceous glands of Zeis, and hair follicles of the surface lanugo hairs also are seen in the lids (see also Figs. 1.12C and 7.1). (**A**, courtesy of Dr. RC Eagle Jr.)

EPIDERMIS TERMINOLOGY

Polarity—normal polarity is the orderly arrangement from basal to squamous to granular to keratin layers

Hyperkeratosis—thickening of the keratin layer

Parakeratosis—incomplete keratinization and retention of nuclei in cells of the keratin layer

Acanthosis—increased thickness of the squamous layer (benign or malignant)

Dyskeratosis—keratinization of individual epithelial cells within the squamous layer

Acantholysis—separation of squamous cells

Bulla—space filled with fluid within or under the epithelium

Atrophy—thinning of the epidermis, diminution of rete pegs, and loss of epidermal appendages

Atypical cell—abnormal cell that, in its extreme, would be cancerous

Leukoplakia—white plaque which has numerous possible causes

FIGURE 6.4

CONGENITAL ANOMALIES

Phakomatous choristoma
Cryptophthalmos
Microblepharon
Coloboma
Epicanthus
Ectopic caruncle
Lid margin anomalies
Eyelash anomalies
Ptosis
Ichthyosis congenita
Xeroderma pigmentosum

FIGURE 6.5

AGING

Atrophy
Dermatochalasis
Herniation of the orbital fat

FIGURE 6.6

INFLAMMATION

Hordeolum
External (stye)
Internal

Chalazion

Acne rosacea

FIGURE 6.7

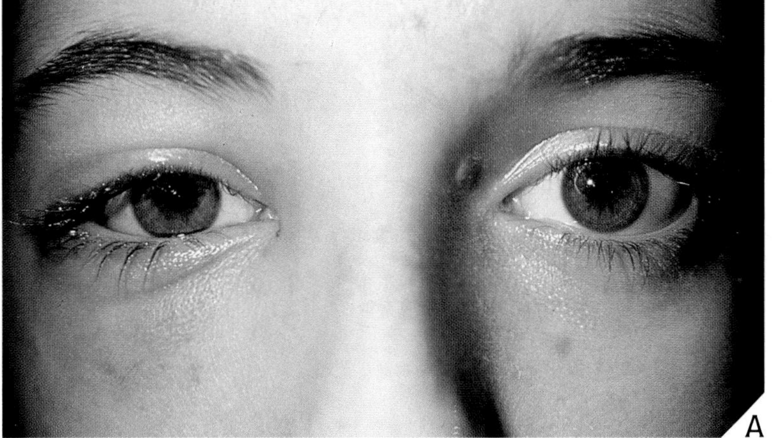

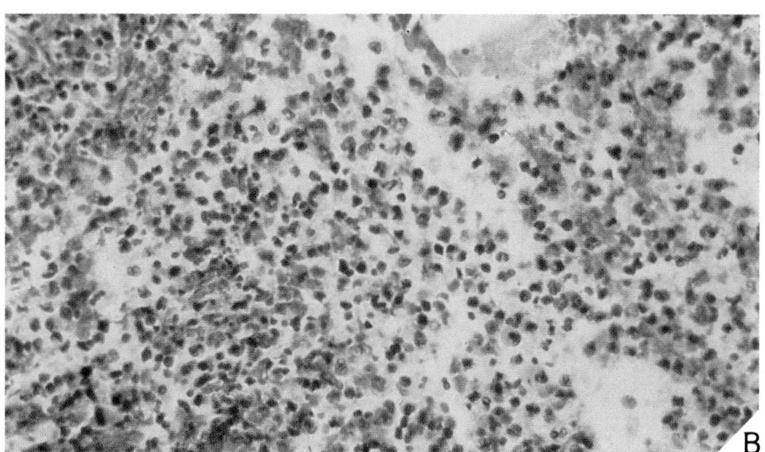

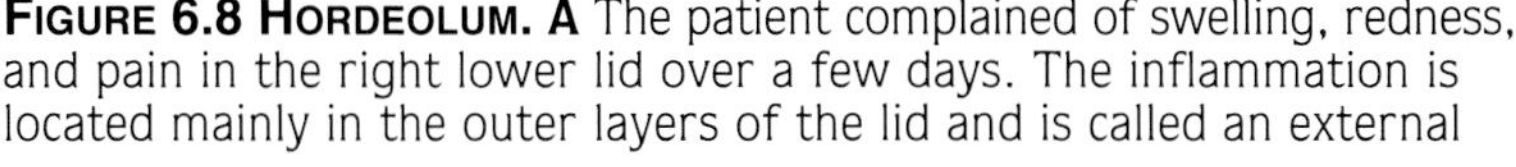

FIGURE 6.8 HORDEOLUM. A The patient complained of swelling, redness, and pain in the right lower lid over a few days. The inflammation is located mainly in the outer layers of the lid and is called an external hordeolum. Similar inflammation in the inner layers is called an internal hordeolum. **B** Histologic section of another case shows a purulent exudate consisting of polymorphonuclear leukocytes and cellular debris.

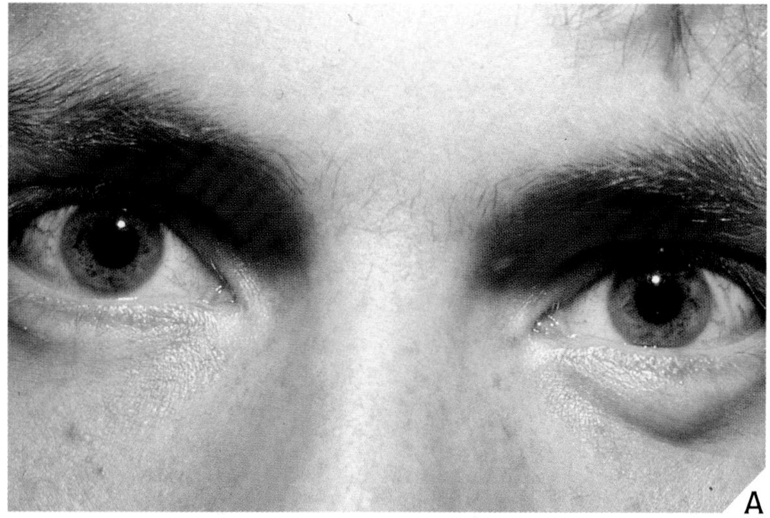

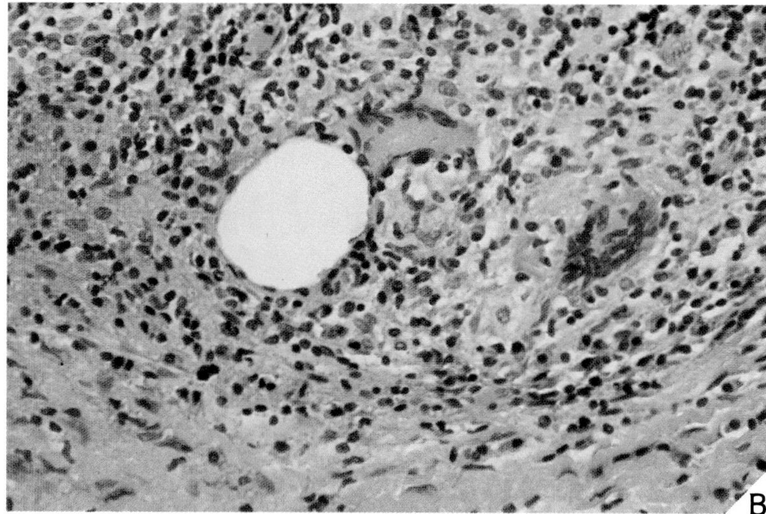

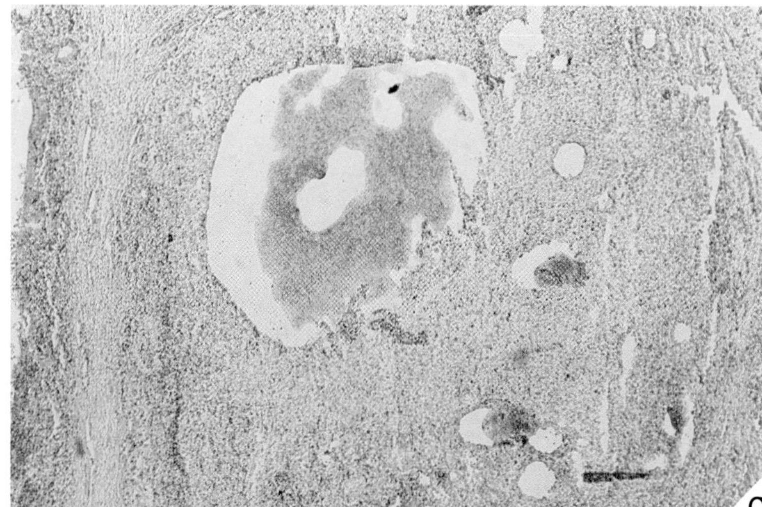

FIGURE 6.9 CHALAZION. A A hard painless lump was present within the left lower lid for at least a few weeks. **B** Histologic section shows a clear circular area surrounded by epithelioid cells and multinucleated giant cells. In processing the tissue, fat is dissolved out, and the area where the fat had been appears clear. **C** Fresh frozen tissue that has not been processed through solvents stains positively for fat in the circular areas. (**C**, oil red-O stain.)

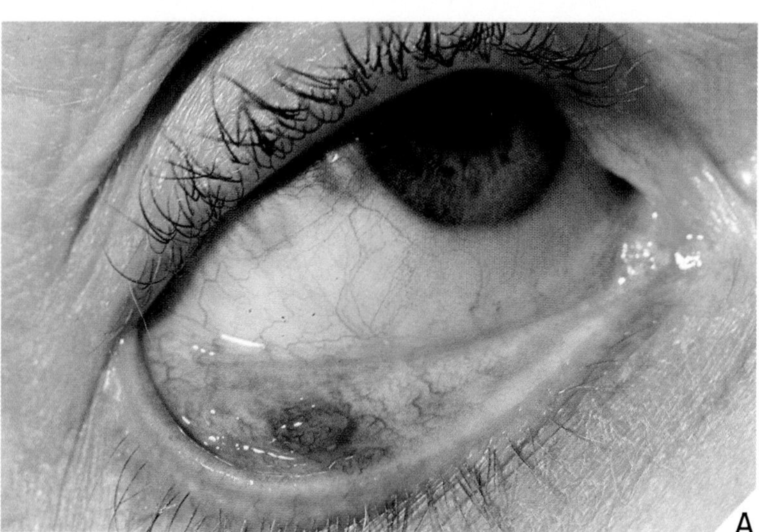

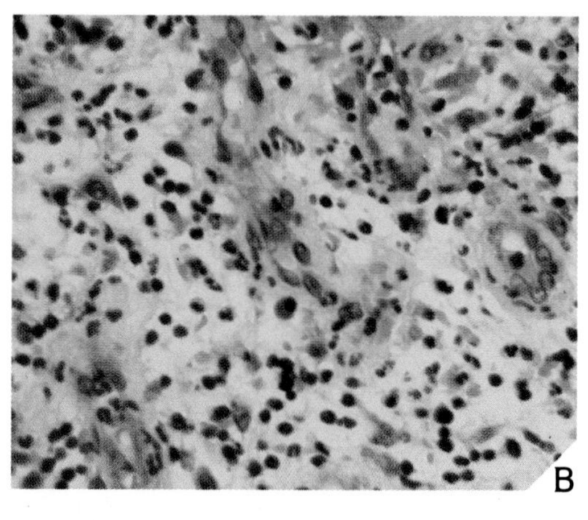

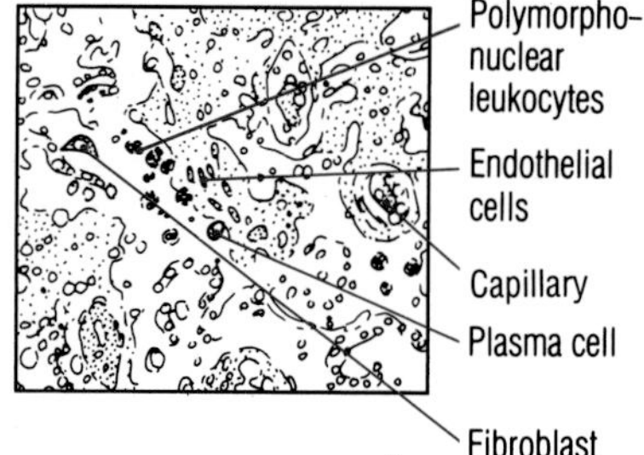

FIGURE 6.10 GRANULOMA PYOGENICUM. A A patient who had a hard painless lump in the right lower lid for over a month came in complaining of a red fleshy area inside the lid. **B** Histologic section shows a vascularized tissue (granulation tissue) that consists of inflammatory cells, fibroblasts, and the endothelial cells of budding capillaries.

Molluscum contagiosum

***Verruca vulgaris* (wart)**

Vesicular lesions
Variola (smallpox)
Varicella (chicken pox)
Herpes zoster (shingles)
Herpes simplex (cold sore)

Trachoma

Lymphogranuloma venereum

FIGURE 6.11

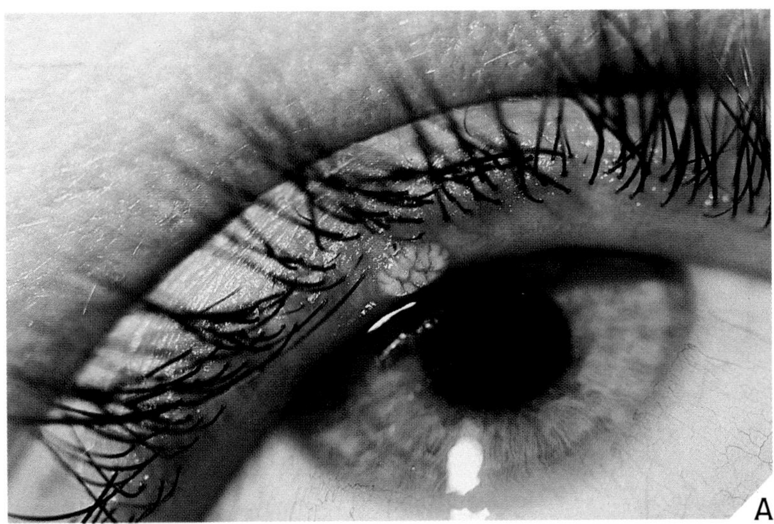

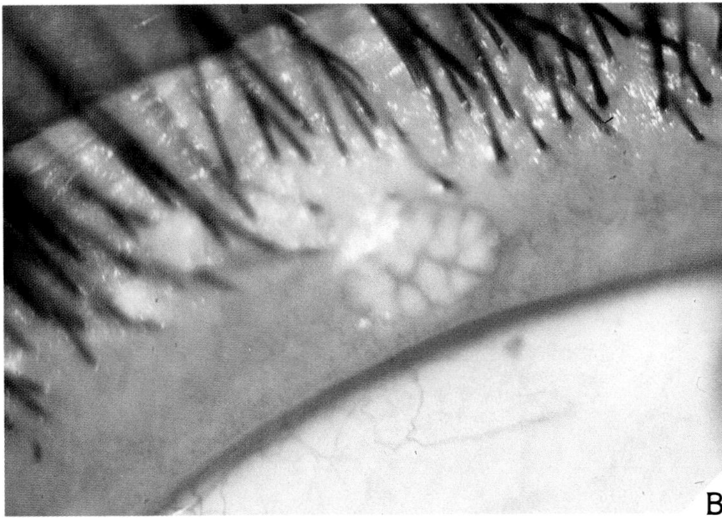

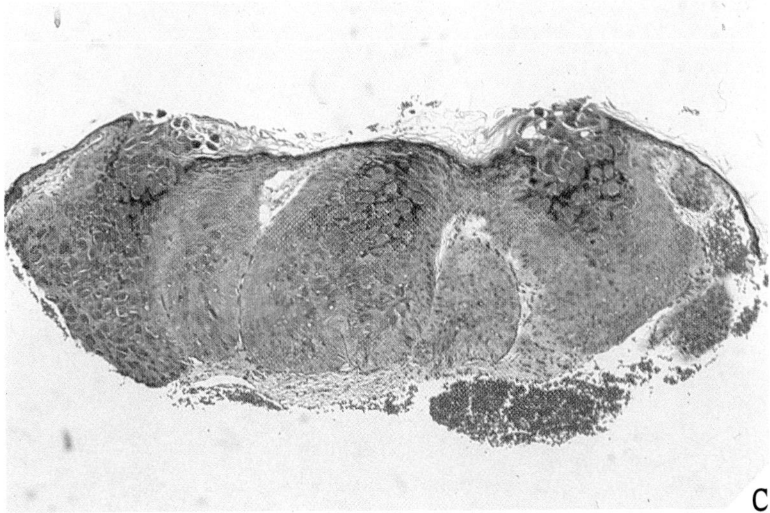

FIGURE 6.12 *MOLLUSCUM CONTAGIOSUM.* A A follicular conjunctivitis is present in the inferior, bulbar conjunctiva. Note the small lesion on the margin of the superior eyelid that is responsible for the follicular conjunctivitis. **B** Increased magnification demonstrates an umbilicated lesion that contains whitish packets of material. **C** Histologic section shows that the epithelium is thickened by intracytoplasmic *Molluscum* bodies that are small and eosinophilic in the deep layers but become enormous and basophilic near the surface. After breaking through the surface epithelium, the *Molluscum* bodies may be shed into the tear film where they cause a secondary, irritative, follicular conjunctivitis. (**A**, **B**, courtesy Dr. WC Frayer.)

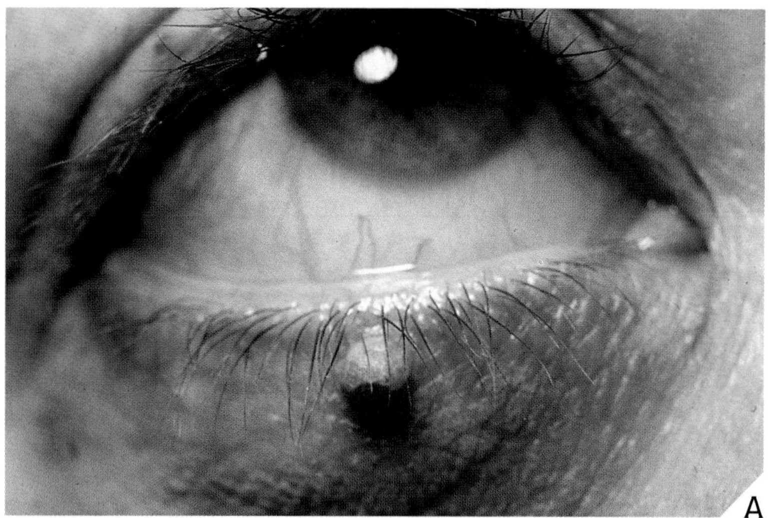

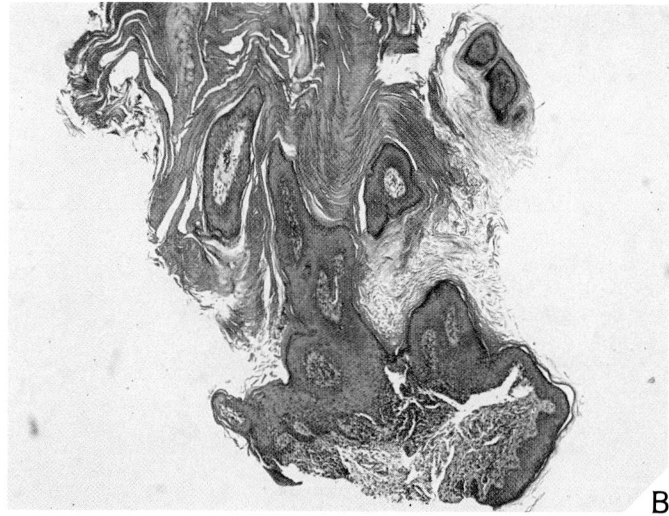

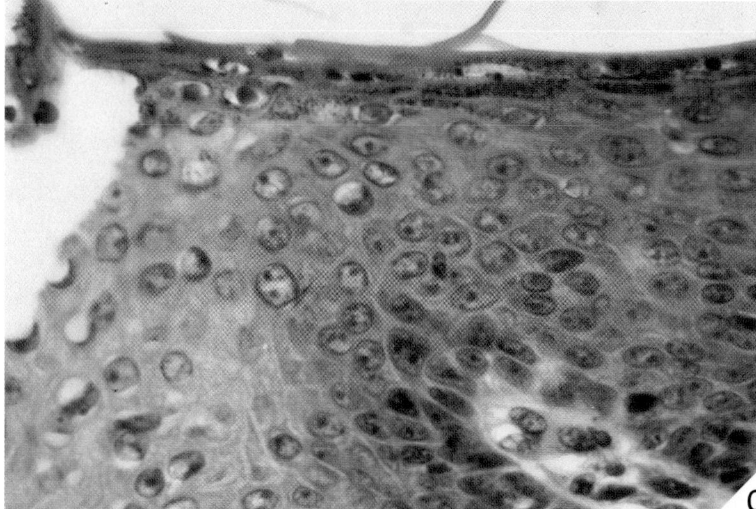

FIGURE 6.13 *VERRUCA VULGARIS.* **A** Clinical appearance of lesion. **B** Histologic section shows marked hyperkeratosis. Note that the rete ridges are elongated and bent inward, a rather typical finding. **C** Another area shows deeply basophilic inclusion bodies and vacuolated cells. Inclusion bodies often are found near the vacuolated cells.

BACTERIAL DISEASES

Impetigo
Staphylococcus
Parinaud oculoglandular syndrome (see Chapter 7)
(Fungal and parasitic diseases, see Chapter 4)

FIGURE 6.14

MANIFESTATIONS OF SYSTEMIC PROBLEMS

Ichthyosis congenita
Xeroderma pigmentosum
Pemphigus
Erythema multiforme
Ehlers-Danlos syndrome
Cutis laxa
Pseudoxanthoma elasticum
Toxic epidermal necrolysis
Contact dermatitis
Collagen diseases
Xanthelasma
Juvenile xanthogranuloma (see Chapter 9)
Amyloidosis (see Chapter 7)
Calcinosis cutis
Lipoid proteinosis
Hemochromatosis
Relapsing febrile nodular nonsuppurative panniculitis

FIGURE 6.15

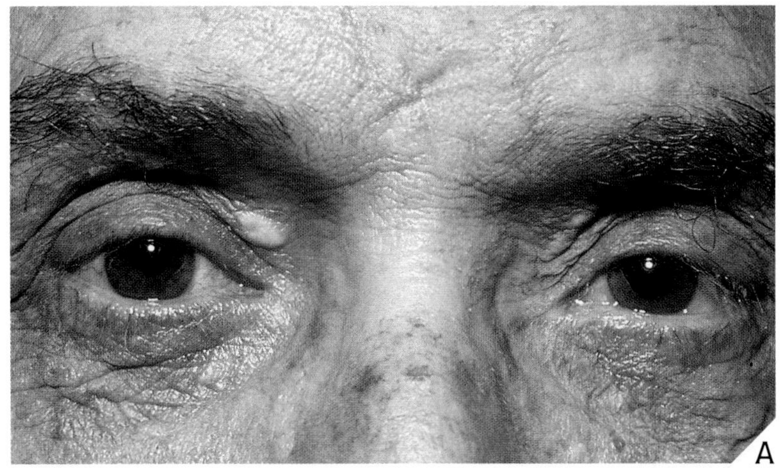

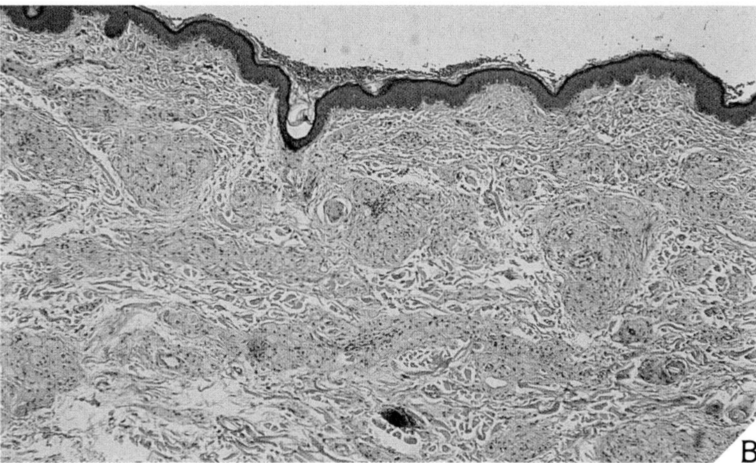

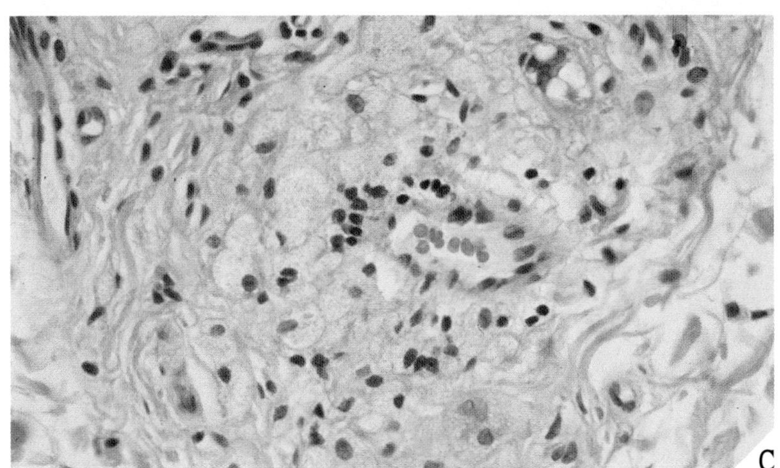

FIGURE 6.16 XANTHELASMA. A The inner aspect of each upper lid (greater on the right upper lid) is thickened by a fatty deposit in the dermis. Xanthelasma may be associated with systemic diseases such as familial lipid diseases or Erdheim-Chester disease (xanthogranulomatous inflammation of many tissues, including the orbit). **B** Histologic section of xanthelasma shows thickening of the dermis by clusters of lipid-filled macrophages. **C** The lipid-filled macrophages tend to cluster around blood vessels. The material within the macrophages stains positively for fat.

BENIGN CYSTIC LESIONS

Epidermoid and dermoid cysts (see Chapter 14)	Epithelial inclusion cyst	Comedo (blackhead)
	Sebaceous cyst	Ductal cysts

FIGURE 6.17

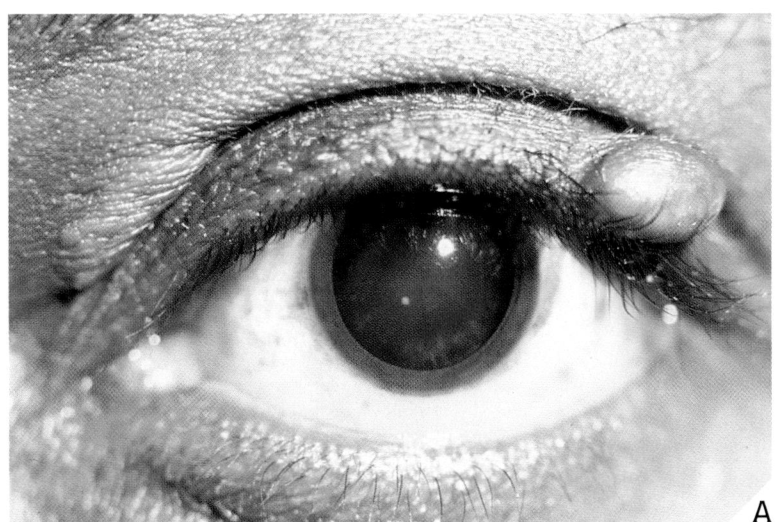

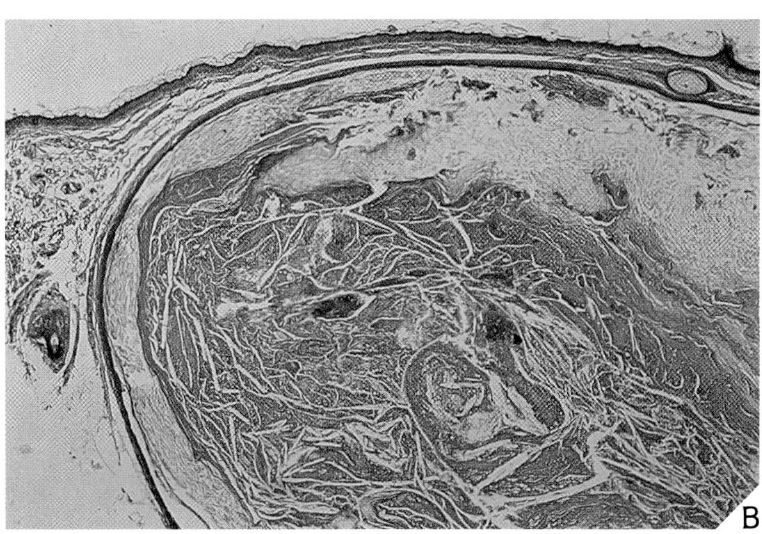

FIGURE 6.18 EPITHELIAL INCLUSION CYST. A The patient has a large epithelial inclusion cyst on the outer third of the left upper lid. Note the xanthelasma at the inner corner of the left upper lid. **B** The cyst is lined by stratified squamous epithelium that desquamates keratin into its lumen.

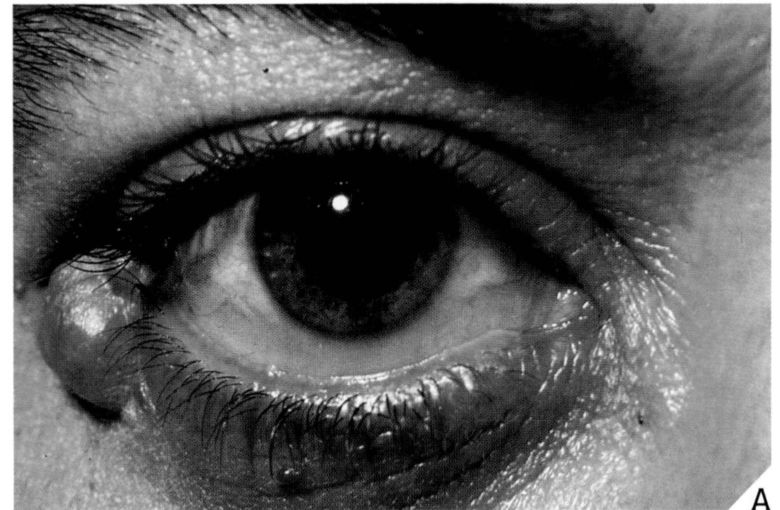

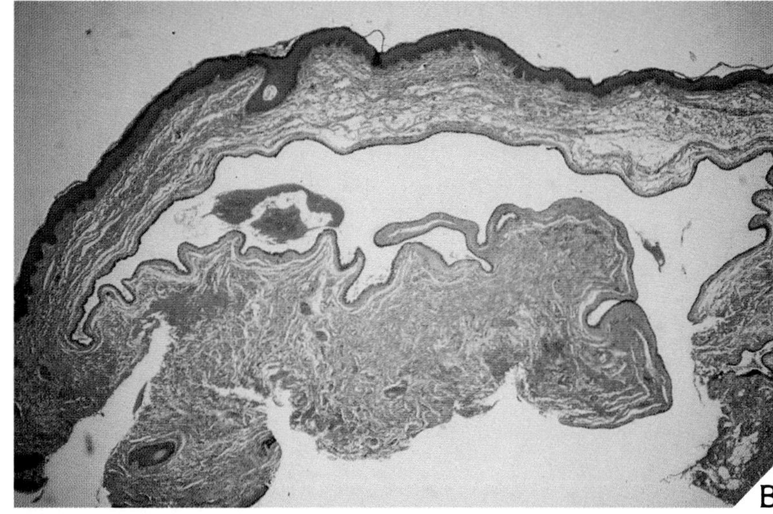

FIGURE 6.19 DUCTAL CYST. A Ductal cyst noted near the outer margin of the right lower lid. **B** The multiloculated cyst is lined by a double-layered epithelium, shown with increased magnification in **C**.

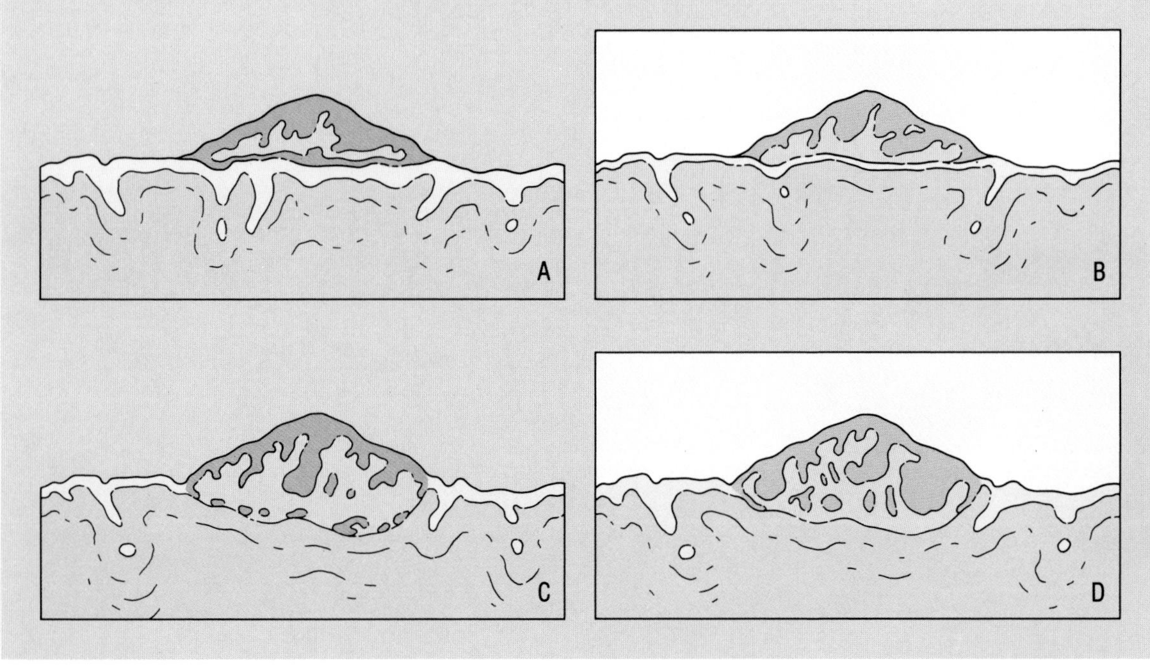

FIGURE 6.20 DIFFERENCES BETWEEN BENIGN AND MALIGNANT SKIN LESIONS. A An elevated lesion sitting as a "button" on the skin surface. This is characteristic of benign papillomatous lesions. When such lesions appear red histologicaly under low magnification, they show acanthosis, as in actinic keratosis. **B** Lesions structurally similar to **A** but that appear blue under low magnification are caused by proliferation of basal cells, as in seborrheic keratosis. **C** An elevated lesion that invades the underlying skin is characteristic of a malignancy. Invasive lesions that appear red under low magnification are caused by a proliferation of the squamous layer (acanthosis), as in squamous cell carcinoma. **D** A lesion structurally similar to **C** but that appears blue under low magnification represents proliferation of basal cells, as seen in basal cell carcinoma.

BENIGN TUMORS OF SURFACE EPITHELIUM

Papilloma
Nevus verrucosis (Jadassohn)
Actinic keratosis
Verruca vulgaris
Seborrheic keratosis
Acanthosis nigricans
Squamous papilloma

Inverted follicular keratosis

Pseudoepitheliomatous hyperplasia
Keratoacanthoma
Others

Benign keratosis

Figure 6.21

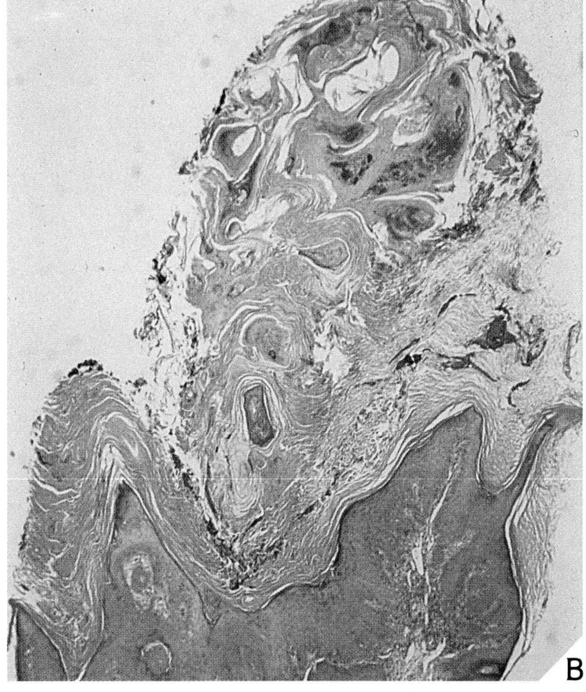

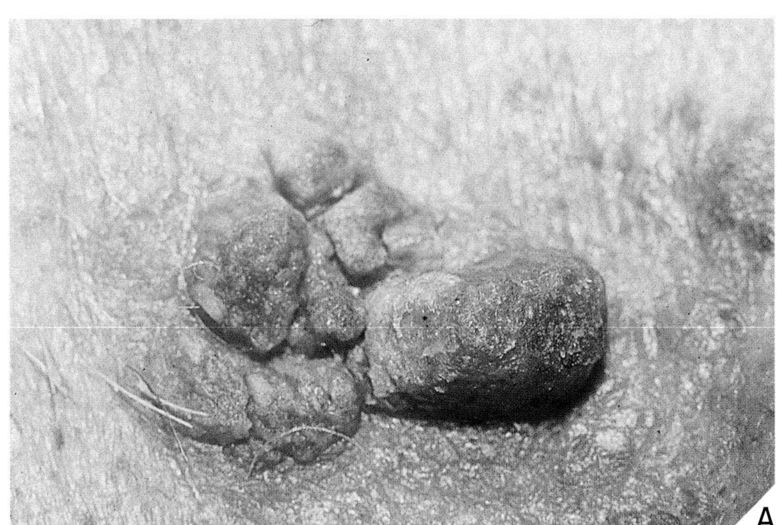

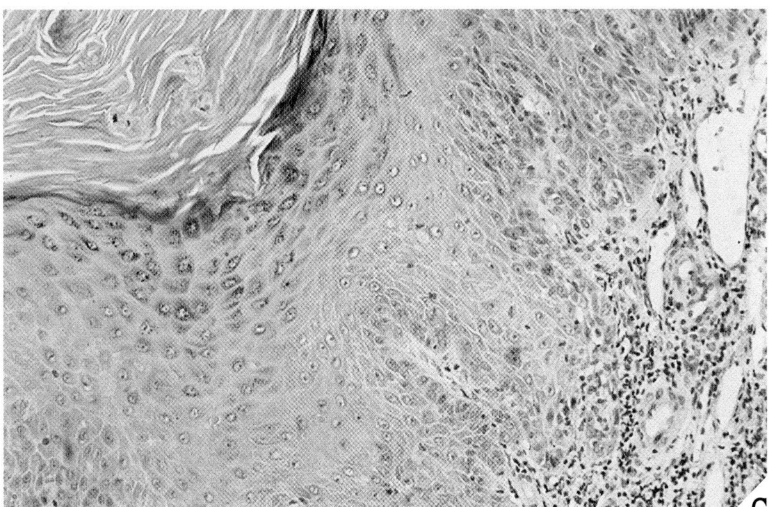

Figure 6.22 Actinic Keratosis. A The clinical appearance of a lesion involving the left upper lid. **B** Histologic section shows a papillomatous lesion that is above the skin surface, appears red, and has marked hyperkeratosis and acanthosis. **C** Although the squamous layer of the skin is increased in thickness (acanthosis) and the basal layer shows atypical cells, the normal polarity of the epidermis is preserved.

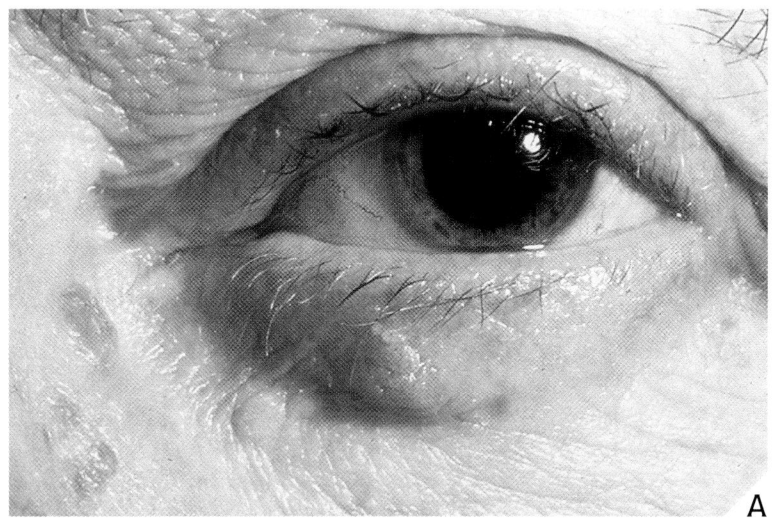

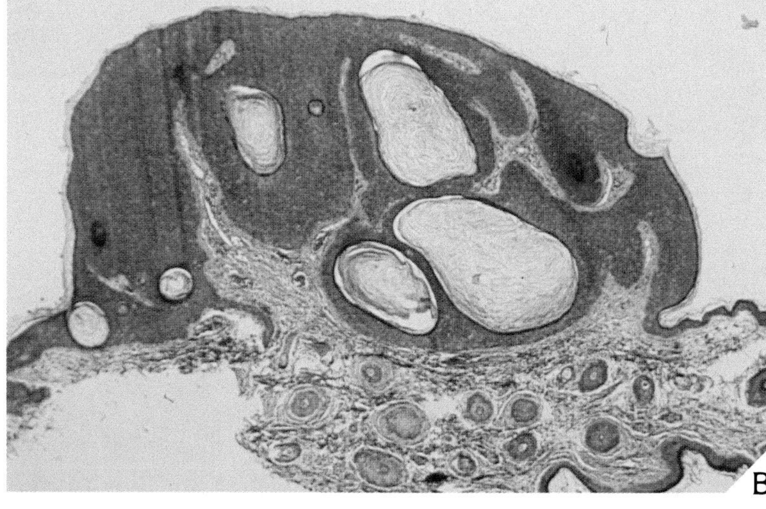

FIGURE 6.23 SEBORRHEIC KERATOSIS. A A "greasy" elevated lesion is present in the middle nasal portion of the left lower lid. Biopsy showed this to be a seborrheic keratosis. The smaller lesion just inferior and nasal to the seborrheic keratosis proved to be a syringoma (see Figure 6.38). Another seborrheic keratosis is present on the side of the nose. **B** Histologic section shows a papillomatous lesion that lies above the skin surface and is blue. The lesion contains proliferated basaloid cells and keratin-filled cysts.

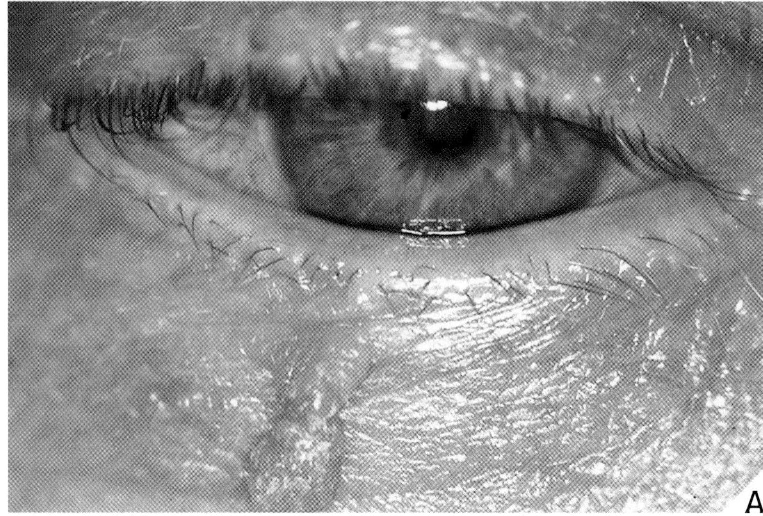

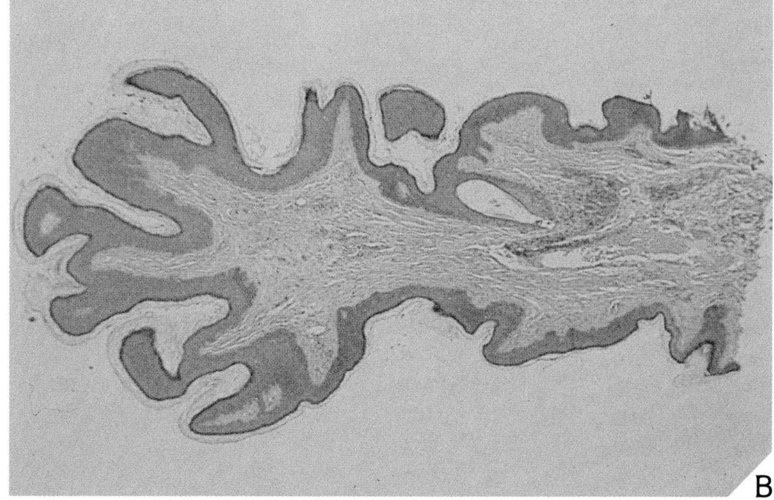

FIGURE 6.24 SQUAMOUS PAPILLOMA. A A skin tag is noted in the middle portion of the lower lid. **B** Histologic section shows a narrow-based papilloma that contains many finger-like processes called fronds. The fronds are covered by an acanthotic, hyperkeratotic epithelium and contain a fibrovascular core.

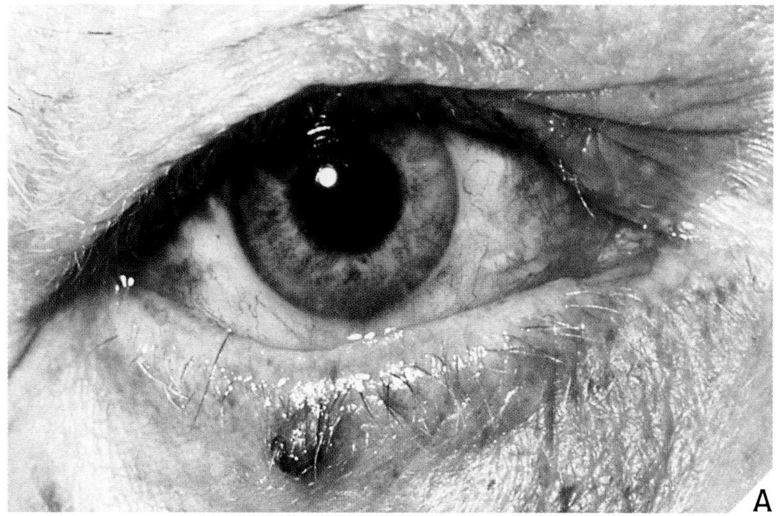

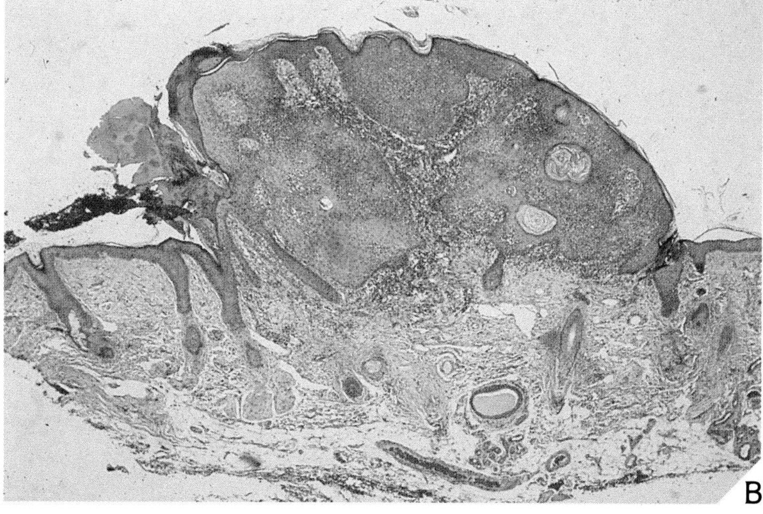

FIGURE 6.25 INVERTED FOLLICULAR KERATOSIS. A Clinical appearance of lesion in the middle of the right lower lid. **B** Histologic section shows a papillomatous lesion above the skin surface composed mainly of acanthotic epithelium. **C** Increased magnification shows separation or acantholysis of individual squamous cells that surround the characteristic squamous eddies.

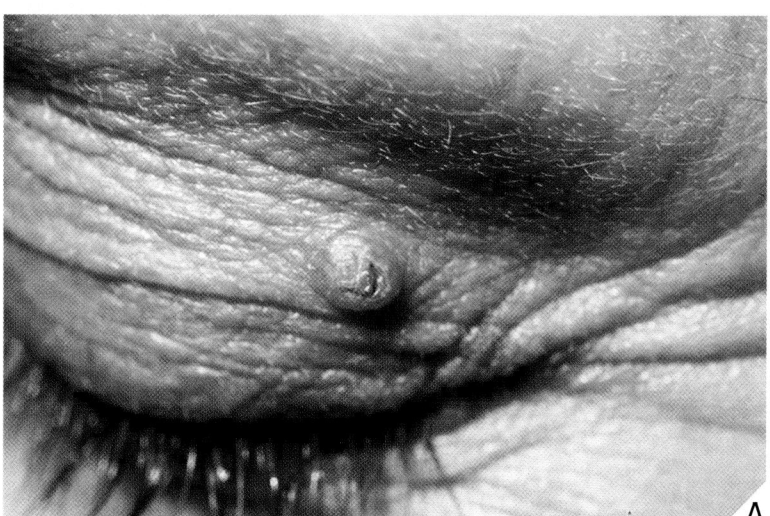

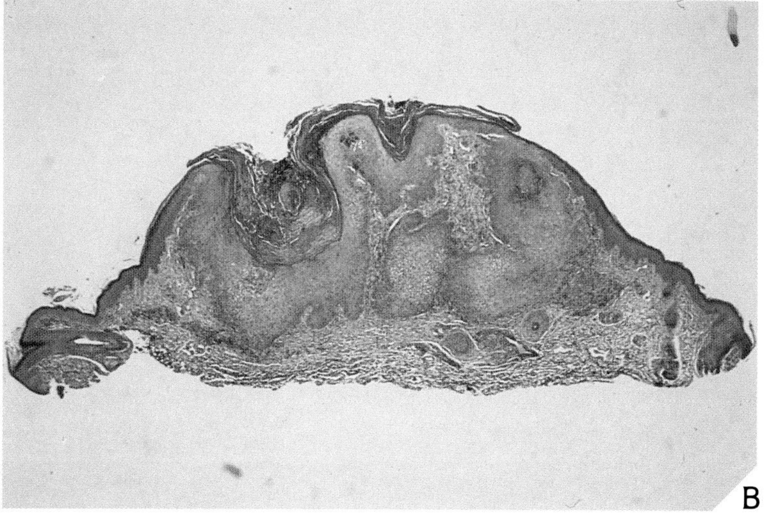

FIGURE 6.26 KERATOACANTHOMA. A This patient had a 6-week history of a rapidly enlarging lesion. Note the umbilicated central area. **B** Histologic section shows that the lesion is above the surface epithelium, has a cup-shaped configuration, and a central keratin core. The base of the acanthotic epithelium is blunted (rather than invasive) at the junction of the dermis.

PRECANCEROUS TUMORS OF SURFACE EPITHELIUM

Xeroderma pigmentosum
Actinic keratosis
Radiation dermatosis

FIGURE 6.27

CANCEROUS TUMORS OF SURFACE EPITHELIUM

Basal cell carcinoma

Squamous cell carcinoma (rare)
Intraepidermal
Invasive

FIGURE 6.28

FIGURE 6.29 BASAL CELL CARCINOMA. A A firm indurated painless lesion had been present for about 8 months. **B** Excisional biopsy shows epithelial proliferation arising from the basal layer of the epidermis. The proliferated cells appear blue and are present in nests of different sizes. Note the sharp demarcation of the pale pink area of stroma supporting the neoplastic cells from the underlying (normal) dark pink dermis. This stromal change, called desmoplasia, is characteristic of neoplastic lesions. Compare with the benign lesions in Figs. 6.23–6.25, where the dermis does not show such a change. **C** The nests are composed of atypical basal cells and show peripheral palisading. Mitotic figures are present. Again, note the pseudosarcomatous change (desmoplasia) of the surrounding supporting stroma, which is light pink and contains proliferating fibroblasts. (**A**, courtesy of Dr. HG Scheie.)

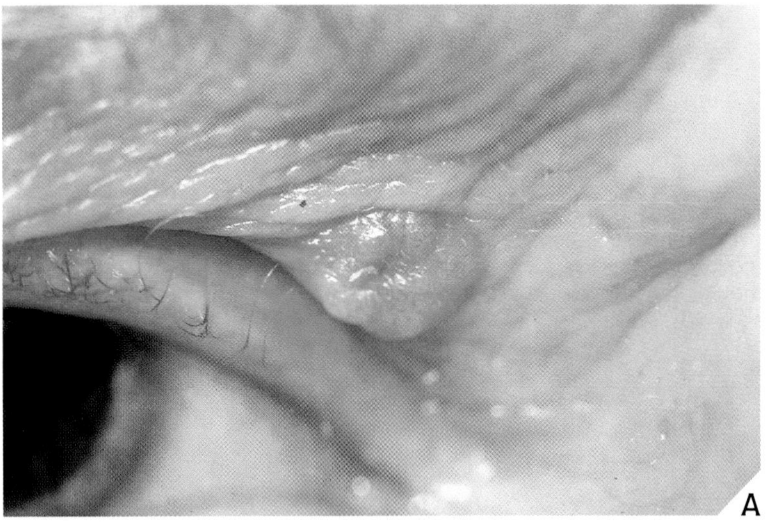
A

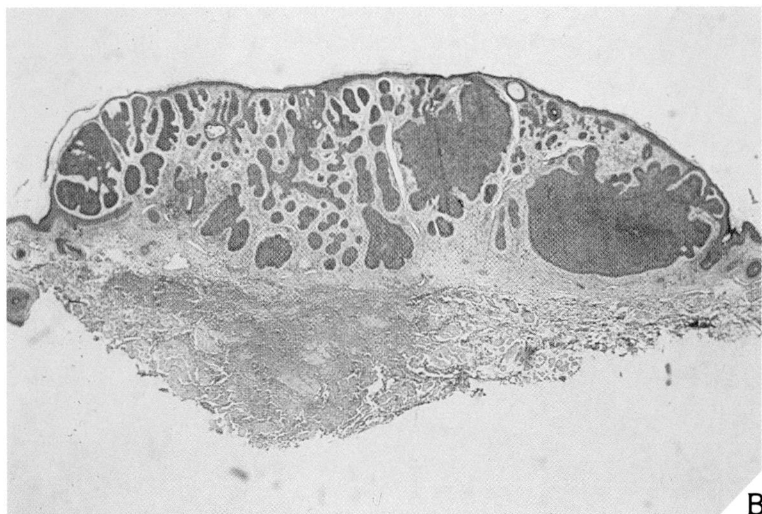
B

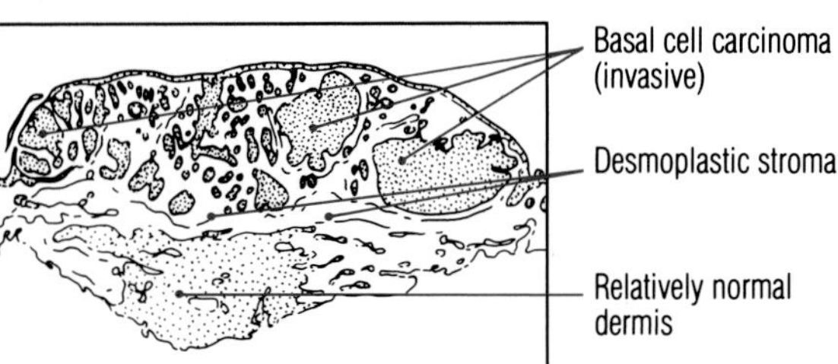

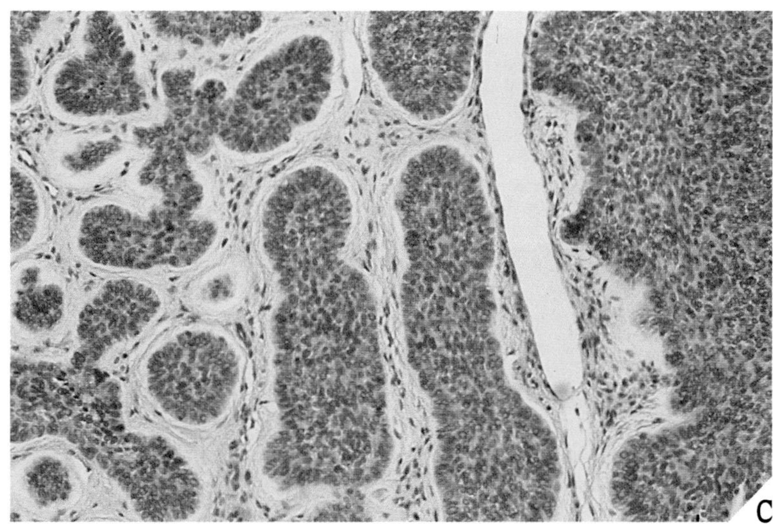
C

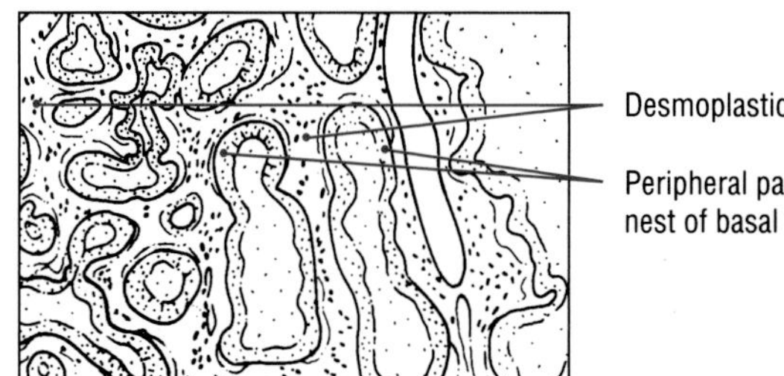

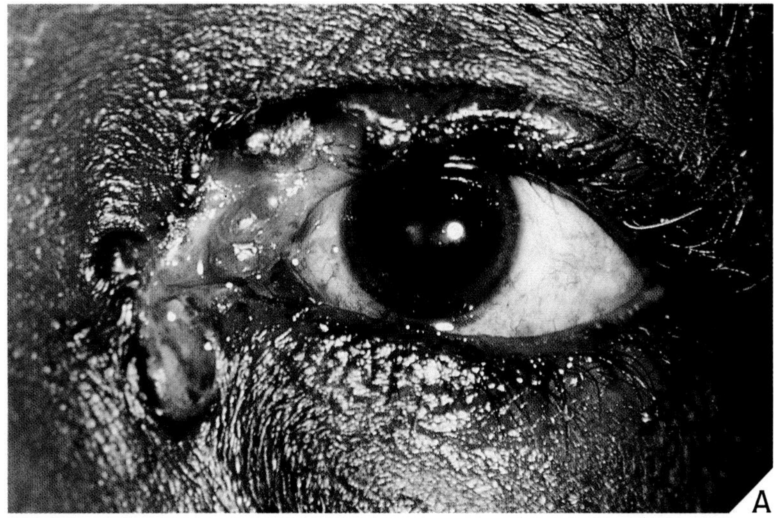

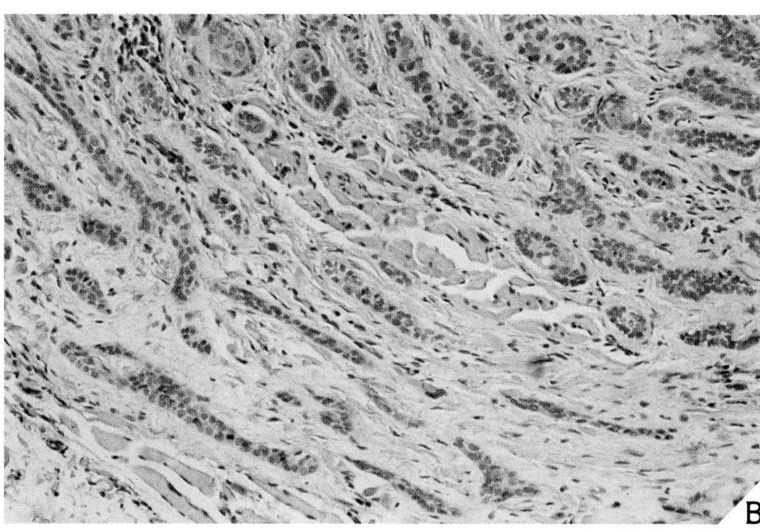

FIGURE 6.30 BASAL CELL CARCINOMA (BCC). A The inner aspect of the eyelids are ulcerated by the infiltrating tumor. **B** Histologic section shows the morphea-like or fibrosing type, where the basal cells grow in thin strands or cords, often only one cell layer thick, closely resembling metastatic scirrhous carcinoma of the breast ("Indian file" pattern). This uncommon type of basal cell carcinoma has a much worse prognosis than the more common types, ie, nodular (Figure 6.29), ulcerative, and multicentric.

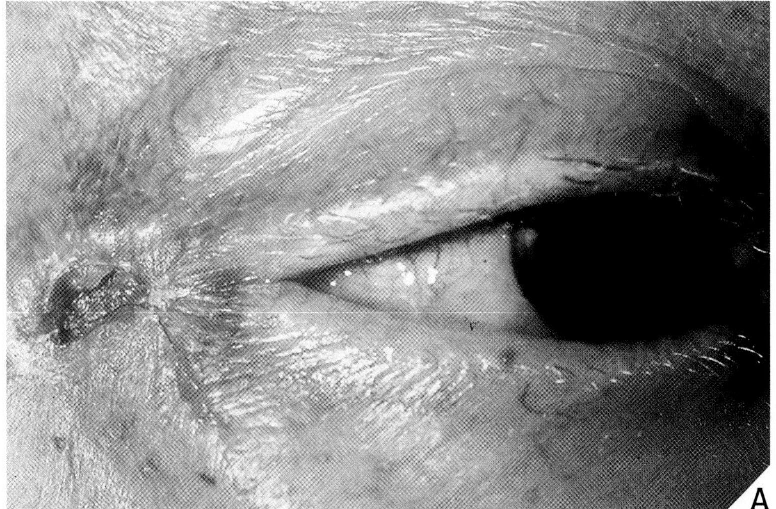

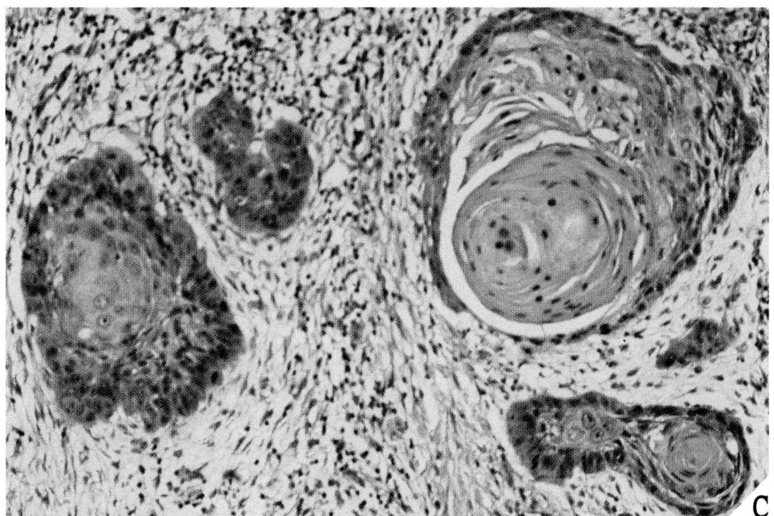

FIGURE 6.31 SQUAMOUS CELL CARCINOMA. A The patient had an ulcerating lesion of the lateral aspect of the eyelids that increased in size over many months. **B** Histologic section of the excisional biopsy shows epithelial cells with an overall pink color that infiltrate the dermis deeply. The overlying region is ulcerated. **C** Increased magnification shows the squamous neoplastic cells making keratin (horn cyst) in an abnormal location (dyskeratosis). Numerous mitotic figures are present. Note the pseudosarcomatous (dysplastic) change in the surrounding stroma.

TUMORS OF SEBACEOUS GLANDS

Congenital sebaceous gland hyperplasia
Acquired sebaceous gland hyperplasia
Adenoma sebaceum of Pringle (angiofibroma of face)
Sebaceous adenoma (may be part of the Muir-Torre syndrome)
Sebaceous gland carcinoma

FIGURE 6.32

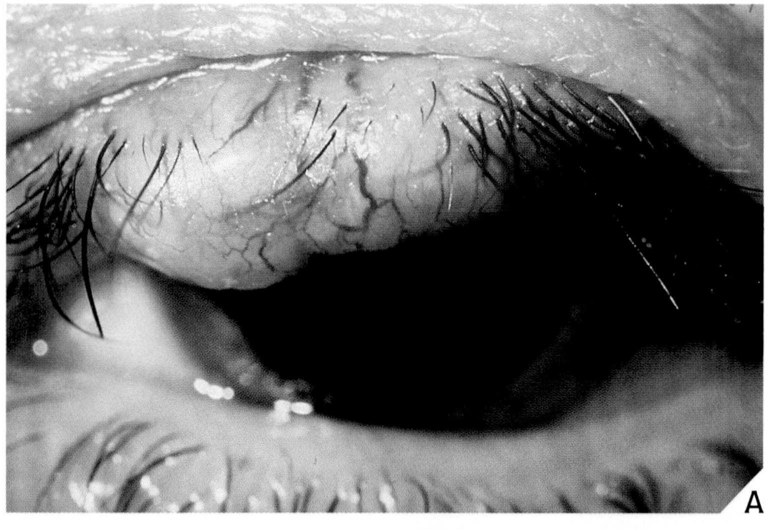
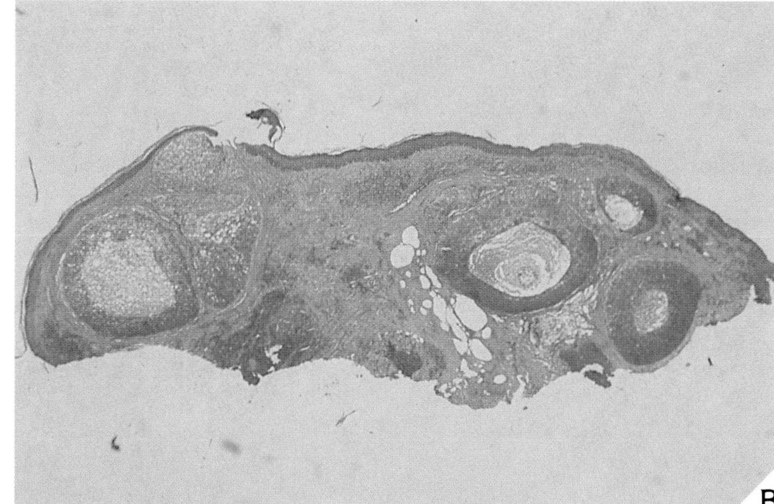
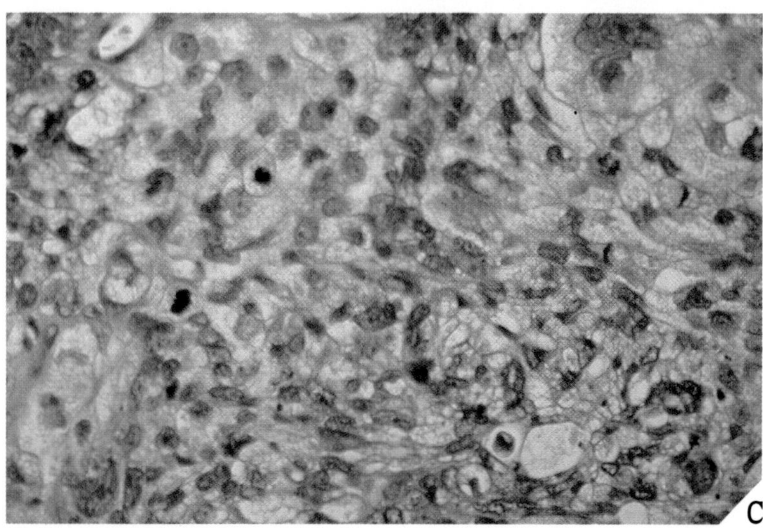
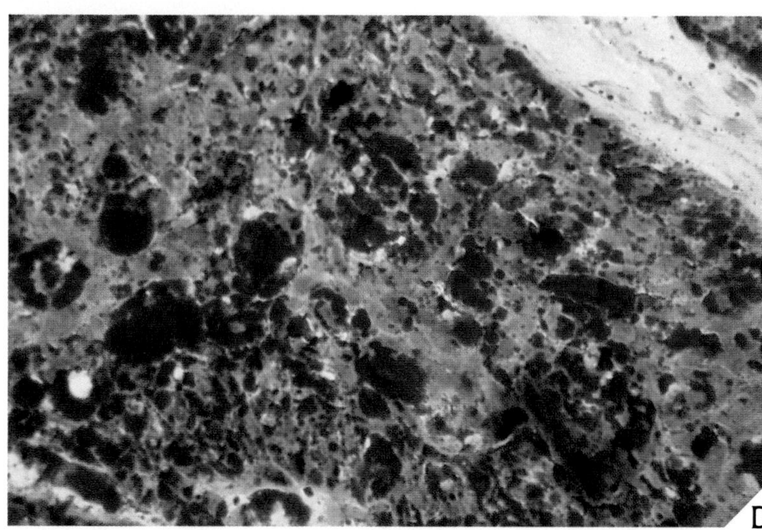
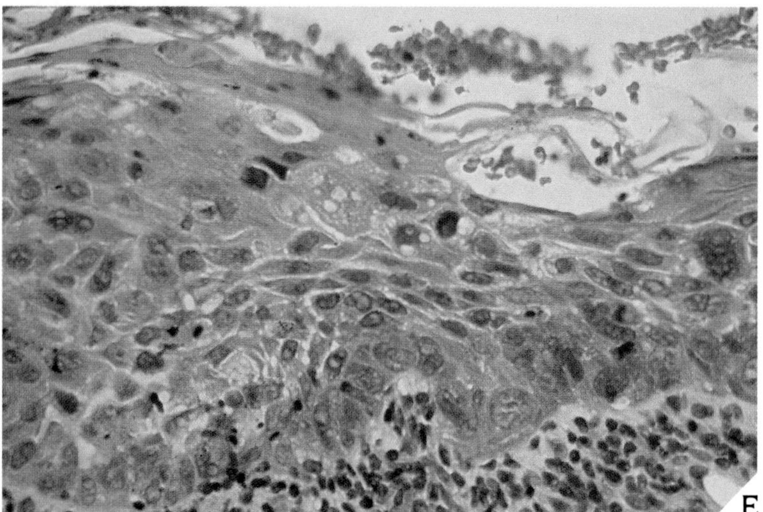

FIGURE 6.33 SEBACEOUS CELL CARCINOMA. A Clinical appearance of lesion that simulates a large chalazion. Note the characteristic loss of hair over the lesion. **B** Histologic section shows large tumor nodules in the dermis, most of which exhibit central necrosis. **C** Increased magnification shows that numerous cells resemble sebaceous gland cells. A number of mitotic figures are present. **D** Many of the cells stain positively for fat. Any recurrent or suspicious chalazion should be biopsied. **E** In another case, large tumor cells are scattered throughout the epithelium, resembling Paget disease and called pagetoid change. The cancerous invasion of the epithelium can cause a chronic nongranulomatous blepharoconjunctivitis (masquerade syndrome). (**D**, oil red-O stain).

TUMORS OF HAIR FOLLICLES

Trichoepithelioma (Brooke tumor)
Trichofolliculoma
Trichilemmoma (may be part of Cowden disease)
Pilomatrixoma (calcifying epithelioma of Malherbe)
Merkel cell tumor
Adnexal carcinoma

FIGURE 6.34

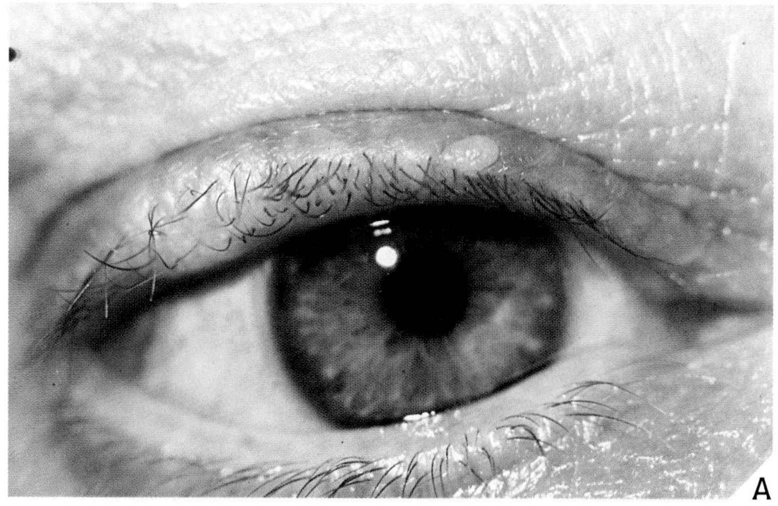

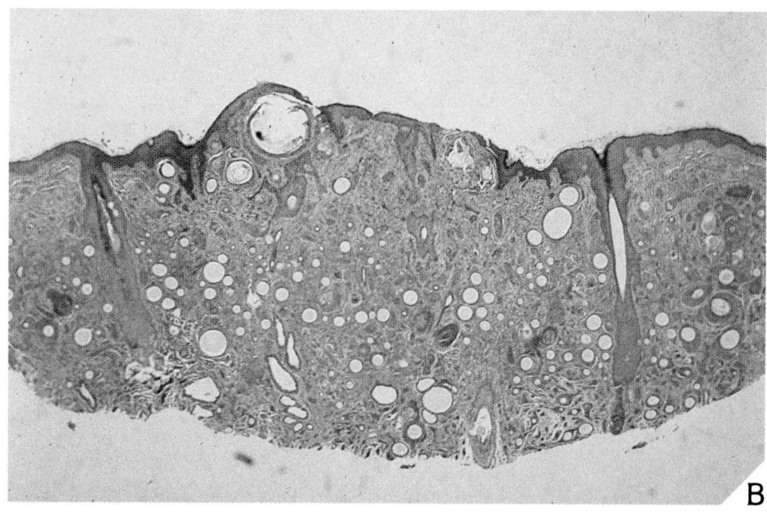

FIGURE 6.35 TRICHOEPITHELIOMA. A Clinical appearance of a lesion in the middle of the right upper lid near the margin. **B** Histologic section shows the tumor diffusely present throughout the dermis. The tumor is composed of multiple squamous cell horn cysts that represent immature hair structures.

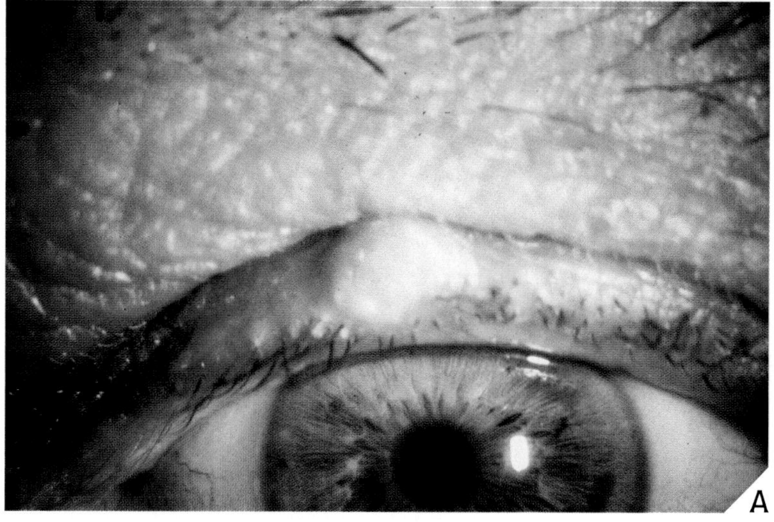

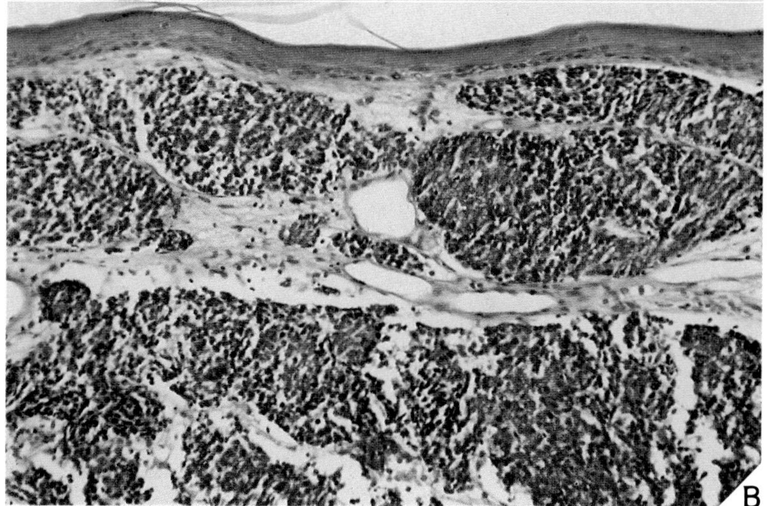

FIGURE 6.36 MERKEL CELL TUMOR. A Clinical appearance of a lesion in the middle portion of the upper lid. **B** Histologic section shows nests of dark, poorly differentiated cells in the dermis. Mitotic figures also are seen. The tumor appears to arise from cells commonly associated with hair follicles that form complexes with terminal neurites, complexes which then act as specific sensory epithelial nerve cell receptors. (Case presented by Dr. DA Morris at the Eastern Ophthalmic Pathology Society, 1985.)

TUMORS OF SWEAT GLANDS

Syringoma
Syringocystadenoma papilleferum
Eccrine spiradenoma
Eccrine mixed tumor
Cylindroma (turban tumor)
Eccrine poroma
Sweat gland carcinoma

FIGURE 6.37

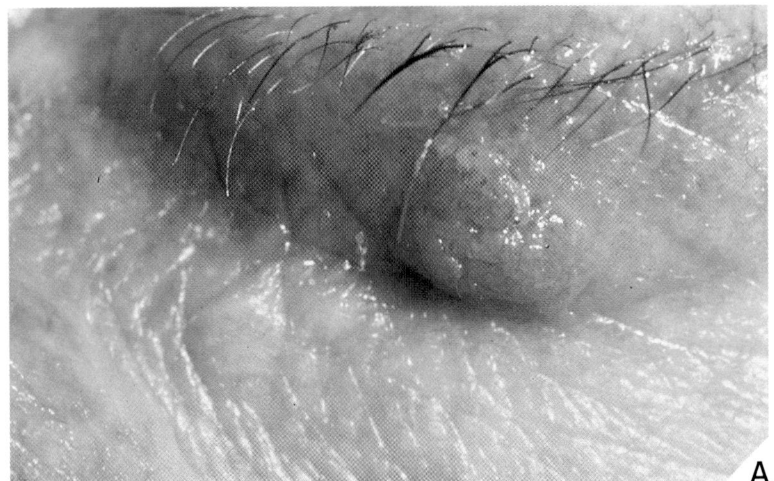

FIGURE 6.38 SYRINGOMA. A Clinical appearance of lesions just below and nasal to seborrheic keratosis of left lower lid (same patient as in Figure 6.23). **B** Histologic section shows that the dermis contains proliferated eccrine sweat structures that form epithelial strands and cystic spaces. **C** Increased magnification demonstrates epithelial strands and cystic spaces that are lined by a double-layered epithelium.

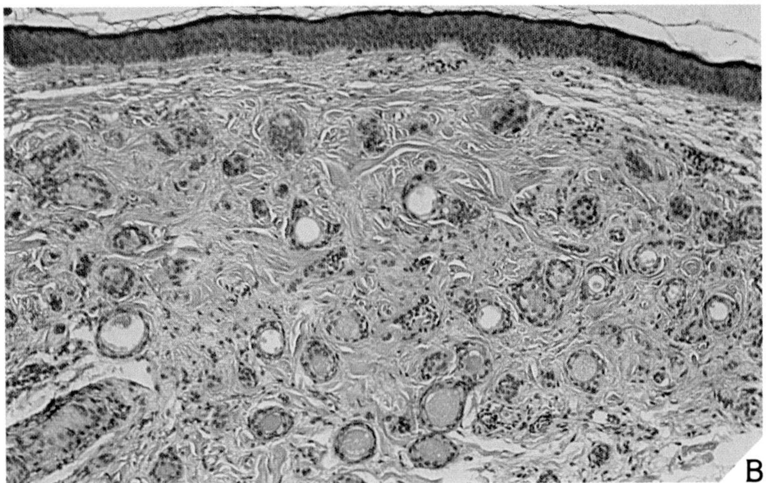

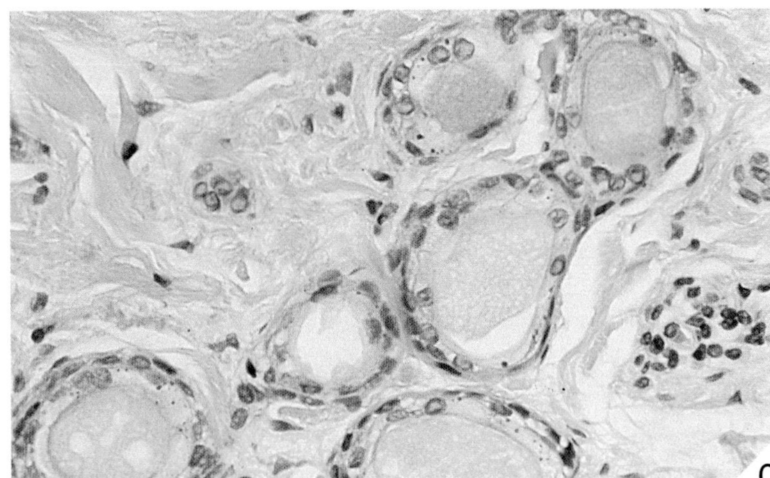

Surface epithelium

Tumor "ducts" and epithelial Strands

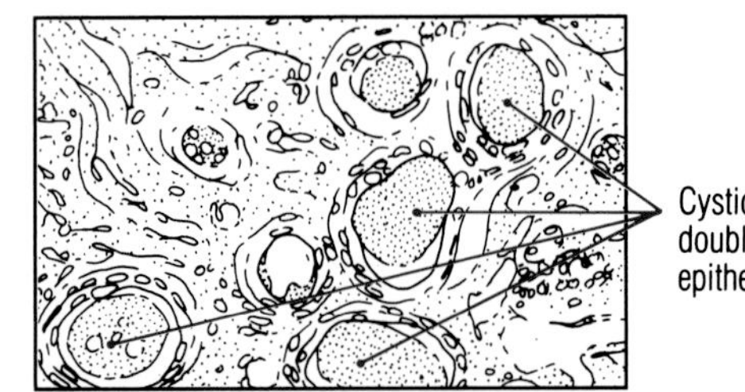

OTHER EYELID TUMORS

Metastatic tumors
Pigmented tumors
(see Chapter 17)
Mesenchymal tumors
(see Chapter 14)

FIGURE 6.39

LACRIMAL DRAINAGE SYSTEM

Congenital abnormalities
Atresia of nasolacrimal duct
Atresia of punctum
Fistula of lacrimal sac

Inflammation

Tumors
Epithelial
- Papillomas: squamous, transitional, or adenoma
- Carcinoma: squamous, transitional, or adenoma

Melanotic (see Chapter 17)
Mesenchymal (see Chapter 14)

FIGURE 6.40

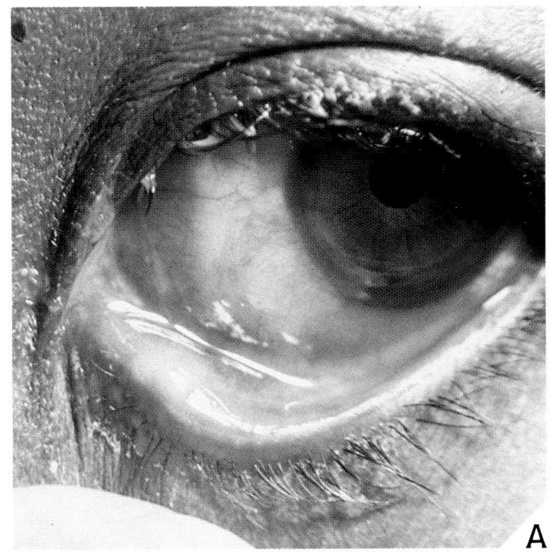

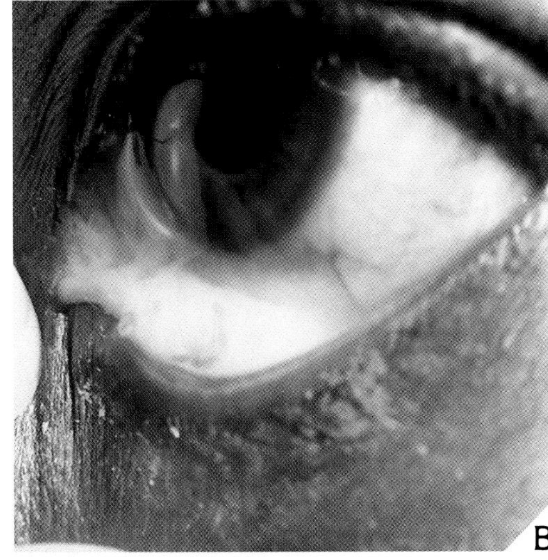

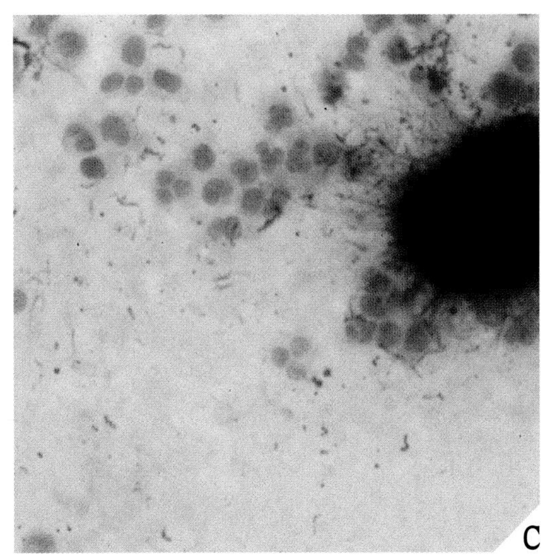

Figure 6.41 Dacryocystitis. A, B The patient had a history of tearing and a lump in the region of the lacrimal sac. Pressure over the lacrimal sac shows increasing amounts of pus coming through the punctum. **C** Another patient had an acute canaliculitis. A smear of the lacrimal cast obtained at biopsy shows large colonies of delicate, branching, intertwined filaments characteristic of *Streptothrix* (*Actinomyces*).

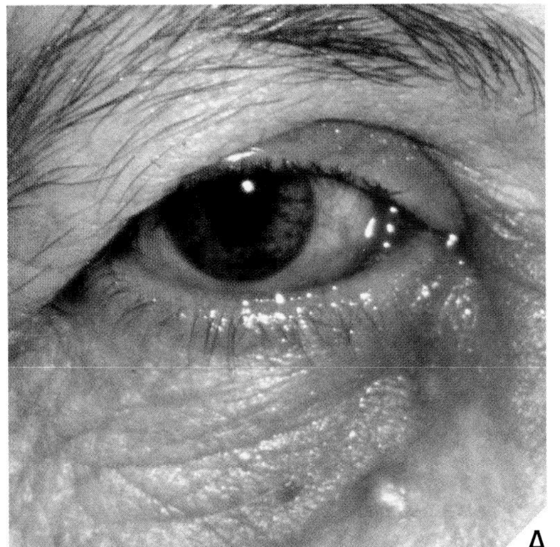

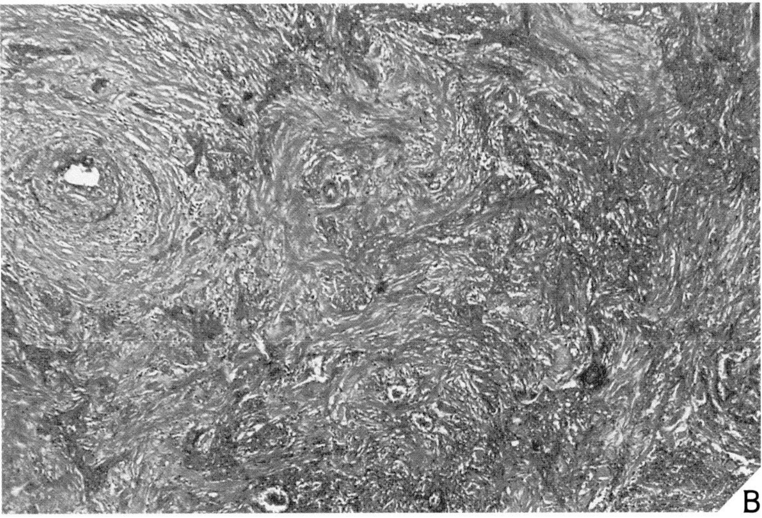

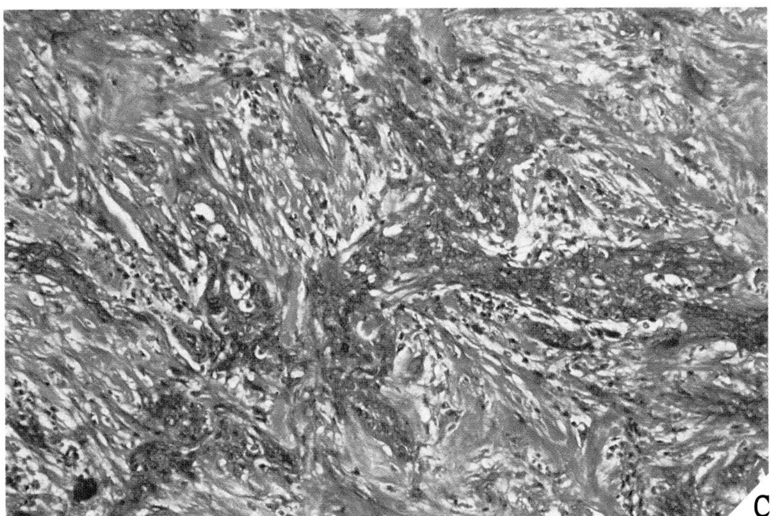

Figure 6.42 Squamous Cell Carcinoma of the Lacrimal Sac. **A** Clinical appearance of tumor in region of right lacrimal sac. **B** Strands and cords of cells are infiltrating the tissues surrounding the lacrimal sac. **C** Increased magnification shows the cells to be undifferentiated malignant squamous cells. (Case presented by Dr. AC Spalding at the Verhoeff Society, 1982.)

Bibliography

Alper MG, Zimmerman LE, LaPiana FG: Orbital manifestations of Erdheim-Chester disease. Trans Am Ophthalmol Soc 81;64, 1983.

Argenyi ZB, Balogh K, Goeken JA: Immunohistochemical characterization of chondroid syringomas. Am J Clin Pathol 90:662, 1988.

Arnold AC, Bullock JD, Foos RY: Metastatic eyelid carcinoma. Ophthalmology 92:114, 1985.

Bardenstein DS, et al: Cowden's Disease. Ophthalmology 95:1038, 1988.

Breuninger H, Black B, Rassner G: Microstaging of squamous cell carcinomas. Am J Clin Pathol 94:624, 1990.

Chu G, Chang E: Xeroderma pigmentosum group E cells lack a nuclear factor that binds to damaged DNA. Science 242:564, 1988.

Ferry AP: Pyogenic granulomas of the eye and ocular adnexa: a study of 100 cases. Trans Am Ophthalmol Soc 87:327, 1989.

Glass SG, Hoover RN: The emerging epidemic of melanoma and squamous cell skin cancer. JAMA 262:2097, 1989.

Grossniklaus HE, Knight SH: Eccrine acrospiradenoma (clear cell hidredenoma) of the eyelid. Immunohistochemical and ultrastructural features. Ophthalmology 98:347, 1991.

Hidyat A, Font RL: Trichilemmoma of eyelid and eyebrow. A clinicopathologic study of 31 cases. Arch Ophthalmol 98:844, 1980.

Jakobiec FA, et al: Unusual eyelid tumors with sebaceous differentiation in the Muir-Torre syndrome. Rapid clinical regrowth and frank squamous tranformation after biopsy. Ophthalmology 95:1543, 1988.

Kass LG, Hornblass A: Sebaceous carcinoma of the ocular adnexa. Surv Ophthalmol 33:477, 1989.

Kivelä T, Tarkkanen A: The Merkel cell and associated neoplasms in the eyelids and periocular region. Surv Opthalmol 35:171, 1990.

Middelkamp JN, Munger BL: Ultrastructure and histogenesis of Molluscum contagiosum. J Pediatr 64:888, 1964.

Perlman GS, Hornblass A: Basal cell carcinoma of the eyelids: a review of patients treated by surgical excision. Ophthal Surg 7:23, 1976.

Rodgers IR, et al: Papillary oncocytoma of the eyelid. A previously undescribed tumor of apocrine gland origin. Ophthalmology 95:1071, 1988.

Ryan SJ, Font RL: Primary epithelial neoplasms of the lacrimal sac. Am J Ophthalmology 76:73, 1973.

Searle SS, et al: Malignant Merkel cell neoplasm of the eyelid. Arch Ophthalmol 102:907, 1984.

Schweitzer JG, Yanoff M: Inverted follicular keratosis. A report of two recurrent cases. Ophthalmology 94:1465, 1987.

Spielvogel RL, Austin C, Ackerman AB: Inverted follicular keratosis is not a specific keratosis but a verruca vulgaris (or seborrheic keratosis) with squamous eddies. Am J Dermatopathol 5:427, 1983.

Stern RS, Boudreaux C, Arndt KA: Diagnostic accuracy and appropriateness of care for seborrheic keratoses. A pilot study of an approach to quality assurance for cutaneous surgery. JAMA 265:74, 1991.

Conjunctiva

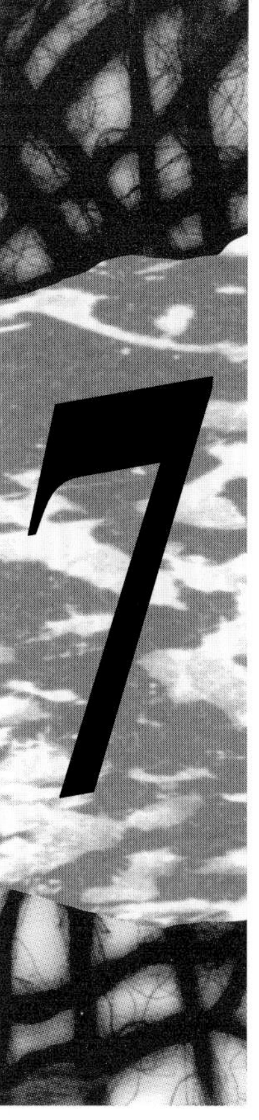

The conjunctiva is a mucous membrane, similar to mucous membranes elsewhere in the body. Congenital anomalies and vascular disorders may involve the conjunctiva, but they are unusual and relatively unimportant from a pathological point of view. Inflammation of the conjunctiva is one of the most common entities that brings patients to the ophthalmologist. The basic principles of the pathology of inflammation have been covered in Chapters 3 and 4 on granulomatous and nongranulomatous inflammation. One group of organisms, the chlamydias (and especially the organism that causes trachoma), is responsible for a significant proportion of human blindness and is illustrated here. Injuries are discussed in Chapter 5, on surgical and nonsurgical trauma.

Manifestations of systemic diseases may be seen in the conjunctiva. For example, metabolic products may be deposited, as in ochronosis. Vitamin A deficiency may cause xerosis or a Bitot spot. Numerous skin diseases also may involve the conjunctiva.

Degenerations, especially pinguecula and pterygium, are extremely common in the conjunctiva. Cysts, either congenital or acquired, also are commonly seen.

The epithelium of the conjunctiva may undergo both benign and malignant proliferations. Stromal neoplasms also may occur, but these are similar to those that occur in the orbit and are considered in Chapter 14. Pigmented lesions of the conjunctiva are discussed with other pigmented lesions in and about the eye in Chapter 17.

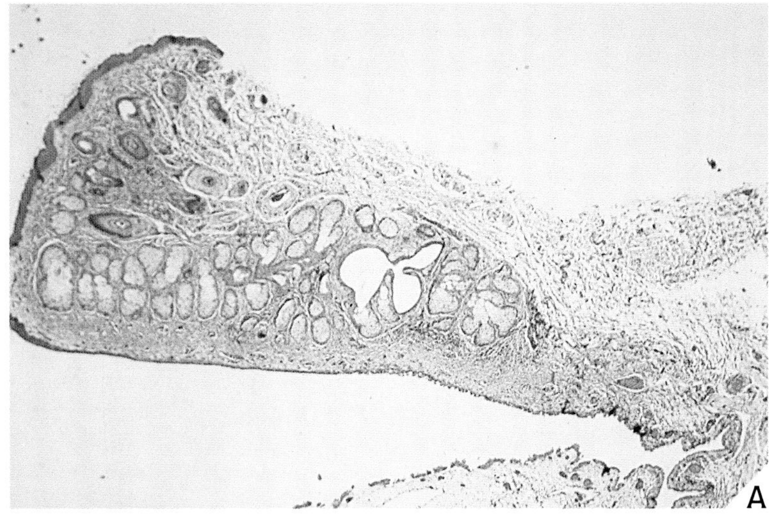

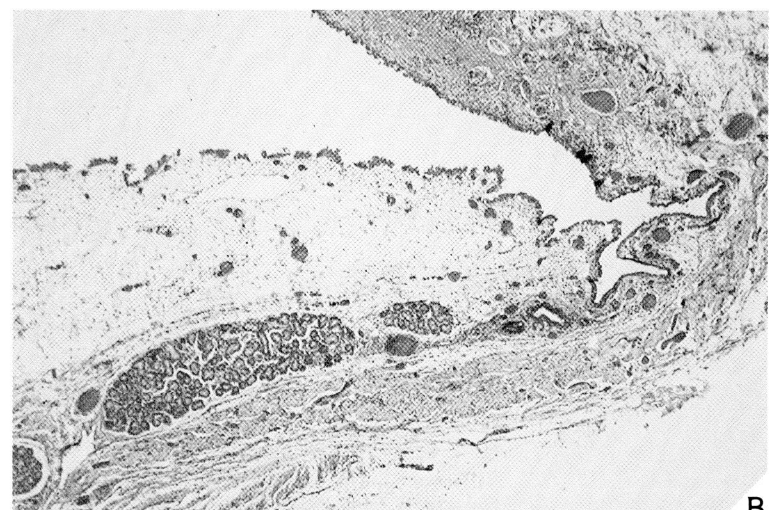

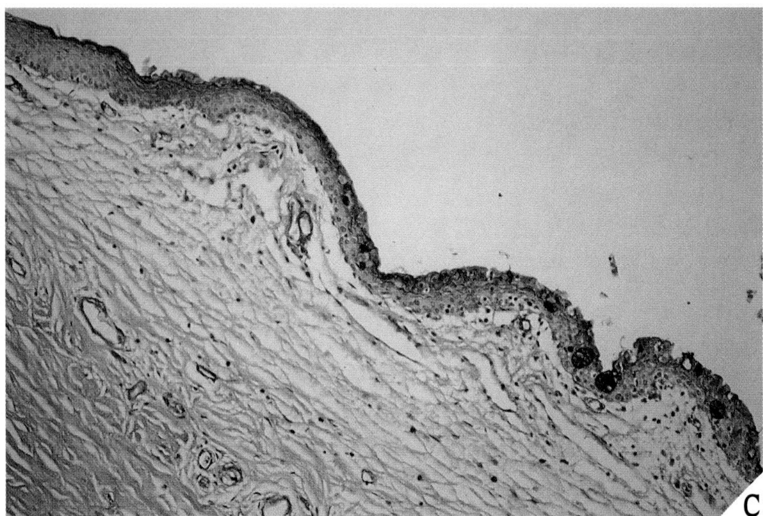

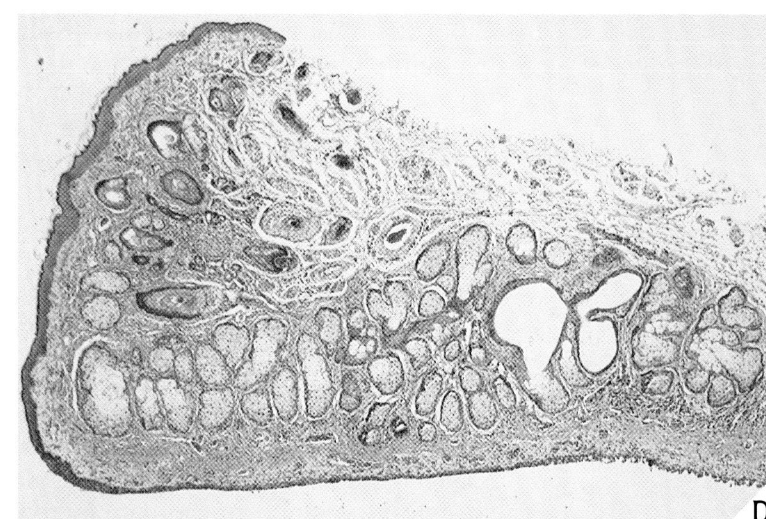

FIGURE 7.1 CONJUNCTIVA. A The normal conjunctiva, a mucous membrane composed of nonkeratinizing squamous epithelium intermixed with goblet cells, sits on a connective tissue substantia propria. It is divided into three zones: tarsal, forneceal-orbital, and bulbar. **B** Increased magnification shows the tight adherence of the substantia propria of the tarsal (palpebral) conjunctival epithelium to the underlying tarsal connective tissue and the loose adherence of the substantia propria of the bulbar conjunctival epithelium to the underlying tissue. **C** The goblet cells of the bulbar conjunctiva are seen easily with this PAS stain. **D** The tarsal conjunctiva becomes keratinized as it becomes continuous with the keratinized squamous epithelium of the skin on the intermarginal surface of the lid near its posterior border.

CONGENITAL ANOMALIES

Cryptophthalmos (ablepharon)
Epitarsus
Hereditary hemorrhagic telangiectasia (Rendu-Osler-Weber syndrome)
Congenital conjunctival lymphedema (Nonne-Milroy-Meige disease)
Dermoids, epidermoids, dermolipomas

FIGURE 7.2

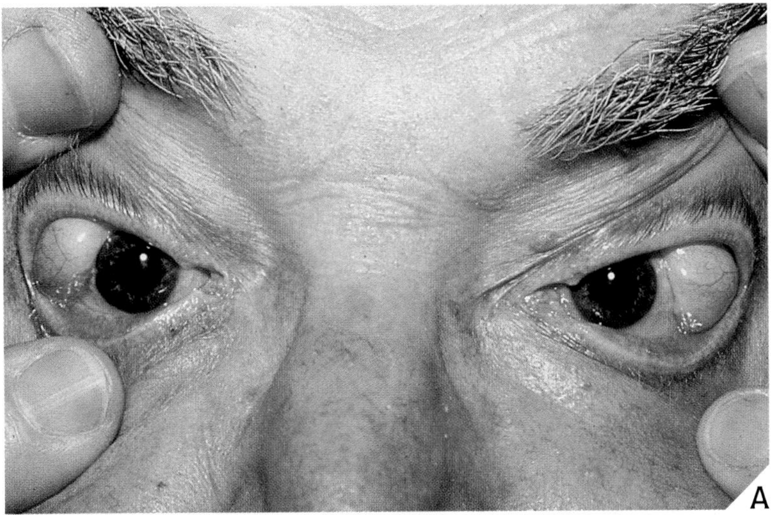

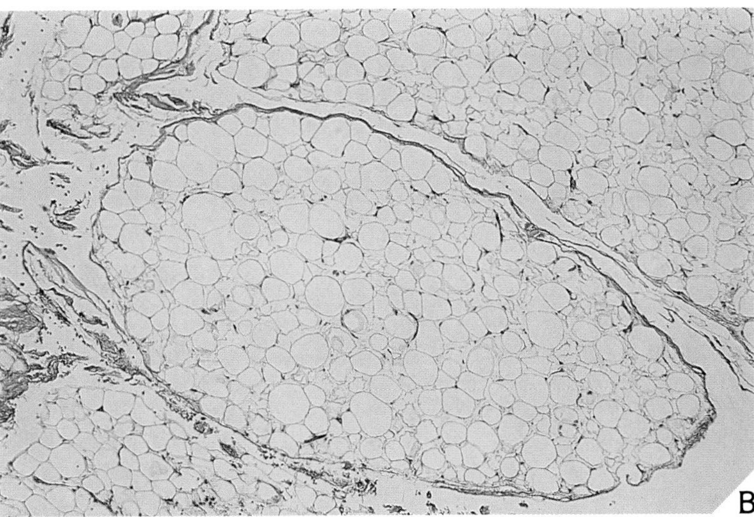

FIGURE 7.3 DERMOLIPOMA. A The patient shows the typical clinical appearance of bilateral, temporal dermolipomas. **B** The histologic specimen shows that the dermolipoma is composed almost completely of fatty tissue. Rarely, dermolipomas also may show structures such as epidermal appendages and fibrous tissue.

INFLAMMATION: CELLS OF CONJUNCTIVITIS

Predominant cells	Type of conjunctivitis
Polymorphonuclear leukocyte	Bacterial
Eosinophils and basophils	Allergic
Mononuclear cells (mainly lymphocytes)	Viral
Multinucleated giant cells	Herpes, rubella, tuberculosis

FIGURE 7.4

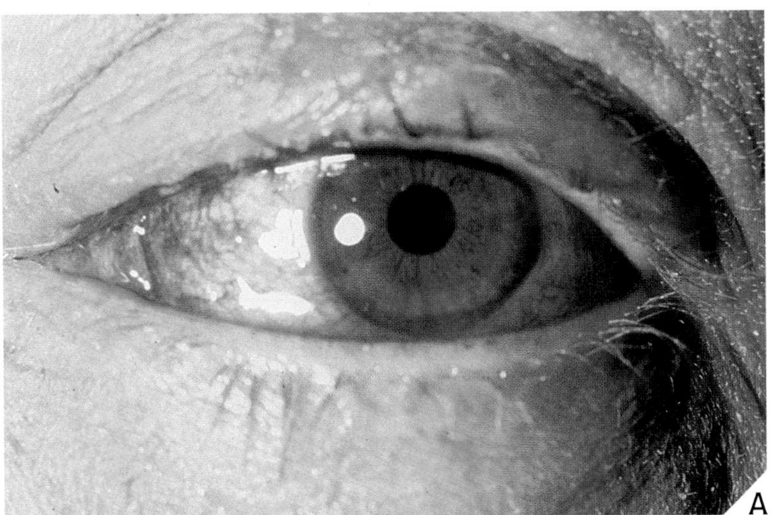

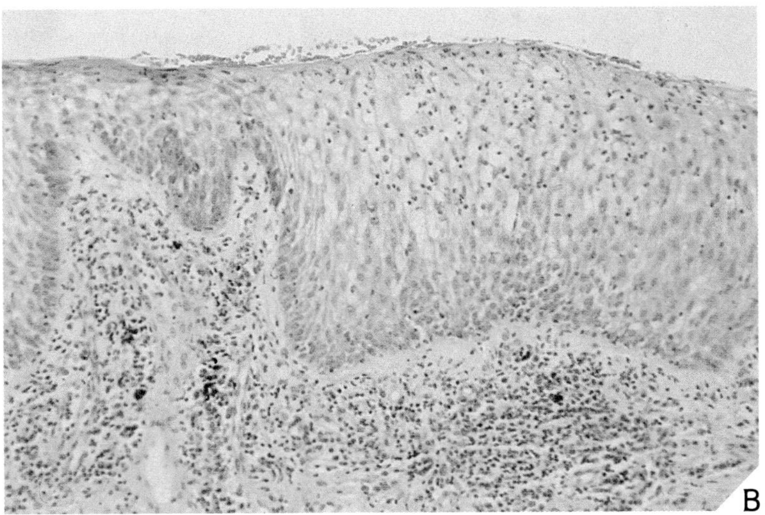

FIGURE 7.5 ACUTE CONJUNCTIVITIS. A Clinical appearance of a mucopurulent conjunctivitis of the left eye. The pupil reacted normally. The conjunctival infection was least at the limbus and increased peripherally. **B** The major inflammatory cell of acute bacterial conjunctivitis is the polymorphonuclear leukocyte, which here infiltrates the swollen edematous epithelium and the substantia propria.

INFLAMMATION: INFLAMMATORY MEMBRANES

True membrane

When removed, epithelium also is removed, leaving a bleeding surface

Seen in epidemic keratoconjunctivitis (EKC), *Corynebacterium diphtheriae,* Stevens-Johnson syndrome, *Pneumococcus,* ligneous conjunctivitis and *Staphylococcus aureus*

Pseudomembrane

When removed, epithelium is not disturbed

Seen in EKC, *Corynebacterium diphtheriae,* Stevens-Johnson syndrome, *Streptococcus hemolyticus,* pharyngoconjunctival fever, vernal conjunctivitis, ligneous conjunctivitis, and alkali burns

FIGURE 7.6

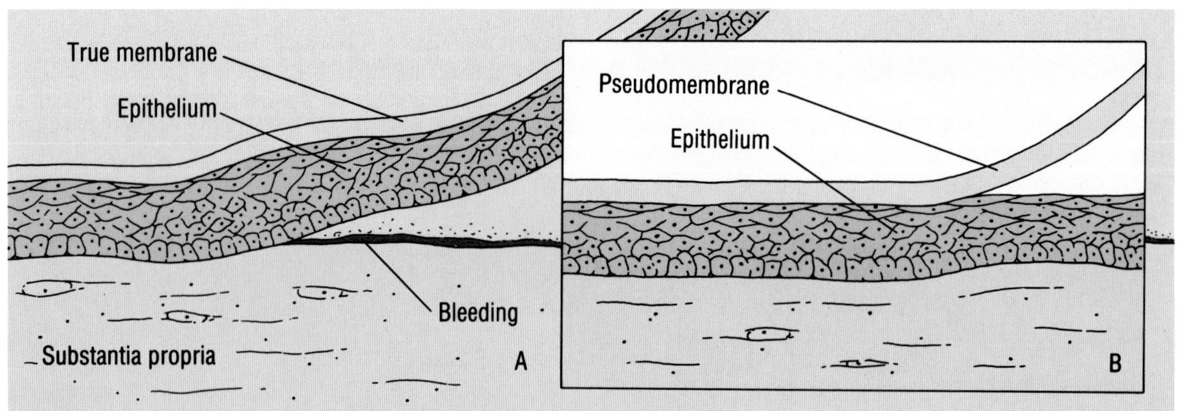

FIGURE 7.7 INFLAMMATORY MEMBRANES. A In a true membrane, when the membrane is stripped off the epithelium also is removed and a bleeding surface is left. **B** In a pseudomembrane, when the membrane is stripped off, it separates from the epithelium, leaving it intact and causing no surface bleeding.

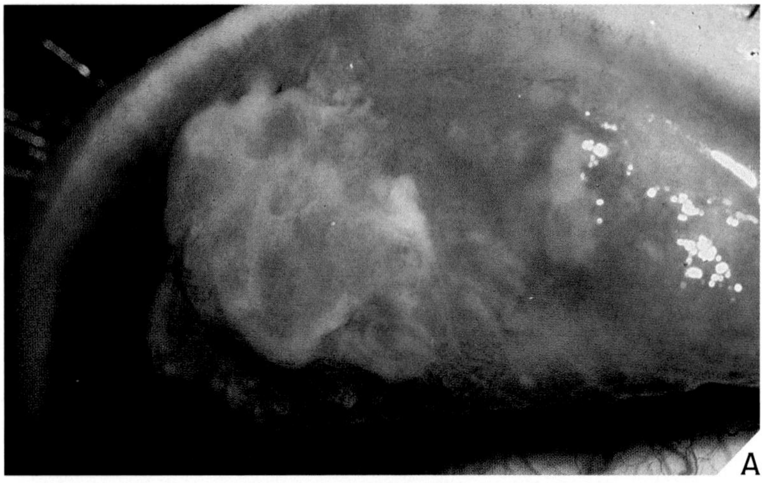

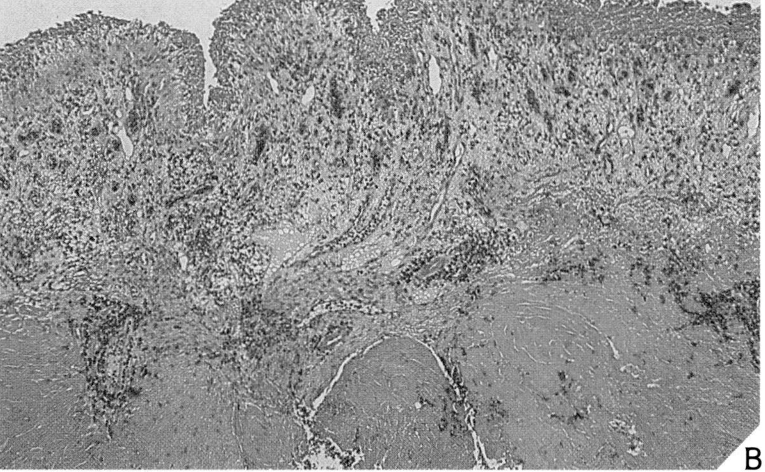

FIGURE 7.8 LIGNEOUS CONJUNCTIVITIS. A A thick membrane covers the upper palpebral conjunctiva. Ligneous conjunctivitis is a chronic bilateral recurrent membranous or pseudomembranous conjunctivitis of childhood of unknown cause. **B** Biopsy shows a thick amorphous material contiguous with an inflammatory membrane composed mostly of mononuclear inflammatory cells, mainly plasma cells and some lymphocytes. (Case presented by Dr. JS McGavic at the Verhoeff Society, 1986.)

INFLAMMATION: CHRONIC CONJUNCTIVITIS

Hyperplastic epithelium
Follicular hypertrophy
Papillary hypertrophy
Granuloma pyogenicum
Granulomatous inflammation

FIGURE 7.9

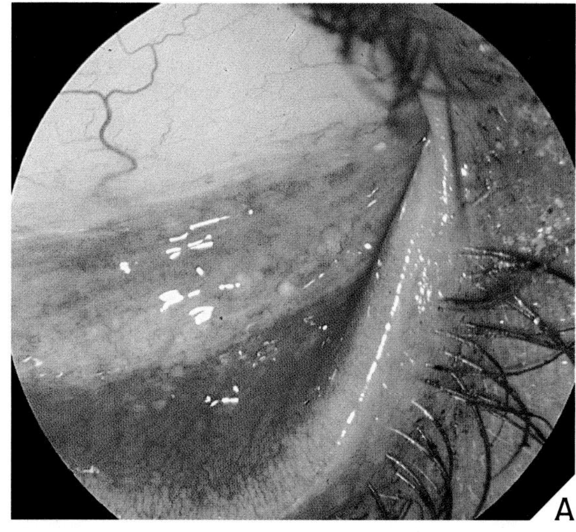

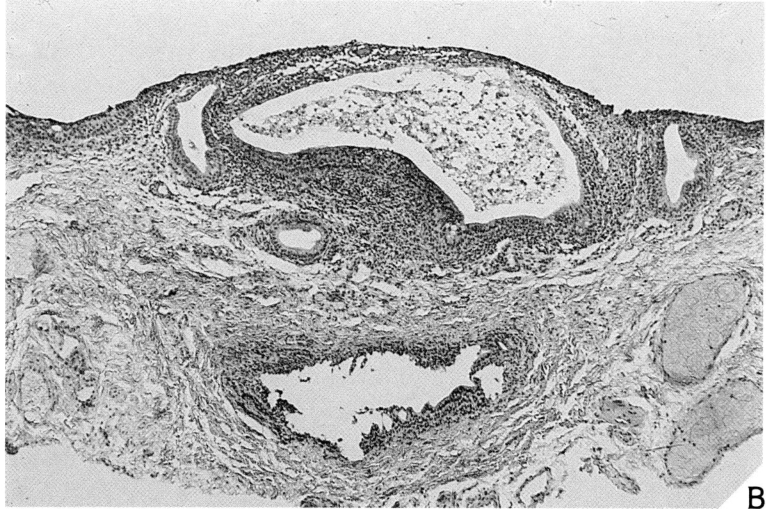

FIGURE 7.10 CHRONIC CONJUNCTIVITIS. A The conjunctiva is thickened and contains tiny yellow cysts. **B** Histologic section of the conjunctiva demonstrates the cyst lined by an epithelium that resembles ductal epithelium and that contains a pink granular material. A chronic non-granulomatous inflammation of lymphocytes and plasma cells surrounds the cyst, along with a proliferation of the epithelium of the palpebral conjunctiva, forming structures which resemble glands and are called pseudoglands (Henle).

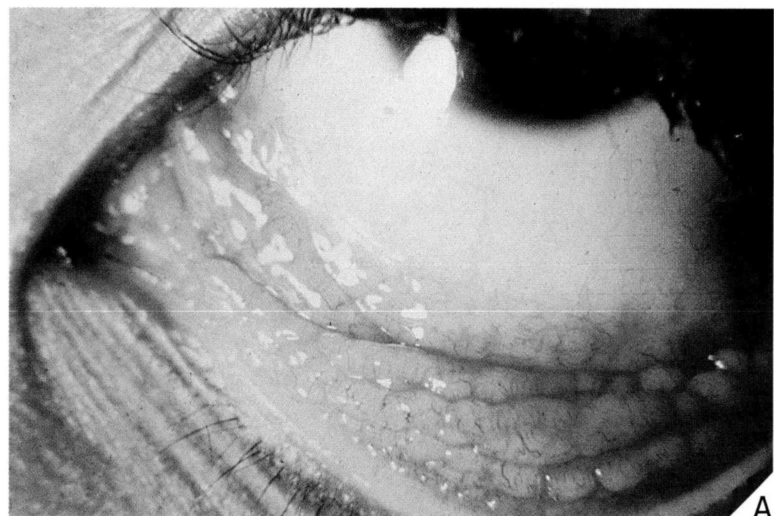

FIGURE 7.11 FOLLICULAR CONJUNCTIVITIS. A The surfaces of the follicles are pale, whereas their bases are red. **B** Histologic section of the conjunctiva shows a lymphoid follicle in the substantia propria.

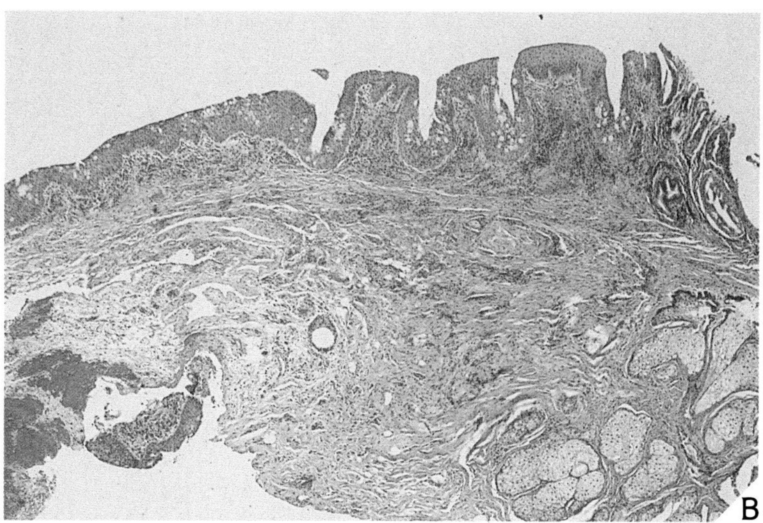

FIGURE 7.12 PAPILLARY CONJUNCTIVITIS. A The surfaces of the papillae are red because of numerous tiny vessels, whereas their bases are pale in color. The yellow staining is caused by fluorescein. **B** Histologic section of the conjunctiva demonstrates an inflammatory infiltrate in the substantia propria and numerous small vessels coursing through the papillae. The inflammatory cells are lymphocytes and plasma cells.

INFLAMMATION: SCARRING

Ocular pemphigoid
Secondary, e.g., to Stevens-Johnson syndrome or alkali burns

INFLAMMATION: SPECIFIC INFLAMMATION

Bacterial

Viral

Chlamydias
Trachoma
Inclusion conjunctivitis
Lymphogranuloma venereum
Ornithosis (psittacosis)

Fungal

Parasitic

Rickettsial

Parinaud oculoglandular syndrome

Chemical injuries

Vernal keratoconjunctivitis

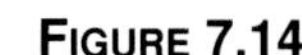

FIGURE 7.13

FIGURE 7.14

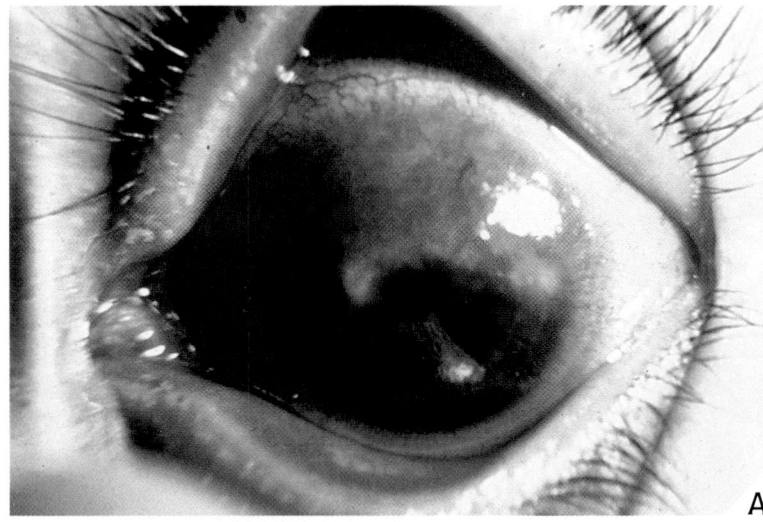

FIGURE 7.15 TRACHOMA. A The patient has a trachomatous pannus growing over the superior conjunctiva. With healing, the follicles disappear from the peripheral cornea, leaving areas filled with a thickened transparent epithelium called Herbert pits. The palpebral conjunctiva scars by the formation of a linear white horizontal line or scar near the upper border of the tarsus, called a von Arlt line. **B** A conjunctival smear from another case of trachoma shows a large cytoplasmic, basophilic initial body. Small cytoplasmic elementary bodies are seen in some of the other cells. **C** Small cytoplasmic elementary bodies are seen in numerous cells. (**A**, courtesy of Dr. AP Ferry.)

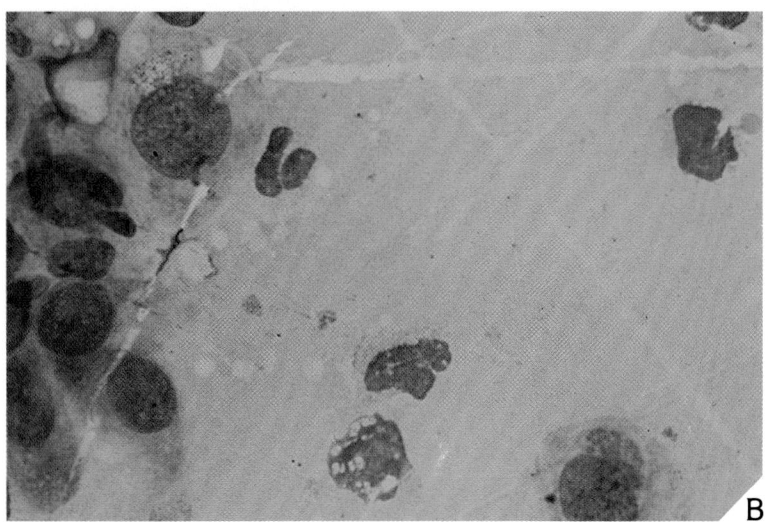

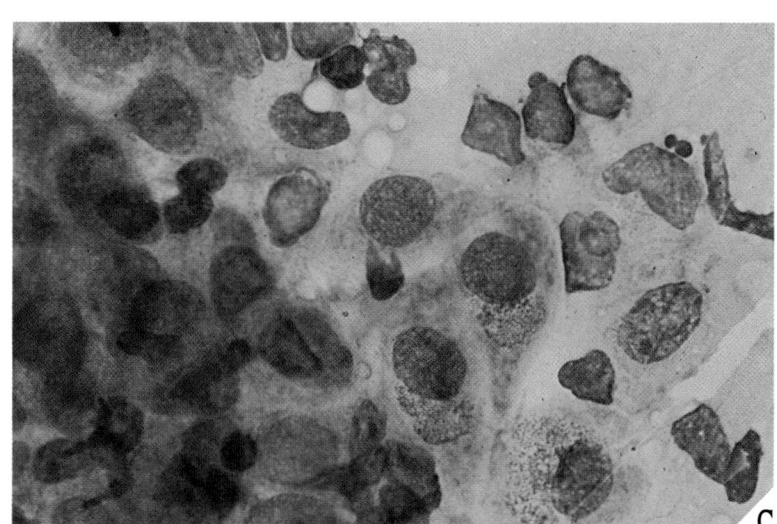

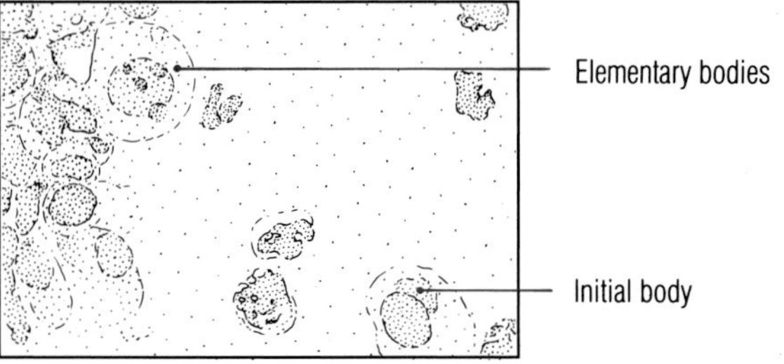

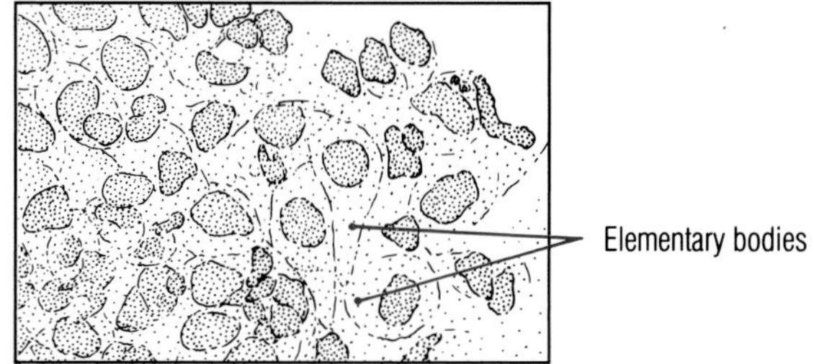

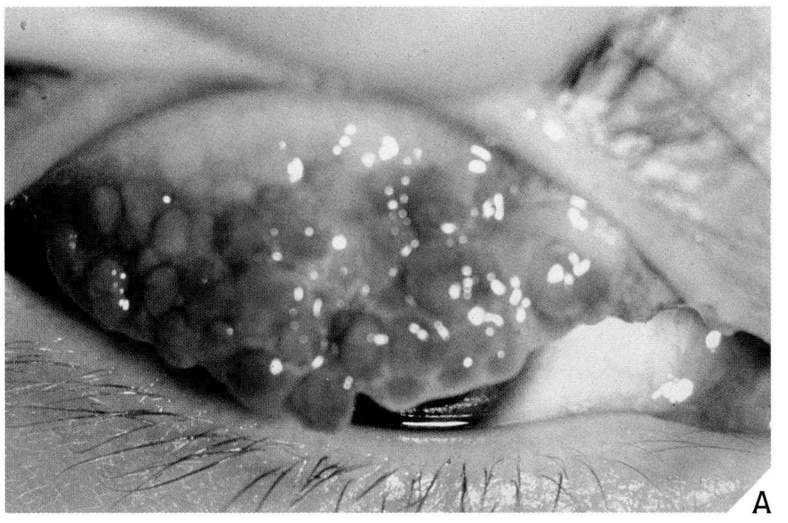

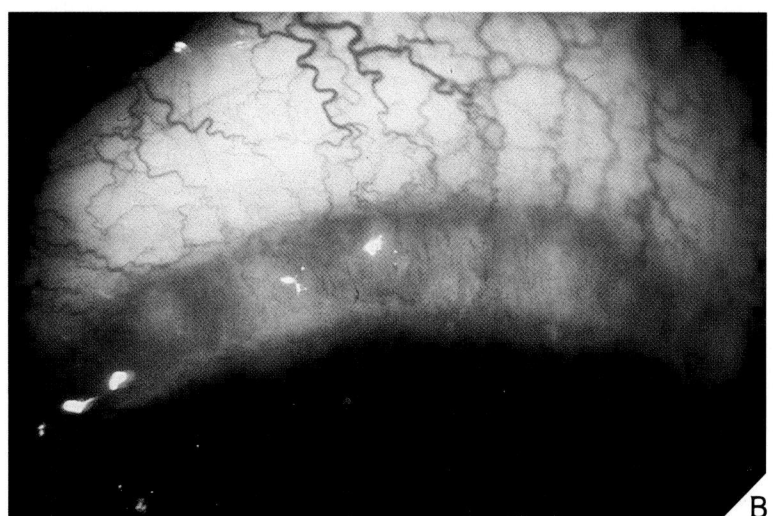

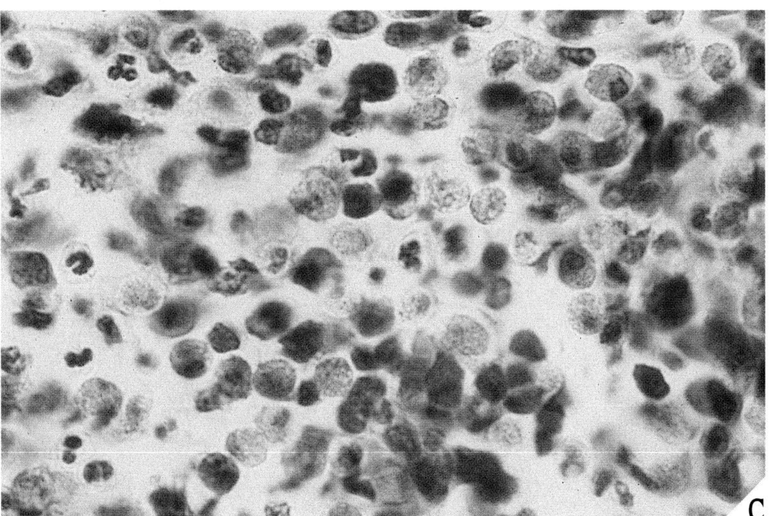

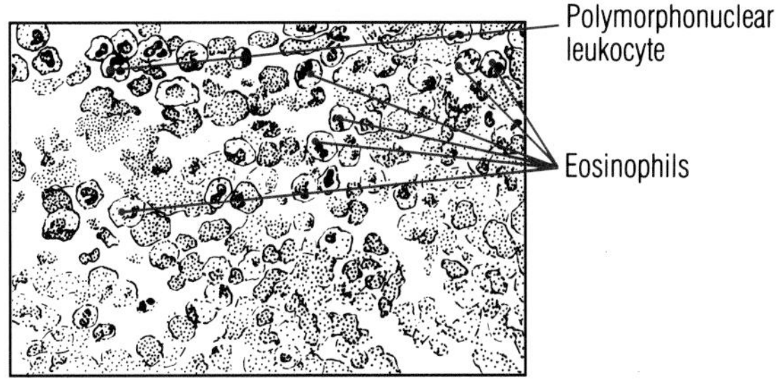

FIGURE 7.16 VERNAL CATARRH. A Clinical appearance of the papillary reaction of the palpebral conjunctiva. **B** Clinical appearance of the less commonly seen limbal reaction. **C** Histologic examination of a conjunctival smear shows the presence of many eosinophils. (**B**, **C**, courtesy of Dr. IM Raber.)

MANIFESTATIONS OF SYSTEMIC DISEASE: DEPOSITION OF METABOLIC PRODUCTS

Cystinosis	Lipoidoses
Ochronosis	Dysproteinemias
Hypercalcemia	Porphyria
Addison disease	Jaundice
Mucopolysaccharidoses	Degos disease

FIGURE 7.17

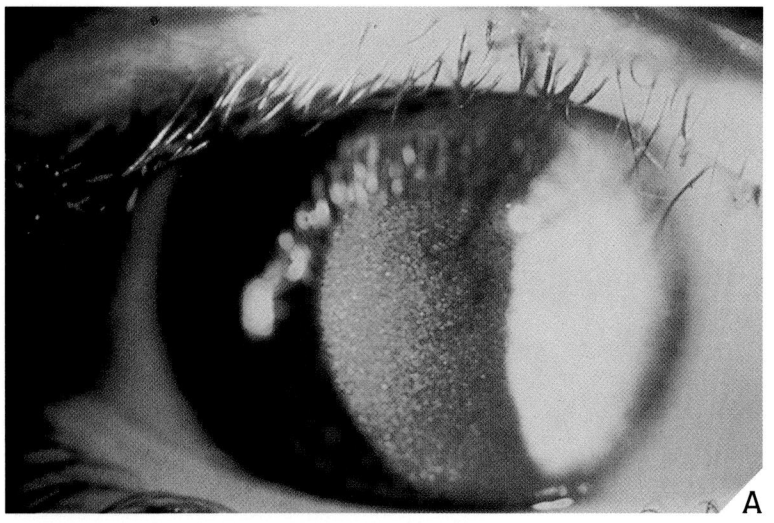

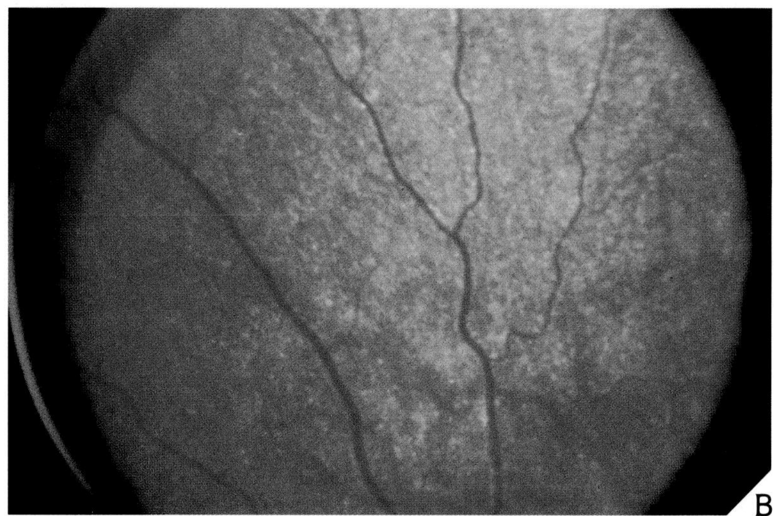

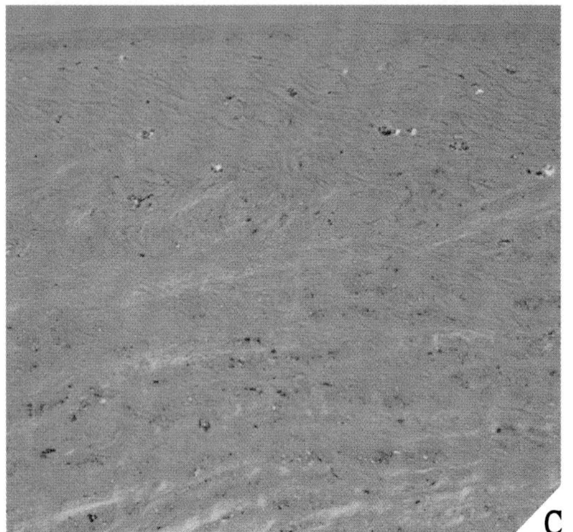

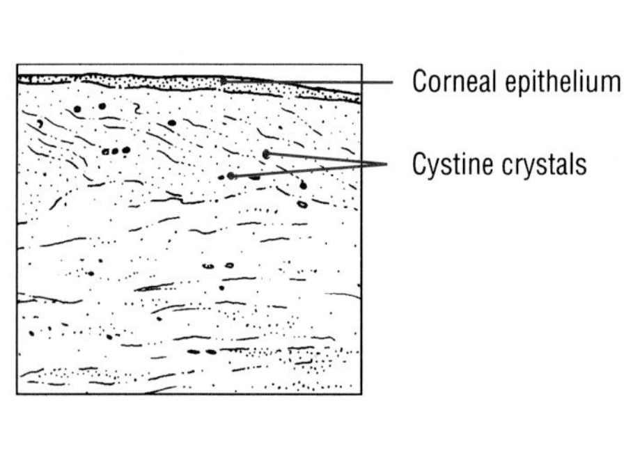

FIGURE 7.18 CYSTINOSIS. A Clinical appearance of cystine crystals in the cornea. **B** Deposition of cystine in the retinal pigment epithelium and choroid gives the fundus a crystalloid appearance. **C** Polarization of an unstained histologic section of cornea shows the birefringent cystine crystals. (**A**, **B**, courtesy of Dr. DB Schaffer.)

MANIFESTATIONS OF SYSTEMIC DISEASE: DEPOSITION OF DRUG DERIVATIVES

Argyrosis	Epinephrine
Chlorpromazine	Mercury
Atabrine	Arsenicals

FIGURE 7.19

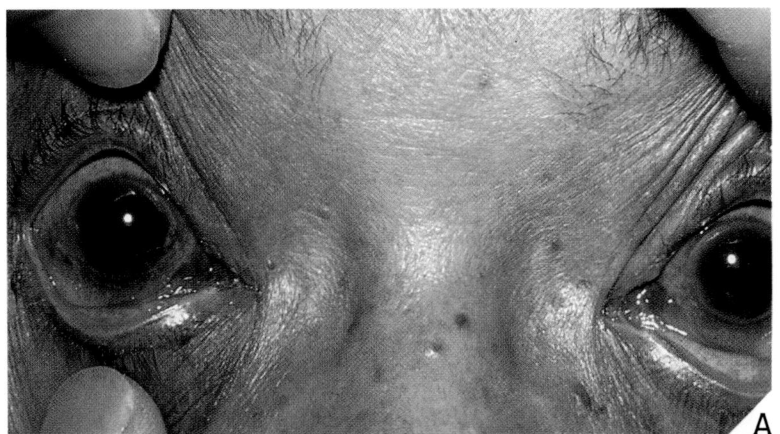

FIGURE 7.20 ARGYROSIS. A Patient had taken silver-containing drops for many years. Note the slate-gray appearance of conjunctiva. **B** The cornea shows a diffuse granular appearance. **C** The granular corneal appearance is caused by silver deposition in the Descemet membrane. **D** Histologic section of another case shows silver deposited in the epithelium and in the mucosal basement membrane of the lacrimal sac. (**D**, modified from Yanoff M, Scheie HG, 1964.)

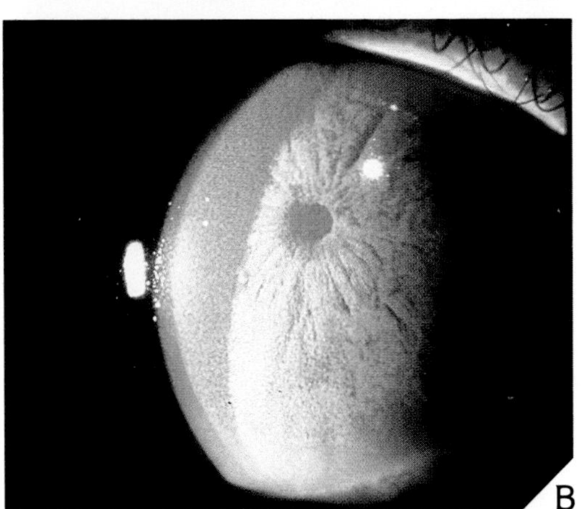

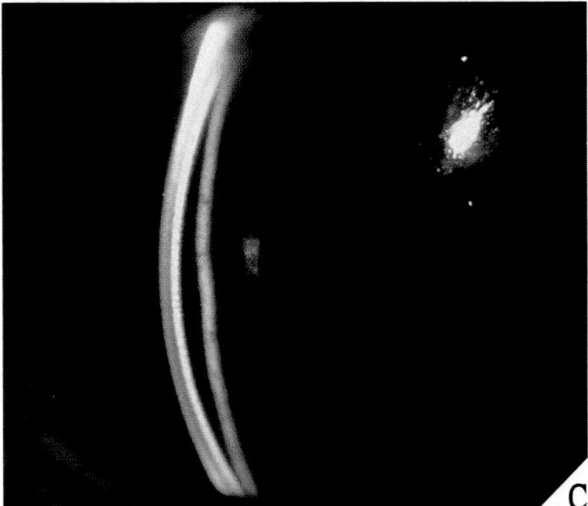

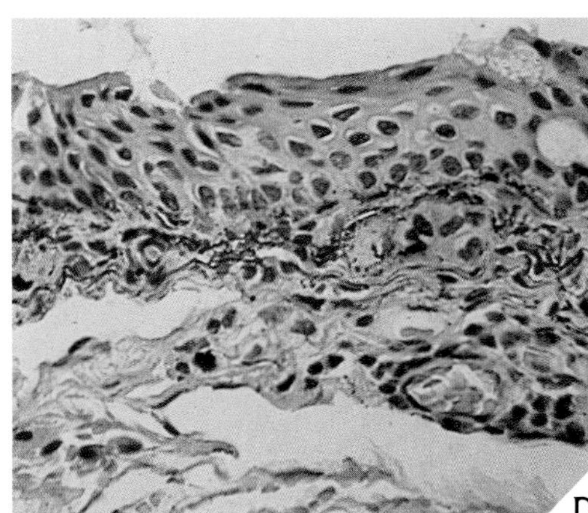

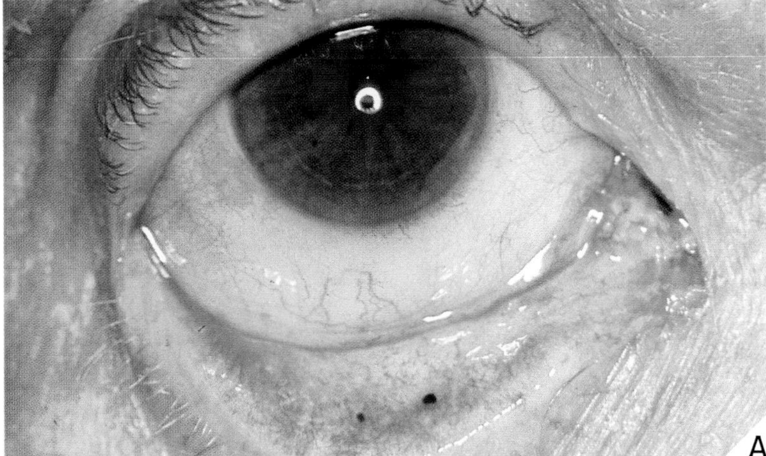

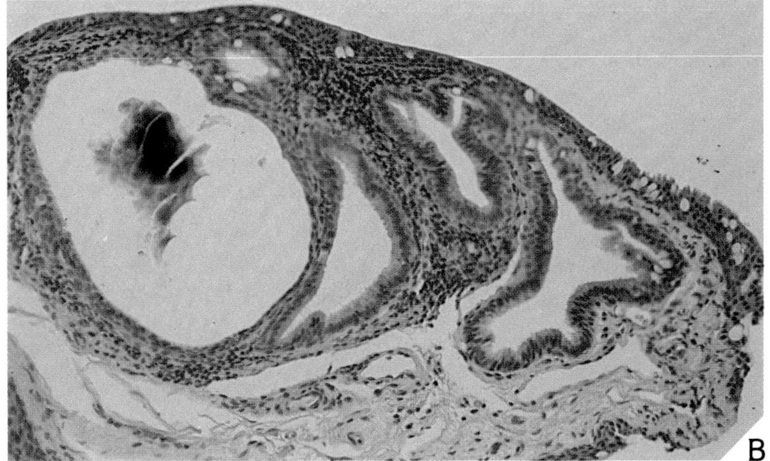

FIGURE 7.21 EPINEPHRINE DEPOSITION. A Black spots in palpebral conjunctiva represent the deposition of epinephrine after long-term use in the treatment of glaucoma. **B** Histologic section shows that the material within a cyst in the epithelium has properties similar to melanin. The stain here is a Fontana stain that characteristically turns melanin dark brown.

DEGENERATIONS

Xerosis
Pterygium (see Chapter 8)
Pinguecula
Lipid deposits
Amyloidosis

FIGURE 7.22

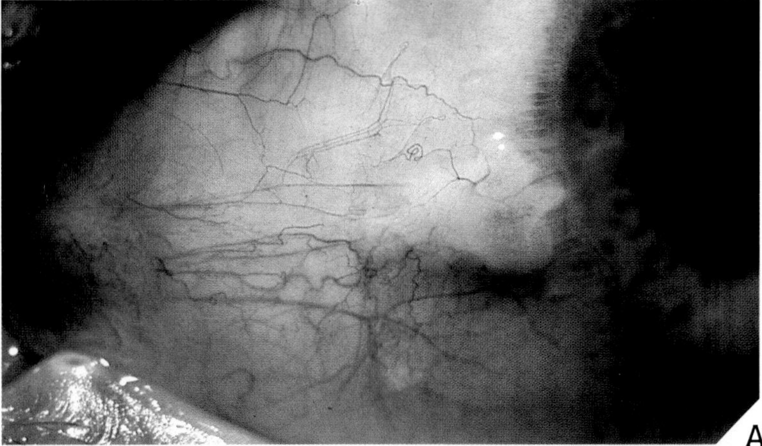

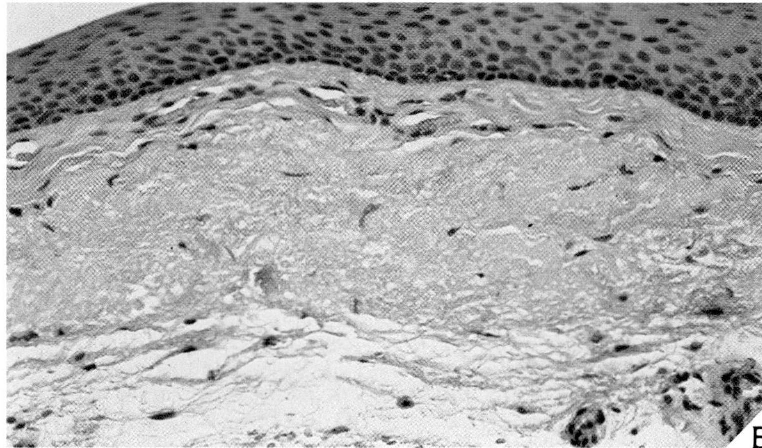

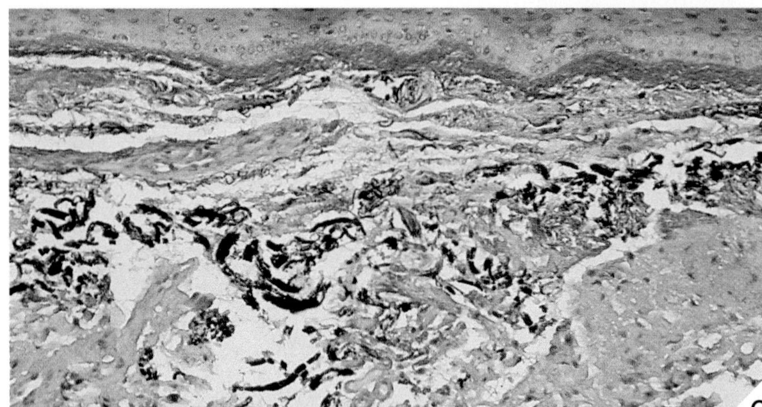

FIGURE 7.23 PINGUECULA. A A pinguecula characteristically involves the limbal conjunctiva, most frequently nasally, and appears as a yellowish-white mound of tissue. **B** Histologic section shows basophilic degeneration of the conjunctival substantia propria. **C** Another case shows even more marked basophilic degeneration that stains heavily black when the Verhoeff elastica stain is used.

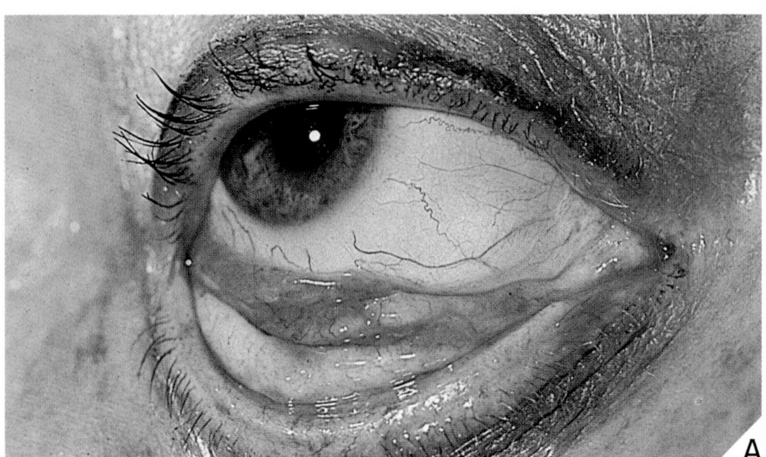

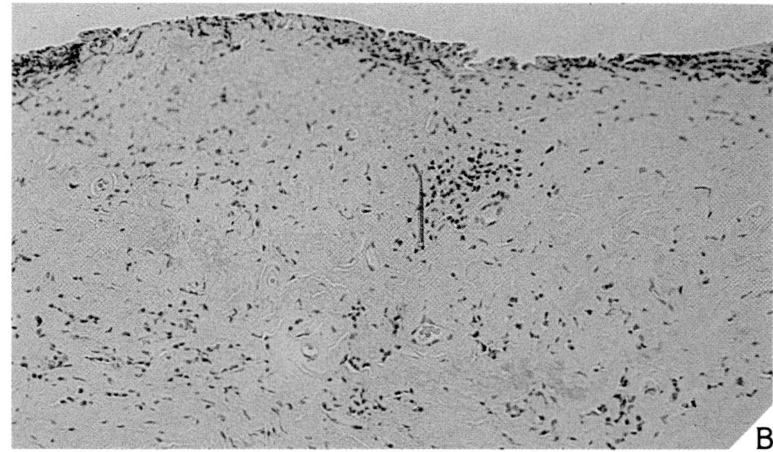

FIGURE 7.24 AMYLOIDOSIS. A The patient has a smooth "fish-flesh" redundant mass in the inferior conjunctiva of both eyes, present for many years. The underlying cause was unknown, and the patient had no systemic involvement. Clinically, this could be lymphoid hyperplasia, lymphoma, leukemia, or amyloidosis. The lesion was biopsied. **B** Histologic section shows an amorphous pale hyaline deposit in the substantia propria of the conjunctiva that stains positively with Congo red stain. The scant inflammatory cellular infiltrate consists mainly of lymphocytes, plasma cells, and mast cells. (**B**, Congo red; reported in Glass R, et al., 1971.)

TUMORS

Epithelial cysts
Epidermoid
Dermoid
Dermolipoma
Ductal
Inflammatory

Hamartomas
Lymphangioma
Hemangioma
Phakomatoses (see Chapter 2)

FIGURE 7.25

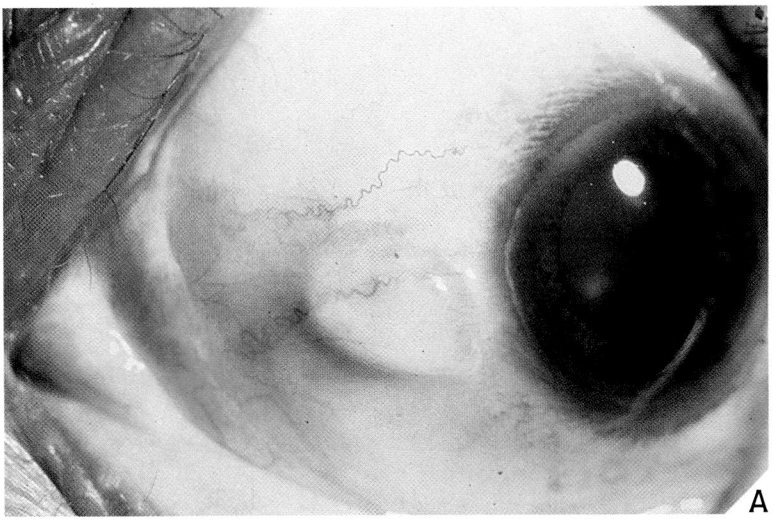

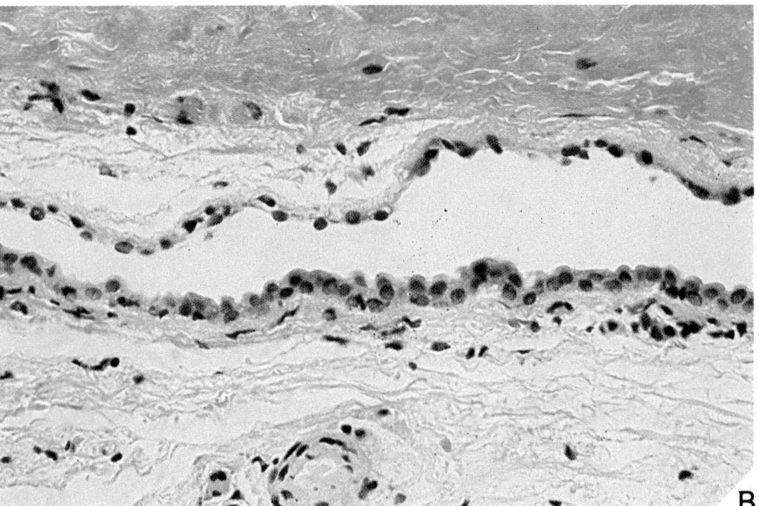

FIGURE 7.26 CONJUNCTIVAL CYST. A A clear cyst is present just nasal to the limbus. **B** Histologic section of another clear conjunctival cyst shows that it is lined by a double layer of epithelium, suggesting a ductal origin.

TUMORS (CONTINUED)

Pseudocancerous epithelial lesions
Hereditary benign intraepithelial dyskeratosis
Pseudoepitheliomatous hyperplasia
Papilloma
Eosinophilic cystadenoma (oncocytoma)

FIGURE 7.27

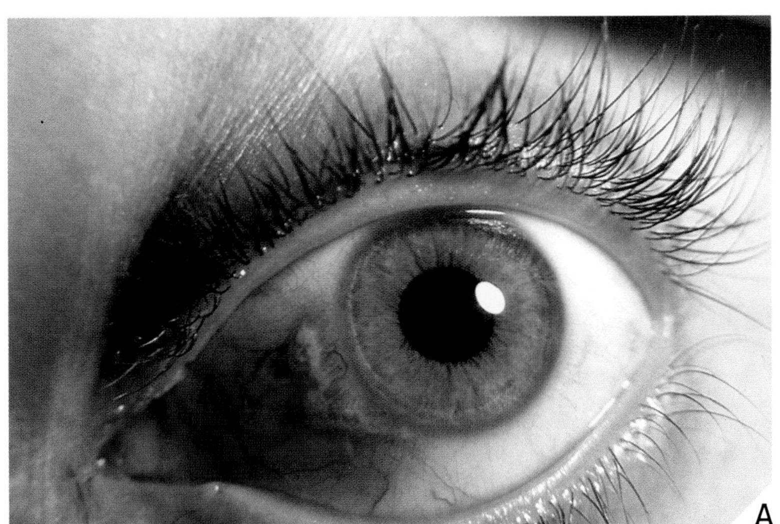

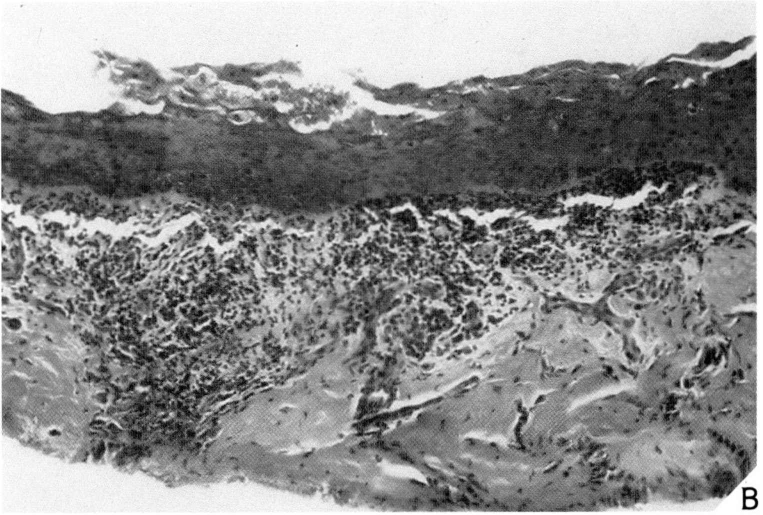

FIGURE 7.28 HEREDITARY BENIGN INTRAEPITHELIAL DYSKERATOSIS (HBID). A The patient has an obvious nasal vascularized pearly lesion in her left eye. The temporal limbal lesion is difficult to see because of the light. The right eye was similar, and the patient's mother also had the lesions. HBID is indigenous to family members of a large triracial (Indian, black, and white) isolate from Halifax County, North Carolina. **B** Histologic section shows an acanthotic epithelium that contains dyskeratotic cells. (**B**, reported in Yanoff M, 1968.)

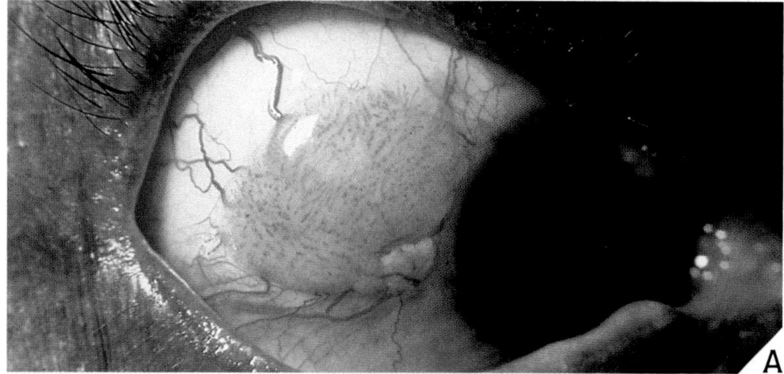

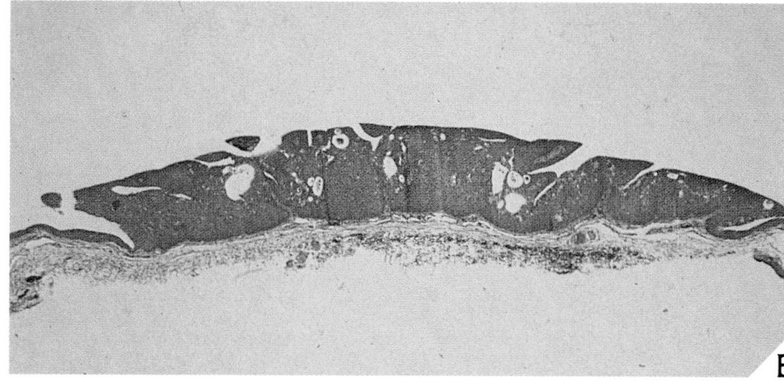

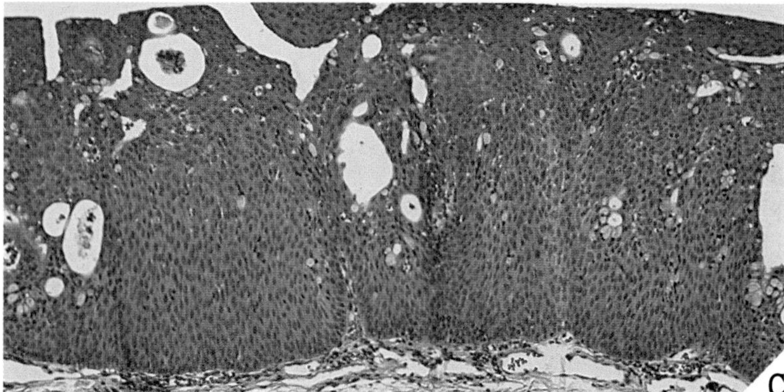

FIGURE 7.29 PAPILLOMA. A A large sessile papilloma of the limbal conjunctiva is present. **B** Histologic section shows a papillary lesion composed of acanthotic epithelium with many blood vessels going into the individual fronds, seen as red dots in the clinical picture in **A**. The base of the lesion is quite broad. **C** Increased magnification shows the blood vessels and the acanthotic epithelium. Although the epithelium is thickened, the polarity from basal cell to surface cell is normal and shows an appropriate transition. (**A**, courtesy of Dr. DM Kozart.)

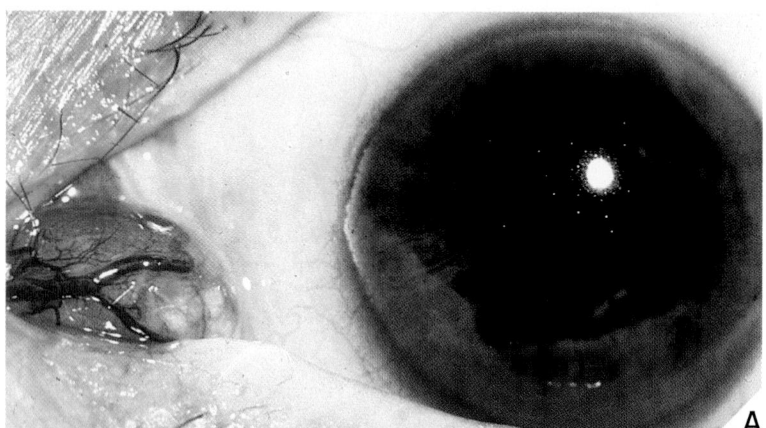

FIGURE 7.30 EOSINOPHILIC CYSTADENOMA (ONCOCYTOMA, OXYPHILIC CELL ADENOMA). A A fleshy vascularized lesion is present at the caruncle. **B** Histologic section shows proliferating epithelium around a cystic cavity. **C** Increased magnification shows large, eosinophilic cells which resemble apocrine cells and are forming gland-like spaces. (**A**, courtesy of Dr. HG Scheie.)

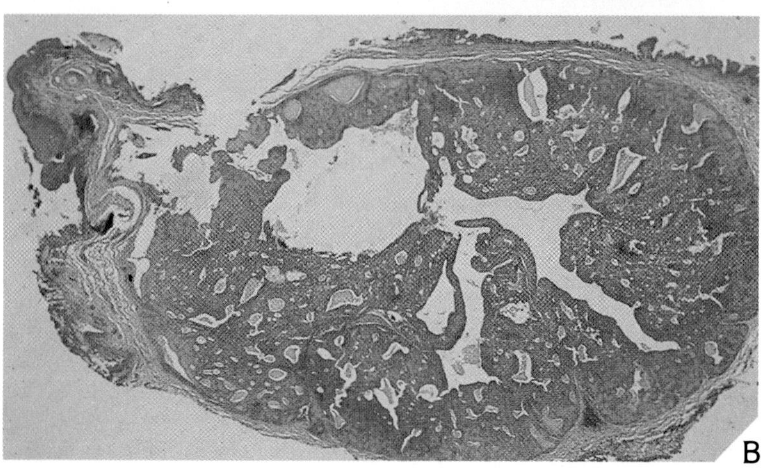

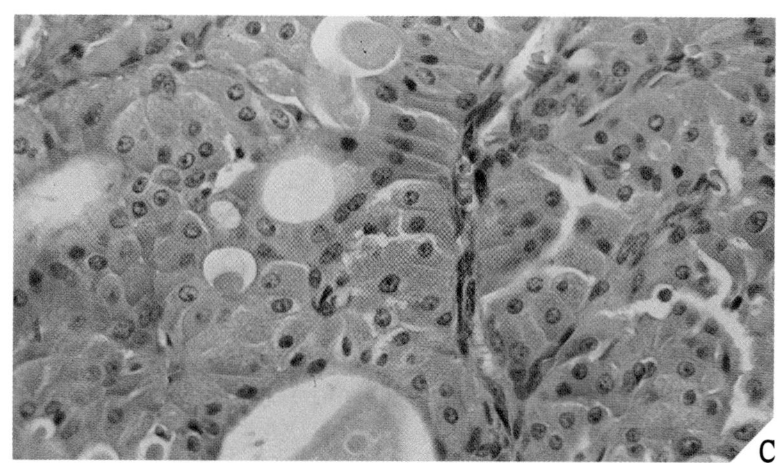

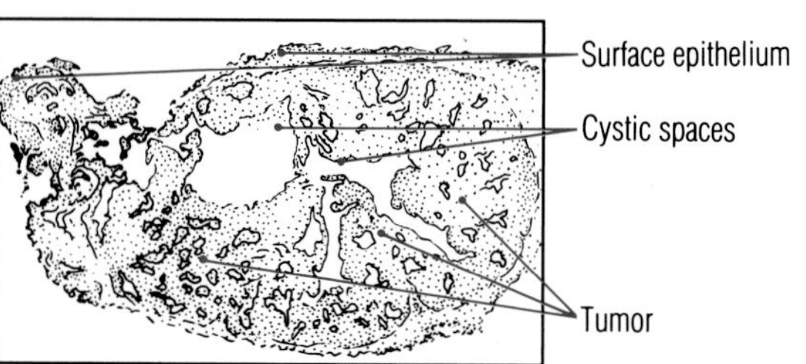

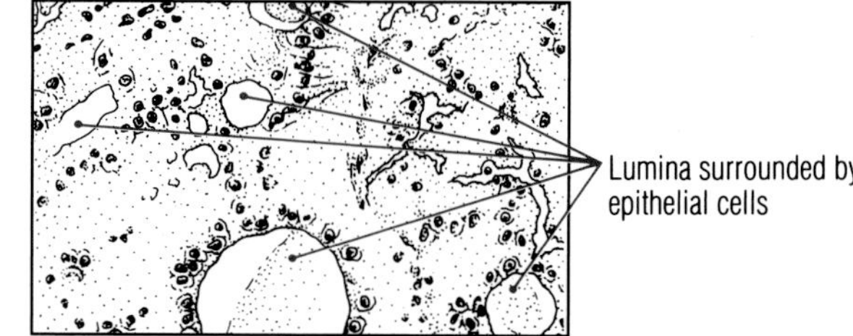

Precancerous epithelial lesions
Xeroderma pigmentosum
Actinic keratosis
Dysplasia

FIGURE 7.31

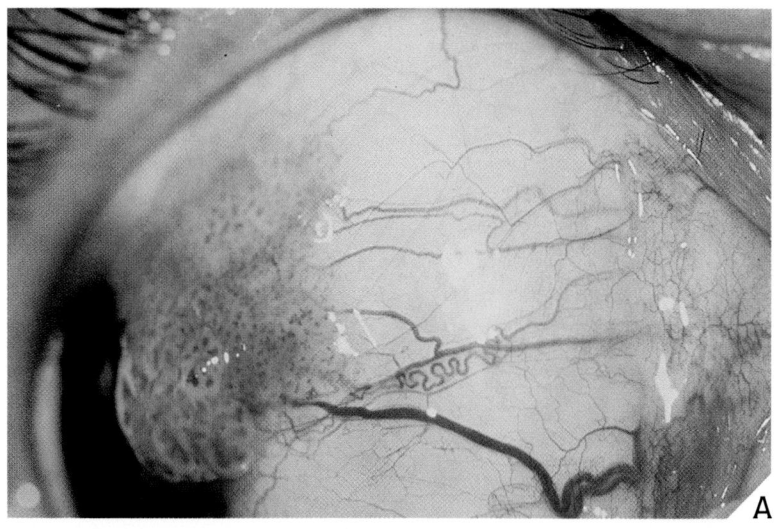

FIGURE 7.32 PAPILLOMA WITH DYSPLASIA. A Clinical appearance of a typical limbal sessile conjunctival papilloma. **B** Histologic section shows a sudden and abrupt transition from the normal conjunctival epithelium to a markedly thickened epithelium. The lesion is broad-based and shows numerous blood vessels penetrating into the thickened epithelium. **C** Increased magnification shows a tissue with normal polarity but which contains atypical cells and individual cells making keratin (dyskeratosis). Because the polarity is normal, a diagnosis of dysplasia was made. About 8% of conjunctival dysplasias or squamous cell carcinomas will contain the human papillomavirus.

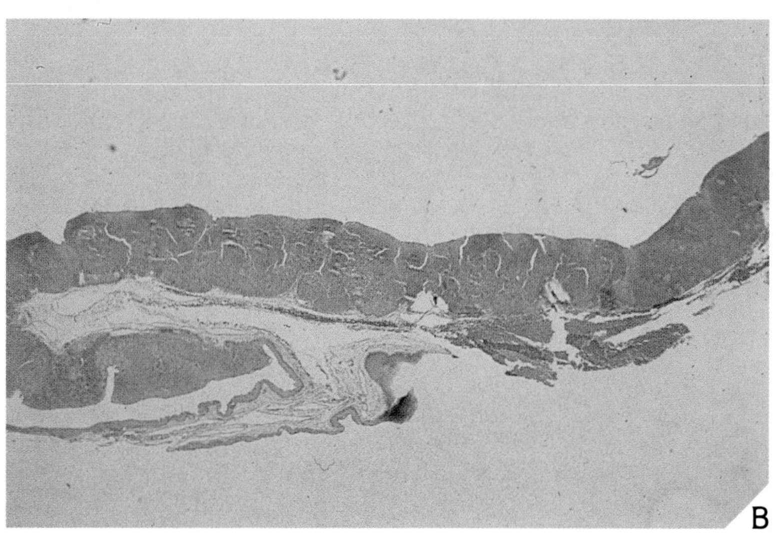

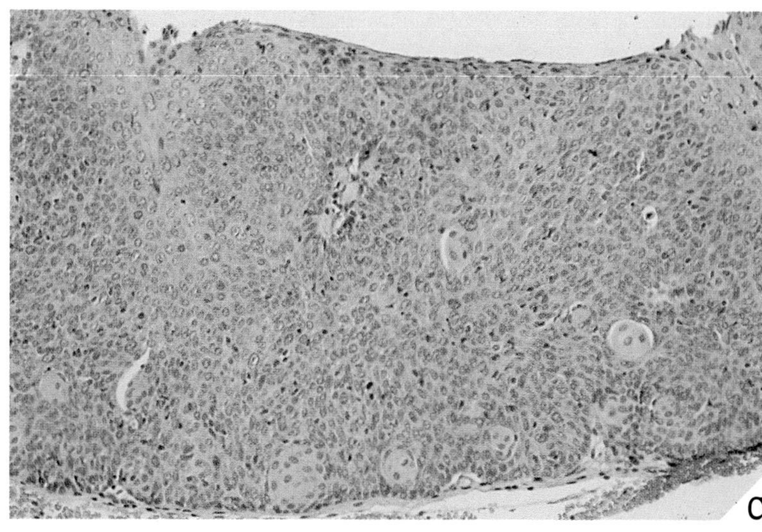

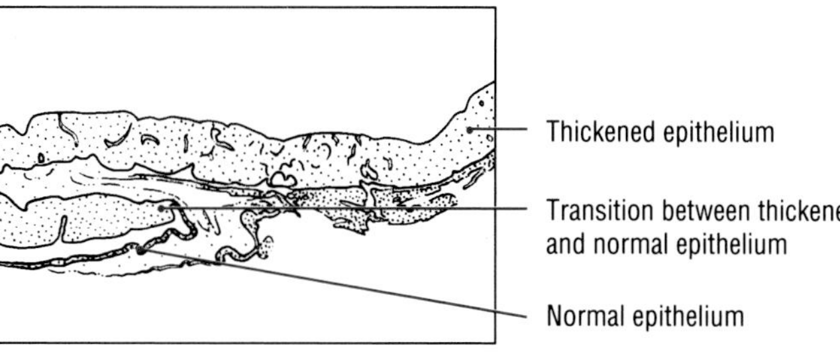

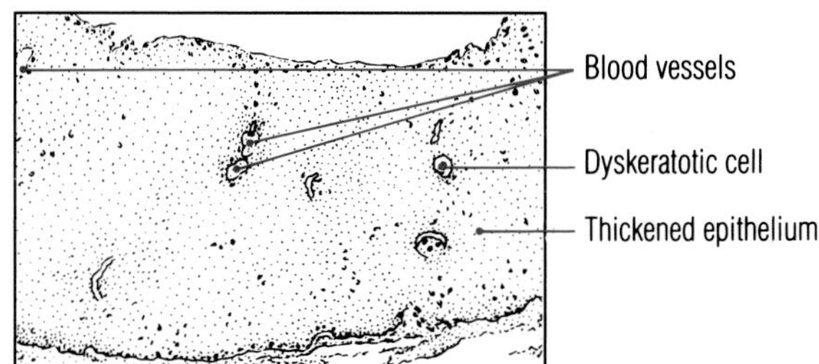

TUMORS (CONTINUED)

Cancerous epithelial lesions
Carcinoma *in situ*
Squamous cell carcinoma, invasive
Basal cell carcinoma (rare)
Carcinoma derived from mucus-secreting cells (rare)

FIGURE 7.33

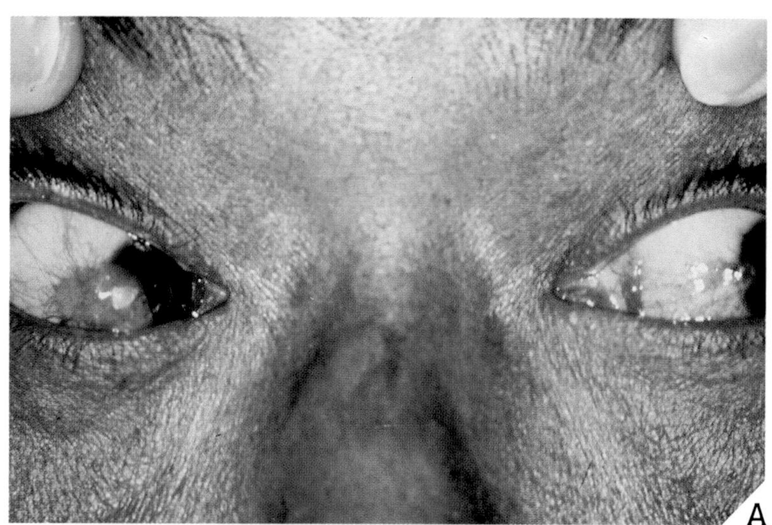

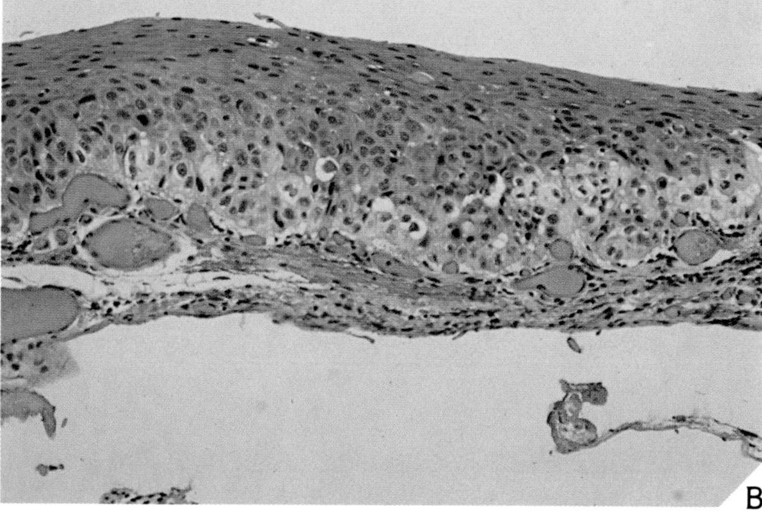

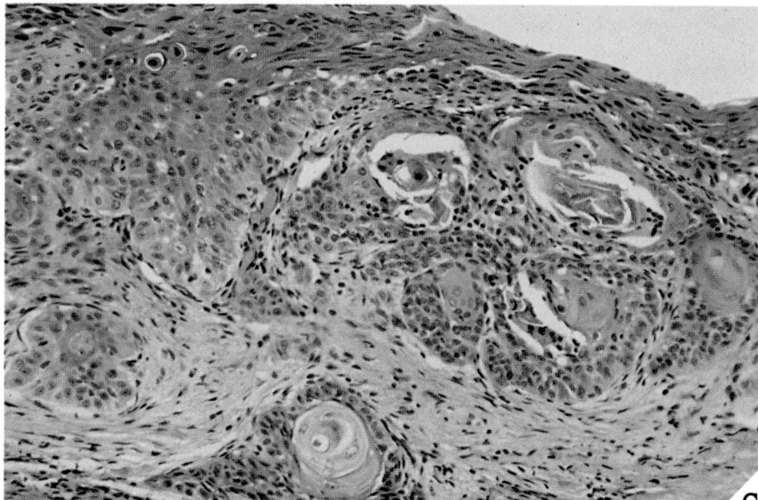

FIGURE 7.34 SQUAMOUS CELL CARCINOMA. A The patient had a vascularized, elevated, pearly lesion at the temporal limbus in the right eye. In addition, he had a pterygium nasally in the left eye. Excisional biopsy of the lesion in the right eye was diagnosed as carcinoma *in situ*. **B** Histologic section of another case shows full thickness atypia and loss of polarity. A diagnosis of carcinoma *in situ* would be made here. **C** Other regions of this case show malignant epithelial cells in the substantia propria of the conjunctiva, forming keratin pearls in some areas representing invasive squamous cell carcinoma.

TUMORS (CONTINUED)

Pigmented tumors (see Chapter 17)

Stromal neoplasms (see Chapter 14)
Angiomatous
Inflammatory pseudotumors, lymphomas, leukemias (see Fig. 9.18)
Juvenile xanthogranuloma (JXG)
Neural, fibrous, and muscle tumors
Metastatic

FIGURE 7.35

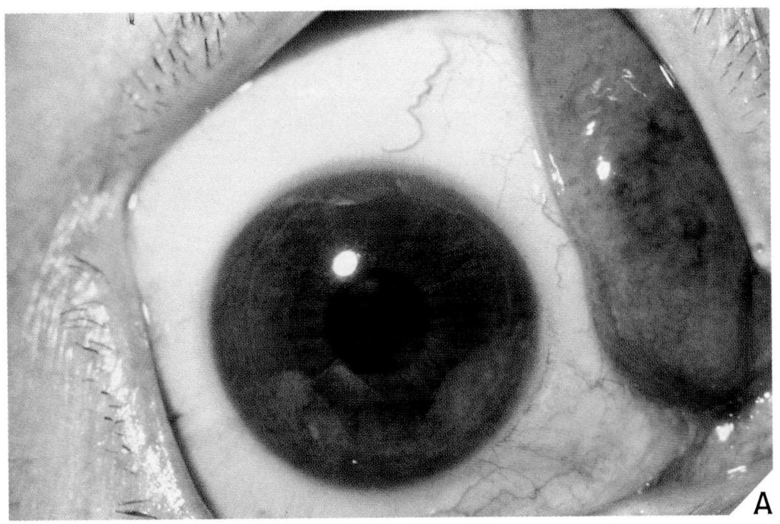

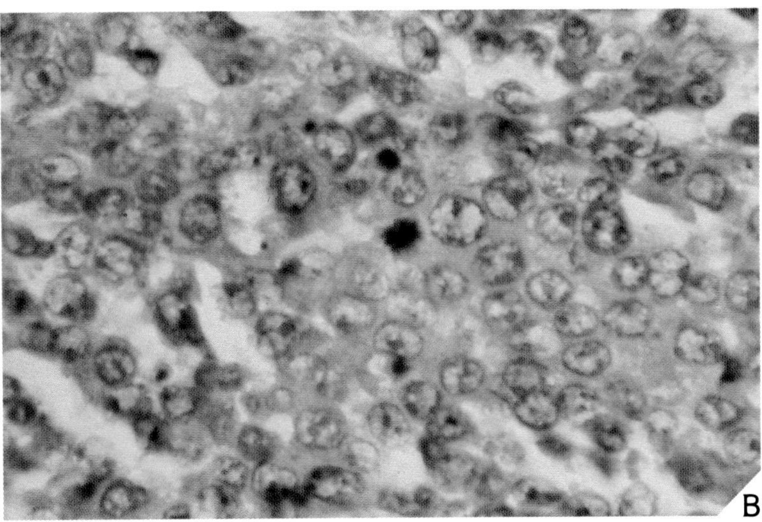

FIGURE 7.36 LEUKEMIA. A The patient has a smooth "fish-flesh" lesion that had appeared a few weeks previously. The lesion resembles that seen in lymphoid hyperplasia, lymphoma, or amyloidosis. A diagnosis of acute leukemia recently had been made. **B** Histologic section shows sheets of immature blastic leukemic cells, many of which exhibit mitotic figures.

Bibliography

Chang S-W, Hou P-K, Chen M-S: Conjunctival concretions. Polarized microscopic, histopathologic, and ultrastructural studies. Arch Ophthalmol 108:405, 1990.

Dark AJ, Streeten BW: Preinvasive carcinoma of the cornea and conjunctiva. Br J Ophthalmol 64:506, 1980.

Ferry AP: Pyogenic granulomas of the eye and ocular adnexa: a study of 100 cases. Trans Am Ophthalmol Soc 87:327, 1989.

Gertz MA, Kyle RA: Primary systemic amyloidosis—a diagnostic primer. Mayo Clin Proc 64:1505, 1989.

Glass R, Scheie HG, Yanoff M: Conjunctival amyloidosis arising from a plasmacytoma. Ann Ophthalmol 3:823, 1971.

Hanna C, Fraunfelder FT, Sanchez J: Ultrastructural study of argyrosis of the cornea and conjunctiva. Arch Ophthalmol 92:18, 1974.

Hogan MJ, Alvarado J: Pterygium and pinguecula: electron microscopic study. Arch Ophthalmol 78:174, 1967.

Huntington AC, Langloss JM, Hidayat AA: Spindle-cell carcinoma of the conjunctiva. An immunohistochemical and ultrastructural study of six cases. Ophthalmology 97:711, 1990.

Lamping KA, et al: Oxyphil cell adenomas. Three case reports. Arch Ophthalmol 102:263, 1984.

Marcus DM, et al: Ligneous conjunctivitis with ear involvement. Arch Ophthalmol 108:514, 1990.

Marsh WM, et al: Localized conjunctival amyloidosis associated with extranodal lymphoma. Ophthalmology 94:61, 1987.

McDonell JM, Mayr AJ, Martin WJ: DNA of human papillomavirus type 18 in dysplastic and malignant lesions of the conjunctiva and cornea. N Engl J Med 320:1442, 1989.

Reacher MH, et al: T cells and trachoma. Their role in cicatricial disease. Ophthalmology 98:334, 1991.

Rice BA, Foster CS: Immunopathology of cicatricial pemphigoid affecting the conjunctiva. Ophthalmology 97:1476, 1990.

Rodgers IR, et al: Papillary oncocytoma of the eyelid. A previously undescribed tumor of apocrine gland origin. Ophthalmology 95:1071, 1988.

Sandstrom I, Kallings I, Melen B: Neonatal chlamydial conjunctivitis. Acta Pediatr Scan 77:207, 1988.

Taylor HR, et al: The epidemiology of infection in trachoma. Invest Ophthalmol Vis Sci 30:1823, 1989.

Wexler SA, Wallow IHL: Squamous cell carcinoma of the conjunctiva presenting with extraocular extension. Arch Ophthalmol 103:1175, 1985.

Yanoff M: Hereditary benign intraepithelial dyskeratosis. Arch Ophthalmol 79:291, 1968.

Yanoff M, Scheie HG: Argyrosis of the conjunctiva and lacrimal sac. Arch Ophthalmol 72:57, 1964.

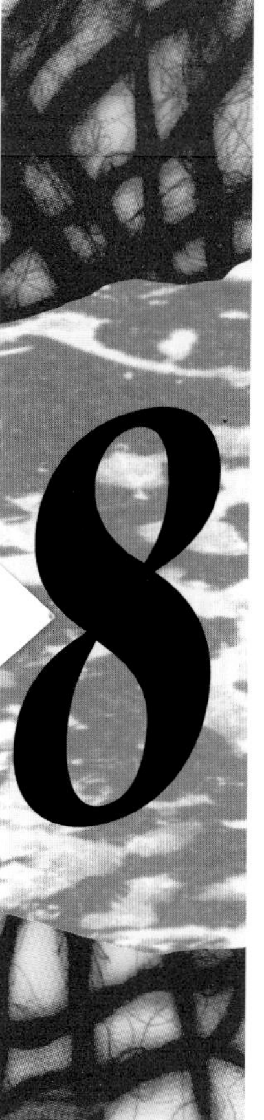

Co[illegible] a[illegible]

The norma[illegible] tinized epithel[illegible] layer of epithelial [illegible] tive layer and is attach[illegible] overlying wing cells by desm[illegible] also attached to its own secretory product, [illegible]what irregular thin basement membrane, by hemidesmosomes. The flattened, nucleated superficial epithelial cells desquamate into the overlying trilaminar (mucoprotein, water, lipid) tear film. Underlying the basal cell basement membrane is a thick acellular collagenous layer known as the Bowman membrane or layer. The bulk of the cornea, called the stroma, consists of collagen lamellae secreted by fibroblasts called keratocytes that lie between the lamellae. The stromal lamellae are arranged as a collapsed honeycomb, the anterior-most lamellae being the most oblique and the posterior-most being the least oblique (i.e., the most parallel) to one another. The posterior surface of the cornea is covered by a single layer of cuboidal cells, the endothelial cells. An unusually thick basement membrane, secreted by the endothelial cells and called the Descemet membrane, lies between the stroma and the endothelial cells.

The cornea is one of the most unusual structures in the body in that it has no blood vessels and is transparent. Any pathological lesions, therefore, are easily seen as an opacification within the cornea. Numerous congenital abnormalities may involve the cornea. The defects range from complete absence of the cornea, to irregularities in the size or shape of the cornea, to congenital opacifications. Opacifications of the cornea may be present as isolated findings (e.g., as a corneal keloid), or may be associated with systemic abnormalities (e.g., in cystinosis). In addition, corneal abnormalities may be associated with other ocular anomalies, especially those of the iris, lens, and anterior chamber angle (e.g., in Peters anomaly and in Rieger syndrome).

Inflammations commonly involve the cornea, and can be broadly divided into two major types: nonulcerative and ulcerative. Both types may be caused by infectious or noninfectious agents. Inflammations generally affect the central cornea or the peripheral cornea. Following inflammation, numerous sequelae may occur that can result in decreased vision.

Degenerations, i.e., lesions that are secondary to previous disease, often involve the cornea. The degenerations may primarily affect the epithelium, as in recurrent erosion, or the stroma, as in arcus senilis.

Dystrophies are primary, usually inherited, bilateral disorders that have approximately equal involvement affecting both corneas. The dystrophy may affect the epithelium, as in Meesmann dystrophy or the Bowman membrane, as in Reis-

Bückler dystrophy. Alternatively, the stroma (e.g., in granular dystrophy) or the endothelium (e.g., in cornea guttata) may be affected. Each dystrophy tends to have easily identifiable clinical and histopathologic characteristics. In addition to the primary corneal dystrophies, systemic disease (often metabolic and inherited, such as the acid mucopoly-saccharidoses), may involve the cornea secondarily.

Because of the clarity of the cornea, pigment deposition is easily seen. Many different types of pigment may be deposited in the cornea. The pigment may arise from local deposition, e.g., from epinephrine drops used in the treatment of glaucoma, or as part of a systemic disease, e.g., from copper in the Kayser-Fleischer ring in Wilson disease (hepatolenticular degeneration).

The sclera is composed of densely packed collagen and is relatively avascular, hence the white color seen clinically. It may be involved in congenital anomalies (e.g., ochronosis), in inflammations (e.g., scleritis), and in tumors (e.g., episcleral osseous choristoma). Some of the more common and important scleral entities will be illustrated.

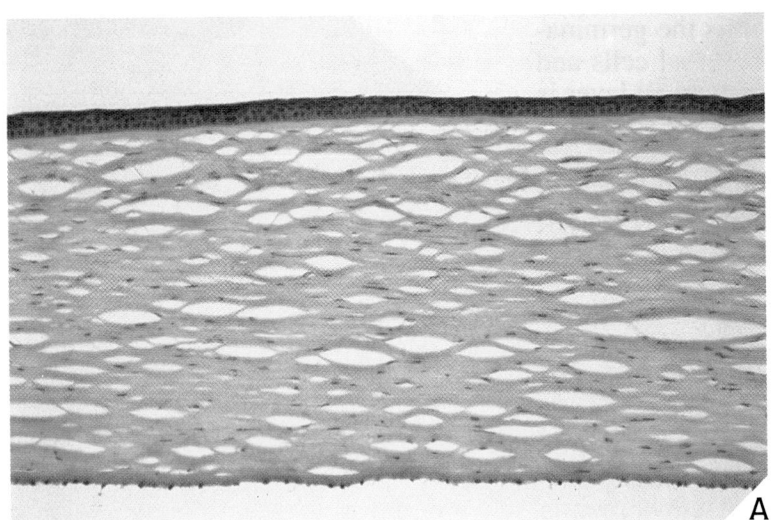

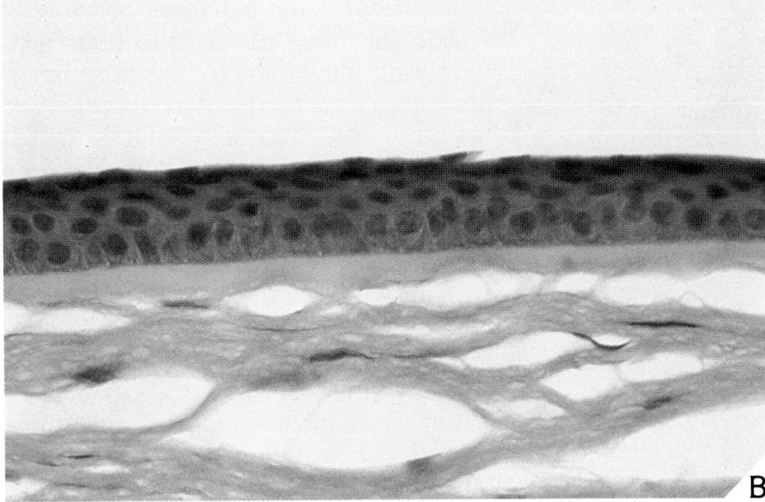

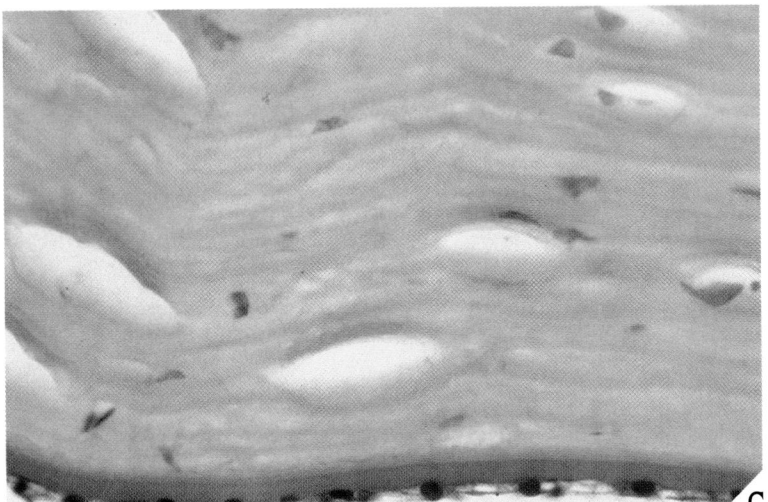

FIGURE 8.1 CORNEA. A The cornea contains five layers: epithelium, Bowman membrane, stroma, Descemet membrane, and endothelium. **B** Increased magnification shows the nonkeratinized, approximately five-layered epithelium, separated from the Bowman membrane (relatively homogeneous) and anterior stroma (numerous large artifactitious clefts) by a thin basement membrane. **C** Descemet membrane and endothelium (a single layer of continuous cells) cover posterior stroma. (**A–C**, PAS stain.)

CONGENITAL DEFECTS

Absence of cornea

Abnormalities of size

Microcornea
(<11 mm in greatest diameter)
Megalocornea
(13> mm in greatest diameter)
Keratoglobus

Aberrations of curvature

Astigmatism
Cornea plana
Keratoconus

FIGURE 8.2

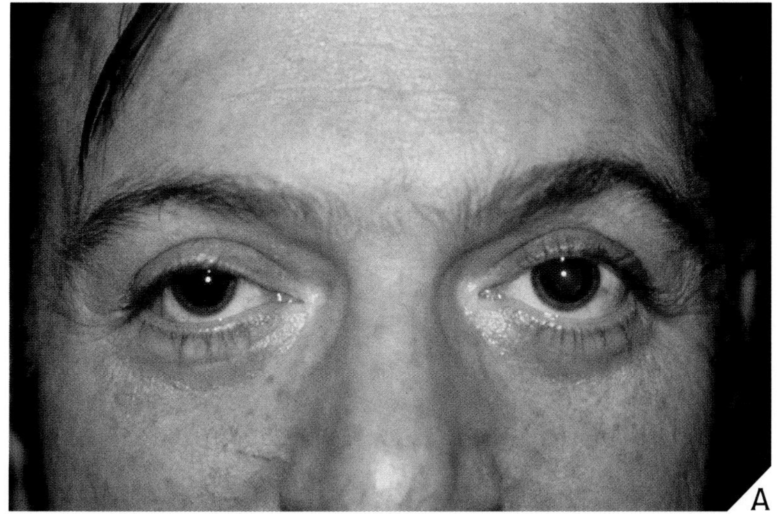

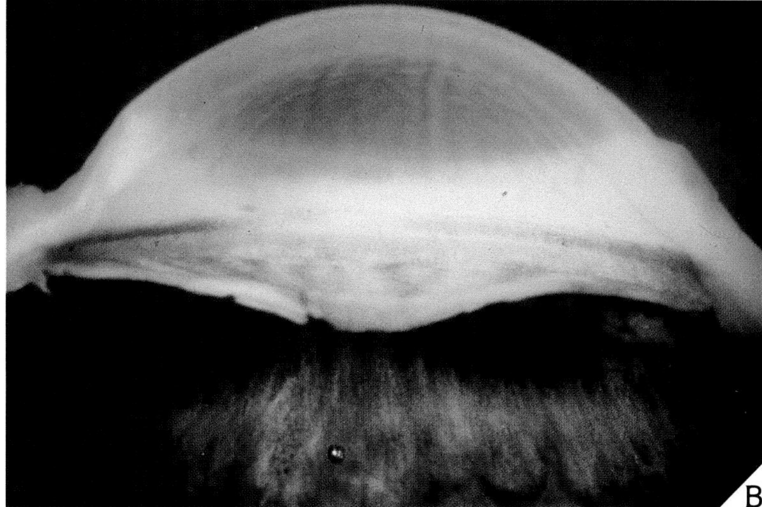

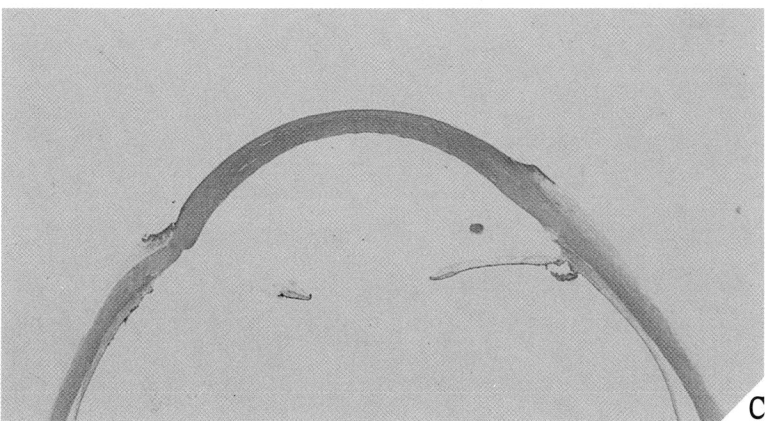

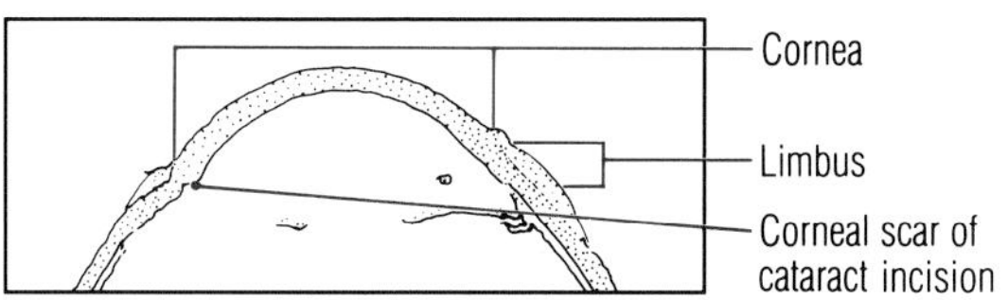

FIGURE 8.3 ABNORMALITIES OF SIZE. **A** The patient has bilateral megalocornea, as do other male members of his family. The patient died from metastatic renal cell carcinoma, and the eyes were obtained at autopsy. **B** Gross examination shows an enlarged cornea and a very deep anterior chamber. **C** Histologic section shows that the cornea itself is of about normal diameter, but the limbal region is enlarged and slightly thicker than normal. The patient had had a cataract extraction and a peripheral iridectomy (**B**, courtesy of Dr. RC Eagle Jr.)

CONGENITAL DEFECTS: CORNEAL OPACITIES

Anterior embryotoxon (arcus juvenilis)

Congenital leukomas (corneal keloids)

Central corneal dysgenesis
Peters anomaly
Localized posterior keratoconus

Peripheral corneal and iris dysgenesis
Posterior embryotoxon (Axenfeld syndrome)
Rieger syndrome

Sclerocornea

Limbal dermoids (may be associated with Goldenhar syndrome)

FIGURE 8.4

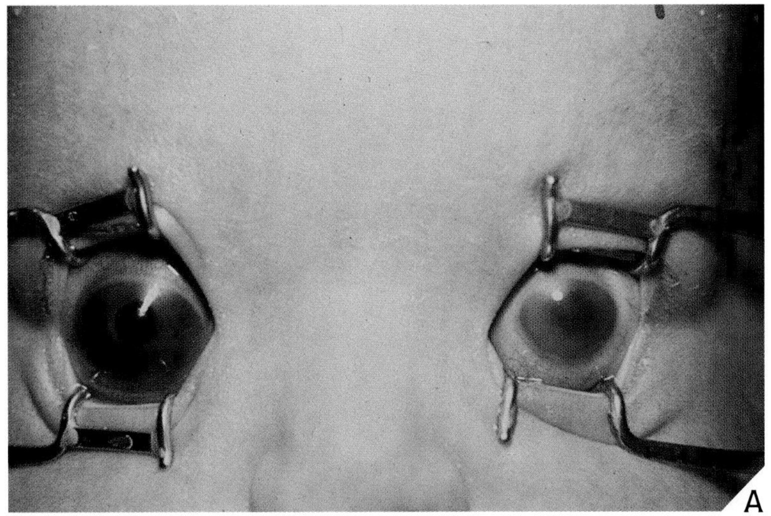

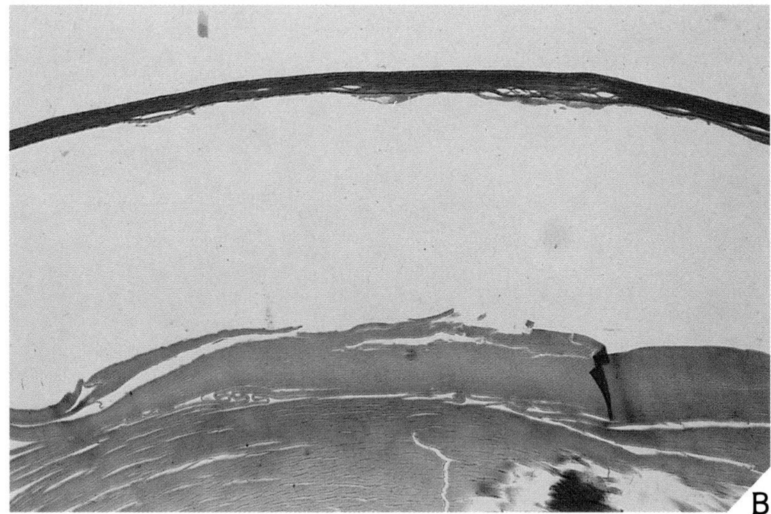

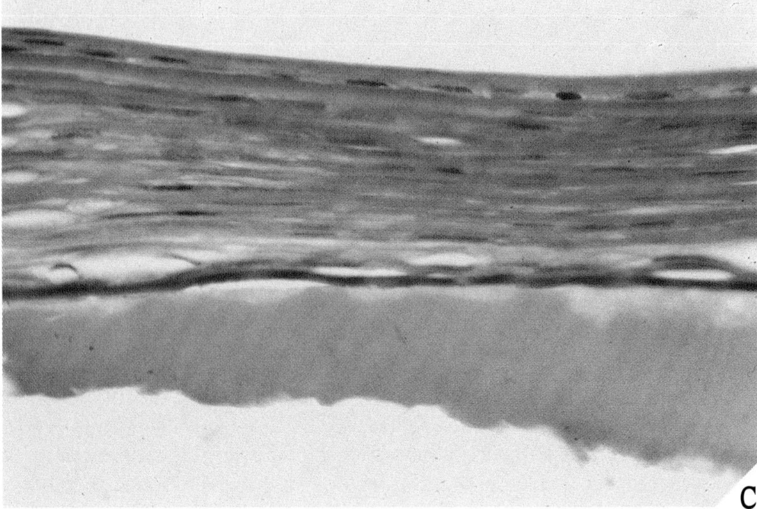

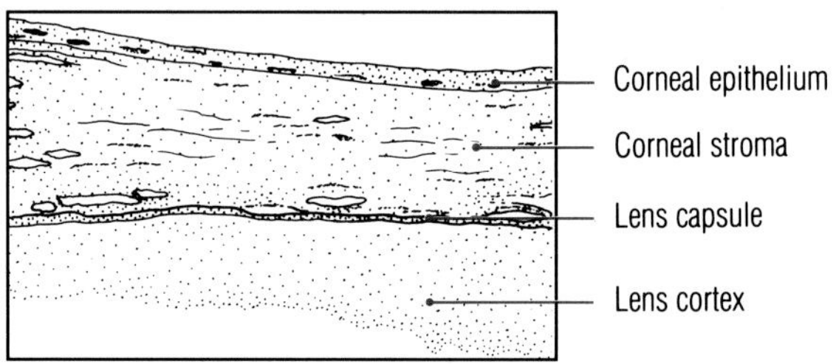

FIGURE 8.5 PETERS ANOMALY. A The right eye shows an enlarged cornea, secondary to glaucoma. The left eye shows a small cornea as part of the anomalous affliction. **B** Histologic section shows considerable corneal thinning centrally. The space between the cornea and the lens material is artifactitious and secondary to shrinkage of the lens cortex during processing of the eye. **C** Increased magnification shows lens material attached to the posterior cornea. Centrally, neither endothelium, Descemet membrane, nor Bowman membrane is present. Lens capsule lines the posterior surface of the cornea. (**B, C**, PAS stain; reported in Scheie HG, Yanoff M, 1972.)

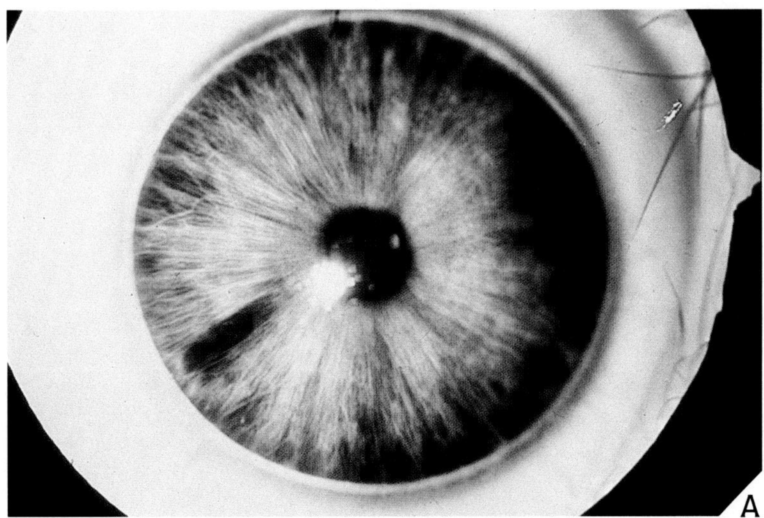

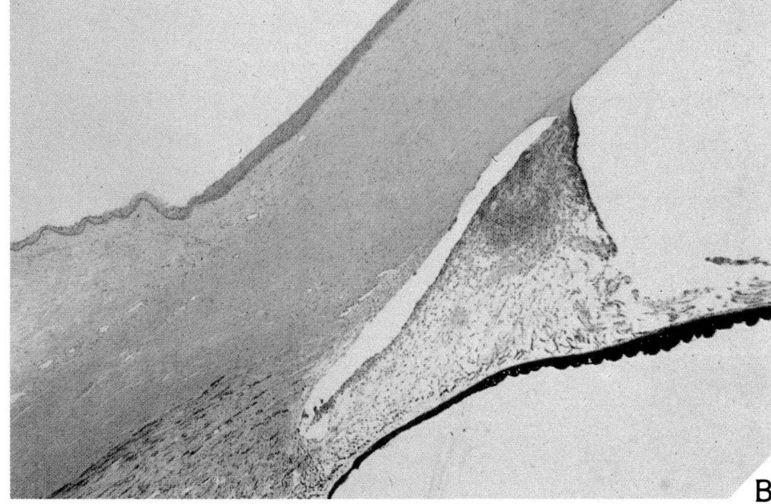

FIGURE 8.6 AXENFELD SYNDROME (POSTERIOR EMBRYOTOXON). A Schwalbe line is anteriorly displaced 360°. **B** Histologic section of another case shows an iris process attached to the anteriorly displaced Schwalbe ring. (**A**, courtesy of Dr. WC Frayer; from Yanoff M, Fine BS: *Ocular Pathology*, 3rd ed.; **B**, courtesy of Dr. RY Foos.)

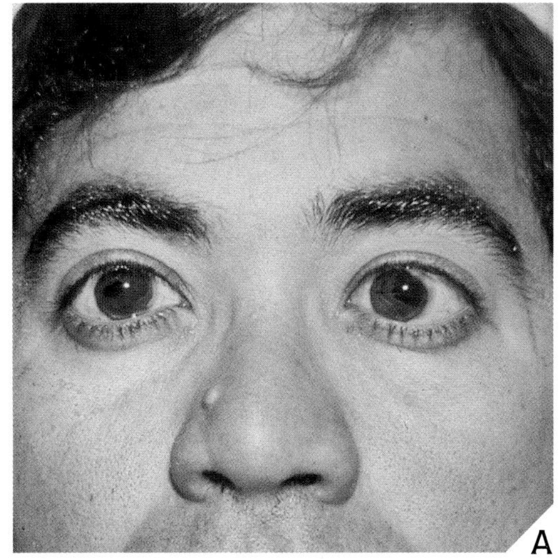

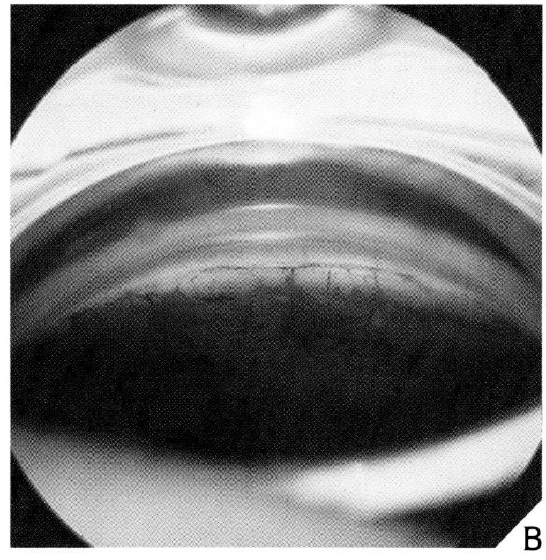

FIGURE 8.7 RIEGER SYNDROME. A The patient has numerous iris abnormalities and bilateral glaucoma. Note the hypertelorism. **B** The patient's daughter has similar abnormalities. Note the iris processes attached to an anteriorly displaced Schwalbe line (anterior embryotoxon). **C** Histologic section of an eye from another patient shows an anteriorly displaced Schwalbe ring. A diffuse abnormality of the iris stroma is present. (**A, B**, courtesy of Dr. HG Scheie; **A**, from Yanoff M, Fine BS: *Ocular Pathology*, 3rd ed.)

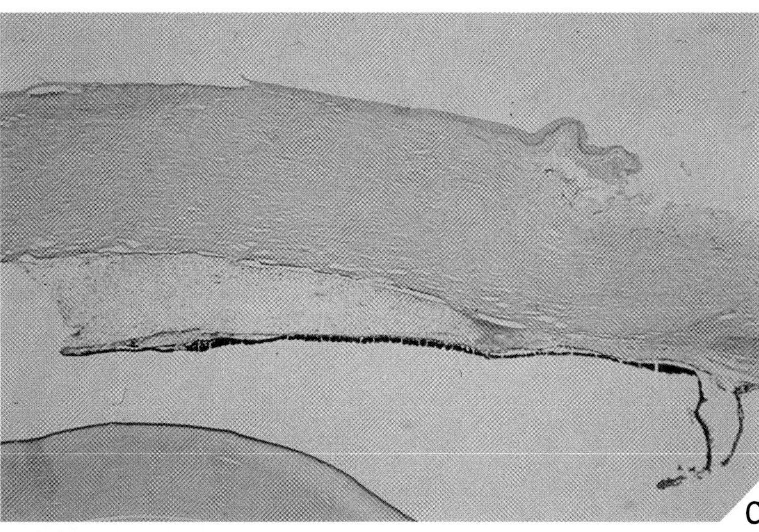

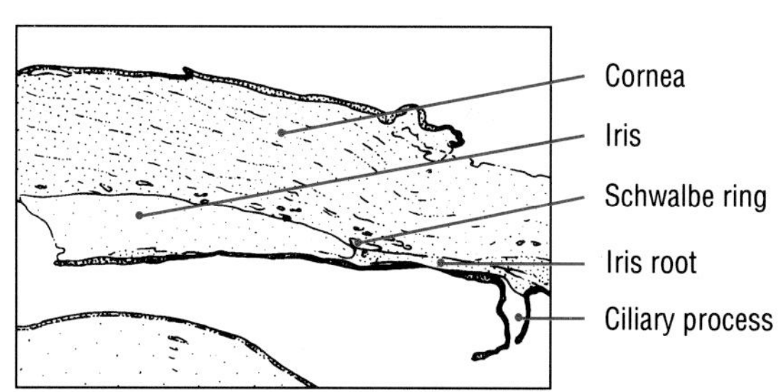

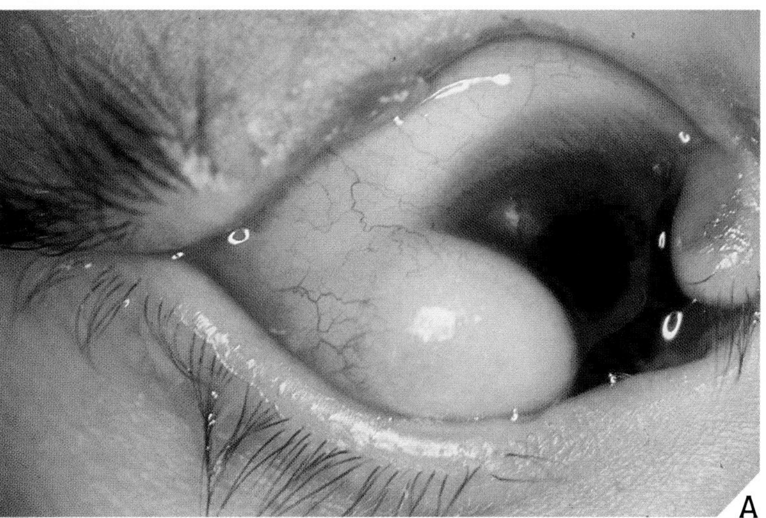

FIGURE 8.8 GOLDENHAR SYNDROME. A The patient has bilateral temporal limbal dermoids and a coloboma of his right upper lid. **B** The dermoid is composed of epidermis, dermis, epidermal appendages, and adipose tissue. (**A,** courtesy of Dr. JA Katowitz)

NONULCERATIVE INFLAMMATIONS

Punctate epithelial keratitis

Subepithelial keratitis
Epidemic keratoconjunctivitis
Trachoma
Leprosy

Superior limbal keratoconjunctivitis

Stromal (interstitial) keratitis
Syphilis
Tuberculosis
Lyme disease
Sarcoidosis
Onchocerciasis
Protozoal
- Leishmaniasis
- Trypanosomiasis

Viral
- Herpes simplex
- Herpes zoster

Cogan syndrome
Hodgkin disease
Mycosis fungoides
Lymphogranuloma venereum
Hypoparathyroidism

FIGURE 8.9

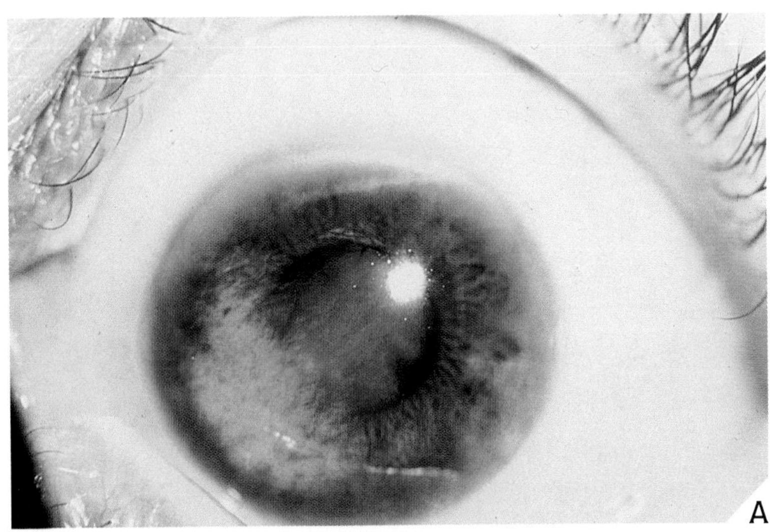

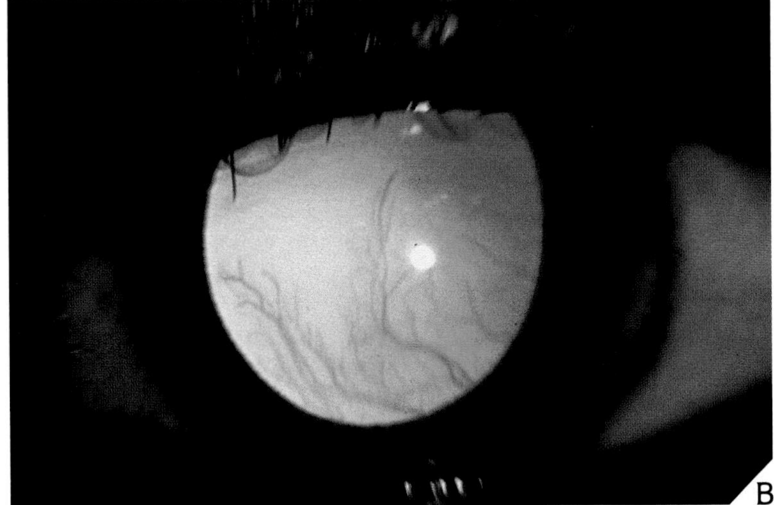

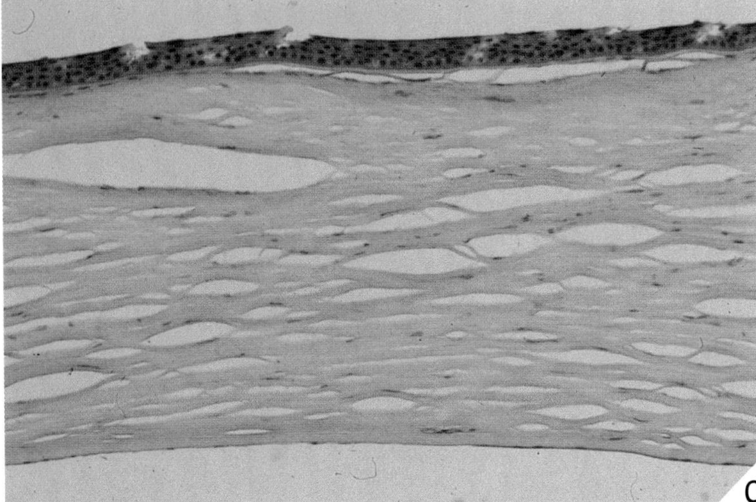

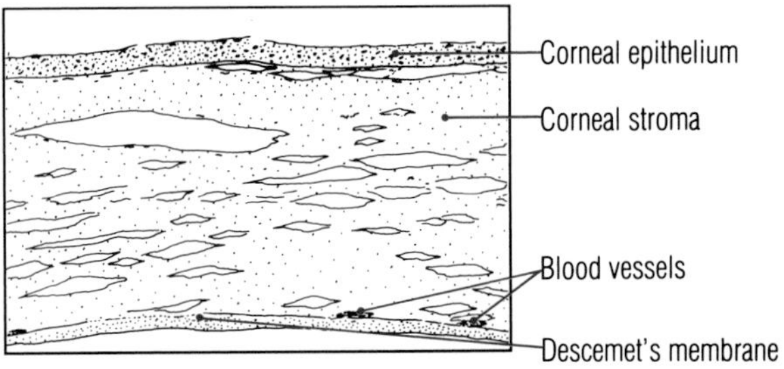

FIGURE 8.10 SYPHILIS. A The cornea shows a range of opacification from a cloud-like nebula, to a moderately dense macula, to a very dense white leukoma. **B** In another case, ghost vessels are easily seen by retroillumination. **C** The vessels are deep in the corneal stroma, just anterior to the Descemet membrane. The stroma shows scarring and thinning. (**A**, courtesy of Dr. WC Frayer; **B** from Yanoff M, Fine BS: *Ocular Pathology*, 3rd ed.)

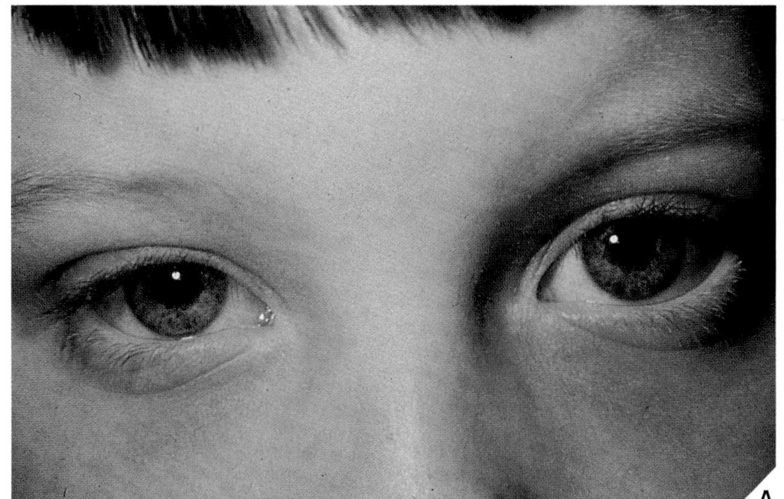

Figure 8.11 Onchocerciasis. A This young girl had just returned from Africa. She had conjunctival injection and small corneal opacities at all levels. During examination at the slit lamp, a tiny thread-like worm was noted in the aqueous. **B** Histologic section of a conjunctival biopsy shows a chronic nongranulomatous inflammation and a tiny segment of the worm in the deep substantia propria; this is shown under higher magnification in **C**. (Case reported in Scheie HG et al., 1971.)

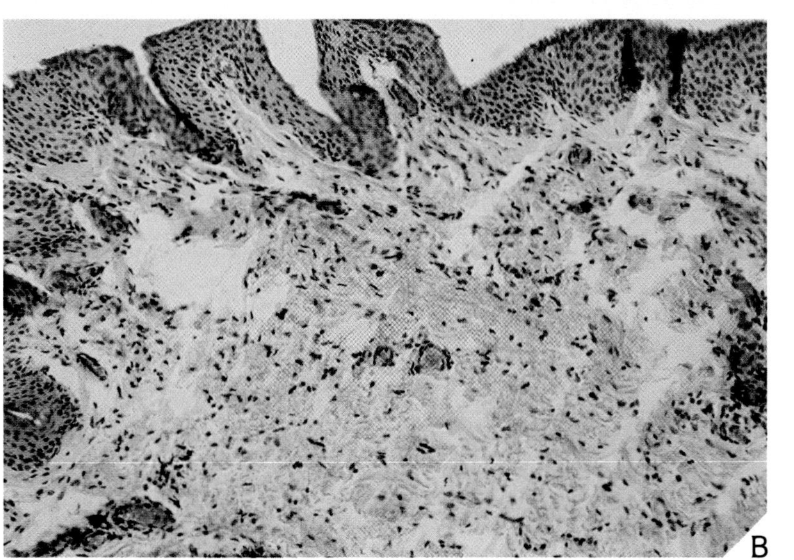

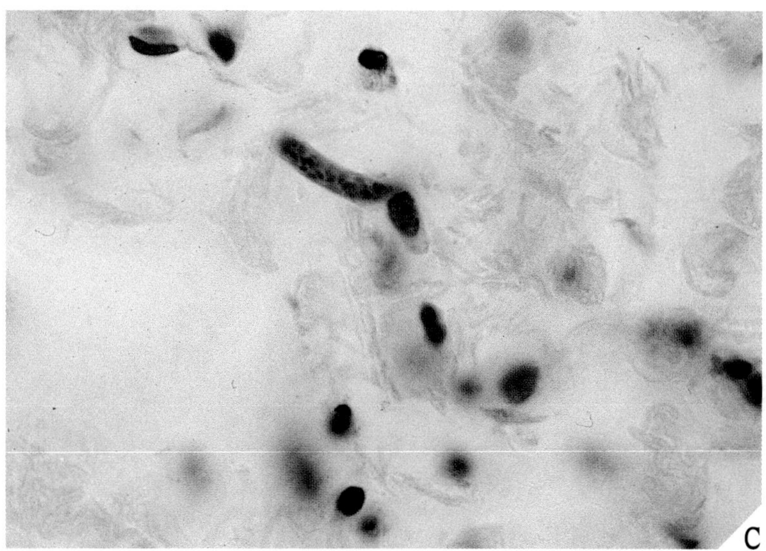

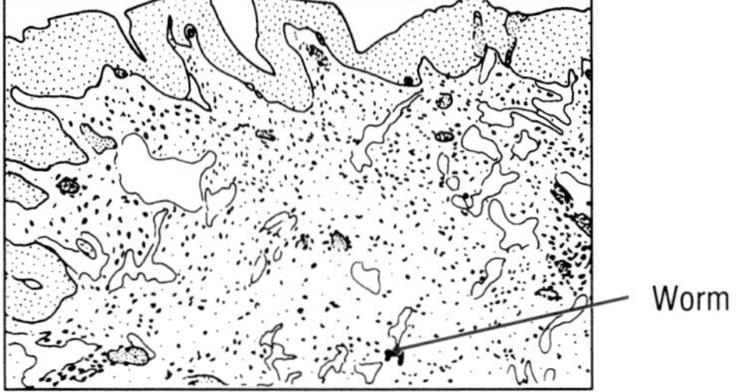

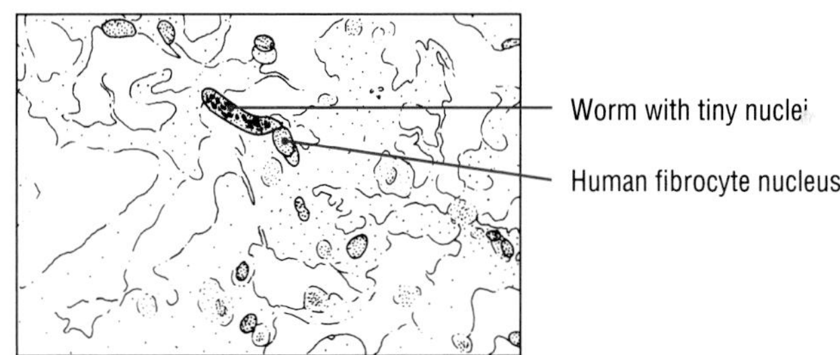

Ulcerative Inflammations

Peripheral	**Central**
Marginal (catarrhal) ulcer	Bacterial
Phlyctenular ulcer	Viral
Ring ulcer	Mycotic
Ring abscess	Parasitic (*Acanthamoeba*)

Figure 8.12

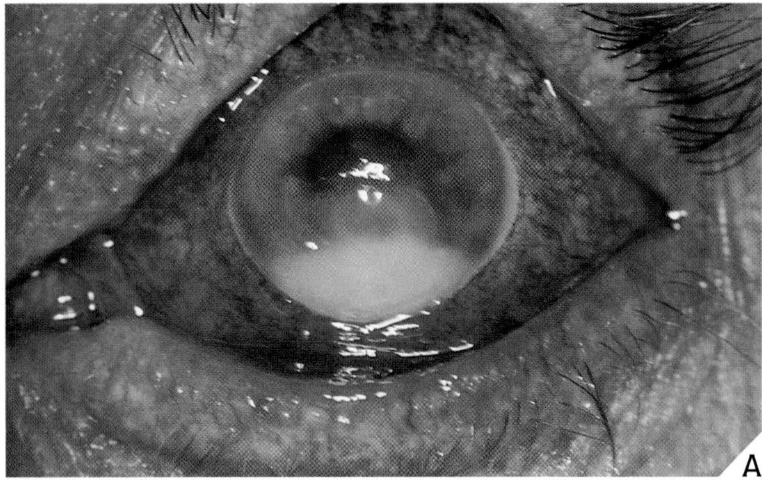

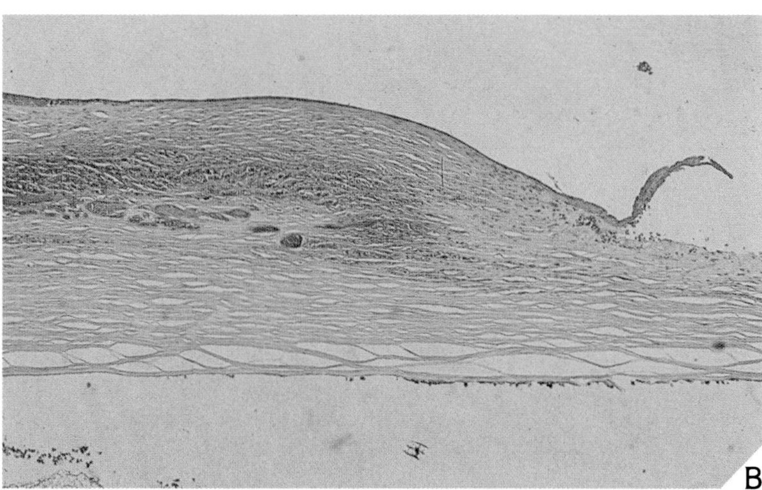

FIGURE 8.13 CENTRAL CORNEAL ULCER. A Note central ulcer and large reactive hypopyon. **B** The right side of the picture shows ulceration. The corneal stroma is infiltrated with polymorphonuclear leukocytes and large purple amorphous collections of material. Special stain of the purple areas showed a collection of many gram-positive bacteria. (**A**, courtesy of Dr. HG Scheie.)

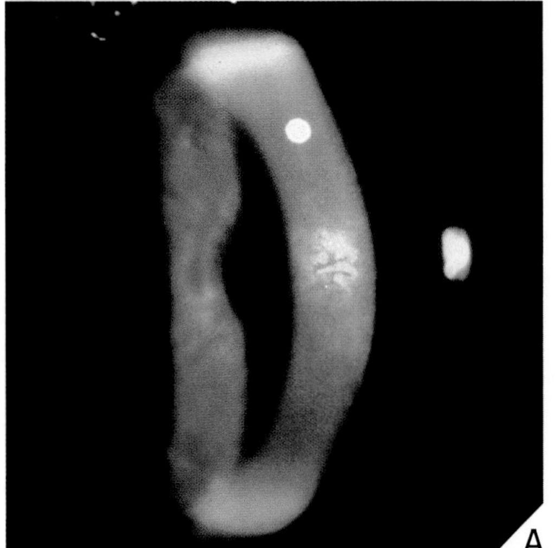

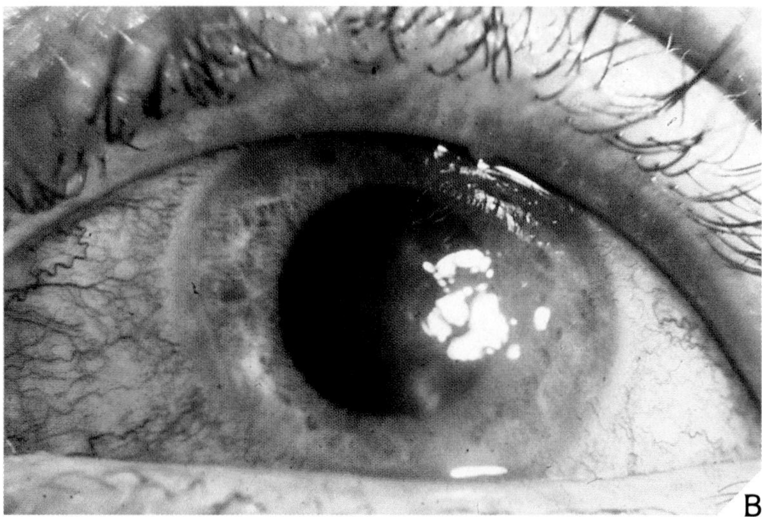

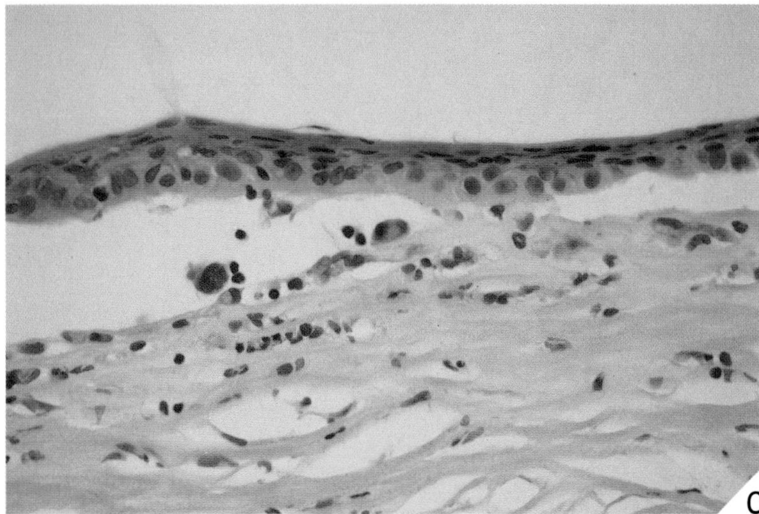

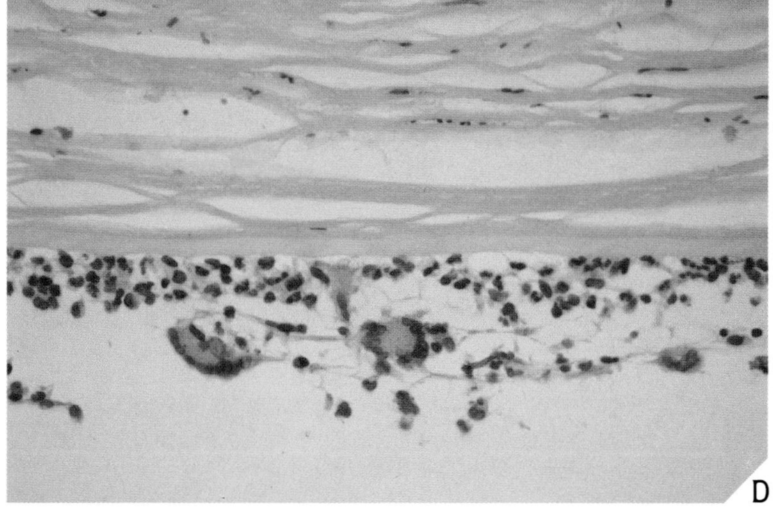

FIGURE 8.14 HERPES SIMPLEX. A Typical dendritic ulcer is present in the central cornea, shown with Rose Bengal stain. Note the characteristic terminal bulbs on the ulcer. **B** The patient had bullous keratopathy following longstanding herpes simplex keratitis (metaherpetic phase). **C** Histologic section shows a large corneal epithelial bleb. Multinucleated giant cells are present in the region of the Bowman membrane. **D** Inflammatory cells and multinucleated giant cells are seen in the anterior chamber in close proximity to the Descemet membrane.

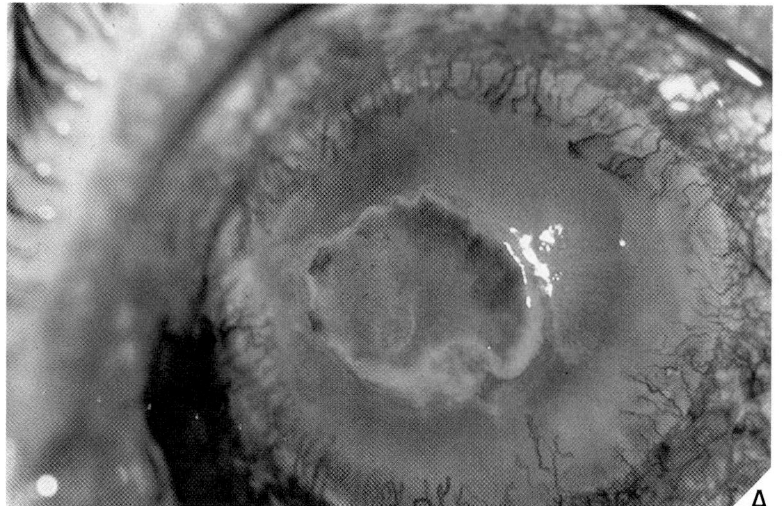

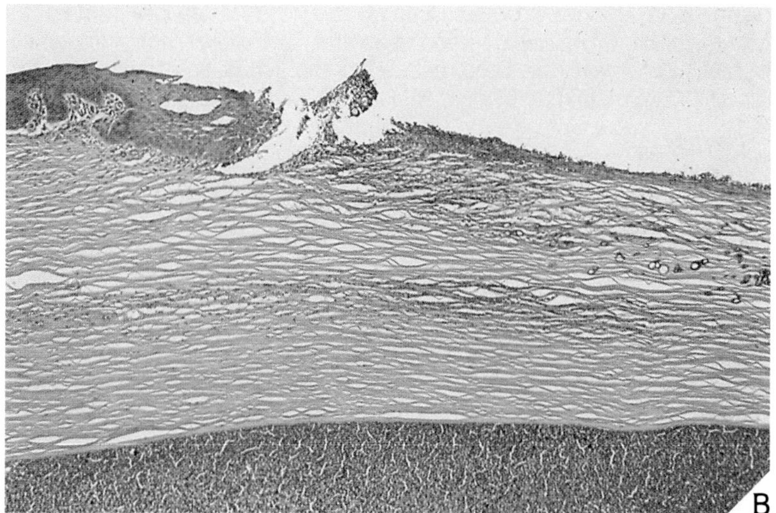

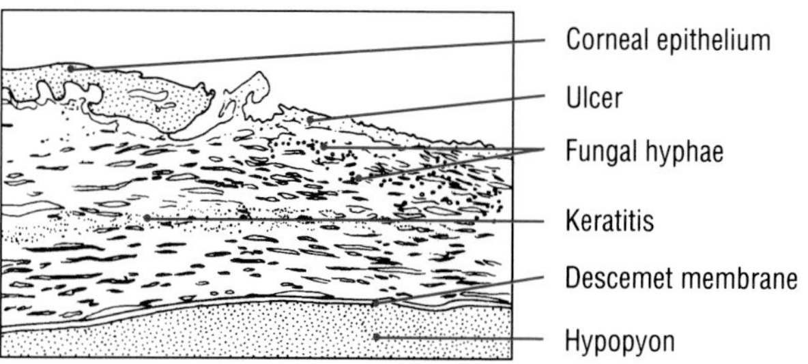

FIGURE 8.15 MYCOTIC ULCER. A The patient developed a central corneal ulcer that was caused by a pigmented fungus. **B** Histologic section of another case shows ulceration of the corneal epithelium and infiltration of the corneal stroma by polymorphonuclear leukocytes and large fungal elements. A hypopyon, consisting of polymorphonuclear leukocytes and cellular debris, is seen in the anterior chamber. Often fungal ulcers have satellite corneal lesions and a hypopyon.

SEQUELAE OF INFLAMMATION

Descemetocele	Staphyloma	Adherent leukoma
Ectasia	Cicatrization	Vascularization

FIGURE 8.16

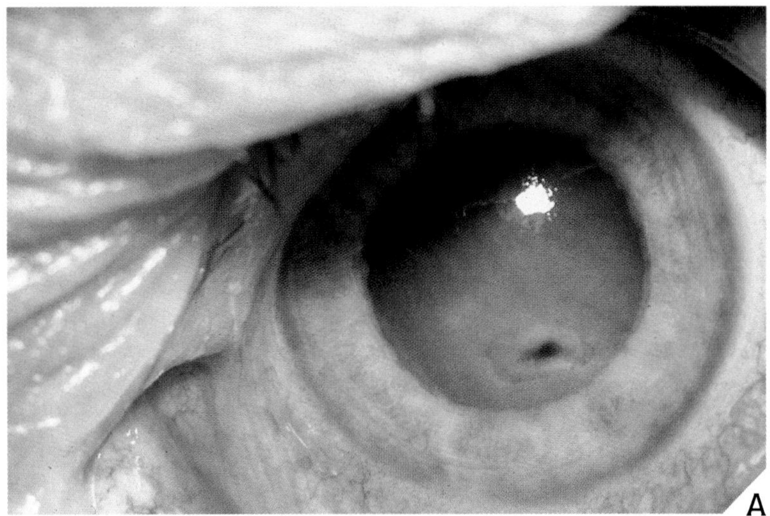

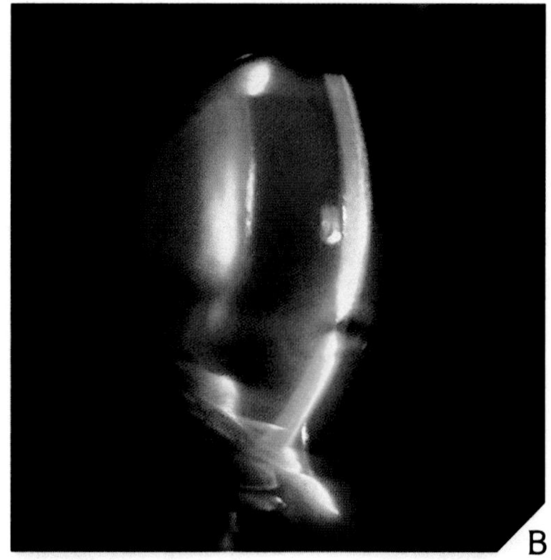

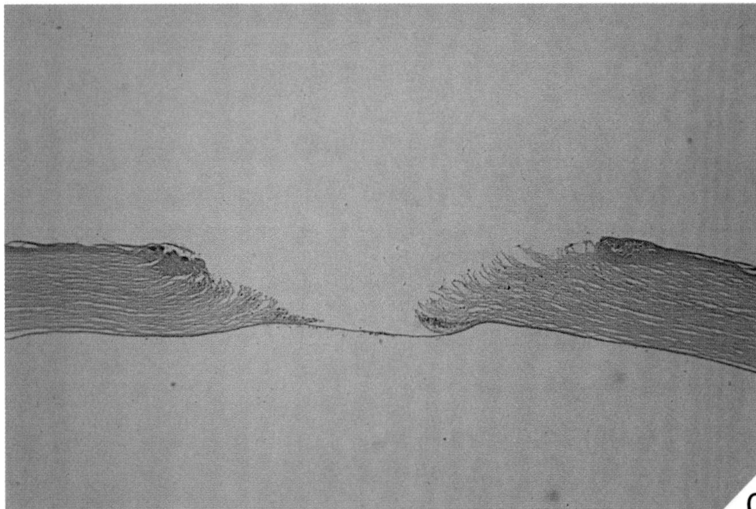

FIGURE 8.17 DESCEMETOCELE. A and **B** show the clinical appearance of a descemetocele. **C** Histologic section of another case shows central loss of all corneal substance except Descemet membrane. (**A, B**, courtesy of Dr. IM Raber; **C**, PAS stain, from Yanoff M, Fine BS: *Ocular Pathology*, 2nd ed.)

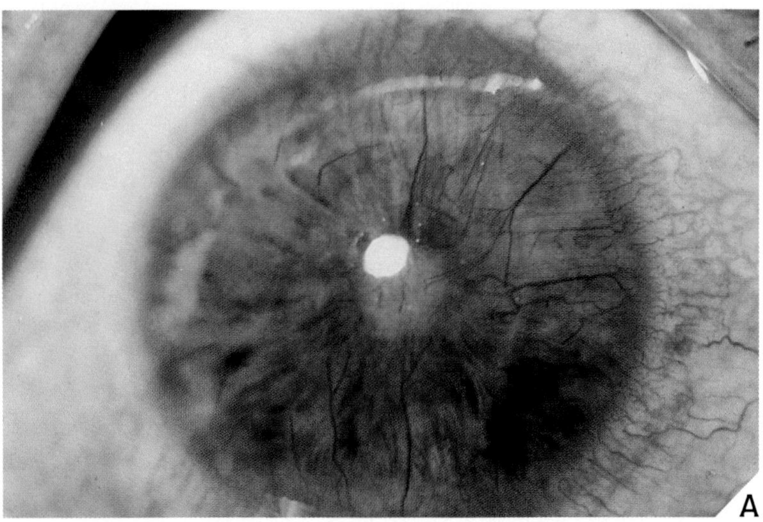

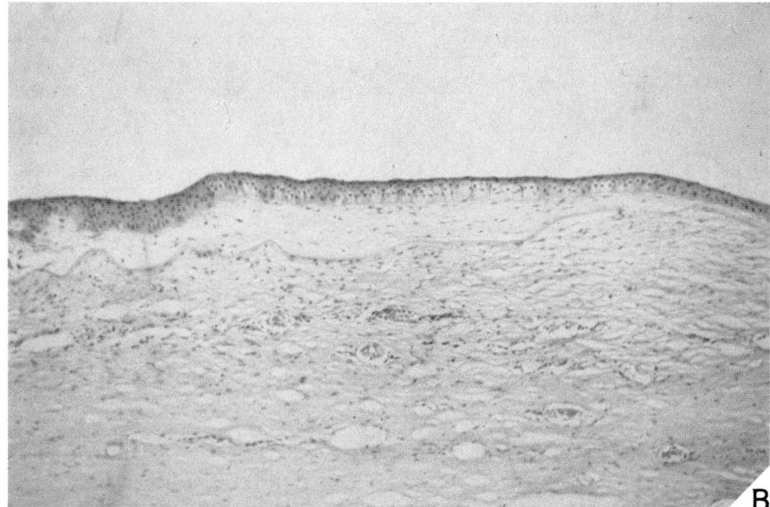

FIGURE 8.18 CORNEAL VASCULARIZATION. A The corneal stroma is vascularized by large trunk vessels. **B** Corneal epithelial edema and stromal inflammation, scarring, and vascularization are present. A fibrotic scar (degenerative pannus) is seen between the Bowman membrane and the epithelium.

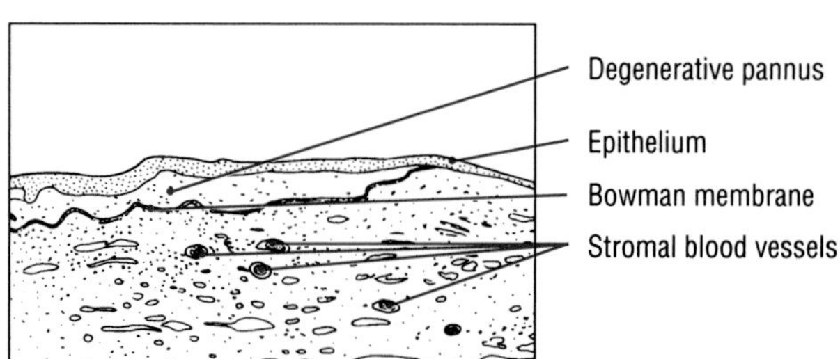

EPITHELIAL DEGENERATIONS

Keratitis sicca
Keratomalacia
Neuroparalytic keratopathy
Exposure keratitis
Recurrent erosion

FIGURE 8.19

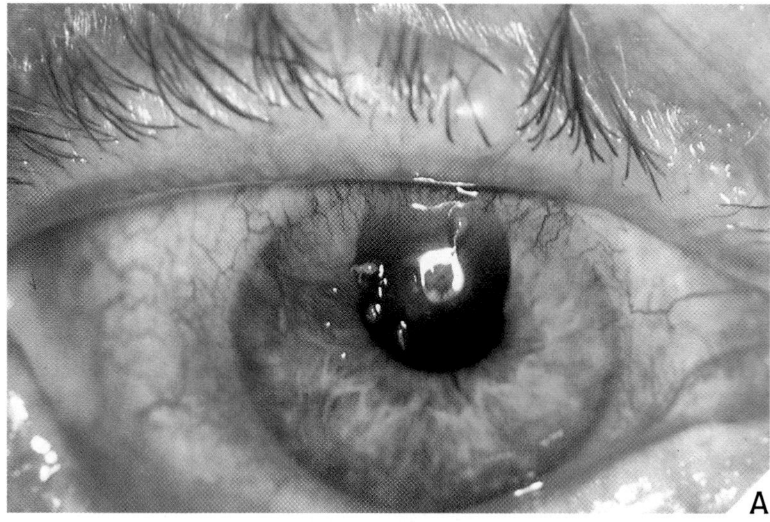

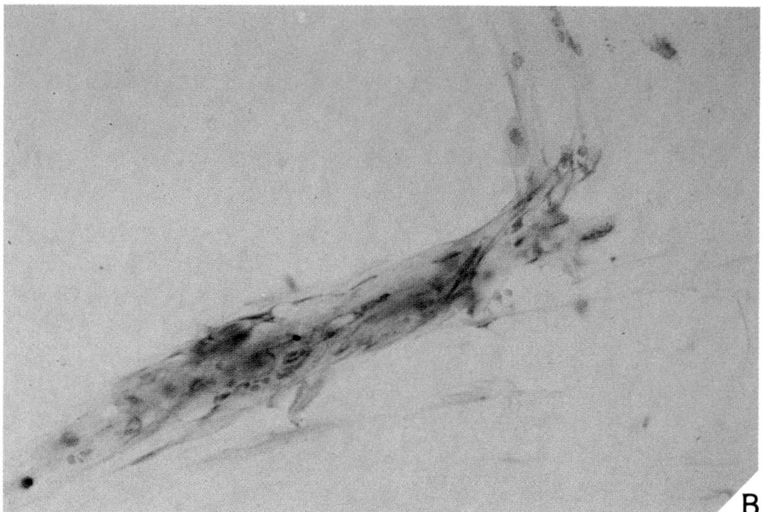

FIGURE 8.20 FILAMENTARY KERATITIS. A Numerous filaments in the form of ropy secretions are present on the cornea, mainly superiorly. **B** Histologic section shows that the filaments are composed of epithelial cells and mucinous material. (**B**, from Yanoff M, Fine BS: *Ocular Pathology*, 2nd ed.)

STROMAL DEGENERATIONS

Arcus senilis
Pterygium
Terrien ulcer
Calcific band keratopathy
Elastotic degeneration
Nodular degeneration (Salzmann)
Lipid keratopathy
Amyloidosis
Limbus girdle (Vogt)
Mooren ulcer
Dellen
Anterior crocodile sheen (Vogt)

FIGURE 8.21

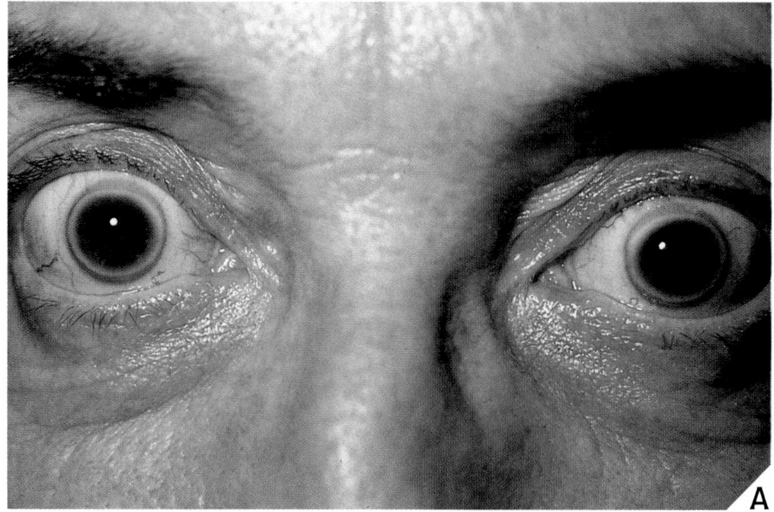

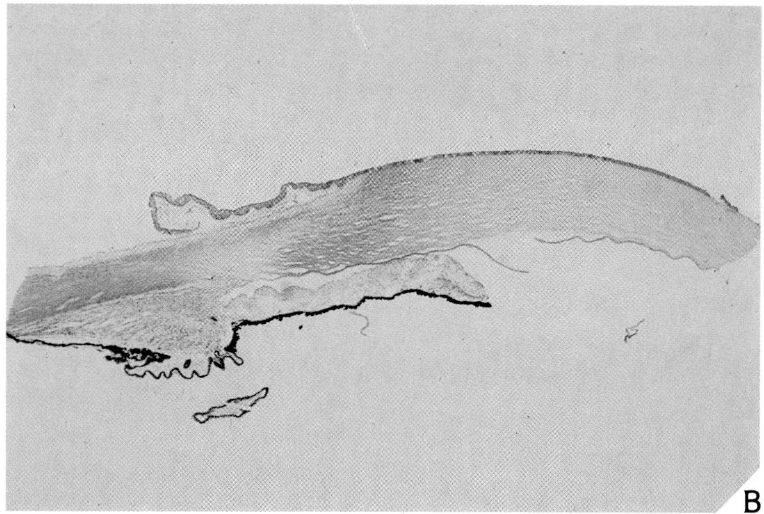

FIGURE 8.22 ARCUS SENILIS. A A white ring is in the peripheral cornea of each eye. The ring is separated from the limbus by a typical tiny clear zone. **B** Histologic section shows that the lipid is concentrated in the anterior and posterior stroma as two red triangles, apex to apex, with the bases being the Bowman membrane and the Descemet membrane, both of which are infiltrated heavily by fat (red staining), as is the sclera. (**B**, oil red-O stain.)

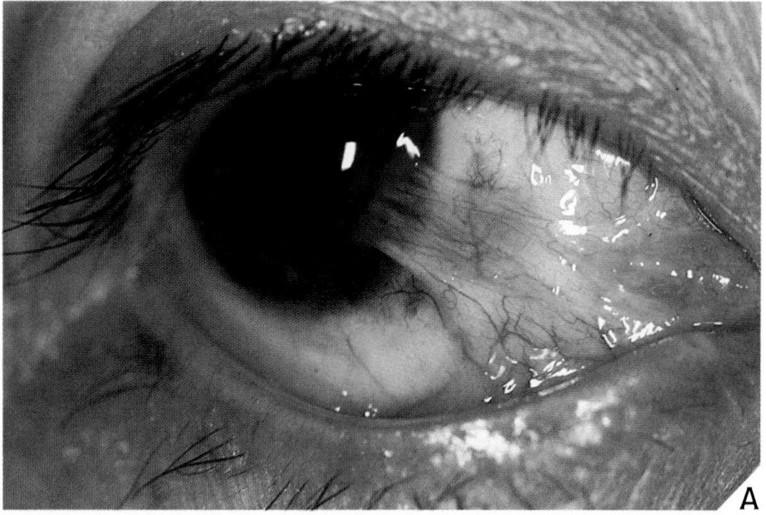

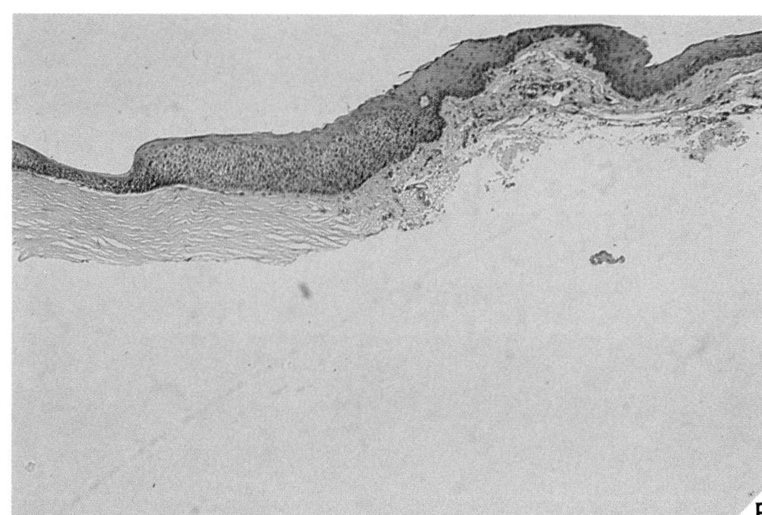

FIGURE 8.23 PTERYGIUM. A The nasal limbal conjunctiva and the contiguous cornea are involved by a vascularized lesion, a pterygium (also see Figure 7.34A). **B** Histologic section of another case shows basophilic degeneration of the substantia propria of the conjunctiva (identical to that seen in a pinguecula) toward the right and invasion of the cornea with destruction of the Bowman membrane toward the left. It is the invasion of the cornea that distinguishes a pterygium from a pinguecula (see Figure 7.23).

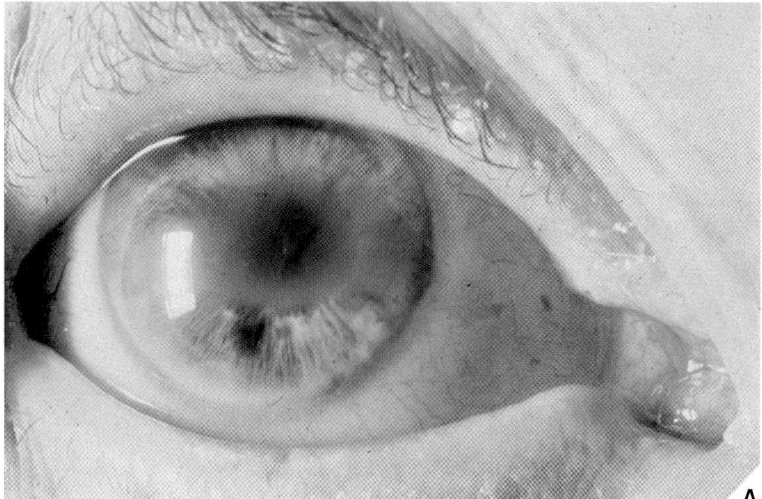

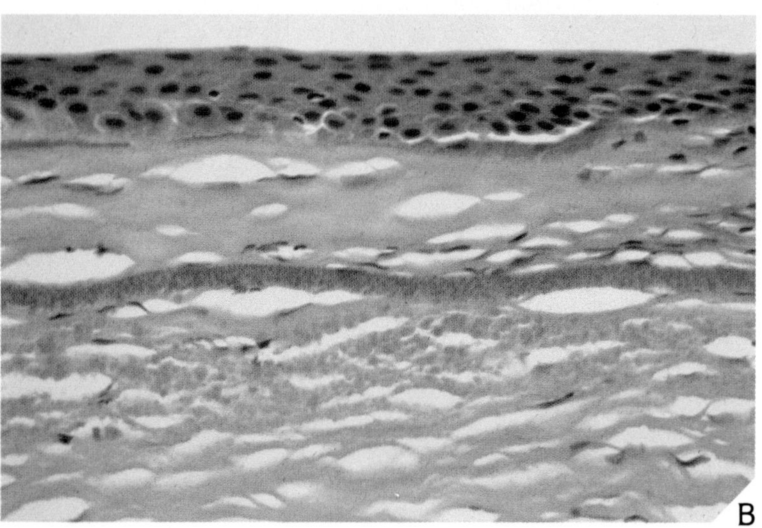

FIGURE 8.24 BAND KERATOPATHY. A Clinical appearance of the band occupying the central horizontal zone of the cornea and typically sparing the most peripheral clear cornea. **B** A fibrous pannus is present between the epithelium and a calcified Bowman membrane. Some deposit also is present in the anterior corneal stroma.

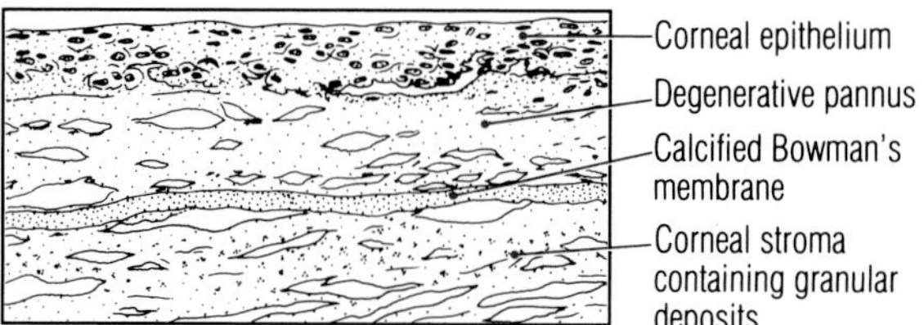

Epithelial
Heredofamilial—primary
- Meesmann (Stocker-Holt)
- Dot (microcystoid), fingerprint, and map (geographic) patterns

Heredofamilial—systemic
- Fabry disease

Bowman membrane
Reis-Bückler dystrophy

FIGURE 8.25

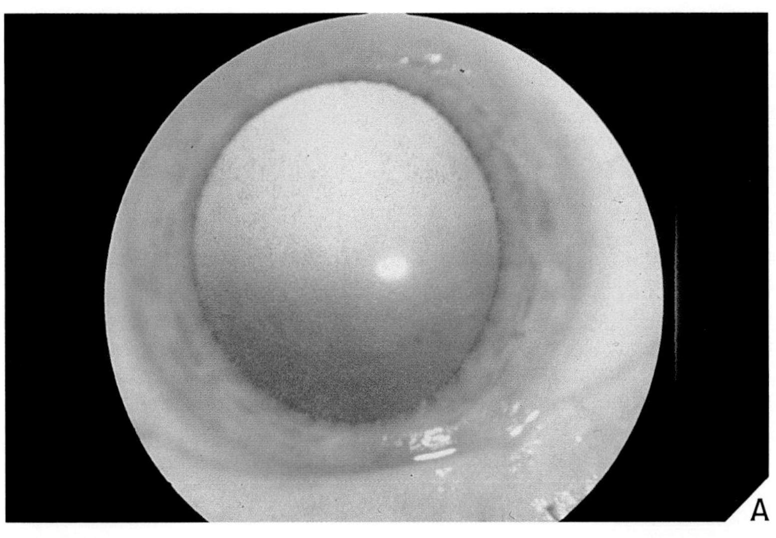

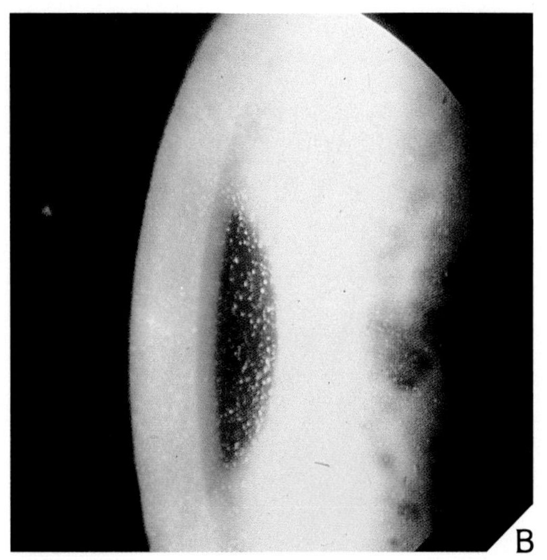

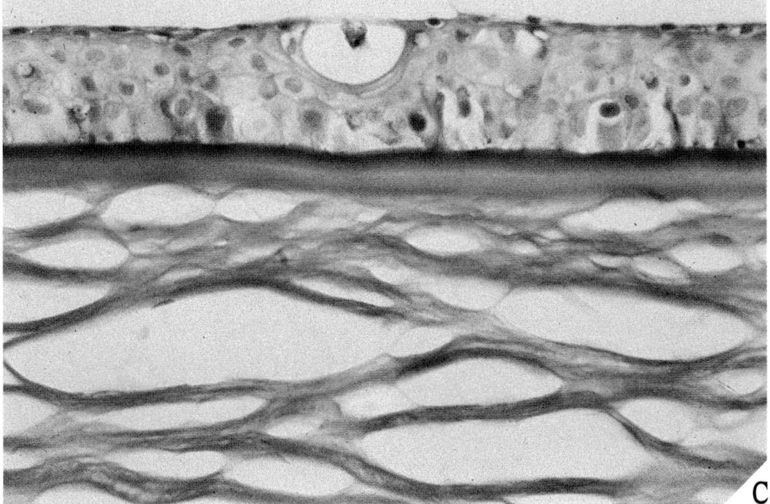

FIGURE 8.26 MEESMANN DYSTROPHY. A and **B** show tiny fine punctate clear vacuoles within the corneal epithelium. **C** Histologic section shows an intraepithelial cyst that contains debris (called "peculiar substance" in electron microscopy). The epithelial basement membrane is thickened here. (**B**, from Yanoff M, Fine BS: *Ocular Pathology*, 2nd ed.; **C**, PAS stain; case reported in Fine BS, et al., 1977.)

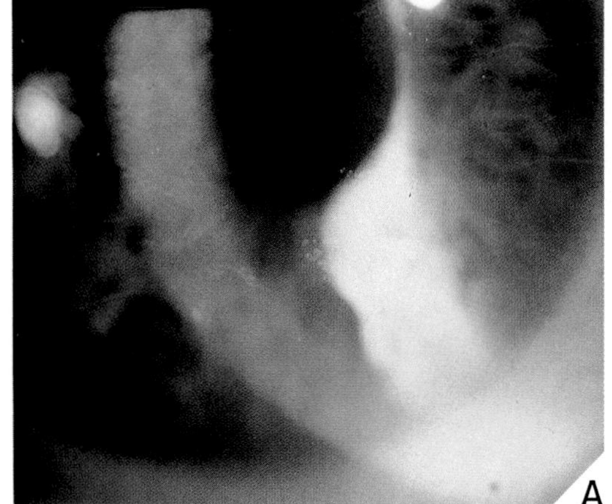

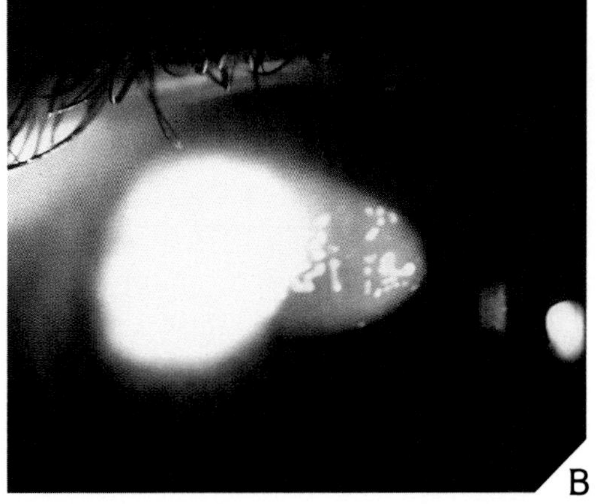

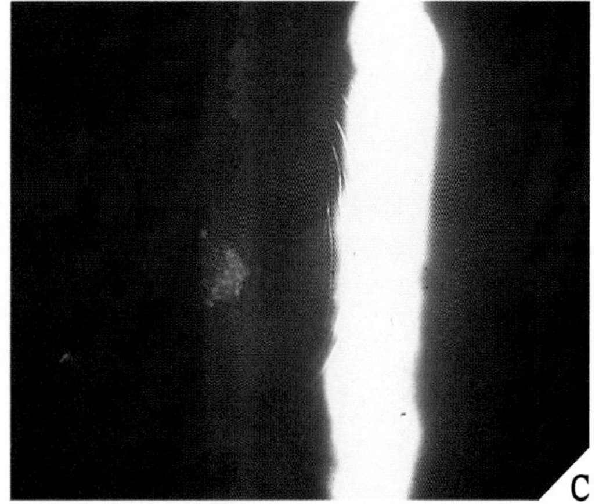

FIGURE 8.27 DOT, FINGERPRINT, AND MAP PATTERNS. A The dot pattern is shown in the lower central cornea. A map pattern is seen above and to the left of the dot pattern. **B** The dot pattern resembles "putty" within the epithelium. **C** The fingerprint pattern, best seen with indirect lighting, is clearly shown. (**B**, courtesy of Dr. WC Frayer.)

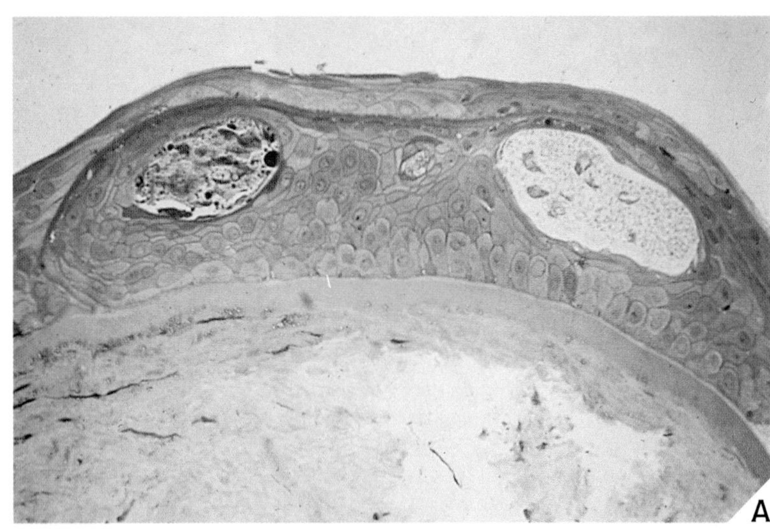

FIGURE 8.28 DOT, FINGERPRINT, AND MAP PATTERNS. A Histologic section shows that the dot pattern is caused by cysts that contain desquamating surface epithelial cells. **B** The fingerprint pattern is caused by extensive aberrant production of basement membrane material within the epithelium (red lines). **C** The map pattern is caused by accumulated subepithelial basement membrane and collagenous tissue that resembles a subepithelial fibrous plaque. (**A**, **B**, PD stain; from Yanoff M, Fine BS: *Ocular Pathology*, 3rd ed.; **C**, PD; cases reported in Rodriques MM, et al., 1974.)

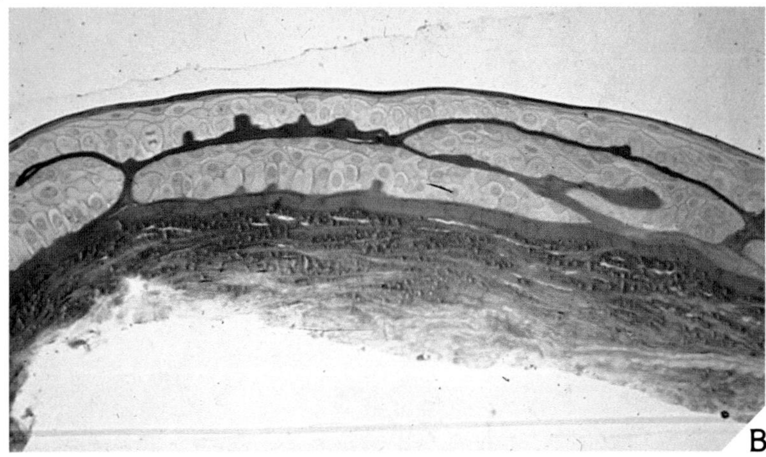

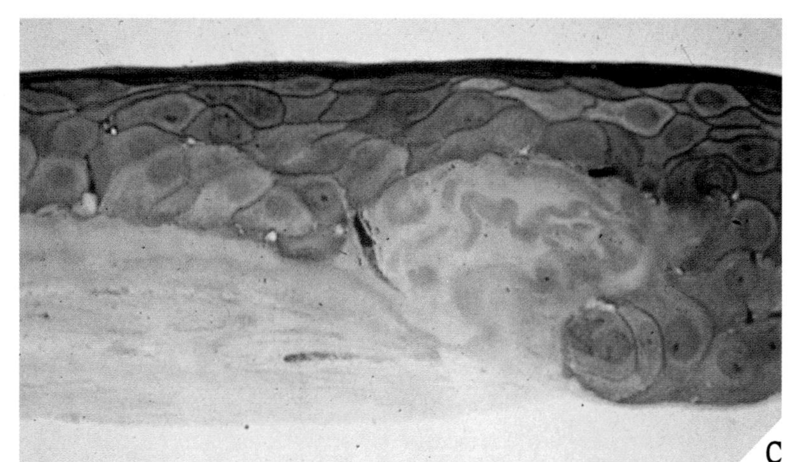

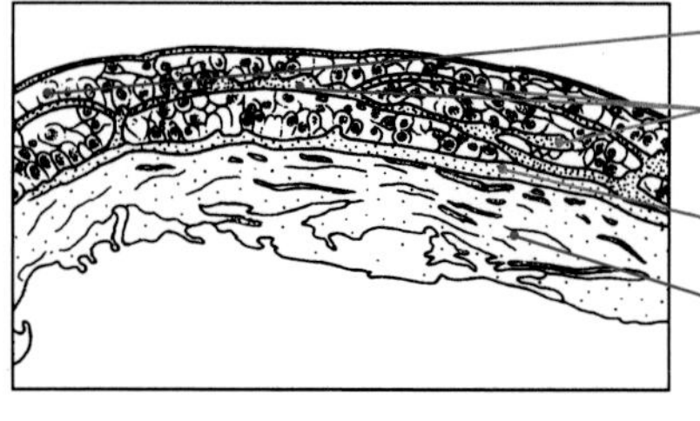

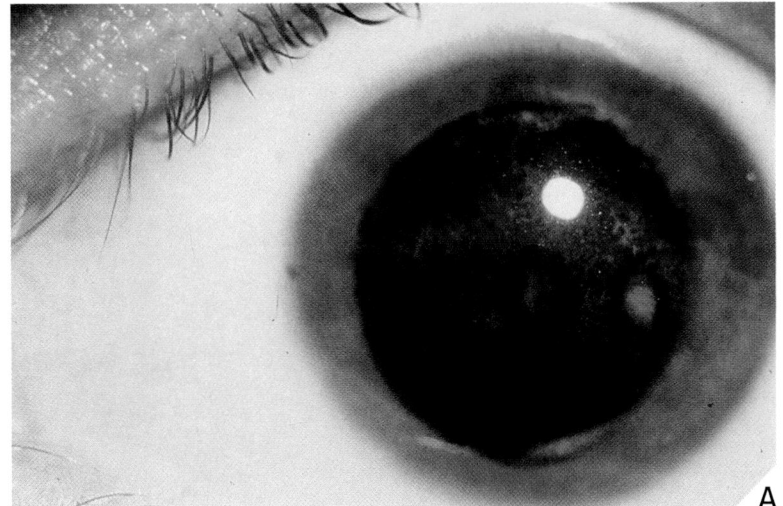

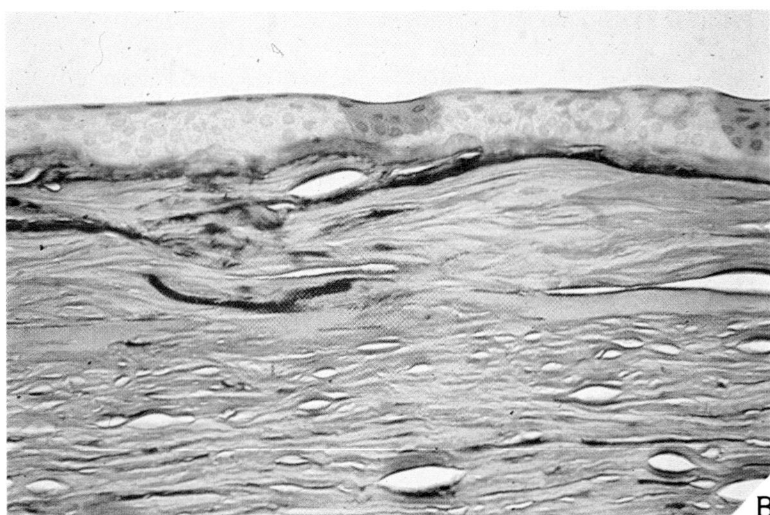

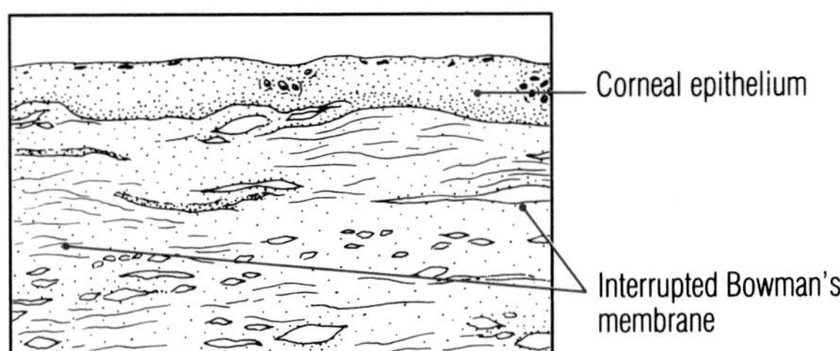

FIGURE 8.29 REIS-BÜCKLER DYSTROPHY.A The characteristic honeycombed corneal pattern is apparent. **B** Histologic section shows disruption of the Bowman membrane by fibrous tissue, along with a fibrous plaque between the Bowman membrane and the epithelium. (**B**, trichrome stain.)

STROMAL DYSTROPHIES

Heredofamilial—primary
Granular
Macular
Lattice
Congenital hereditary stromal dystrophy
Hereditary fleck dystrophy
Central stromal crystalline corneal dystrophy (Schnyder)

Heredofamilial—systemic
Mucopolysaccharidoses
Mucolipidoses
Sphingolipidoses
Ochronosis
Cystinosis
Hypergammaglobulinemia

Nonheredofamilial
Keratoconus
Keratoglobus
Pellucid marginal degeneration

FIGURE 8.30

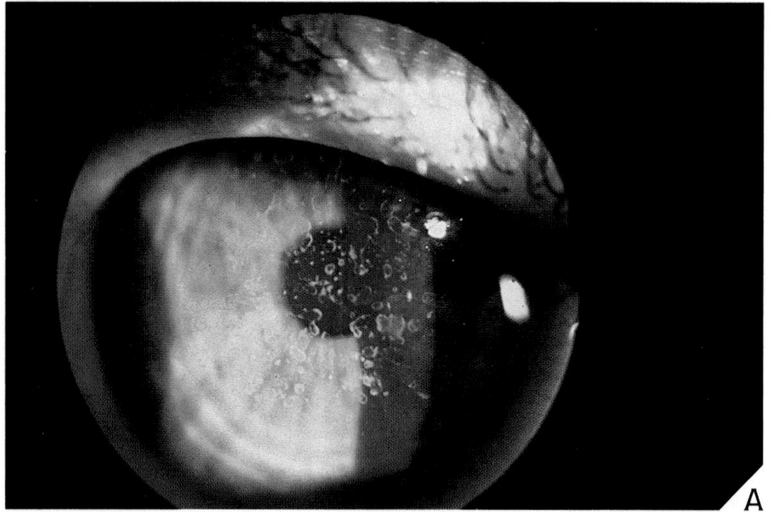

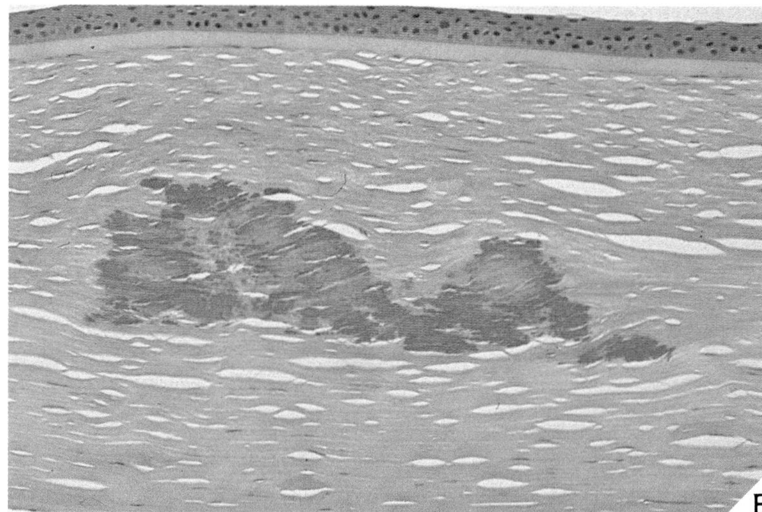

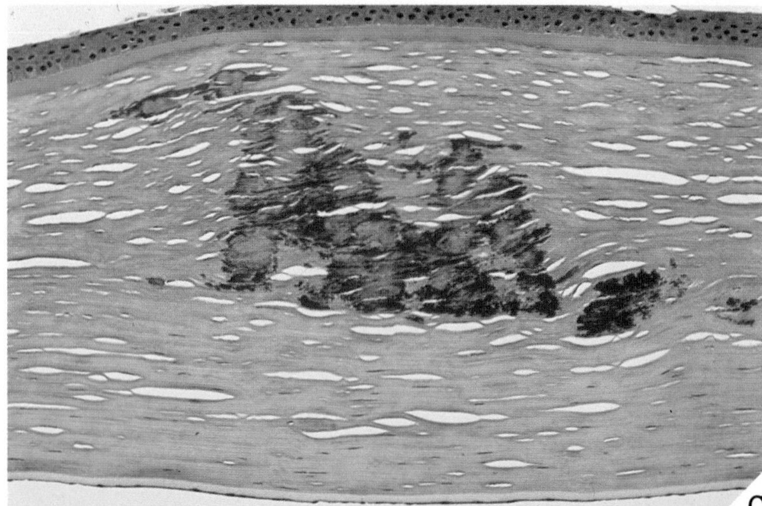

FIGURE 8.31 GRANULAR DYSTROPHY. A Clear cornea is present between the small, sharply outlined, white stromal granules. **B** Histologic section shows that the granules stain deeply with H&E and **C** stain red with the trichrome stain. The PAS stain and stains for both acid mucopolysaccharides and amyloids are negative. The condition is inherited as an autosomal-dominant trait.

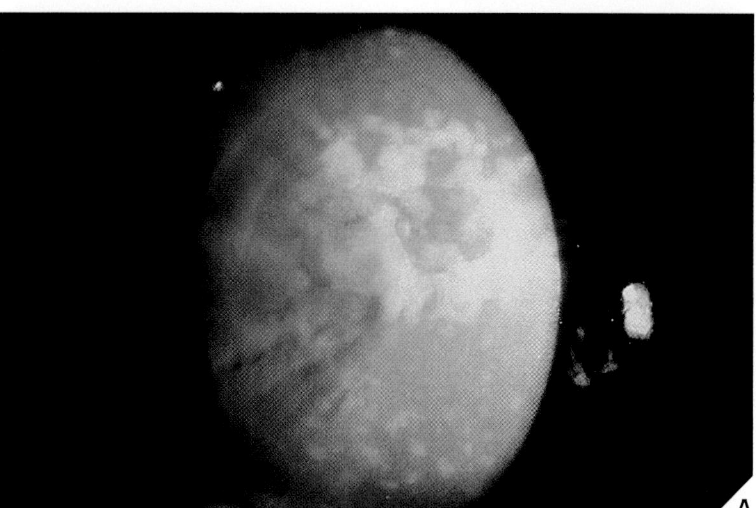

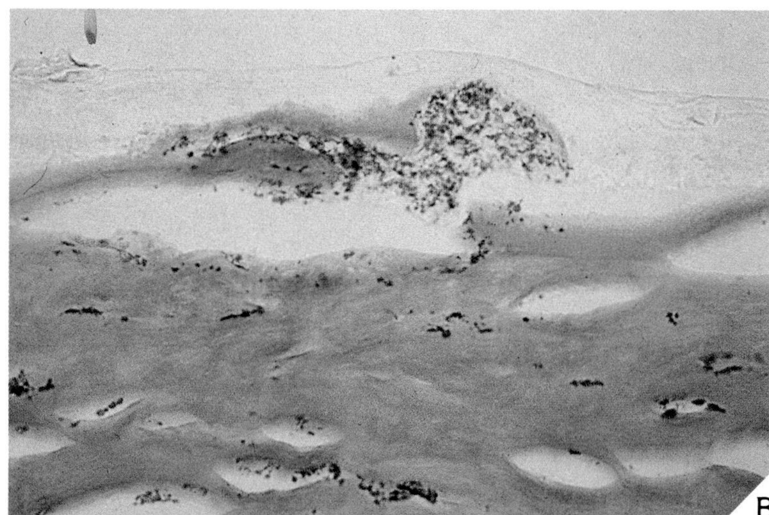

FIGURE 8.32 MACULAR DYSTROPHY. A The corneal stroma between the opacities is cloudy. **B** Histologic section shows that keratocytes and vacuolated cells beneath the epithelium are filled with acid mucopolysaccharide. In this condition, the trichrome stain and stains for amyloid are negative, but the PAS stain is positive. The condition is inherited as an autosomal-recessive trait. The cornea and serum of most patients who have type 1 macular dystrophy lack detectable antigenic keratan sulfate, whereas it is present in the cornea and serum in type 2. (**B**, AMP.)

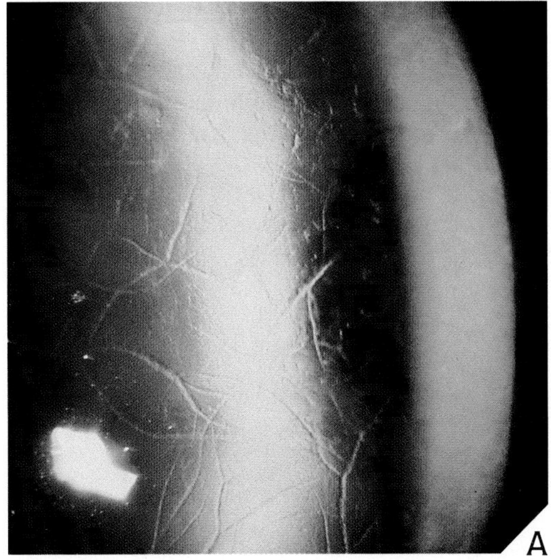

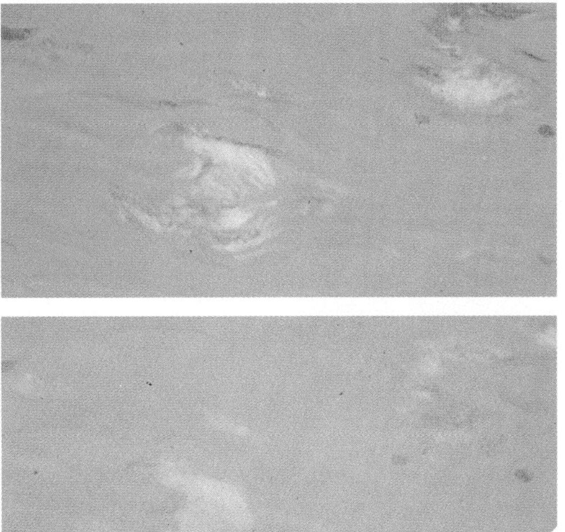

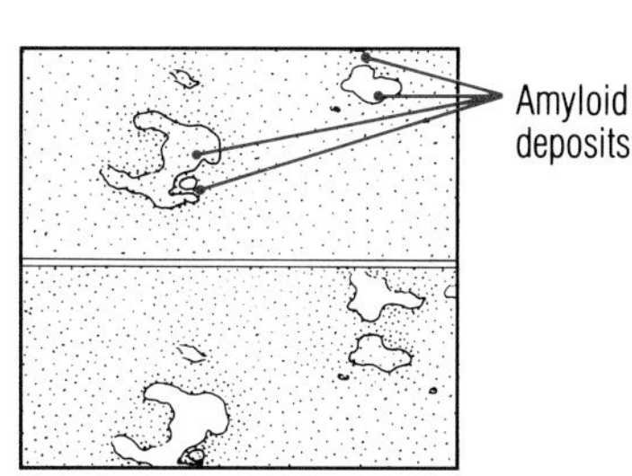

FIGURE 8.33 LATTICE DYSTROPHY. A The lattice network is apparent in the corneal stroma. Three types of lattice corneal dystrophy (LCD) exist: LCD type I, childhood onset; LCD type II, associated with Meretoja syndrome; LCD type III, adult onset; and a variant of III, LCD type IIIA. **B** Histologic section shows positive staining with Congo red and positive birefringence. The color of the birefringence changes as the polarizer is moved 90° (bottom). Stains for acid mucopolysaccharides are negative, whereas the trichrome and PAS stains are positive. The condition is inherited as an autosomal-dominant trait. (**A**, courtesy of Dr. JH Krachmer; **B**, Congo red, polarized; **A, B**, from Yanoff M, Fine BS: *Ocular Pathology*, 3rd ed.)

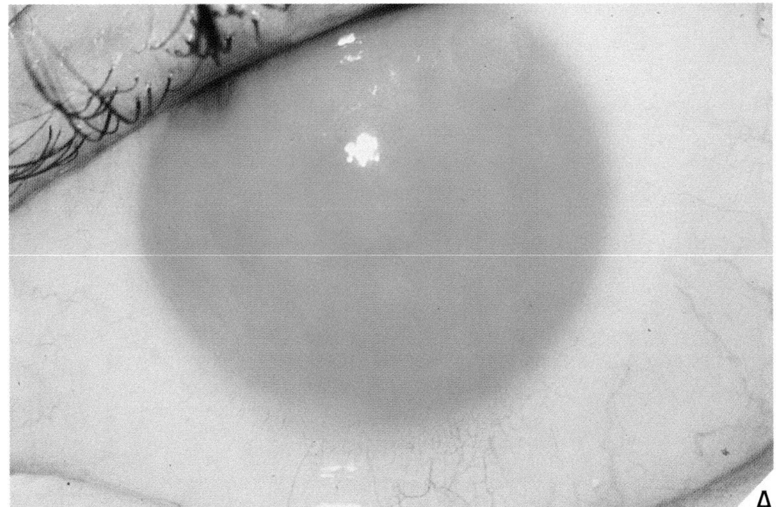

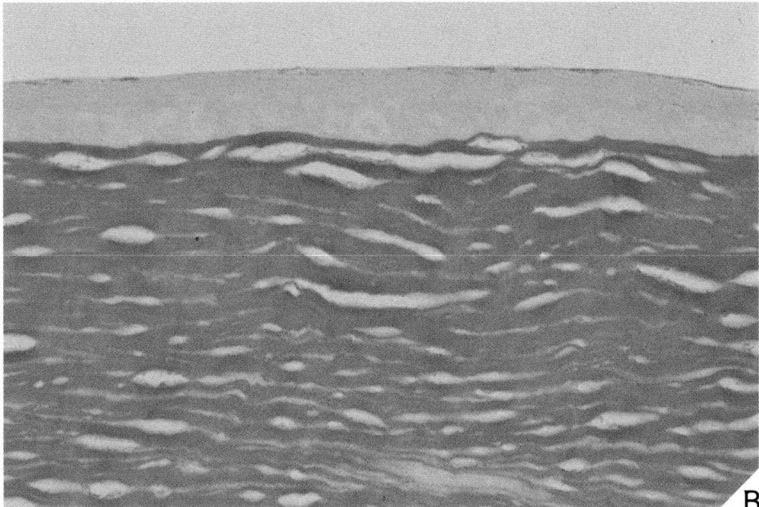

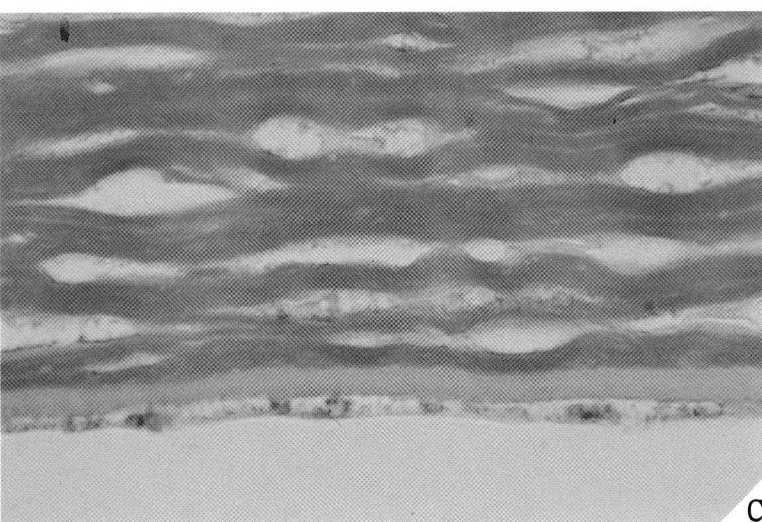

FIGURE 8.34 ACID MUCOPOLYSACCHARIDOSES. A The cornea is diffusely clouded in a case of Hurler-Scheie syndrome. **B** Histologic section of a case of Maroteaux-Lamy syndrome shows acid mucopolysaccharides deposited in epithelial cells, in stromal keratocytes, and **C** in endothelial cells.(**B, C**, AMP; **A**, courtesy of Dr. HG Scheie; **B, C**, courtesy of Dr. GOS Naumann.)

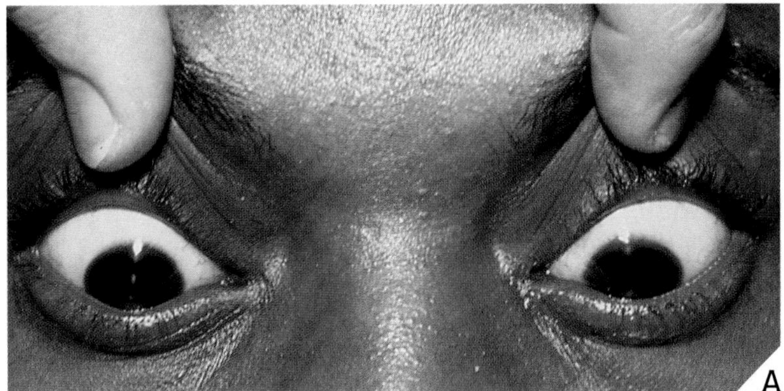

FIGURE 8.35 KERATOCONUS. A When the patient looks down, the cone in each eye causes the lower lids to bulge (Munson sign). **B** Histologic section shows the central thinning of the cornea. **C** Increased magnification of the central cone shows stromal scarring and breaks in the Bowman membrane. **D** A brown Fleischer ring is noted in the cornea at the level of the epithelium, seen in the blue light. **E** Histologic section shows that the ring is caused by a deposition of iron in the corneal epithelium. Note the typical thinning of the cornea in the region of the cone to the right of the iron deposition. (**B**, PAS; **E**, Perl stain.)

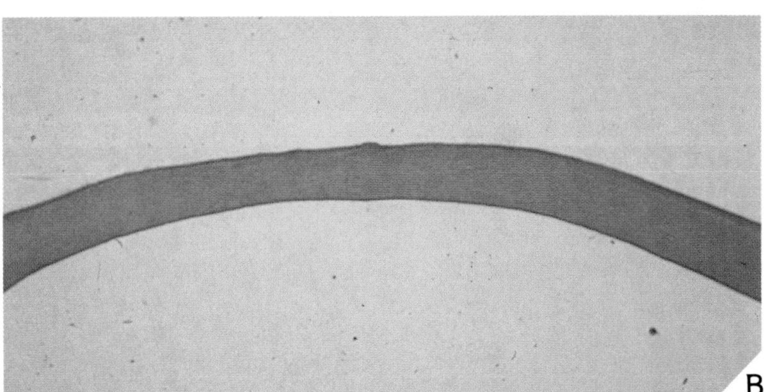

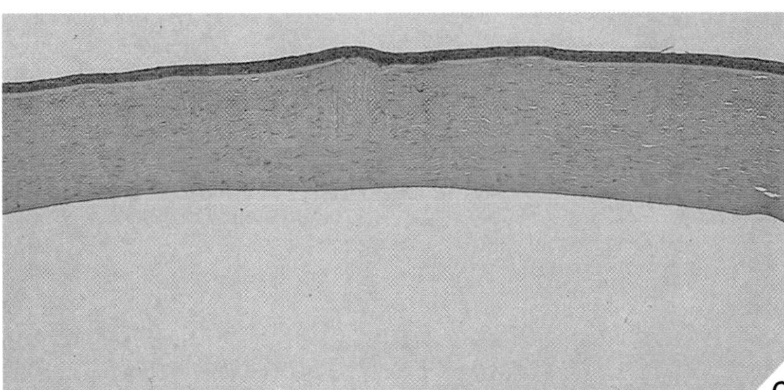

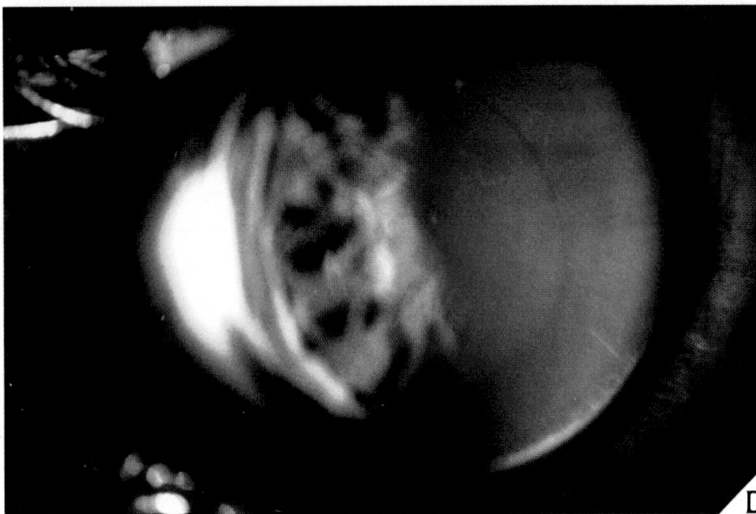

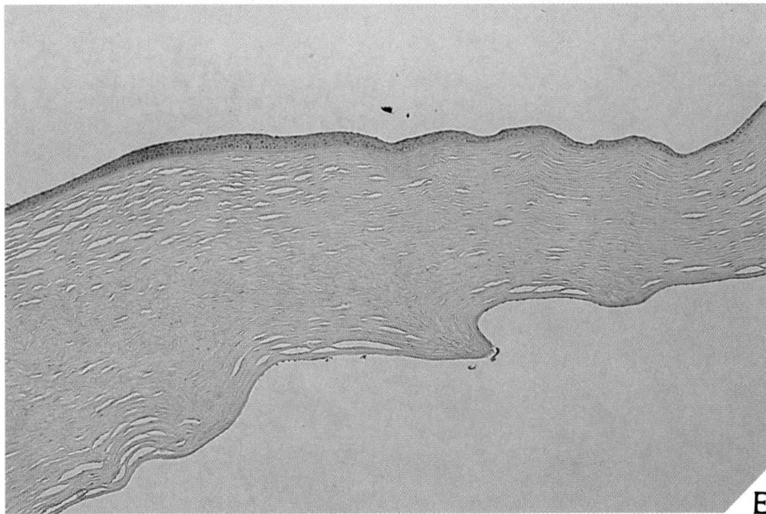

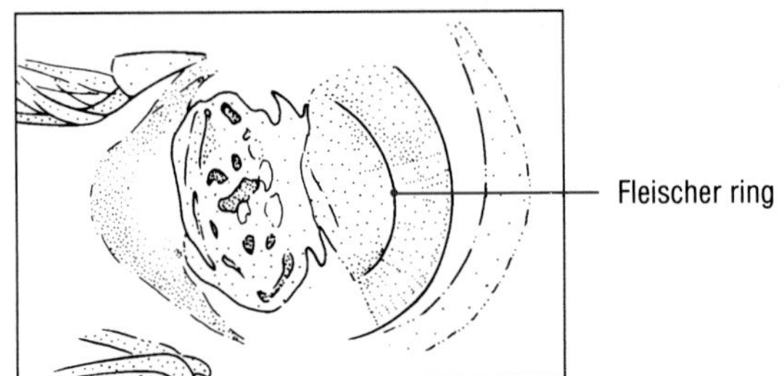

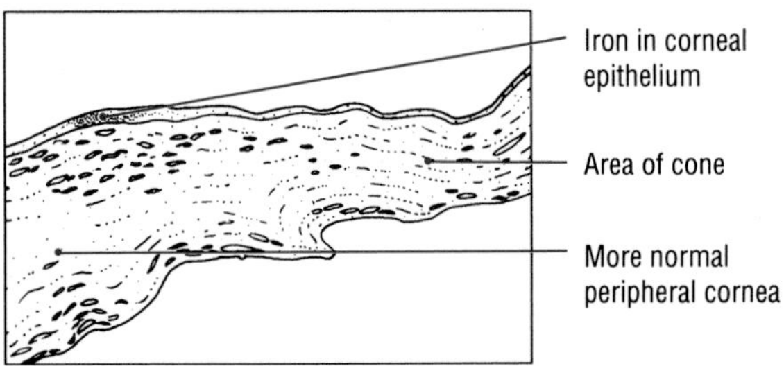

ENDOTHELIAL DYSTROPHIES

Cornea guttata (Fuchs)
Posterior polymorphous dystrophy
Congenital hereditary endothelial dystrophy (CHED)
Nonguttate corneal endothelial degeneration

FIGURE 8.36

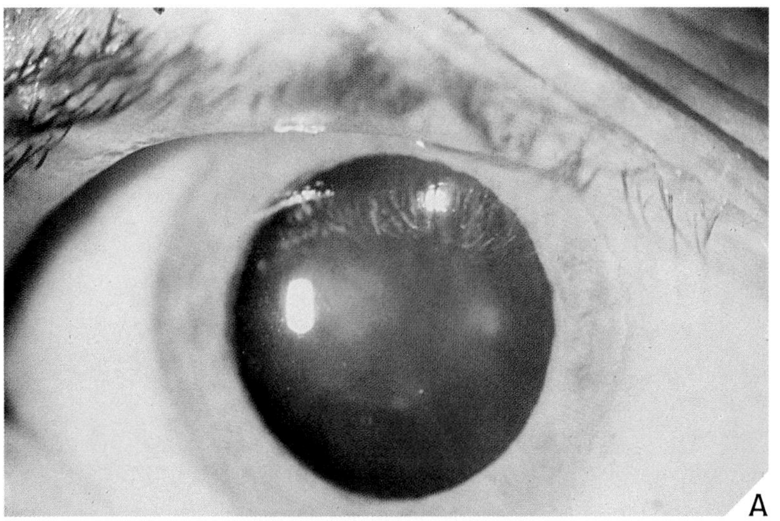

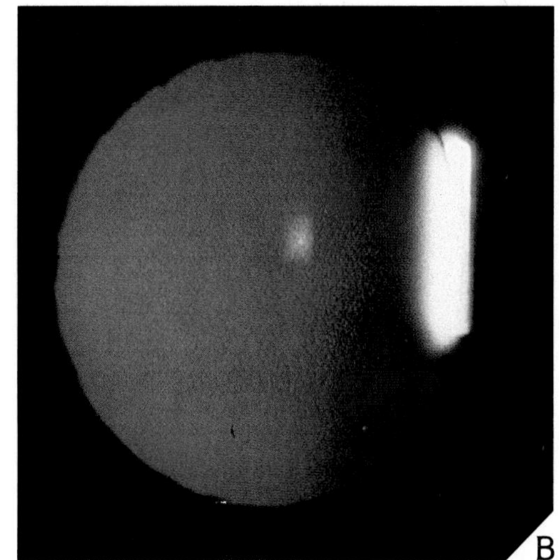

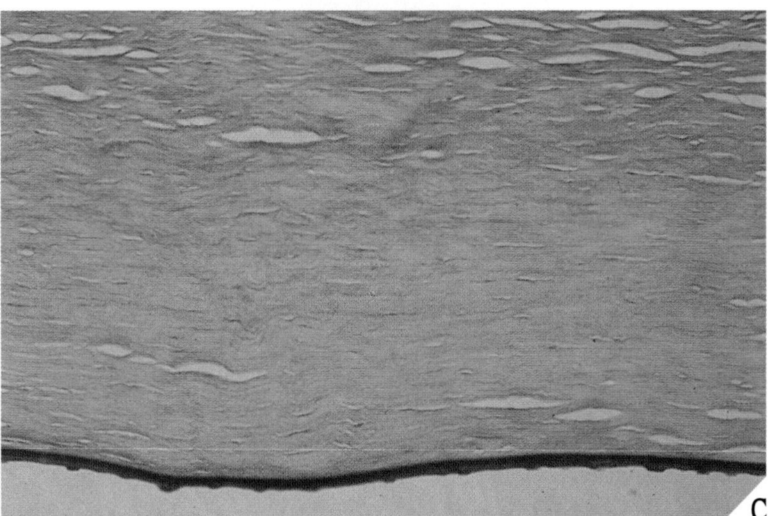

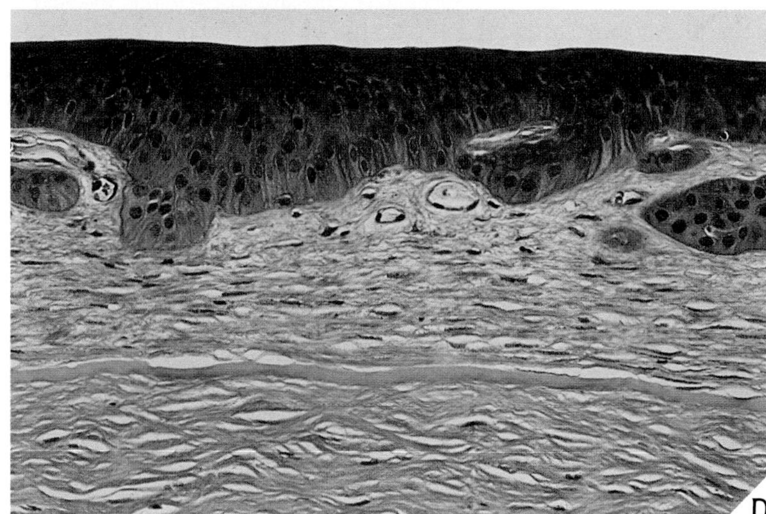

Figure 8.37 Cornea Guttata. **A** The cornea shows central thickening and haze. **B** The characteristic appearance of cornea guttata is shown in the fundus reflex. **C** Typical wart-like bumps are present on the Descemet membrane. The primary endothelial defect leads to secondary epithelial, subepithelial, and stromal edema and to degeneration. The epithelial edema may spread between and under the epithelial cells, resulting in bleb formation (bullous keratopathy). **D** Fibrous tissue has formed between the epithelium and the Bowman membrane, forming a degenerative pannus. (**B**, from Yanoff M, Fine BS: *Ocular Pathology*, 3rd ed.; **C**, PAS stain; **D**, trichrome stain.)

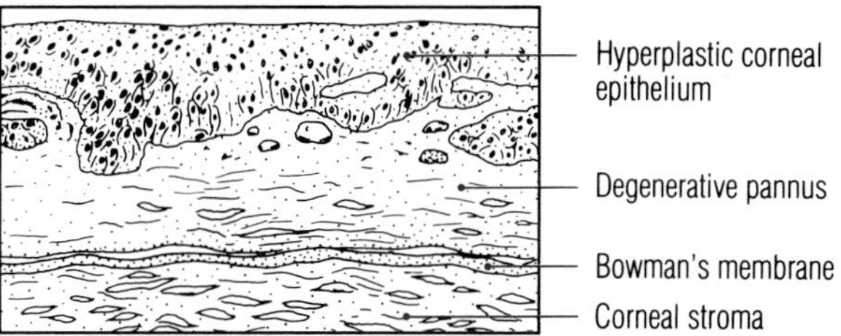

PIGMENTATIONS

Melanin

Blood

Iron lines
Fleischer ring (keratoconus)
Hudson-Stahli line (palpebral fissure)
Stocker line (pterygium)
Ferry line (filtering bleb)

Kayser-Fleischer ring

Tattoo

Drug-induced

Silver (see Fig. 7.20)

Figure 8.38

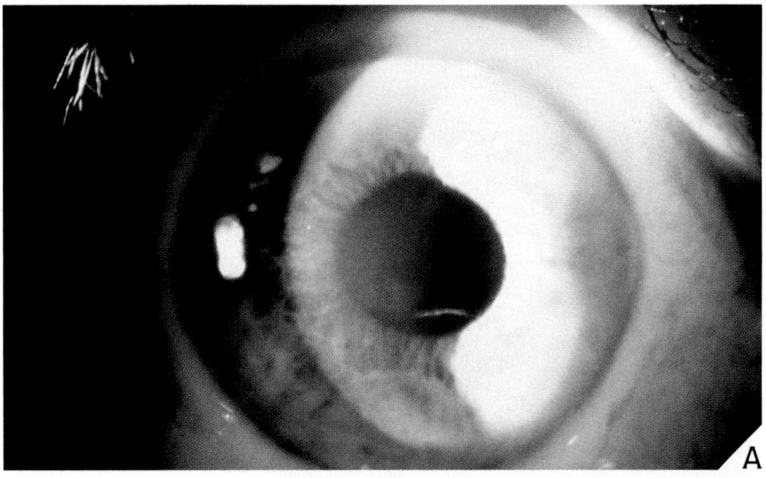

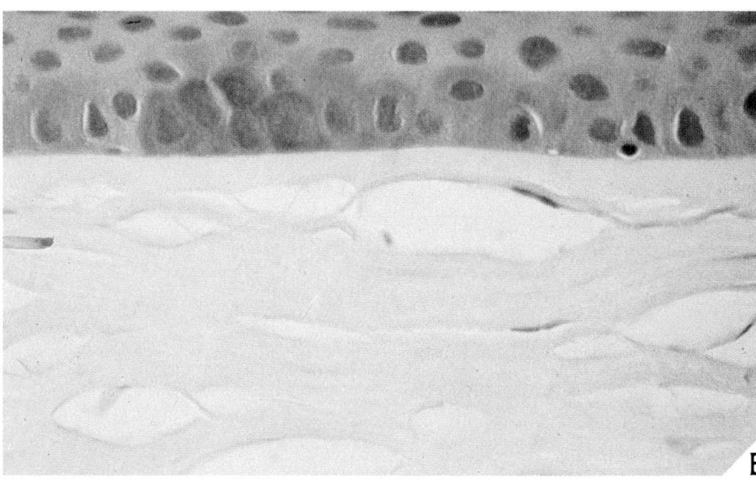

FIGURE 8.39 HUDSON-STAHLI LINE. A A curved horizontal brown line is seen just below the central cornea (lower pupillary space) within the epithelium. **B** Histologic section shows that the line is caused by iron deposition within the epithelium. The other iron lines (Fleischer, Stocker, and Ferry) have a similar histologic appearance. (**B**, Perl stain.)

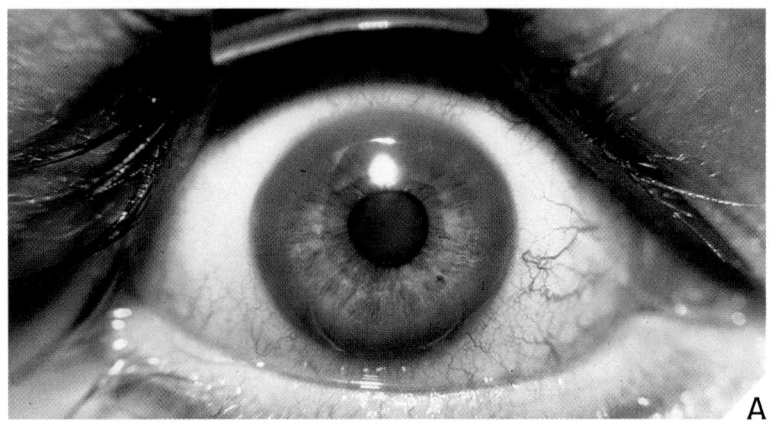

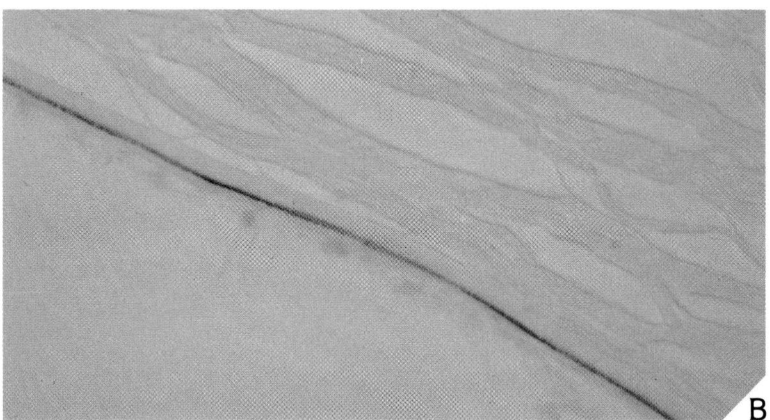

FIGURE 8.40 KAYSER-FLEISCHER RING. A The deposition of copper in the Descemet membrane peripherally causes a brown color that obstructs the view of the underlying iris, especially superiorly. A "sunflower" cataract is seen in the lens. **B** An unstained histologic section shows the deposition of copper in the inner portion of the Descemet membrane. A similar deposition of copper in the inner portion of the lens capsule centrally, both anteriorly and posteriorly, results in the sunflower cataract. (**A**, courtesy of Dr. MOM Tso; case in **A, B** reported in Tso MOM et al., 1975.)

CORNEAL AND CONJUNCTIVAL CRYSTALS

Bietti dystrophy (cornea and retina)
Chronic renal failure
Cystinosis (cornea, conjunctiva, and retina)
Dieffenbachia plant
Drugs (gold, chlorpromazine, chloroquine, clofazimine)
Dysproteinemias (gammopathies, malignant lymphomas, multiple myeloma)
Gout
Hypercalcemia
Keratitis (*Streptococcus*)
Lipid keratopathy
Schnyder corneal dystrophy

FIGURE 8.41

SCLERA

Congenital anomalies
Blue sclera
Ochronosis

Inflammations
Episcleritis
Anterior scleritis
Posterior scleritis

Tumors
Fibrous
Nodular fasciitis
Hemangiomas
Neurofibromas
Contiguous tumors
Episcleral osseous choristoma
Ectopic lacrimal gland

FIGURE 8.42

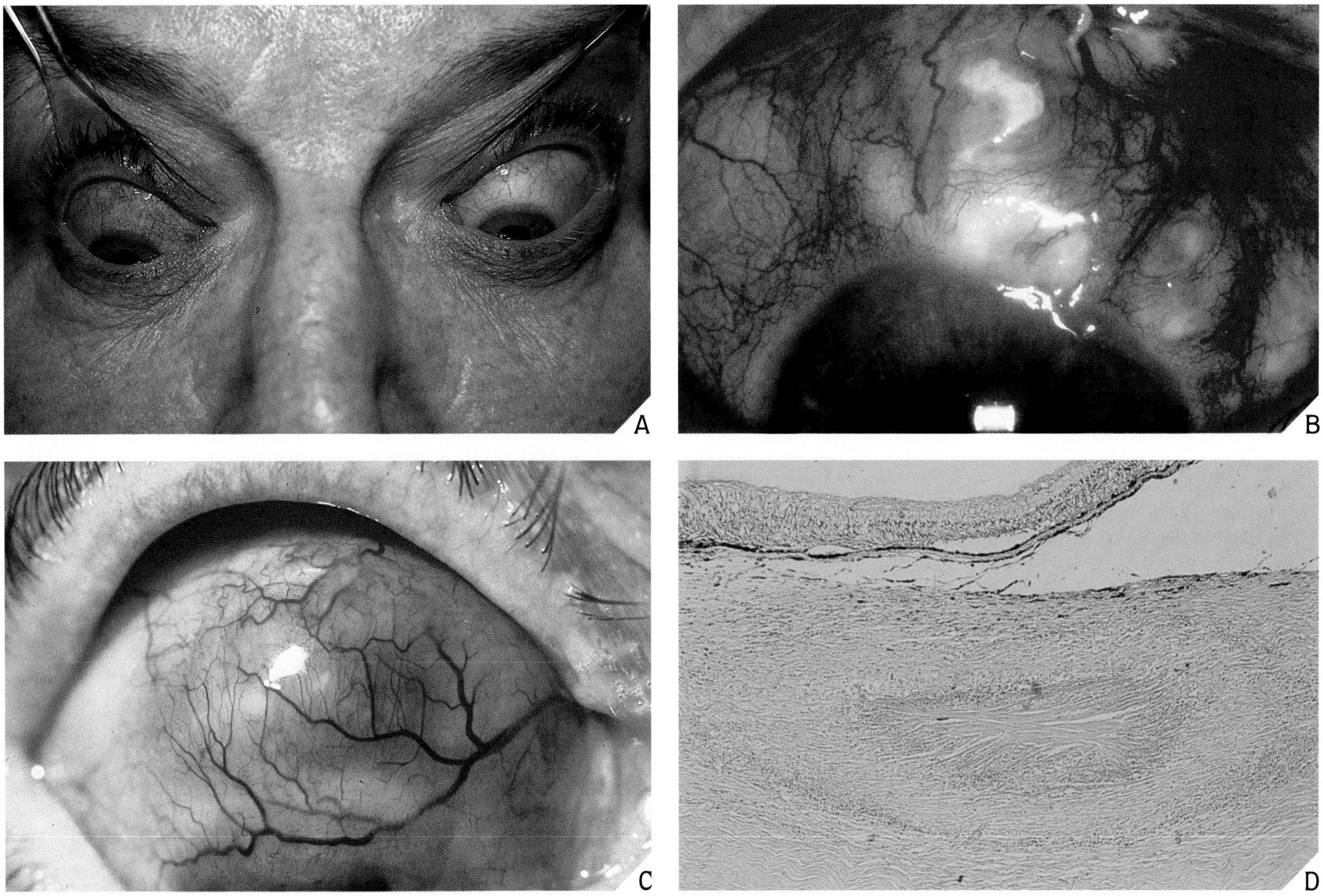

FIGURE 8.43 SCLERITIS. Scleritis can go on to **A** thickening (brawny scleritis) and **B** necrosis. **C** Healing of the necrotic area leads to scleromalacia perforans. **D** Histologic section shows a zonal granulomatous reaction around necrotic scleral collagen. (**D**, presented by Dr. IW McLean to the AFIP Alumni, 1973.)

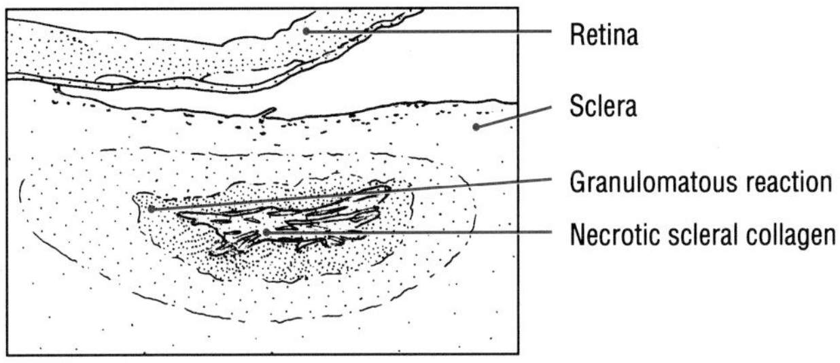

Retina
Sclera
Granulomatous reaction
Necrotic scleral collagen

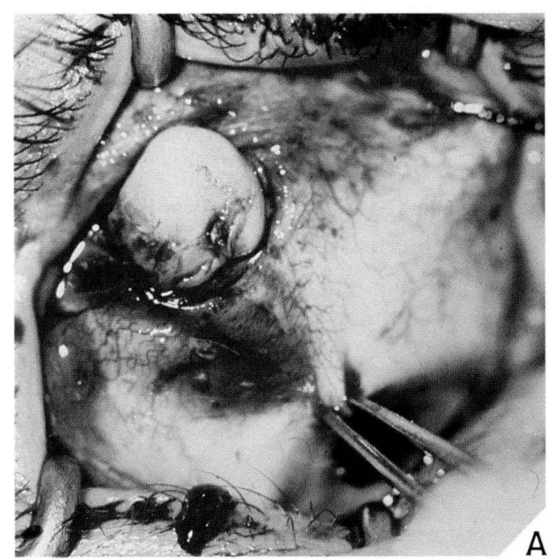

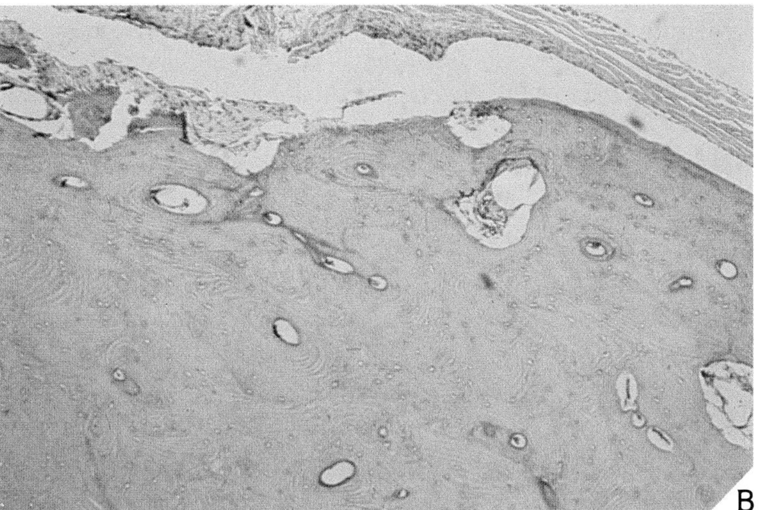

FIGURE 8.44 EPISCLERAL OSSEOUS CHORISTOMA. **A** The tumor, exposed at surgery, is located in its characteristic position, superotemporally. **B** Histologic section shows compact bone. (**B**, reported in Ortiz JM, Yanoff M, 1979.)

Bibliography

Benson WE: Posterior scleritis. Surv Ophthalmol 32:297, 1988.

Brooks AM, Grant G, Gillies WE: Differentiation of posterior polymorphous dystrophy from other posterior opacities by specular microscopy. Ophthalmology 96:1639, 1989.

Cogan DG, Kuwabara T: Arcus senilis. Its pathology and histochemistry. Arch Ophthalmol 61:353, 1959.

Contreras F, Pereda J: Congenital syphilis of the eye with lens involvement. Arch Ophthalmol 96:1052, 1978.

Eagle RE Jr, Laibson PR, Arensten JJ: Epithelial abnormalities in chronic corneal edema: a histopathological study. Trans Am Ophthalmol Soc 87:107, 1989.

Edward DP, et al: Macular dystrophy of the cornea. A systemic disorder of keratan sulfate metabolism. Ophthalmology 97:1194, 1990.

Fine BS, Yanoff M, Pitts E, Slaughter FD: Meesmann's epithelial dystrophy of the cornea. Report of two families with discussion of the pathogenesis of the characteristic lesion. Am J Ophthalmol 83:633, 1977.

Font RL, Sobol W, Matoba A: Polychromatic corneal and conjunctival crystals secondary to clofazamine therapy in a leper. Ophthalmology 96:311, 1989.

Holbach LM, Font RL, Naumann GOH: Herpes simplex stromal and endothelial keratitis. Granulomatous cell reactions at the level of Descemet's membrane, the stroma, and Bowman's layer. Ophthalmology 97:722, 1990.

Kincaid MC, Fouraker BD, Schanzlin DJ: Infectious crystalline keratophay after relaxing incisions. Am J Ophthalmol 111:374, 1991.

Kornmehl EW, et al: Bilateral keratitis in Lyme disease. Ophthalmology 96:1194, 1989.

Krachmer JH, Feder RS, Belin MW: Keratoconus and related noninflammatory corneal thinning disorders. Review. Surv Ophthalmol 28:293, 1984.

Lee C-F, et al: Immunohistochemical studies of Peters' anomaly. Ophthalmology 96:958, 1989.

Lipman RM, Rubenstein JB, Torczynski E: Keratoconus and Fuchs' corneal dystrophy in a patient and her family. Arch Ophthalmol 108:993, 1990.

Mansour AM, et al: Ocular choristomas. Surv Ophthalmol 33:339, 1989.

Mansour AM, et al: Ocular findings in the facioauriculovertebral sequence (Goldenhar-Gorlin syndrome). Am J Ophthalmol 100:555, 1985.

Matta CS, et al: Climatic droplet keratopathy with corneal amyloidosis. Ophthalmology 98:192, 1991.

Meisler DM, Fine M: Recurrence of the clinical signs of lattice corneal dystrophy (Type I) in corneal transplants. Am J Ophthalmol 97:210, 1984.

Naumann G: Clearing of cornea after perforating keratoplasty in mucopolysaccharidosis type VI (Maroteaux-Lamy syndrome). N Engl J Med 312:995, 1985.

Naumann GOH, Küchle M: Unilateral arcus lipoides corneae with traumatic cyclodialysis in two patients. Arch Ophthalmol 107:1121, 1989.

Ormerod LD, et al: Infectious crystalline keratopathy. Role of nutritionally variant streptococci and other bacterial factors. Ophthalmol 98:159, 1991.

Ortiz JM, Yanoff M: Epipalpebral conjunctival osseous choristoma. Br J Ophthalmol 63:173, 1979.

Pepose JS, et al: Mononuclear cell phenotypes and immunoglobulin gene rearrangements in lacrimal gland biopsies from patients with Sjögren's syndrome. Ophthalmology 97:1599, 1990.

Pflugfelder SC, et al: Conjunctival cytologic features of primary Sjögren's syndrome. Ophthalmology 97:985, 1990.

Rao NA, Marak GE, Hidayat AA: Necrotizing scleritis. A clinicopathologic study of 41 cases. Ophthalmology 92: 1542, 1985.

Richler M, et al: Ocular manifestations of nephropathic cystinosis. The French-Canadian experience in a genetically homogeneous population. Arch Ophthalmol 109:359, 1991.

Rodriques MM, et al: Disorders of the corneal epithelium—a clinicopathologic study of dot, geographic and fingerprint patterns. Arch Ophthalmol 92:475, 1974.

Rodriques MM, Gaster RN, Pratt MV: Unusual superficial confluent form of granular cornea dystrophy. Ophthalmology 90:1507, 1983.

Scheie HG, Shannon RE, Yanoff M: Onchocerciasis (ocular). Ann Ophthalmol 3:697, 1971.

Scheie HG, Yanoff M: Peters anomaly and total posterior coloboma of retinal pigment epithelium and choroid. Arch Ophthalmol 87:525, 1972.

Semba RD, et al: Longitudinal study of lesions of the posterior segment in onchocerciasis. Ophthalmology 97:1334, 1990.

Sharma S, Srinivasan M, George C: *Acanthamoeba* keratitis in non-contact lens wearers. Arch Ophthalmol 108:676, 1990.

Shields MB, et al: Axenfeld-Rieger syndrome. A spectrum of developmental disorders. Review. Surv Ophthalmol 29:387, 1985.

Stein R, Lazar M, Adam A: Brittle cornea. A familial trait associated with blue sclera. Am J Ophthalmol 66:67, 1968.

Steul K-P, et al: Paraprotein corneal deposits in plasma cell myeloma. Am J Ophthalmol 111:312, 1991.

Stock EL, et al: Lattice corneal dystrophy type IIIA. Clinical and histologic correlations. Arch Ophthalmol 109:354, 1991.

Suan EP, et al: Corneal perforation in patients with vitamin A deficiency in the United States. Arch Ophthalmol 108:350, 1990.

Tso MOM, Fine BS, Thorpe HE: Kayser-Fleischer ring and associated cataract in Wilson's disease. Am J Ophthalmol 79:479, 1975.

Zaidman GW, et al: The histopathology of filamentary keratitis. Arch Ophthalmol 103:1178, 1985.

Uvea

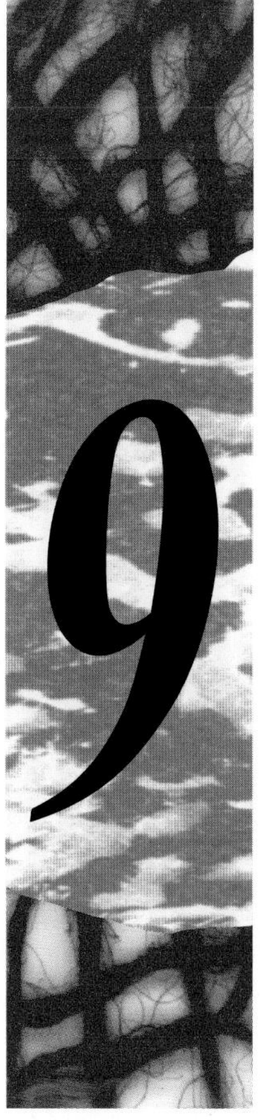

The uvea is composed of the iris, the ciliary body, and the choroid. The iris is a circular diaphragm that separates the anterior from the posterior chamber. The iris can be subdivided from pupil to ciliary body into three zones: pupillary, mid, and iris root. From front to back it can be divided into a thin anterior border layer, the stroma (the bulk of the iris), the partially pigmented anterior pigment epithelium (which contains the dilator muscle), and the completely pigmented posterior pigment epithelium. The sphincter muscle, like the dilator muscle and pigment epithelium, is of neuroectodermal origin and lies as a ring in the pupillary stroma.

The ciliary body is divisible into an anterior ring, the pars plicata, and a wider posterior ring, the pars plana. From outside (toward the sclera) to inside it can be divided into the suprachoroidal (potential) space, the ciliary muscle, a layer of vessels, the external basement membrane, the outer pigmented and inner nonpigmented epithelium, and the internal basement membrane.

The choroid, the largest part of the uvea, is divided from outside to inside into the suprachoroidal (potential) space and lamina fusca; the choroidal stroma (which contains uveal melanocytes, fibrocytes, collagen, blood vessels, and nerves); the choriocapillaris; and the outer aspect of the Bruch membrane.

Congenital and developmental defects may involve any part of the uveal tract. The defects may be as simple as a persistent pupillary membrane or as complex as some colobomas of the choroid that contain contiguous orbital cystic structures. The uveal anomaly may be associated with systemic findings, such as in the Miller oculocerebrorenal syndrome in which Wilms tumor, genitourinary anomalies, and aniridia are found.

Inflammation of the uvea is quite common. The specific entities have been discussed in the appropriate chapters on nongranulomatous (Chapter 3) and granulomatous (Chapter 4) inflammations.

Systemic diseases often affect the uvea. Perhaps the most common association is with diabetes mellitus. In addition, juvenile xanthogranuloma (JXG), which is found mainly in children under 6 months of age, characteristically involves the iris and may cause a spontaneous hyphema. When confronted with an infant who has a spontaneous hyphema, one must consider JXG, retinoblastoma (iris neovascularization here can cause bleeding into the anterior chamber), and trauma (histories are unreliable in infants and, although the parent may think the hemorrhage was spontaneous, it could have been caused by trauma).

Many atrophies and degenerations affect the uvea. Macular degeneration, one of the leading causes of blindness, is described separately in Chapter 11.

The uvea may be involved in a number of dystrophies. Most of these are inherited. Our knowledge of both the underlying causes and the pathology of these entities is still in its infancy.

The most common primary malignant tumor of the eye is the malignant melanoma found in the choroid. Melanomas will be described separately with pigmented tumors of the eye (Chapter 17). Other tumors can arise from the pigment epithelium, from the mesenchymal tissue of the uvea, from the vascular tissue, and so forth. Some of the more important examples are shown below. In addition to primary tumors of the uvea, systemic tumors may involve the uvea secondarily, e.g., as metastases or in multifocal entities such as leukemias and lymphomas.

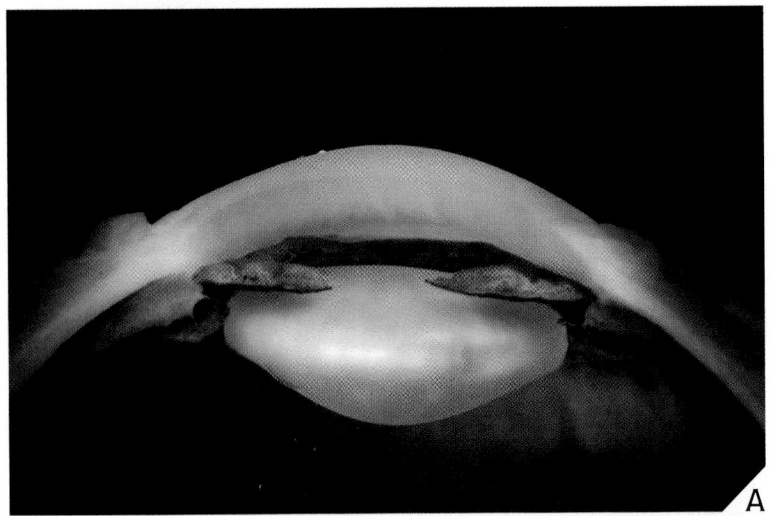

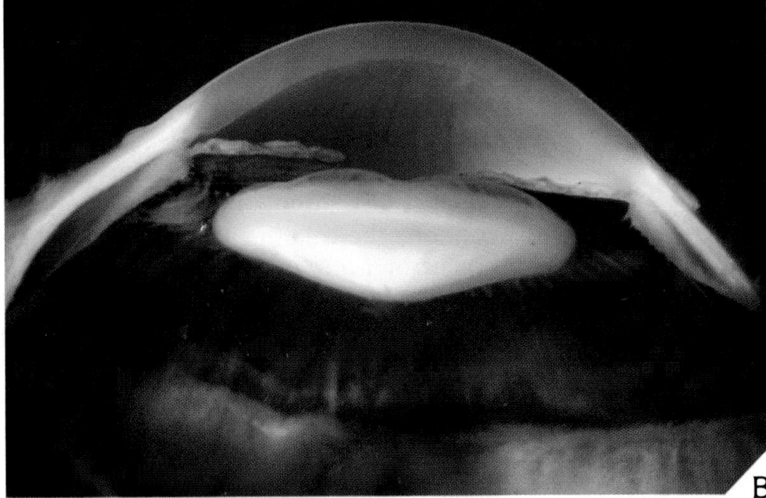

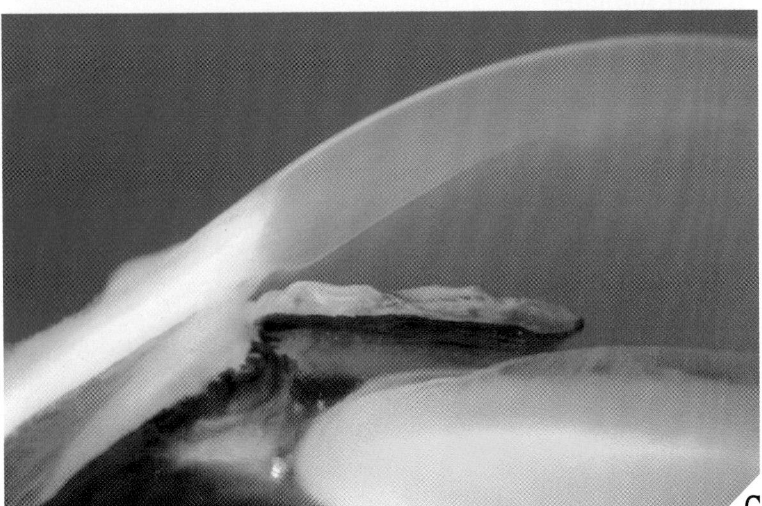

FIGURE 9.1 IRIS AND CILIARY BODY. A, B The iris is lined posteriorly by its pigment epithelium and anteriorly by the avascular anterior border layer. The bulk of the iris is made up of vascular stroma. Considerable pigment is present in the anterior border layer and stroma in the brown iris (**A**), as contrasted to little pigment in the blue eye (**B**). The iris pigment epithelium is maximally pigmented in both **A** and **B**; the color of the iris, therefore, is determined only by the amount of pigment in the anterior border layer and stroma. **A,B,C** The ciliary body is wedge-shaped and has a flat anterior end, continuous with the iris root, and a pointed posterior end, continuous with the choroid. (**A–C**, courtesy of Dr. RC Eagle Jr.)

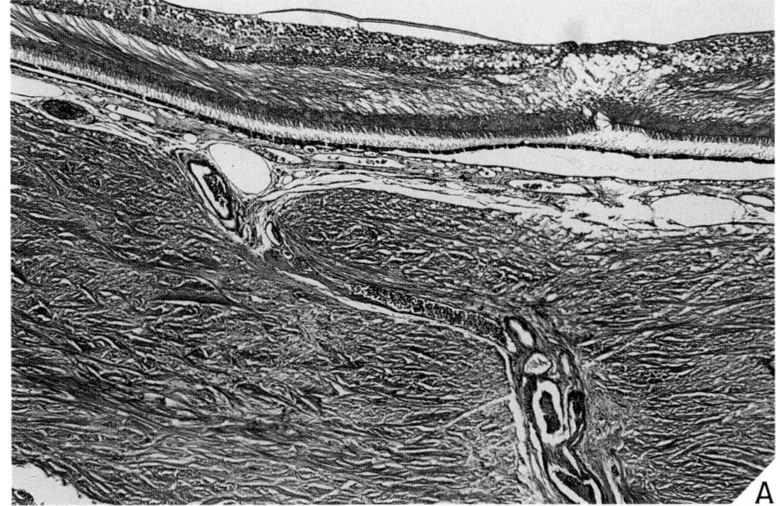

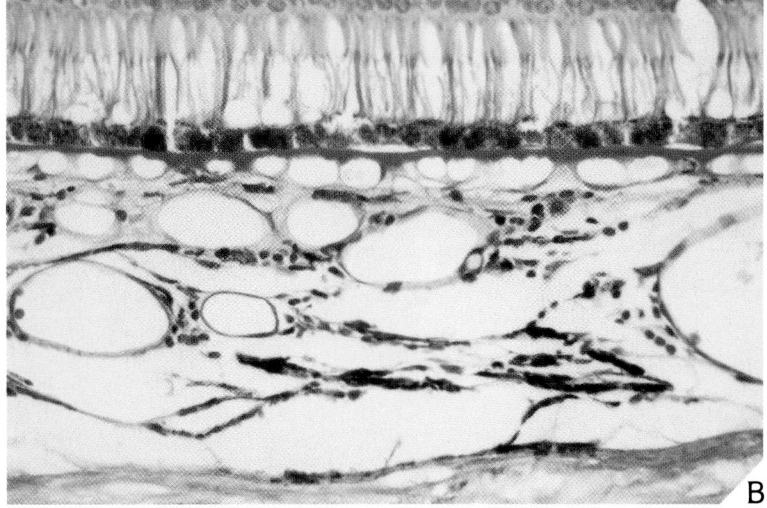

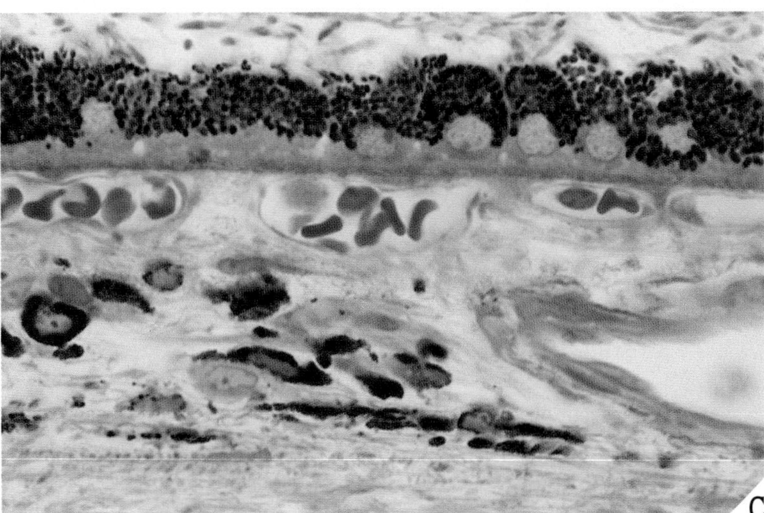

FIGURE 9.2 CHOROID. A The choroid lies between the sclera (blue in this trichrome stain) and the retinal pigment epithelium. Uveal tissue spills out into most scleral canals, as into this scleral canal of the long posterior ciliary artery. **B** The choroid is composed of, from outside to inside, the suprachoroidal (potential) space and lamina fusca; the choroidal stroma, which contains uveal melanocytes, fibrocytes, collagen, blood vessels, and nerves; the fenestrated choriocapillaris; and the outer aspect of the Bruch membrane. **C** Whereas the normal capillary in the body is large enough for only one erythrocyte to pass through, the capillaries of the choriocapillaris, the largest capillaries in the body, permit passage of numerous erythrocytes. The choriocapillaris' basement membrane and associated connective tissue compose the outer half of the Bruch membrane, while the inner half is composed of the basement membrane and associated connective tissue of the retinal pigment epithelium. Note that the pigment granules are larger in the retinal pigment epithelial cells than the uveal melanocytes (also see Fig. 17.1**C**).

CONGENITAL ABNORMALITIES

- Persistent pupillary membrane (if minor, considered a normal finding)
- Persistent tunica vasculosa lentis
- Heterochromia iridis
- Hematopoiesis (normal finding in infant)
- Ectopic lacrimal gland
- Hypoplasia of iris
- Dysgenesis of cornea and iris
- Coloboma
- Cyst (see Fig. 2.14**B**)

FIGURE 9.3

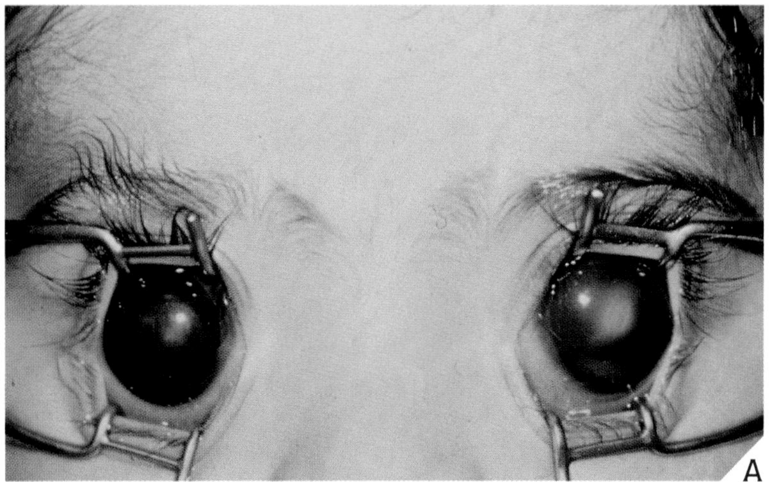

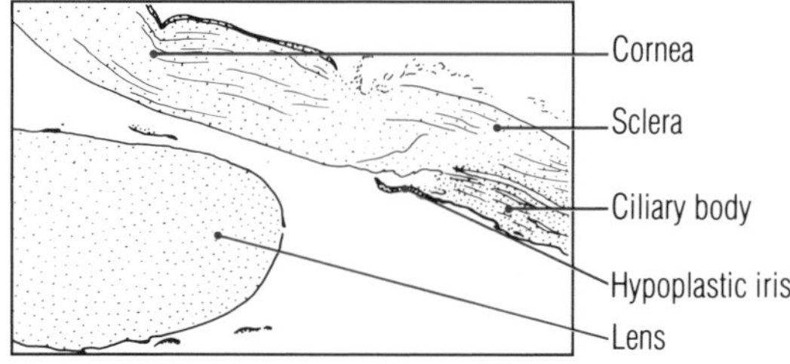

Figure 9.4 Aniridia. A This child has bilateral aniridia and glaucoma. **B** A histologic section of another case shows that true aniridia is not present, but rather a marked hypoplasia of the iris is indicated by the rudimentary iris. True aniridia does not exist; seen clinically, "apparent aniridia" always is found histologically to be hypoplasia (hypoiridia). The condition of apparent aniridia may be associated with glaucoma, as in **A** and **B** or with Wilms tumor (caused by deletion of chromosome 11p13), which did not occur in this case. (**B**, courtesy of Dr. HG Scheie, from Yanoff M, Fine BS: *Ocular Pathology*, 3rd ed.)

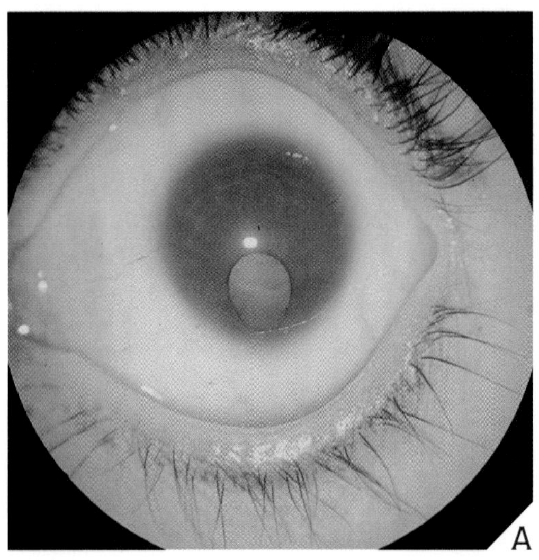

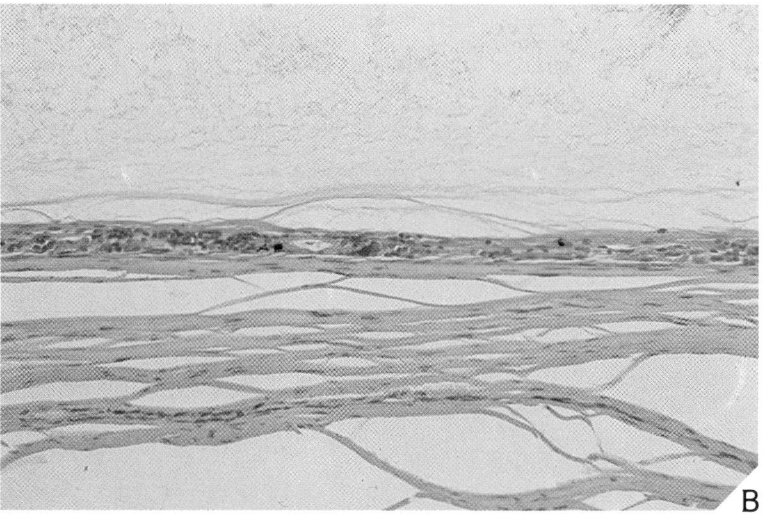

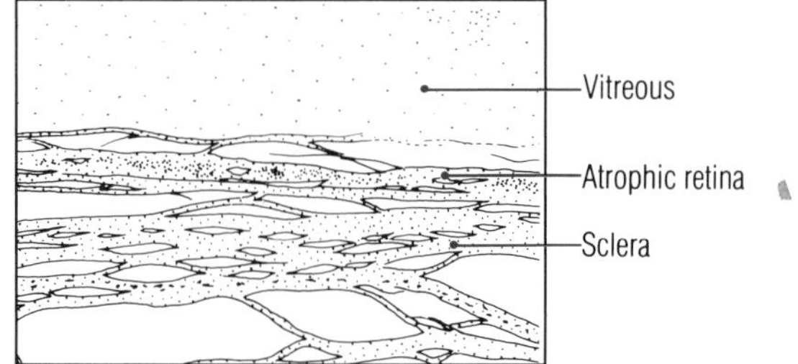

Figure 9.5 Coloboma of Iris and Choroid. A The patient is looking down, causing the light reflex to be centered in the choroidal coloboma, resulting in a white pupillary reflex (leukokoria). Note the small cornea and the microphthalmic eye. **B** A histologic section of another case of choroidal coloboma shows that the major defect is an absence of the retinal pigment epithelium. The overlying neural retina is atrophic and the underlying choroid is absent, so that the retina lies directly on the sclera. (**A**, courtesy of Dr. RC Lanciano Jr.)

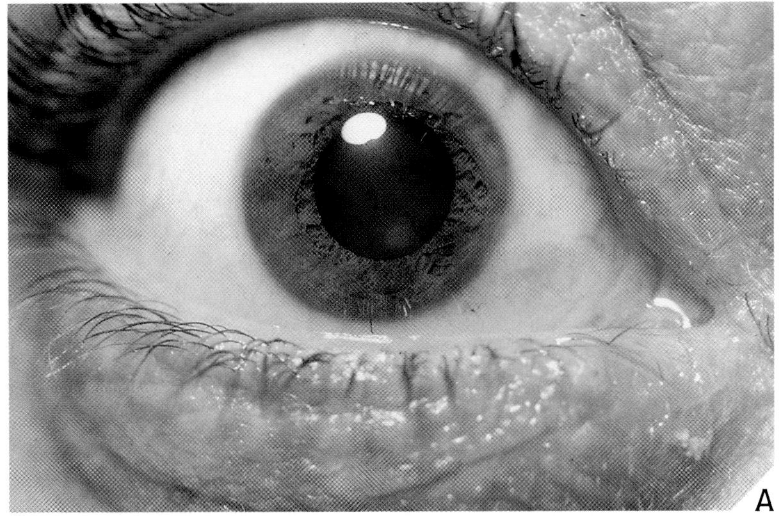

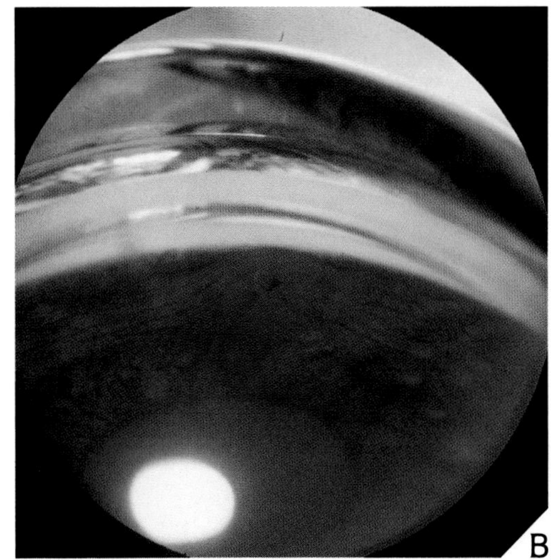

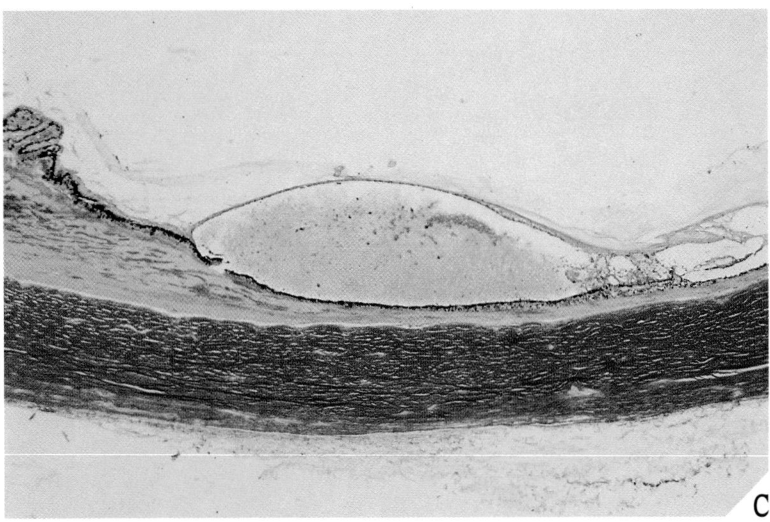

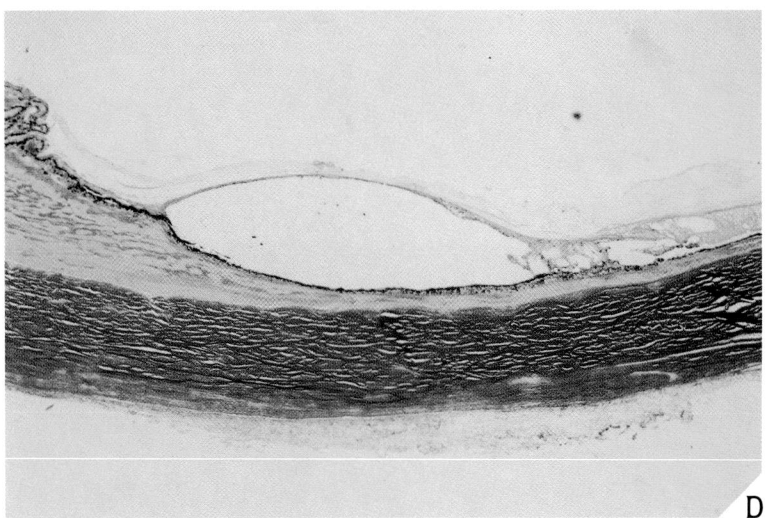

FIGURE 9.6 CYSTS OF THE IRIS AND CILIARY BODY. A A bulge is present in the iris from the 9- to 10-o'clock position. The stroma in this area is slightly atrophic. **B** Gonioscopic examination of the region clearly delineates a bulge caused by an underlying cyst of the pigment epithelium of the peripheral iris. **C** A histologic section of another case shows a large cyst of the pars plana of the ciliary body. A special stain, which stains acid mucopolysaccharides blue, shows that the material within the cyst stains positively. **D** If the section is first digested with hyaluronidase and then stained as in **C**, the cyst material is absent, demonstrating that the material is hyaluronic acid.

SYSTEMIC DISEASES

Diabetes mellitus
Vascular diseases
Cystinosis
Homocystinuria
Amyloidosis
Juvenile xanthogranuloma
Histiocytosis X (Langerhans granulomatoses)
Collagen diseases
Mucopolysaccharidoses

FIGURE 9.7

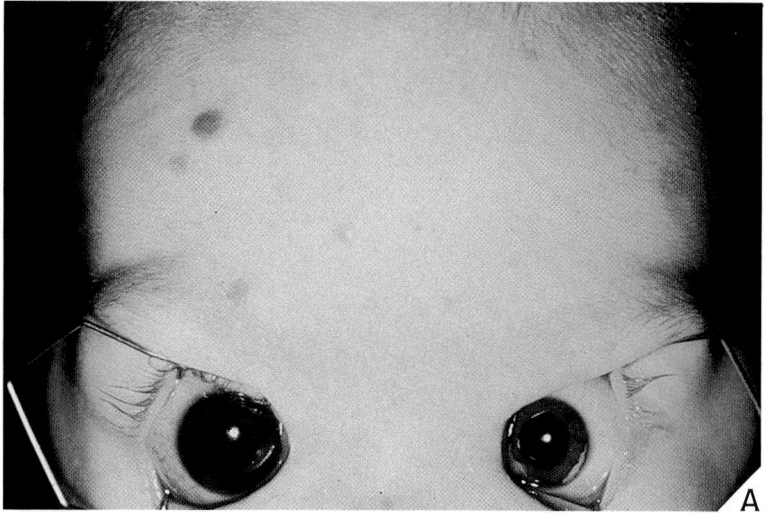

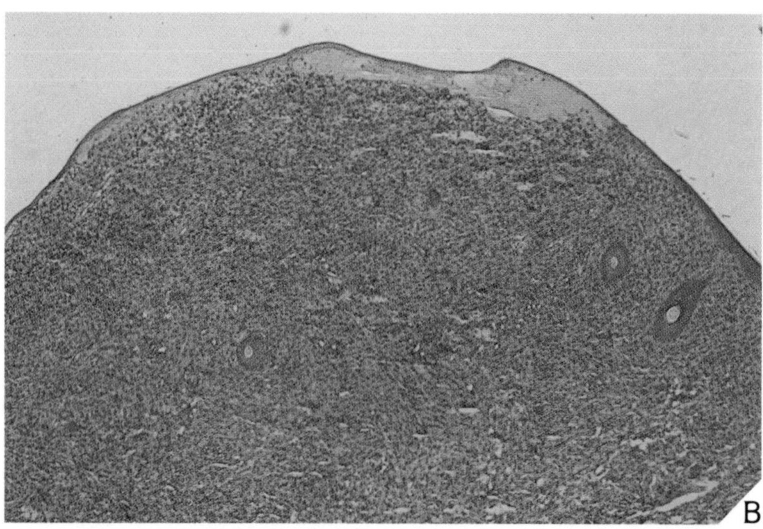

Figure 9.8 Juvenile Xanthogranuloma (JXG). A The patient has multiple orange skin lesions (note those on the right side of the patient's forehead), characteristic of JXG. Both eyes are involved. A spontaneous hyphema in the right eye has resulted in glaucoma and enlargement of the globe (buphthalmos). **B** Biopsy of the skin lesion shows that the dermis is largely replaced by histiocytes. The characteristic Touton giant cells were not found in these sections. However, the clinical picture and the histologic features were so characteristic that the diagnosis of JXG was not in doubt. (**B**, from Yanoff M, Fine BS: *Ocular Pathology*, 3rd ed.)

ATROPHIES AND DEGENERATIONS

Iris neovascularization (rubeosis iridis)
Choroidal folds

Figure 9.9

DYSTROPHIES

Iridocorneal endothelial (ICE) syndrome (see Chapter 16)

Iridoschisis

Choroidal dystrophies

Regional choroidal dystrophies
Central areolar choroidal sclerosis
Serpiginous degeneration
Malignant myopia

Diffuse choroidal dystrophies
Diffuse choriocapillaris atrophy
Gyrate atrophy
Choroideremia

Figure 9.10

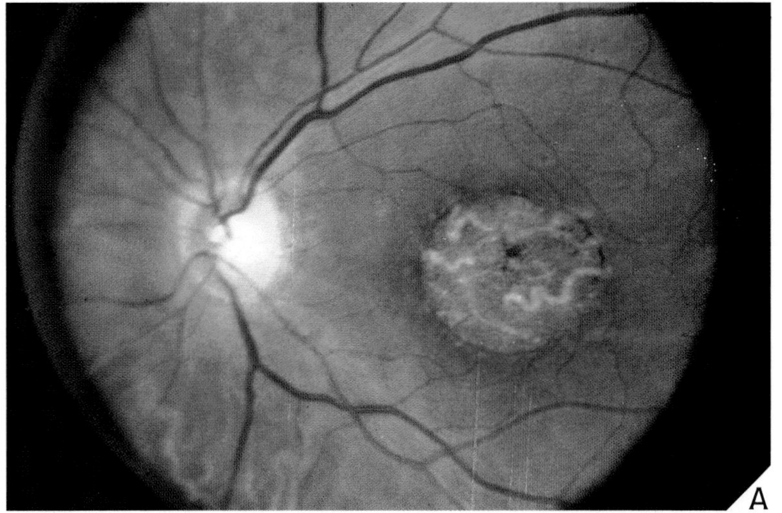

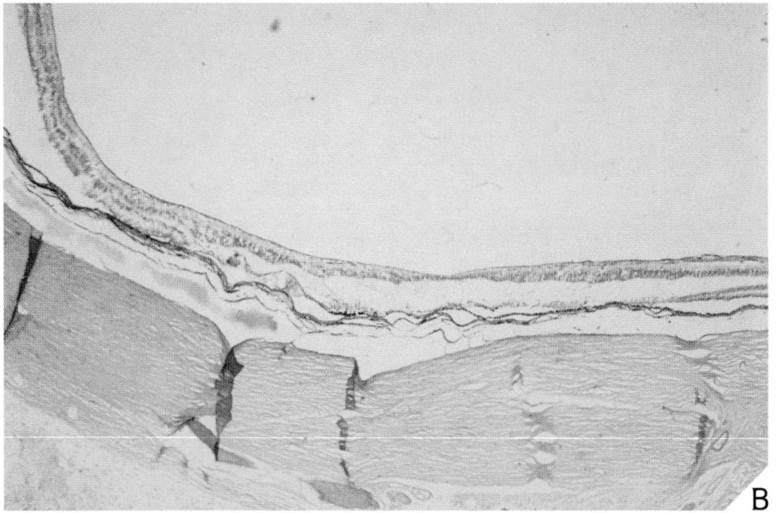

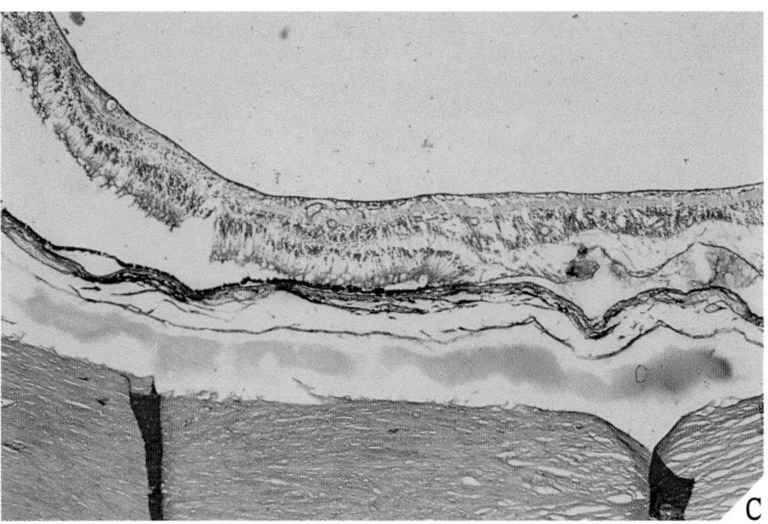

FIGURE 9.11 CENTRAL AREOLAR CHOROIDAL SCLEROSIS. A The patient has bilateral "punched-out" lesions of the macula. **B** A histologic section of another case shows loss of the pigment epithelium just temporal to the fovea (on the left side), shown under higher magnification in **C**. The photoreceptors are atrophic in the area of pigment epithelial loss. (**A**, courtesy of Dr. WE Benson, from Yanoff M, Fine BS: *Ocular Pathology,* 3rd ed.; **B**, **C**, presented by Dr. AP Ferry at the Eastern Ophthalmic Pathology Society, 1969 and reported in Ferry AP et al., 1972.)

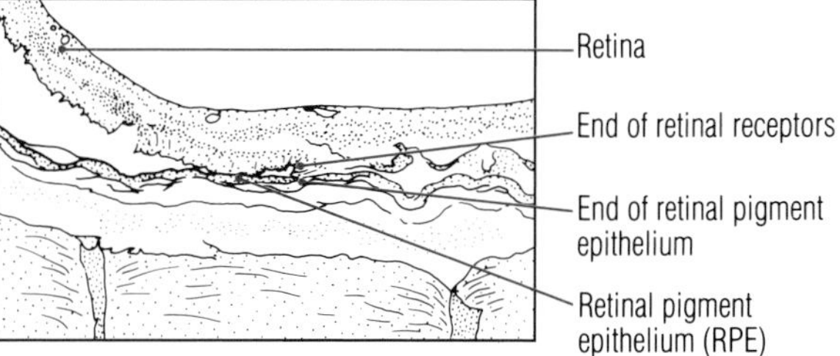

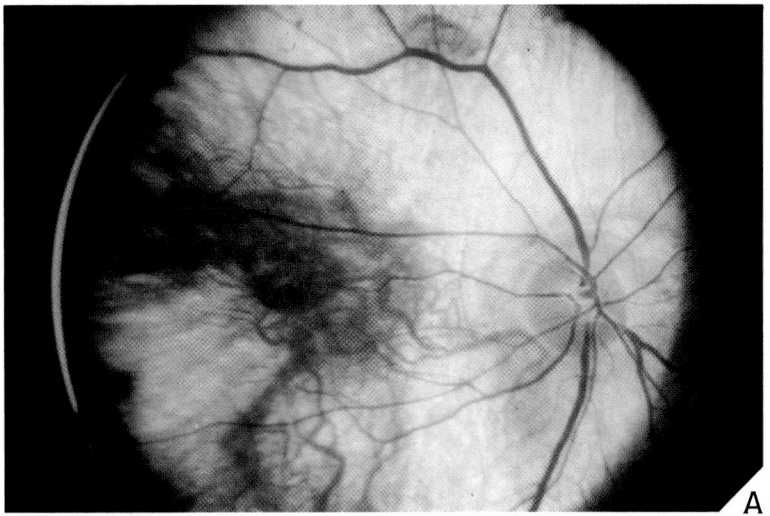

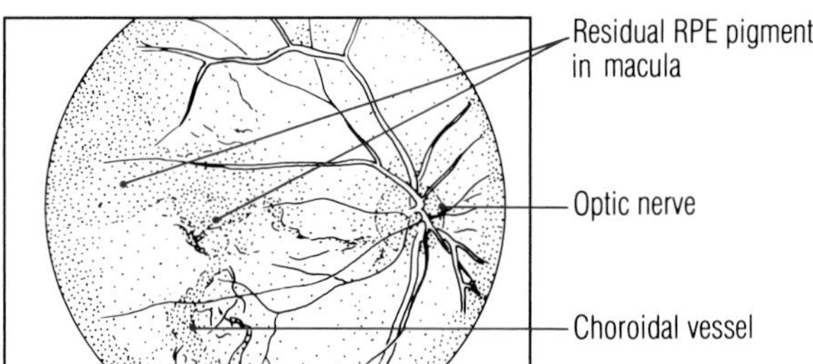

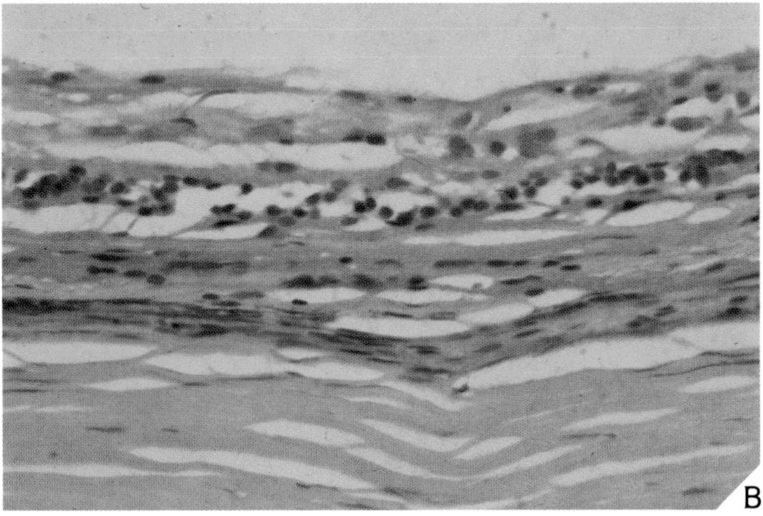

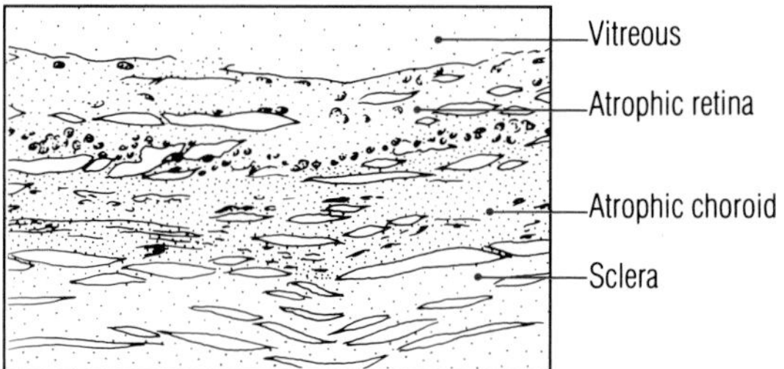

FIGURE 9.12 CHOROIDEREMIA. A Often in choroideremia a diffuse loss of the peripheral retinal pigment epithelium (RPE) occurs, leaving an island of RPE in the central macular region. **B** Histologic section of another case shows absence of RPE and atrophy of both the overlying retina and the underlying choroid. (**A**, courtesy of Dr. WE Benson, from Yanoff M, Fine BS: *Ocular Pathology*, 3rd ed.; **B**, presented by Dr. WS Hunter at the AOA-AFIP meeting, 1969.)

TUMORS

Epithelial
Hypertrophy of retinal pigment epithelium (RPE)
Hyperplasia of RPE
Benign epithelioma (adenoma) of Fuchs

Muscular
Leiomyoma
Rhabdomyosarcoma

Vascular
Hemangioma

Osseous
Osseous choristoma

Melanoma (see Chapter 17)

Leukemias and lymphomas (see Fig. 7.36)

Neural

Secondary neoplasms

FIGURE 9.13

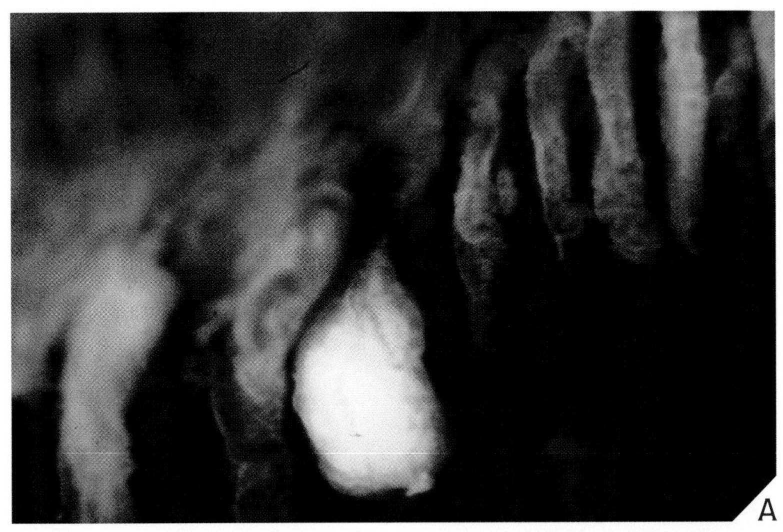

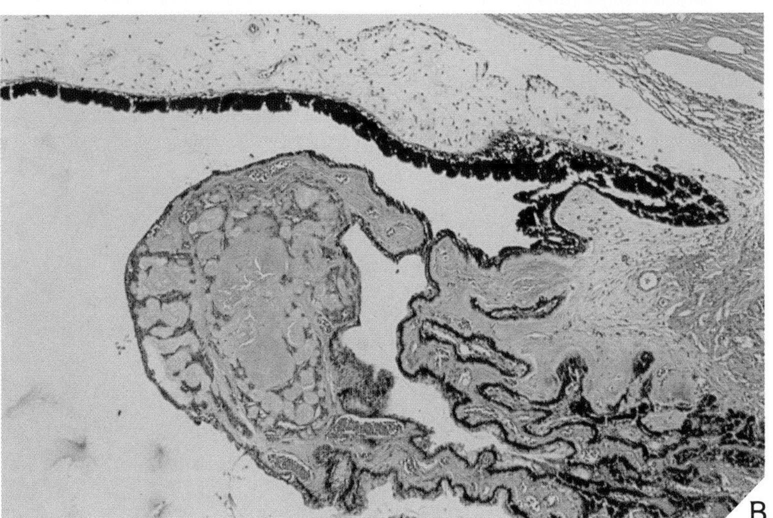

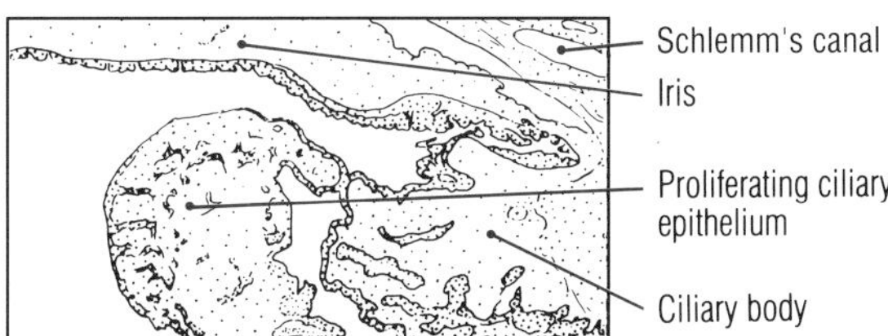

FIGURE 9.14 FUCHS ADENOMA. A The lesion is seen grossly as a white tumor within the pars plicata of the ciliary body. **B** Histologic section shows a proliferation of nonpigmented ciliary epithelium that is elaborating considerable basement membrane material. (**A**, from Yanoff M, Fine BS: *Ocular Pathology*, 3rd ed.)

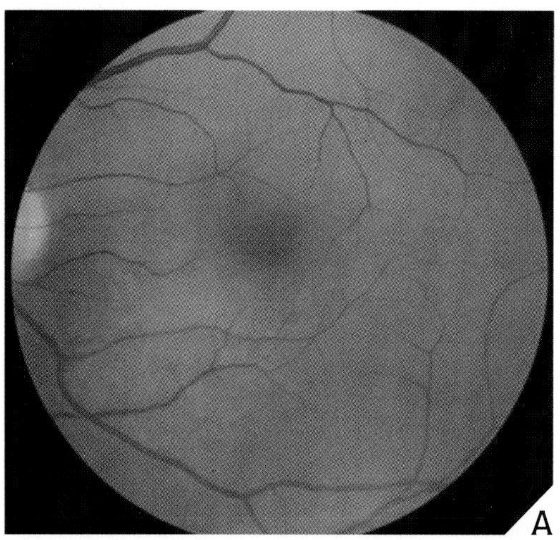

FIGURE 9.15 HEMANGIOMA. A An elevated lesion, which shows a characteristic orange color, is seen in the inferior nasal macular region. **B** A histologic section of another case shows a total retinal detachment and an extensive hemangioma of the choroid in the macular area. **C** Increased magnification of the temporal edge of the hemangioma shows it is blunted and well demarcated from the adjacent normal choroid to the left. **D** Similarly, the nasal edge of the hemangioma is blunted and easily demarcated from the adjacent choroid. This hemangioma was not associated with any systemic findings; in Sturge-Weber syndrome, the choroidal hemangioma is diffuse and not clearly demarcated from the adjacent choroid.

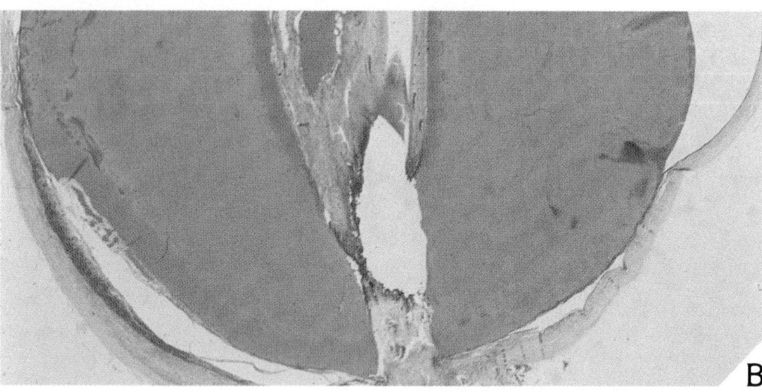

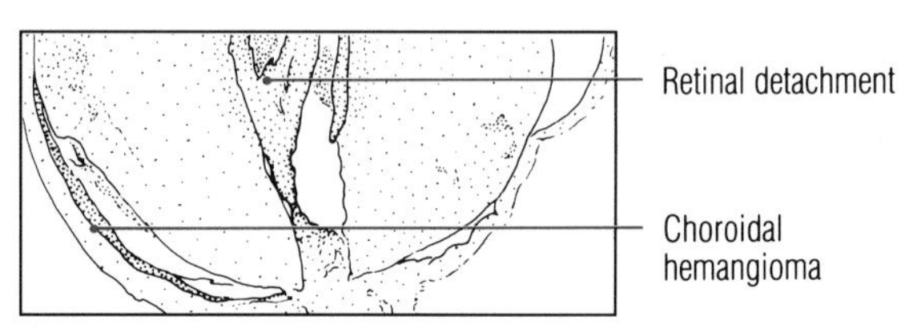

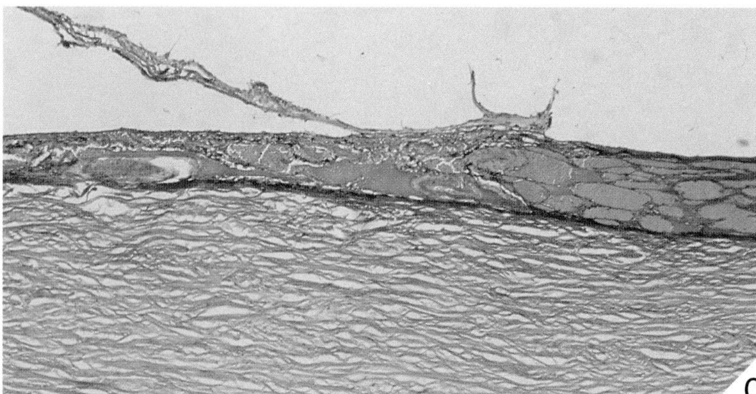

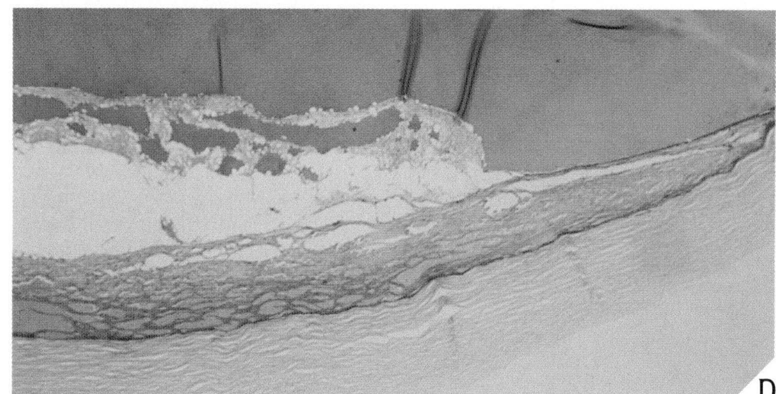

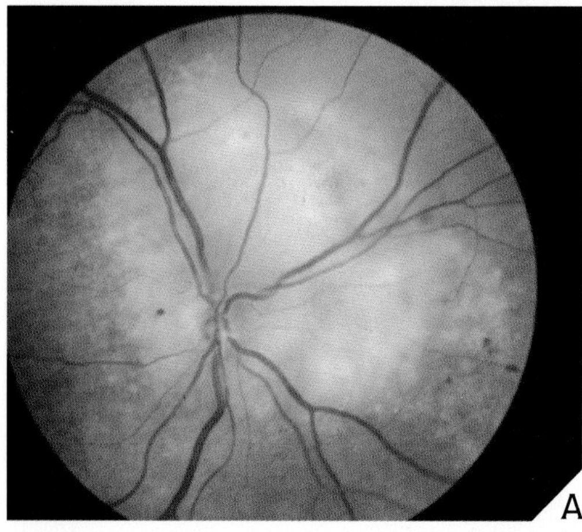

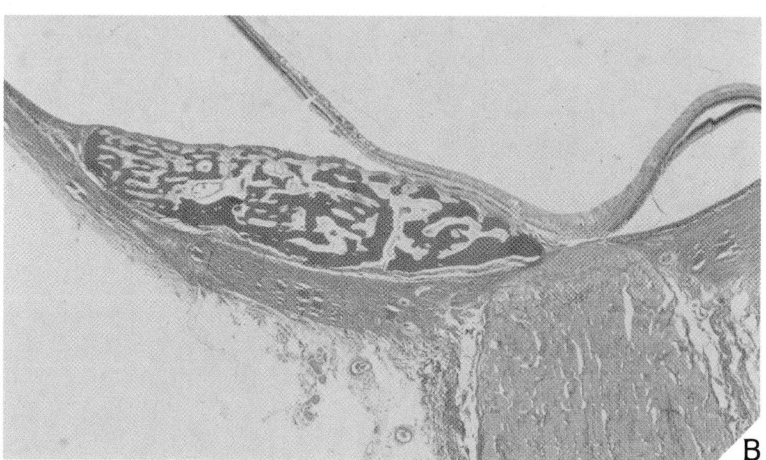

FIGURE 9.16 CHOROIDAL OSTEOMA. A The patient has an irregular, slightly elevated yellow-white juxtapapillary lesion. Ultrasound showed the characteristic features of bone in the choroid. **B** A histologic section of another case shows that the choroid is replaced by mature bone that contains marrow spaces. (**A**, courtesy of Dr. WE Benson, from Yanoff M, Fine BS: *Ocular Pathology*, 2nd ed.; **B**, presented by Dr. RL Font at the Eastern Ophthalmic Pathology Society, 1976.)

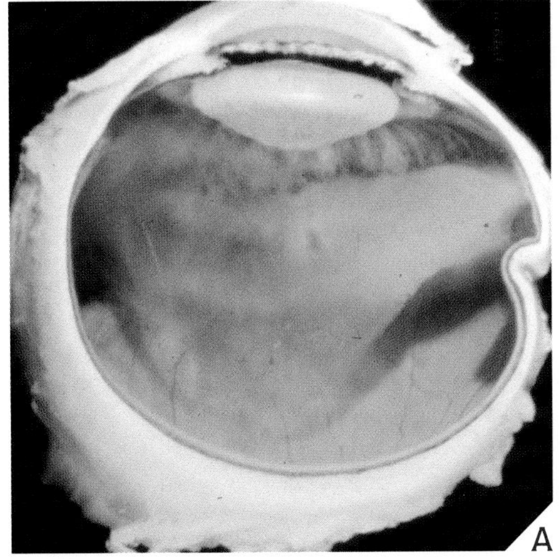

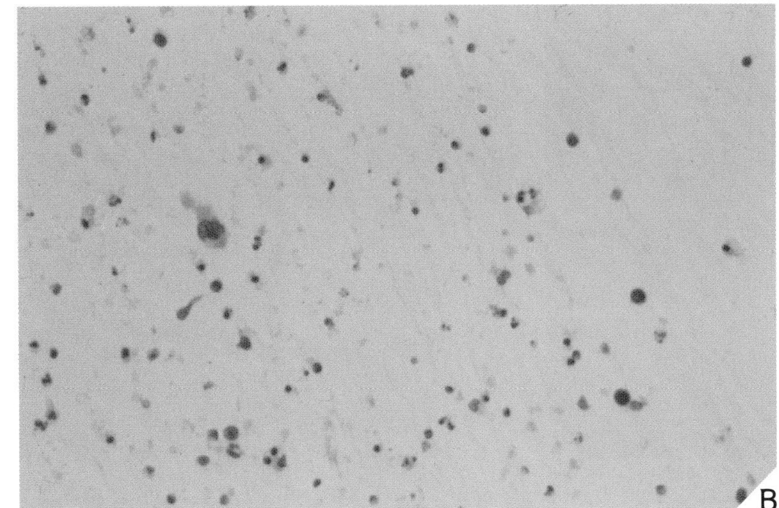

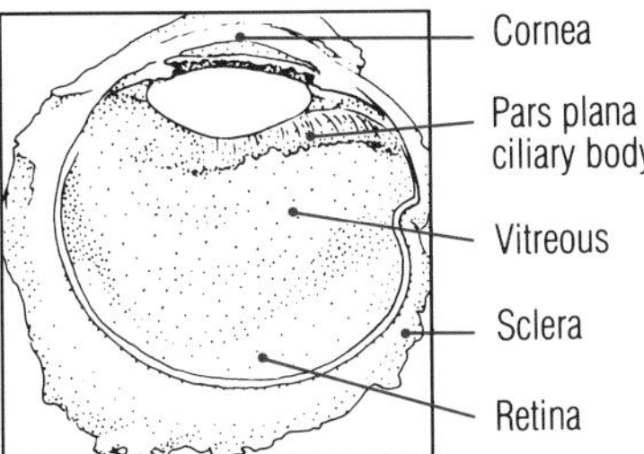

FIGURE 9.17 RETICULUM CELL SARCOMA. A The gross specimen shows a cloudy and prominent vitreous body. The patient had been treated for posterior uveitis in both eyes for over a year when symptoms of a central nervous system disorder developed. **B** The vitreous body contains cells that show pleomorphism and hyperchromatic nuclei. The cells are quite abnormal and malignant. Although the cells in this entity are not reticulum cells but lymphoblasts, the term reticulum cell sarcoma is still useful in evoking a clinical picture. (**A**, from Yanoff M, Fine BS: *Ocular Pathology*, 2nd ed.; case presented by Dr. M Yanoff at the Verhoeff Society Meeting, 1974.)

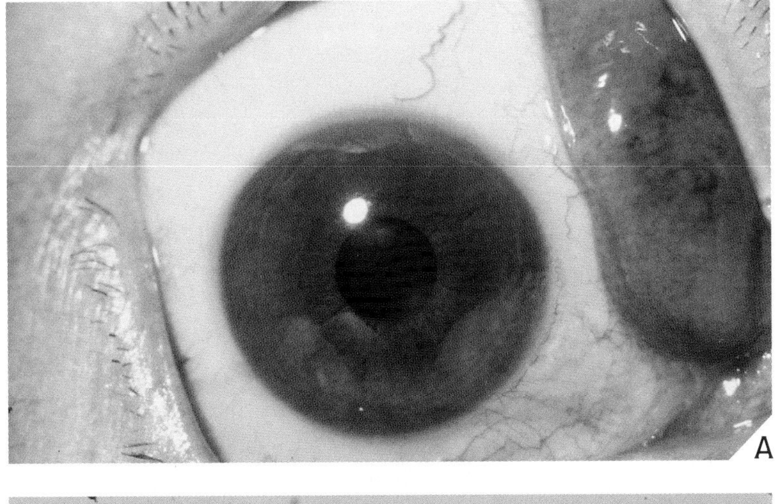

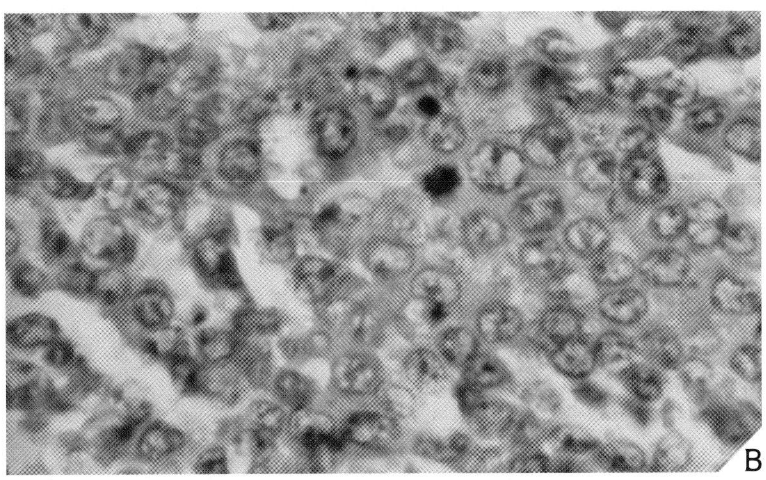

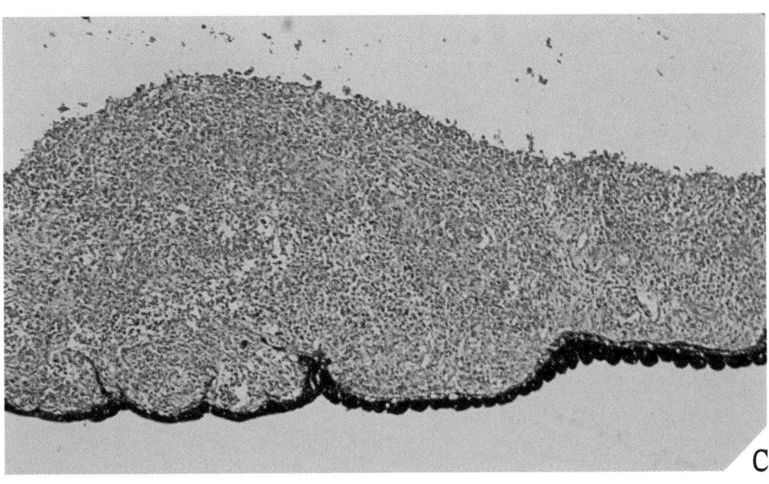

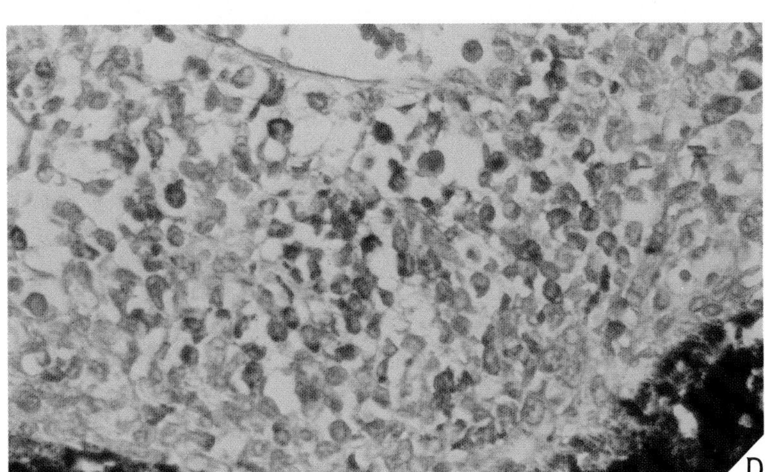

FIGURE 9.18 LEUKEMIA. A A patient presented with a large infiltrate of leukemic cells positioned nasally within the conjunctiva of the right eye, giving this characteristic clinical picture. These lesions look similar to those caused by benign lymphoid hyperplasia, lymphoma, or amyloidosis. **B** A biopsy of the lesion shows primitive blastic leukocytes. **C** In another case, the iris is infiltrated by leukemic cells. A special stain (Lader stain) shows that some of the cells stain red, better seen when viewed under increased magnification in **D**. This red positivity is characteristic of myelogenous leukemic cells.

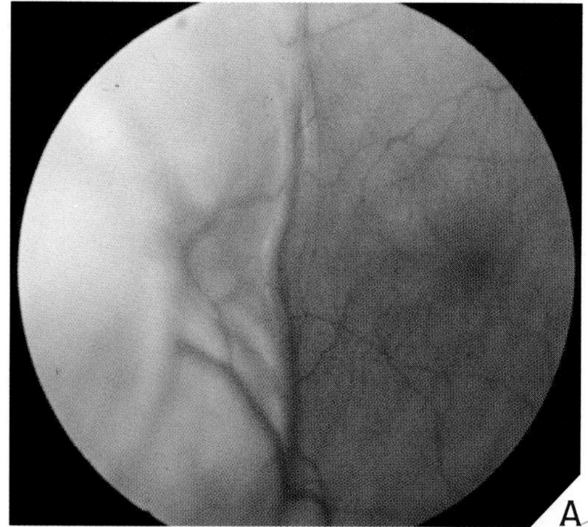

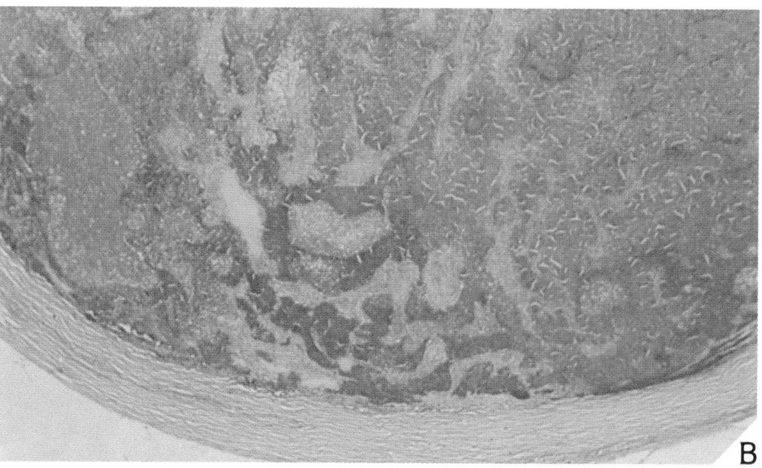

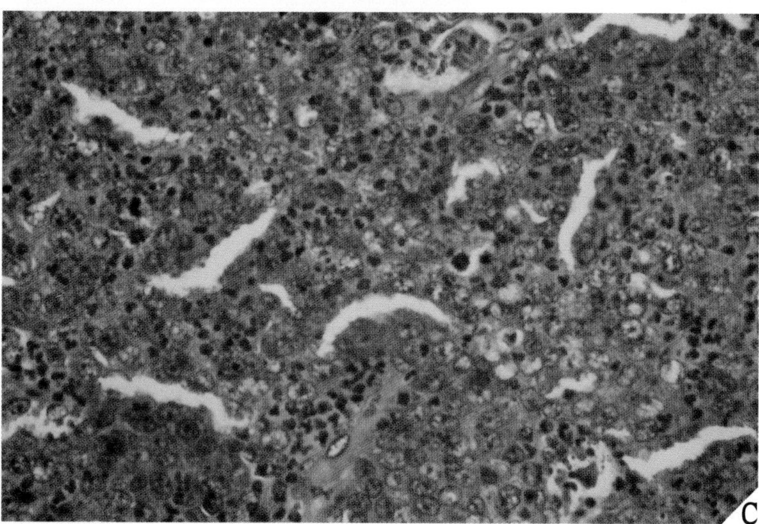

FIGURE 9.19. METASTATIC CARCINOMA. A The patient had an adenocarcinoma of the lung that metastasized to the eye. **B** A histologic section shows dark and light areas. The dark areas represent the cellular tumor, and the light areas represent stroma. Even under low magnification, a choroidal malignant melanoma can be ruled out because a melanoma does not have any stroma. **C** Increased magnification shows the malignant epithelial cells, many of which show mitotic figures. (**A**, from Yanoff M, Fine BS: *Ocular Pathology*, 2nd ed.)

Bibliography

Buettner H: Spontaneous involution of a choroidal osteoma. Arch Ophthalmol 108:1517, 1990.

Cameron JD, Fine BS, Shapiro I: Histopathologic observations in choroideremia with emphasis on vascular changes of the uveal tract. Ophthalmology 94:187, 1987.

Cremers FPM, et al: Cloning of a gene that is rearranged in patients with choroideremia. Nature 347:674, 1990.

Ferry AP, Llovera I, Shafer DM: Central areolar choroidal dystrophy. Arch Ophthalmol 88:39, 1972.

Gass JDM et al: Multifocal pigment epithelial detachments by reticulum cell sarcoma: a characteristic funduscopic picture. Retina 4:135, 1984.

Johnson MW, Gass JDM: Surgical management of the idiopathic uveal effusion syndrome. Ophthalmology 97:778, 1990.

Lang GK et al: Ocular reticulum cell sarcoma. Clinicopathologic correction of a case with multifocal lesions. Retina 5:79, 1985.

Leonardy NJ, et al: Analysis of 135 autopsy eyes for ocular involvement in leukemia. Am J Ophthalmol 109:436, 1990.

Nelson LB, et al: Aniridia. A review. Surv Ophthalmol 28:621, 1984.

Noble KG: Bilateral choroidal osteoma in three siblings. Am J Ophthalmol 109:656, 1990.

Trochme SD, et al: Extracellular deposition of eosinophil major basic protein in orbital histiocytosis X. Ophthalmology 98:353, 1991.

Waeltermann JM, Hettinger ME, Cibis GW: Congenital cysts of the iris stroma. Am J Ophthalmol 100:549, 1985.

Wilson DJ, Weleber RG, Green WR: Ocular clinicopathologic study of gyrate atrophy. Am J Ophthalmol 111:24, 1991.

Wu J-S, et al: Clinicopathologic findings in a patient with serpiginous choroiditis and treated choroidal neovascularization. Retina 9:292, 1989.

Yanoff M, Fine BS: *Ocular Pathology: A Text and Atlas*, 2nd ed. Philadelphia, JB Lippincott, 1982 and 3rd ed., 1989.

Zimmerman LE: Ocular lesions of juvenile xanthogranuloma. Nevoxanthoendothelioma. Trans Am Acad Ophthalmol Otolaryngol 69:412, 1965.

Lens

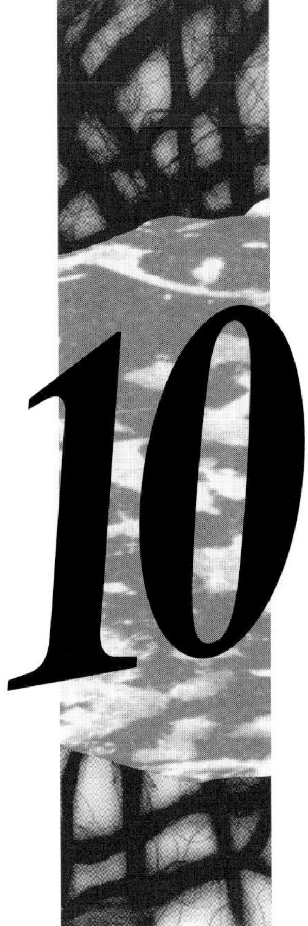

The lens is an unusual tissue for a number of reasons. It is not only transparent, but it also has an inverted surface epithelium that grows inward at the equator. Unable to desquamate or shed as does corneal or dermal epithelium, the proliferating, elongating lens cells become inwardly compacted with advancing age. This compaction often is accompanied by formation of intracellular yellow pigment of varying density. On one hand, accumulating yellow pigment together with increasing cellular compaction decreases the penetration of light and so decreases vision; on the other hand, the same aging changes filter out ultraviolet light preferentially, which may help protect the foveal macular region of the retina from light damage.

Lens epithelial cells are quite reactive and participate in the formation of certain kinds of cataract, but do not seem to have the ability to undergo neoplastic change, a characteristic they share to some extent with retinal pigment epithelium cells.

Many congenital abnormalities of the lens have been described. These range from very simple abnormalities such as a Mittendorf dot, to very complex abnormalities that may be secondary to a metabolic defect, such as occur in galactosemia.

The capsule of the lens is secreted by the lens epithelium and is the thickest basement membrane in the body (the second thickest is the Descemet membrane). The capsule may participate in ocular lesions such as true exfoliation and the pseudoexfoliation syndrome.

The epithelium may be damaged by a noxious stimulus such as trauma or inflammation, and then may proliferate to form either an anterior or posterior subcapsular cataract, or both. Following trauma the epithelium may form abnormal lens cells that result in the development of Elschnig pearls, or may form a secondary thickening on the posterior lens capsule.

With aging, the cortex of the lens tends to become denatured and undergoes degeneration, forming globules of liquefied cortex that are called morgagnian globules. Materials such as cholesterol may become deposited in the cortex. Also, fluid clefts (water clefts) may form. The process may continue to such a degree that all of the cortex becomes liquefied and milky white, resulting in a mature or morgagnian cataract. The fluid may escape through the intact lens capsule and result in a shrinking of the lens substance and a redundancy or folding of the capsule, called a hypermature cataract.

The nucleus of the lens, in contrast to the "soft" cortex, tends to be "hard." With aging, in addition to the accumulation of pigment, other substances such as calcium oxalate may be deposited. Cortical and nuclear cataracts may occur at any age, but tend to have two peaks: one peak under 10 years of age and caused mainly by congenital factors, and the other after 60 years as part of the normal aging process.

Cataracts may be secondary to a variety of local and systemic abnormalities, as well as to metabolic diseases and trauma. Whatever the cause of the cataract, a number of complications may occur. Through a variety of mechanisms, the cataract may cause glaucoma or inflammation. An ectopic lens may arise due to a congenital condition (e.g., Marfan syndrome) or an acquired one (e.g., traumatic subluxation or dislocation).

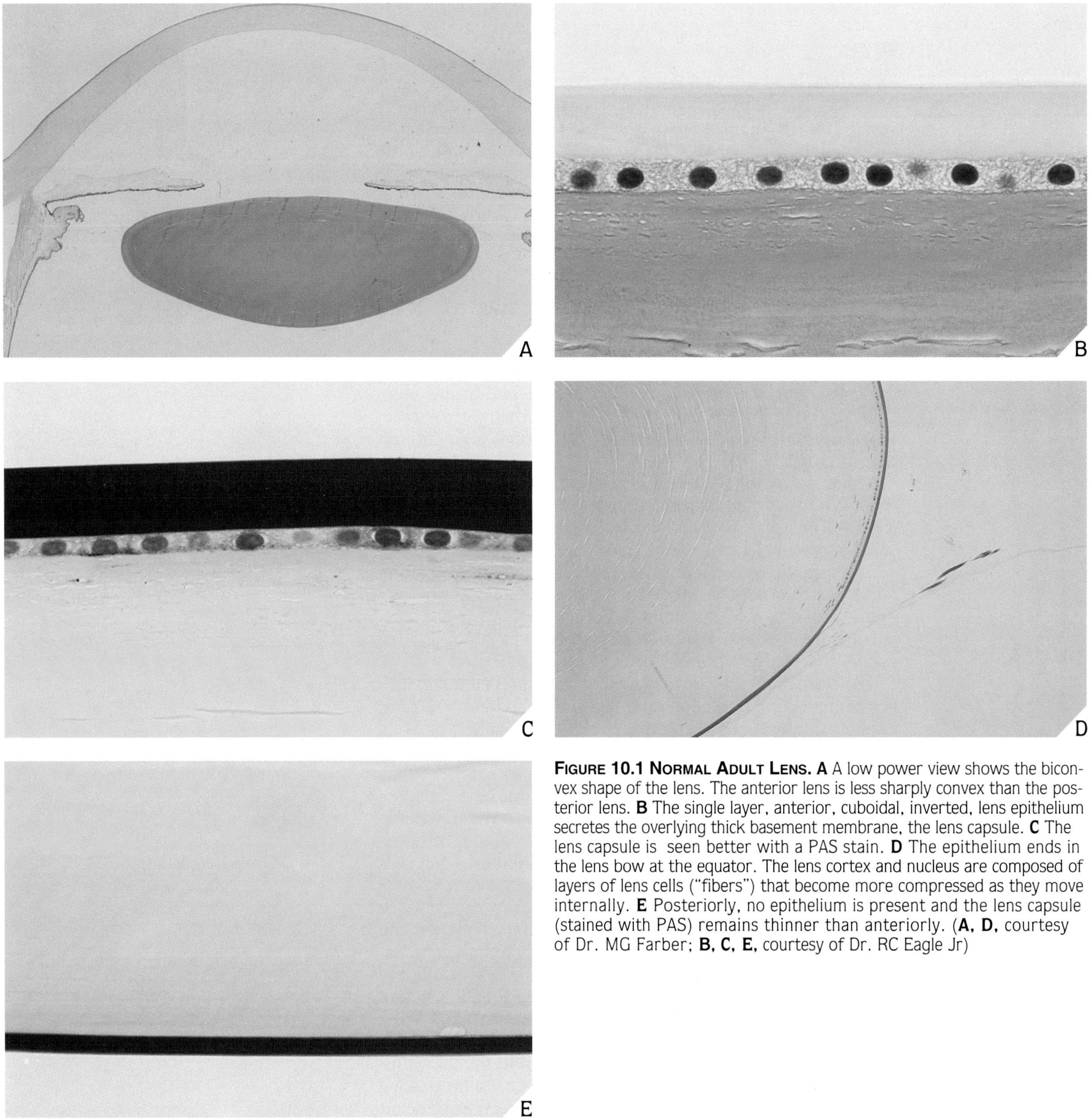

FIGURE 10.1 NORMAL ADULT LENS. A A low power view shows the biconvex shape of the lens. The anterior lens is less sharply convex than the posterior lens. **B** The single layer, anterior, cuboidal, inverted, lens epithelium secretes the overlying thick basement membrane, the lens capsule. **C** The lens capsule is seen better with a PAS stain. **D** The epithelium ends in the lens bow at the equator. The lens cortex and nucleus are composed of layers of lens cells ("fibers") that become more compressed as they move internally. **E** Posteriorly, no epithelium is present and the lens capsule (stained with PAS) remains thinner than anteriorly. (**A, D,** courtesy of Dr. MG Farber; **B, C, E,** courtesy of Dr. RC Eagle Jr)

CONGENITAL ABNORMALITIES

Mittendorf dot

Aphakia

Duplication

Fleck cataract

Anterior polar cataract

Posterior polar cataract

Anterior lenticonus

Posterior lenticonus

Congenital cataract
Zonular
Sutural
Axial
Membranous
Filiform
Secondary to intrauterine infection

Galactosemia

Transient neonatal lens vacuoles

FIGURE 10.2

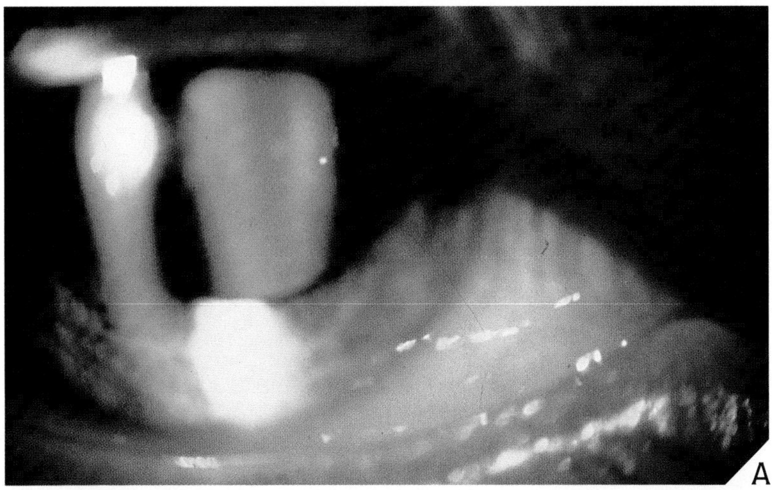

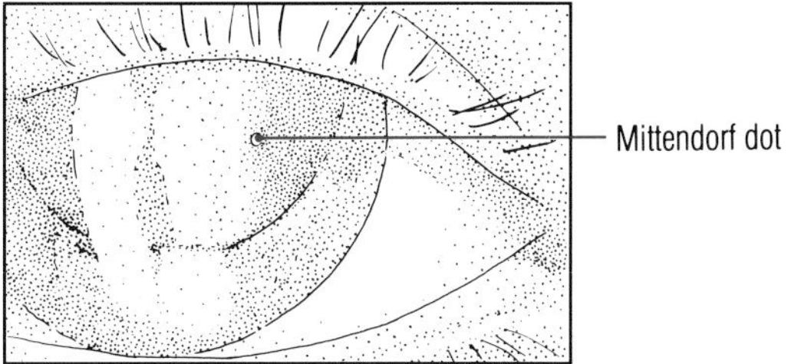

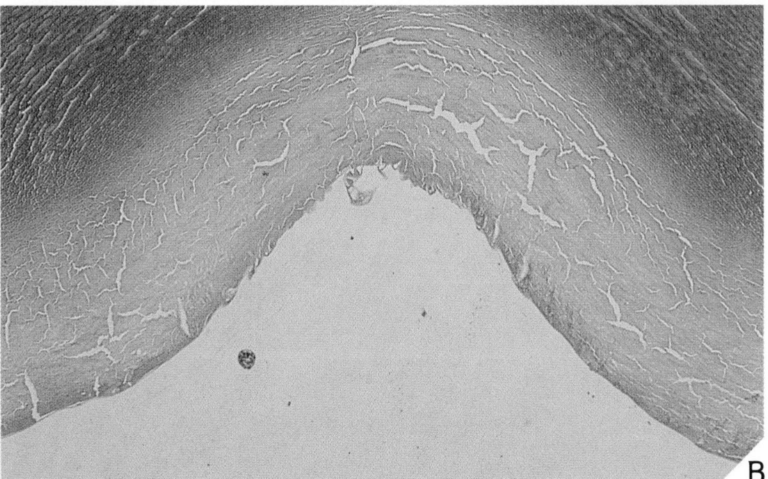

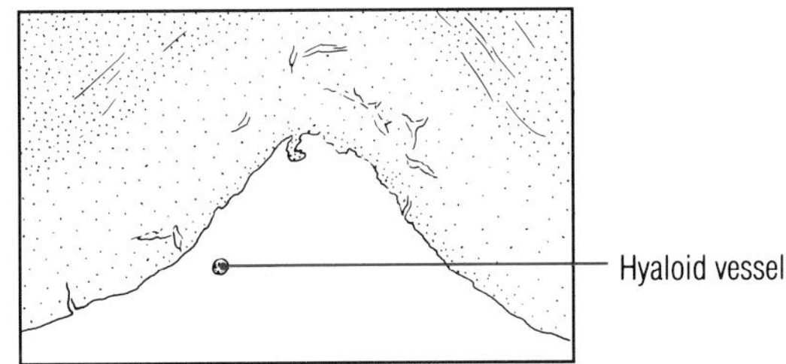

FIGURE 10.3 MITTENDORF DOT. A The hyaloid vessel remnant is seen as a small white dot on the posterior surface of the lens, slightly nasal to the posterior pole of the lens. The attachment site is called a Mittendorf dot. **B** A histologic section shows the hyaloid vessel approaching the posterior surface of the lens. The posterior umbilication of the lens is an artifact of fixation, often seen in infants and young children. (**A**, from Yanoff M, Fine BS: *Ocular Pathology*, 3rd ed.)

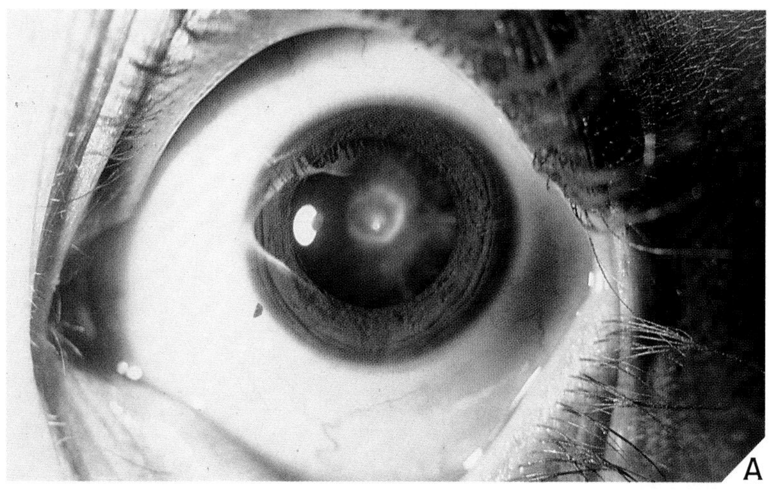

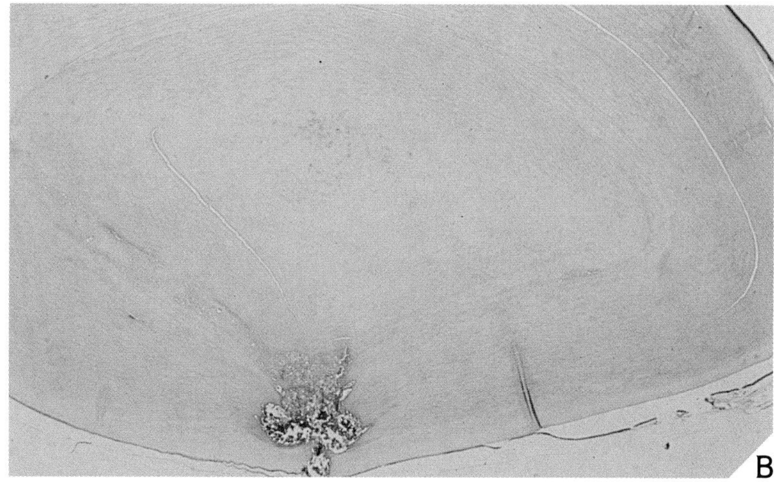

FIGURE 10.4 CONGENITAL POLAR CATARACT. A This patient had both anterior and posterior congenital polar cataracts. **B** Histologic section of another lens that contained a congenital posterior polar cataract shows degeneration of the posterior subcapsular cortex.

CAPSULE

General reactions
Elasticity
Thickening
Thinning
Rupture

"True" exfoliation

Pseudoexfoliation syndrome (exfoliation syndrome, basement membrane exfoliation syndrome)

FIGURE 10.5

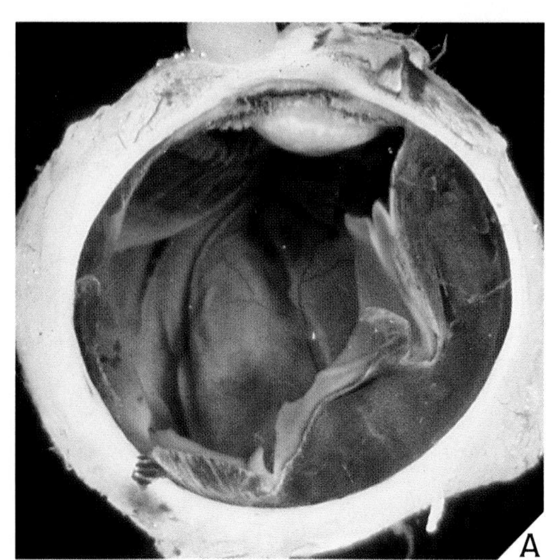

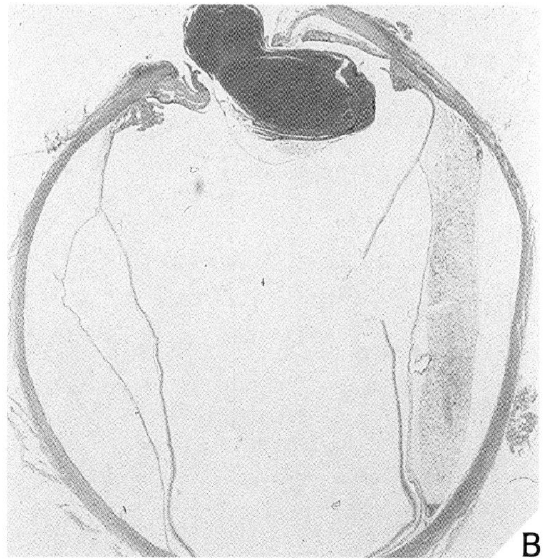

FIGURE 10.6 LENS CAPSULE ELASTICITY. A This patient had developed bullous keratopathy, secondary to glaucoma. The cornea then became ulcerated and perforated, resulting in an expulsive choroidal hemorrhage. The eye was enucleated. Gross examination shows the massive choroidal hemorrhage and the lens protruding through the ruptured cornea. **B** A histologic section demonstrates the molding of the lens through the corneal opening. The lens capsule is intact.

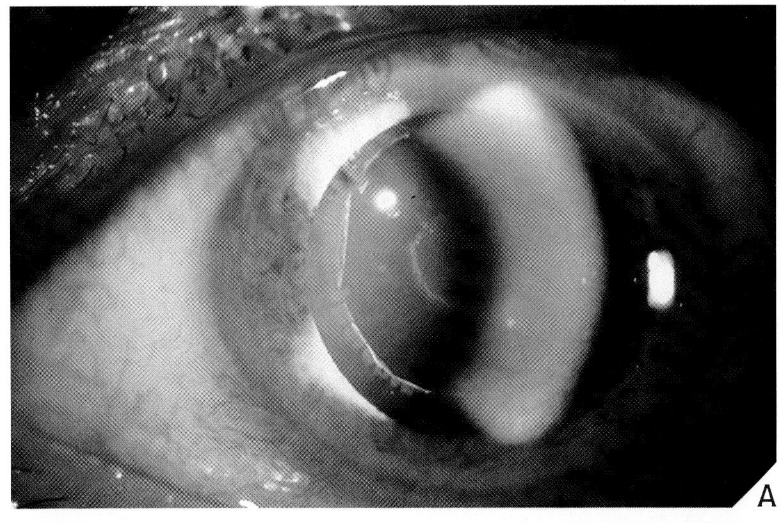

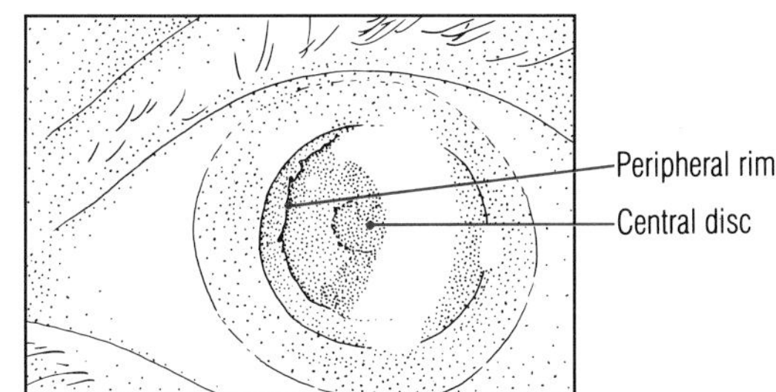

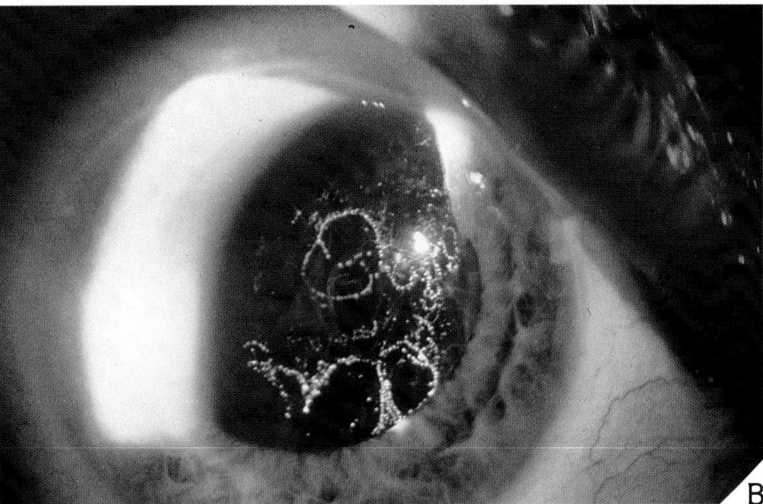

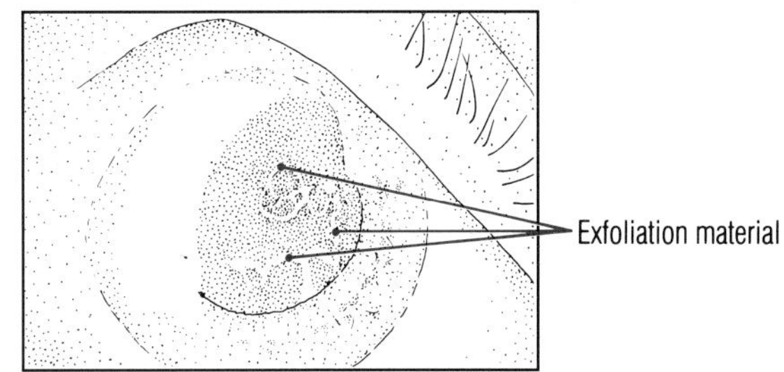

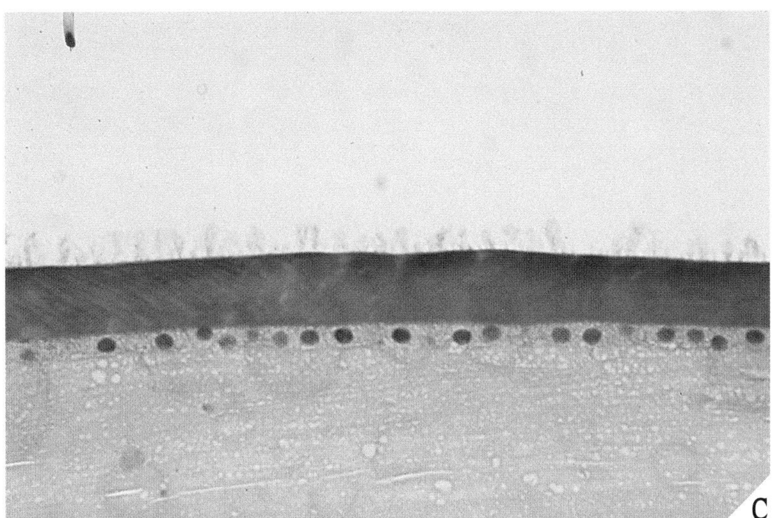

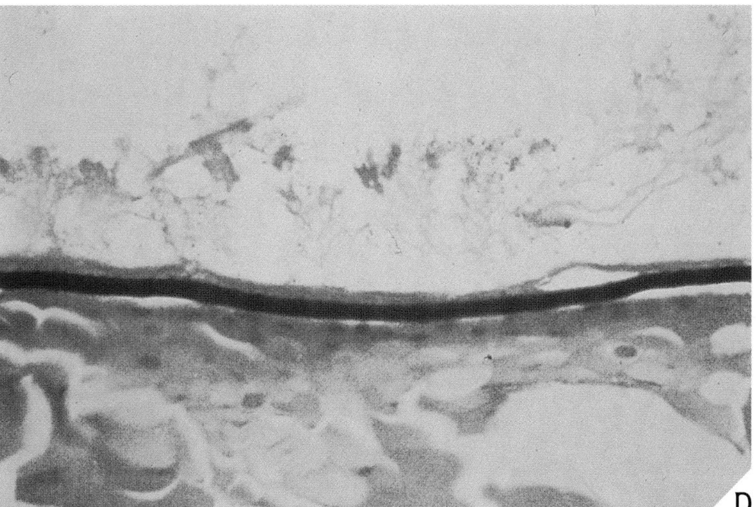

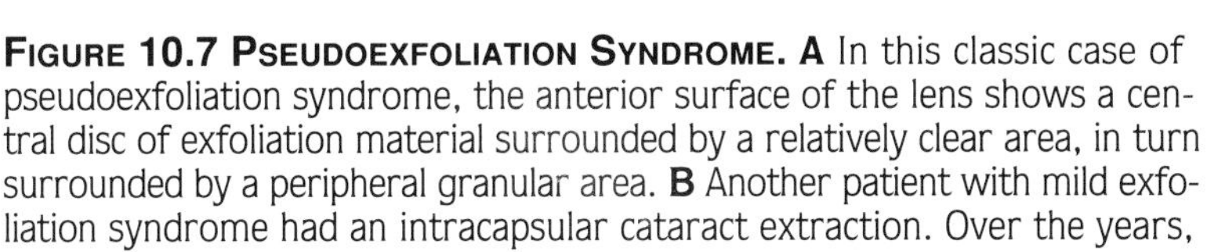

Figure 10.7 Pseudoexfoliation Syndrome. A In this classic case of pseudoexfoliation syndrome, the anterior surface of the lens shows a central disc of exfoliation material surrounded by a relatively clear area, in turn surrounded by a peripheral granular area. **B** Another patient with mild exfoliation syndrome had an intracapsular cataract extraction. Over the years, the exfoliation material was deposited on the anterior face of the vitreous. **C** In the central disc area, the exfoliation material is deposited as small slivers that line up parallel to each other and perpendicular to the lens capsule. **D** In the peripheral granular area, the material is abundant and has a thick dendritic appearance. (**C**, **D**, PAS stain.)

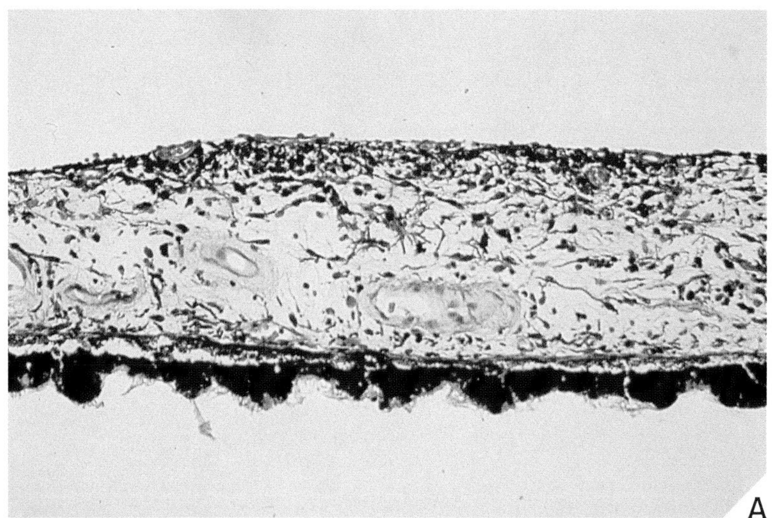

FIGURE 10.8 PSEUDOEXFOLIATION SYNDROME. A The exfoliation material deposits on the posterior surface of the iris, causing the iris to have a saw-tooth posterior configuration. The deposited material often acts as a strut, limiting dilatation of the iris. The material also can be seen deposited on the zonular fibers of the lens **B** and on the ciliary epithelium **C**. (**B**, courtesy of Dr. RC Eagle Jr; **C**, PAS stain.)

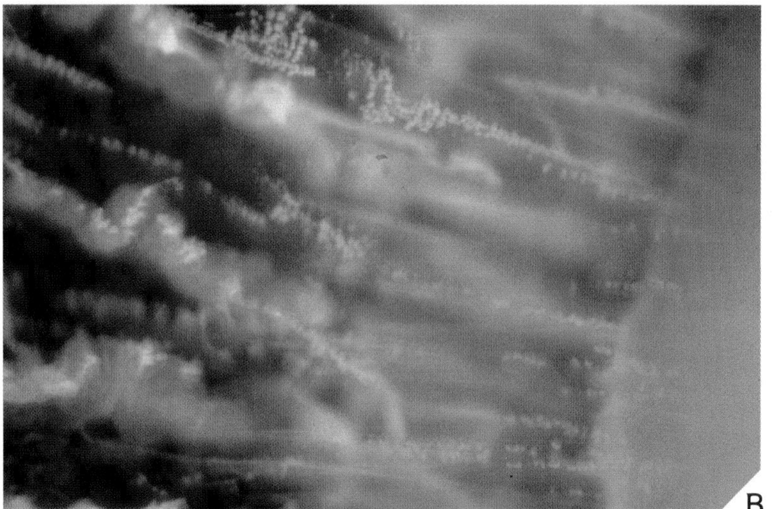

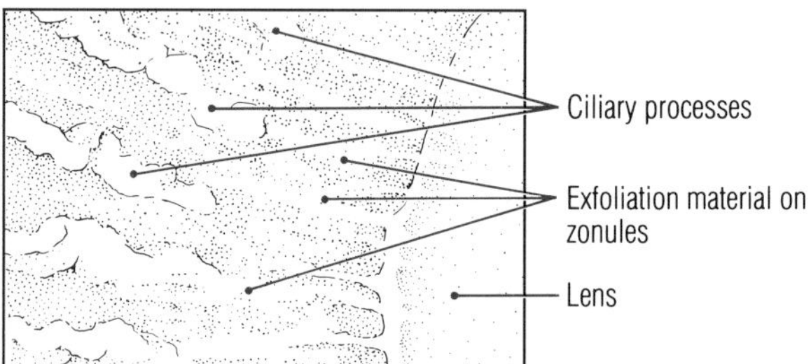

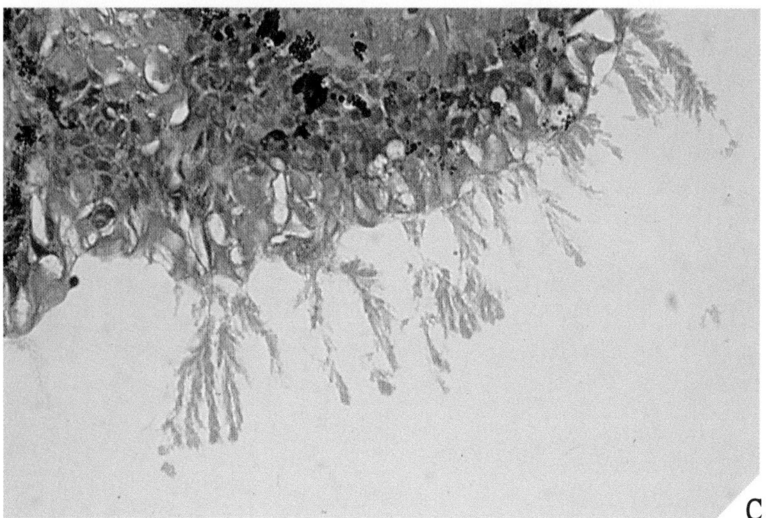

EPITHELIUM

Anterior subcapsular cataract
Posterior subcapsular cataract
Elschnig pearls
Degeneration and atrophy
"After cataract" (after ECCE)

FIGURE 10.9

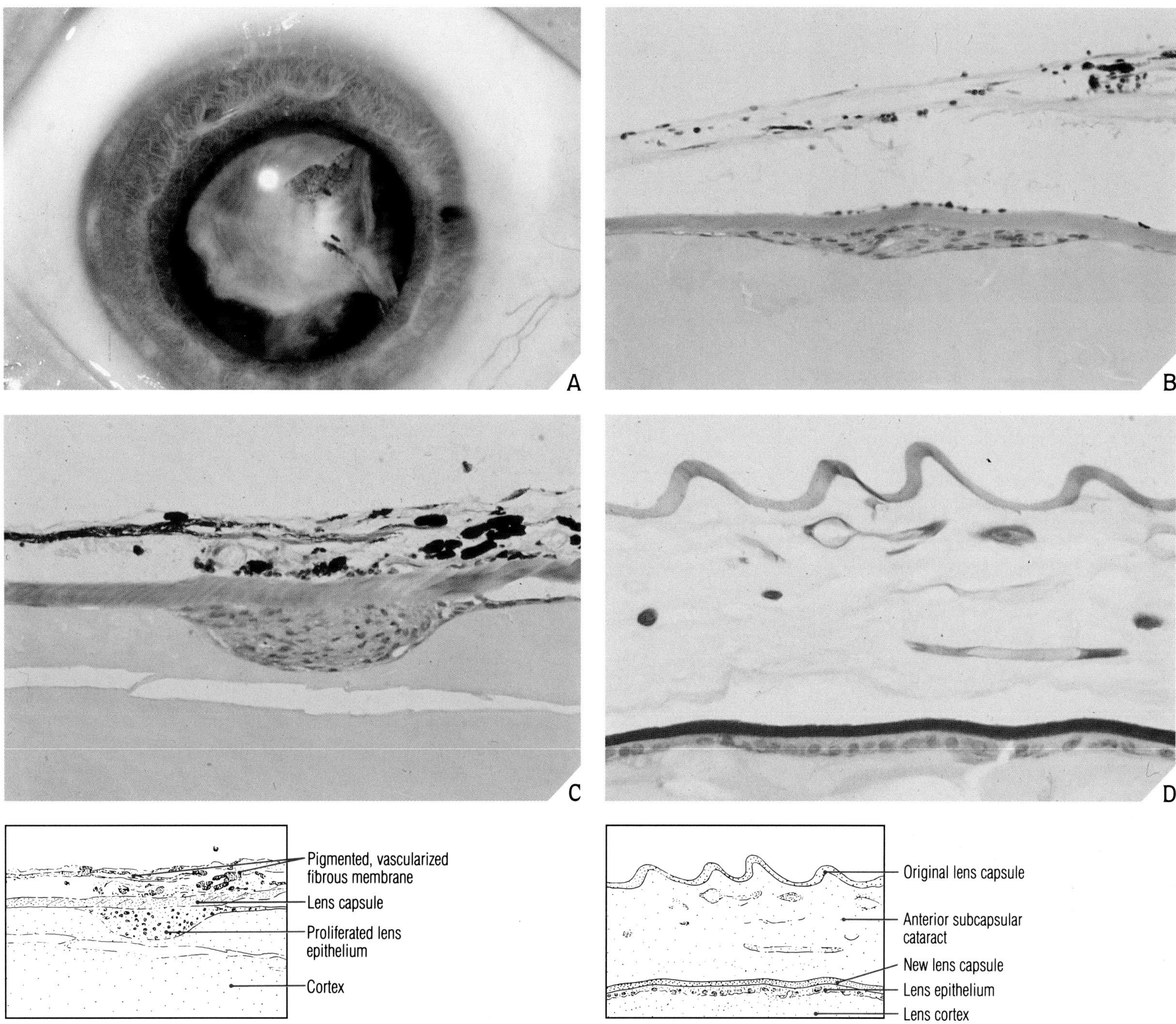

FIGURE 10.10 ANTERIOR SUBCAPSULAR CATARACT. A The patient developed an anterior subcapsular cataract some years after blunt trauma to the eye. **B** A histologic section of another case shows early proliferation of the lens epithelium beneath the capsule. **C** In yet another case, continued proliferation of the lens epithelium has occurred along with fibroblastic metaplasia. **D** The proliferated epithelium has largely disappeared and has laid down collagen tissue. The original lens capsule is thrown into folds and the original lens epithelium has laid down a new lens capsule. The underlying cortex shows globular degeneration forming a duplication cataract, i.e., an anterior subcapsular and a cortical cataract. (**B, C**, from Yanoff M, Fine BS: *Ocular Pathology*, 3rd ed.; **B–D**, PAS stain)

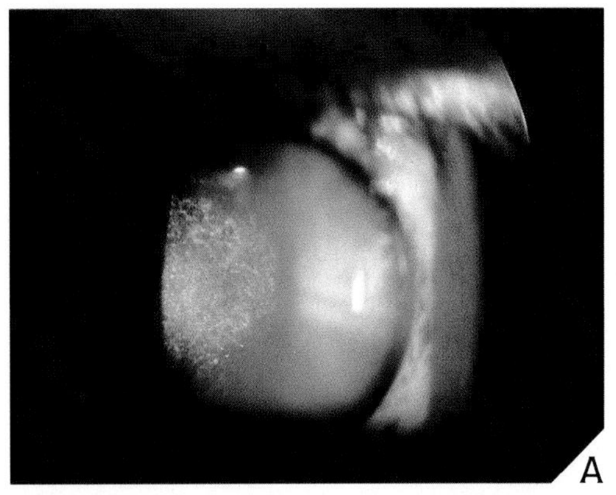

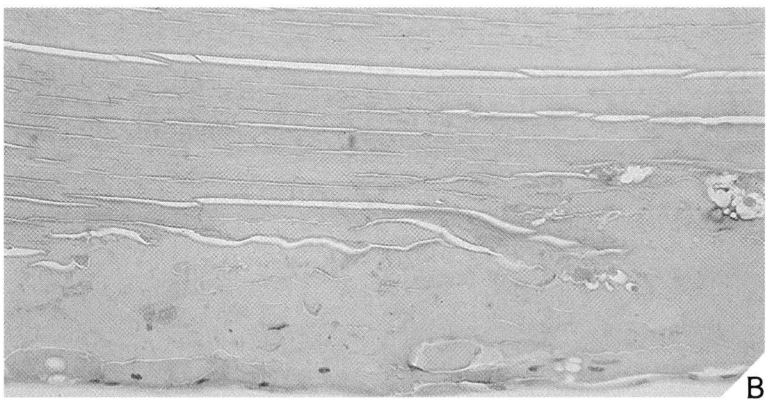

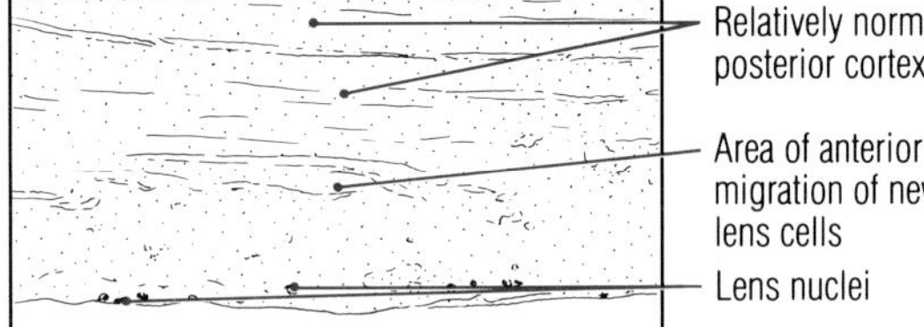

FIGURE 10.11 POSTERIOR SUBCAPSULAR CATARACT. A The patient had been on long-term systemic steroid therapy following a renal transplant. Over the years, a cataract developed just anterior to the posterior surface of the lens. **B** A histologic section of another case shows migration of the lens epithelium to the posterior pole. Here the epithelial cells tend to form new, but abnormal, lens cells (bladder cells) that migrate anteriorly into the posterior lens cortex. This lens was removed from a patient who had retinitis pigmentosa.

CORTEX AND NUCLEUS

Cortex: soft cataract	Nucleus: hard cataract

FIGURE 10.12

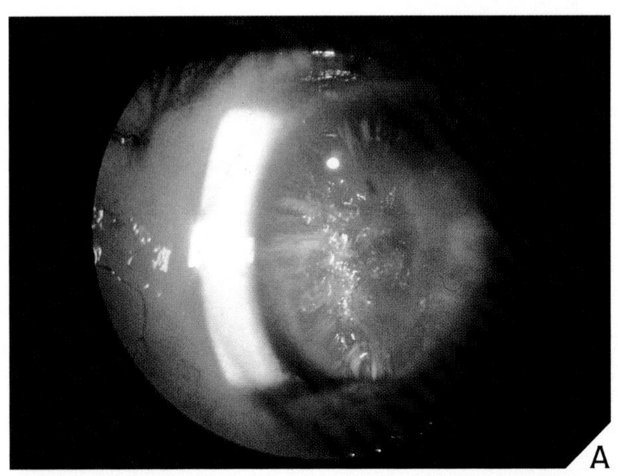

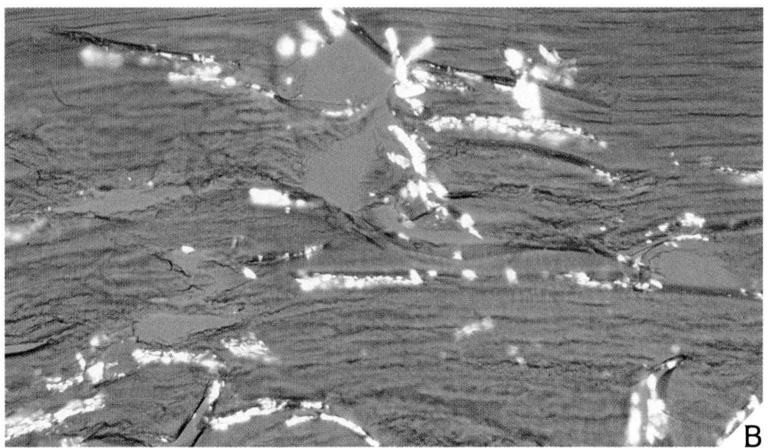

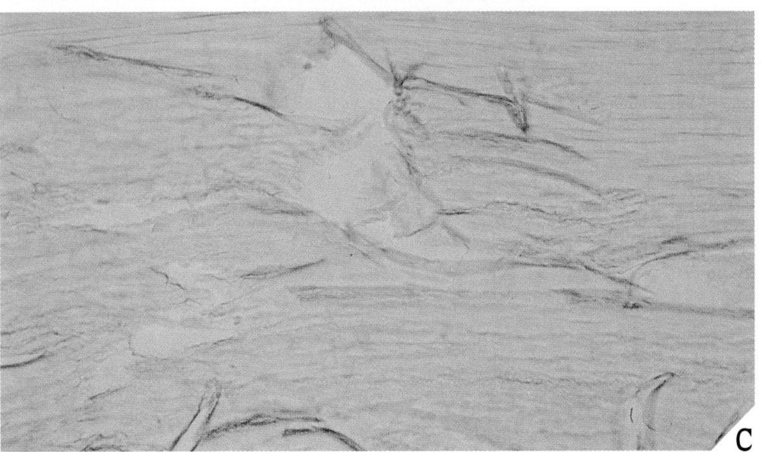

FIGURE 10.13 CHOLESTEROLOSIS LENTIS. A The patient had glistening crystals in the lens cortex of both eyes. **B** Frozen sectioning of the removed lens shows clear areas. **C** Polarization of the clear areas demonstrates birefringent material, characteristic of cholesterol.

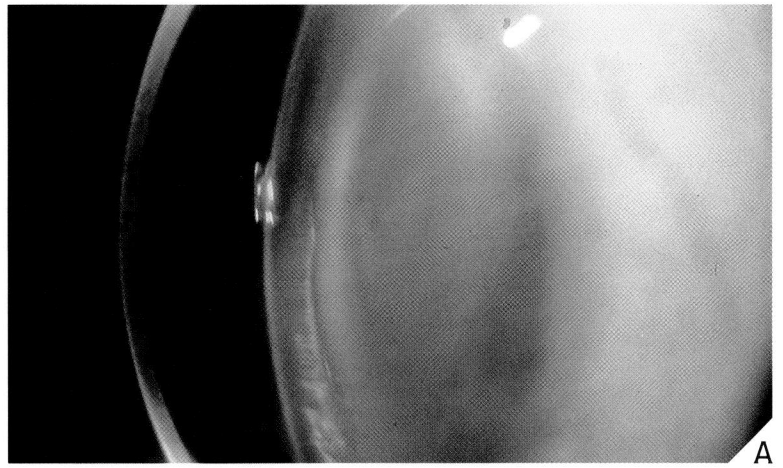

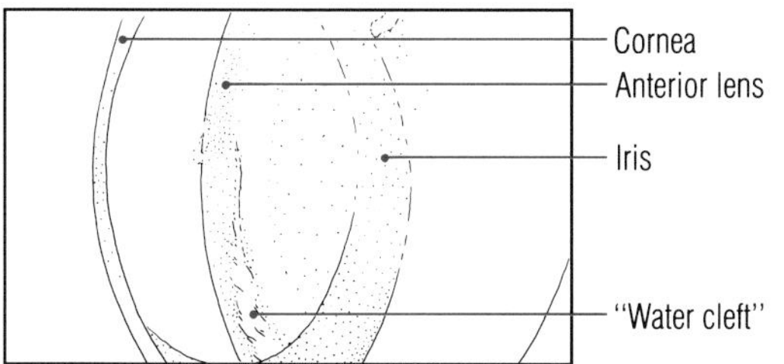

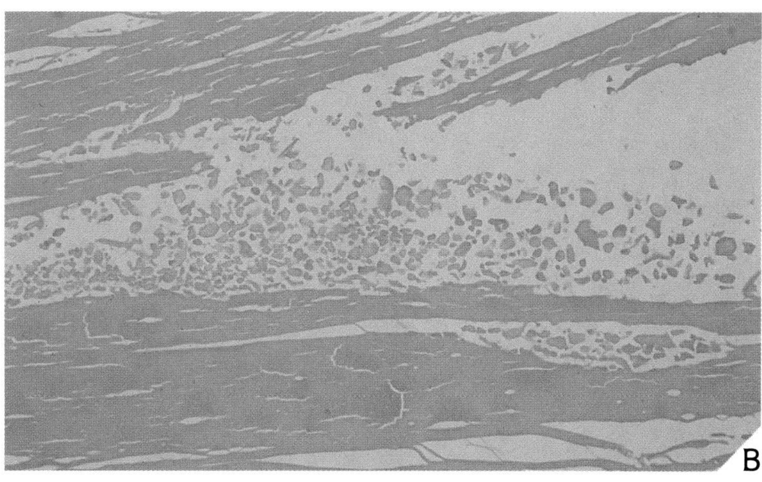

FIGURE 10.14 MORGAGNIAN DEGENERATION. A Slit-lamp examination of the lens shows a water cleft that is composed of liquefied cortex in the form of morgagnian degeneration. **B** A histologic section of another case shows the morgagnian globules between fragmented cortical lens "fibers."

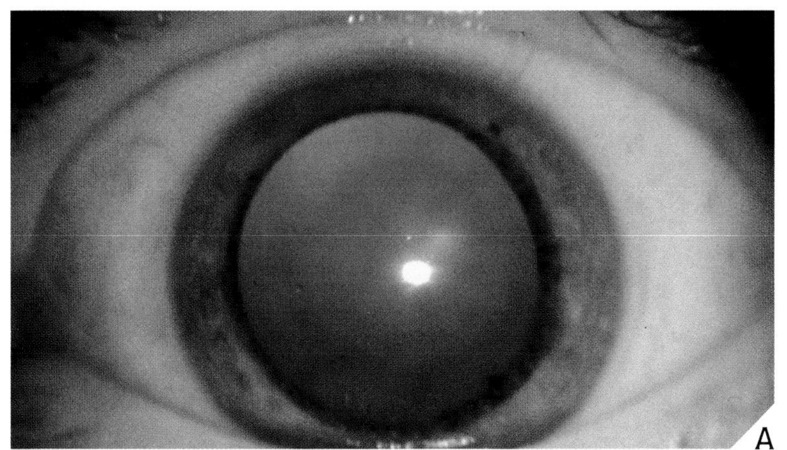

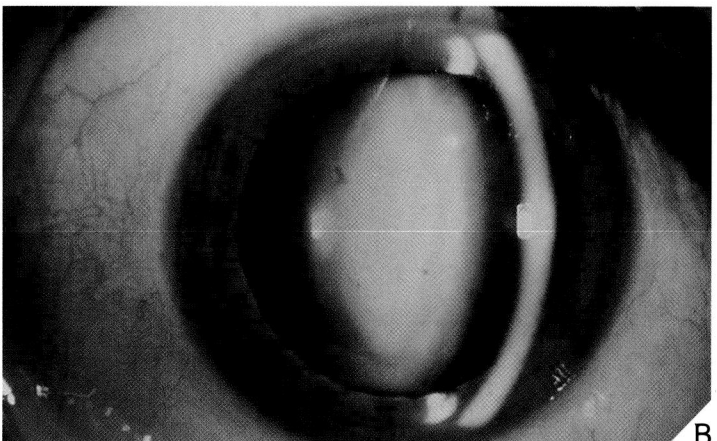

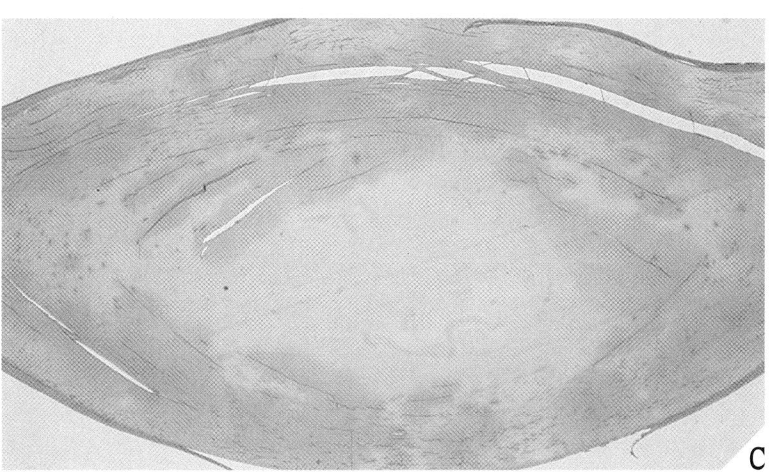

FIGURE 10.15 NUCLEAR CATARACT. A The red reflex shows the "oil droplet" effect of the nuclear cataract. **B** Slit-lamp examination of another case shows the cataractous yellow-pigmented nucleus. **C** A histologic section of yet another case shows the homogeneous appearance of the compacted cells within the nuclear cataract. (**B**, from Yanoff M, Fine BS: *Ocular Pathology*, 3rd ed.)

SECONDARY CATARACTS

Intraocular disease	Toxic	Endocrine and metabolic

FIGURE 10.16

COMPLICATIONS OF CATARACTS

Glaucoma

Mechanical

Phacolytic

Phacoanaphylactic endophthalmitis

Ectopic lens

Congenital with systemic diseases

- Homocystinuria
- Marfan syndrome
- Weill-Marchesani syndrome
- Cutis hyperelastica (Ehlers-Danlos syndrome)
- Proportional dwarfism
- Oxycephaly
- Crouzon disease
- Sprengel deformity
- Sturge-Weber syndrome

Congenital without systemic disease

- Simple ectopic lens
- Ectopic lens and pupil

Acquired ectopic lens

- Nontraumatic
- Traumatic

FIGURE 10.17

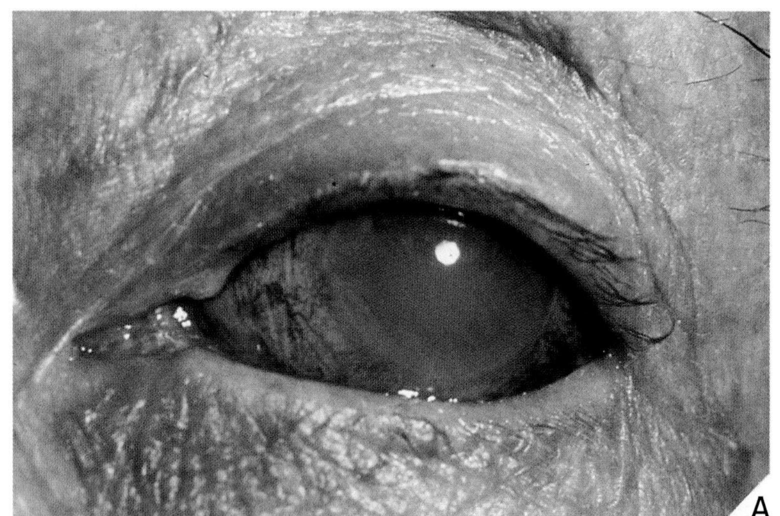

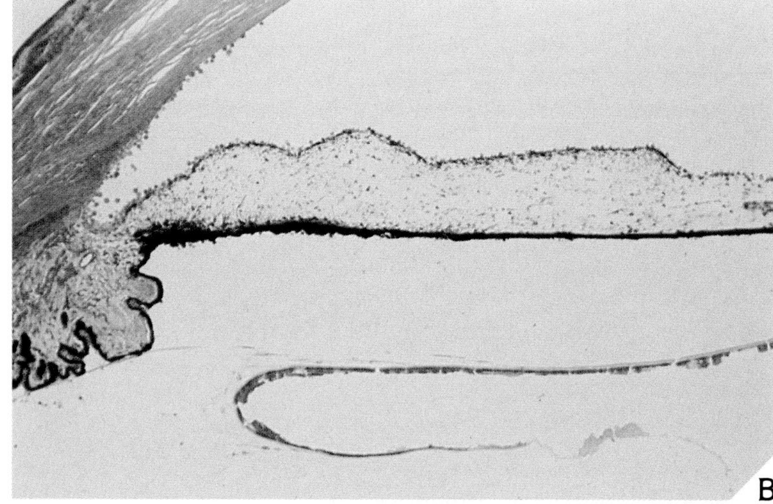

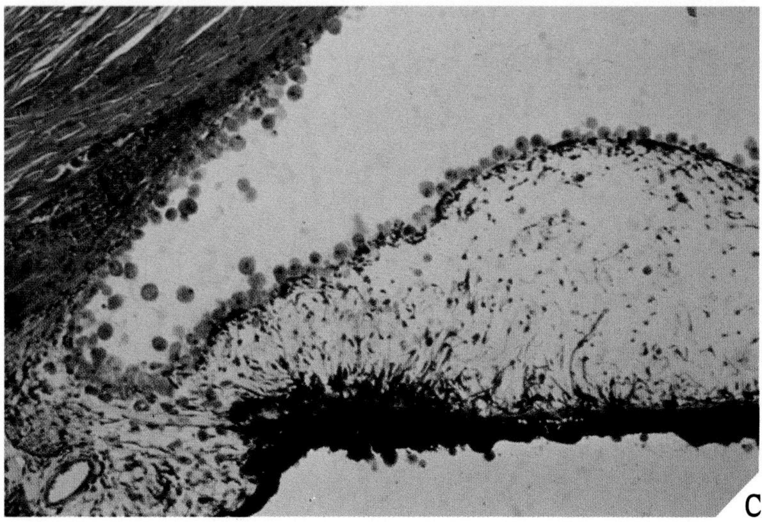

FIGURE 10.18 PHACOLYTIC GLAUCOMA. A The patient presented with signs and symptoms of acute closed-angle glaucoma. Chalky material was present in the anterior chamber. **B** A histologic section of another eye shows that no lens cortex is present within the lens. The liquefied cortex had leaked out through an intact capsule, resulting in a hypermature cataract. The lens material was then phagocytosed by macrophages, present on the anterior surface of the iris and within the open angle of the anterior chamber. **C** Increased magnification of another section better shows the macrophages. The macrophages are swollen by the ingested lens material.

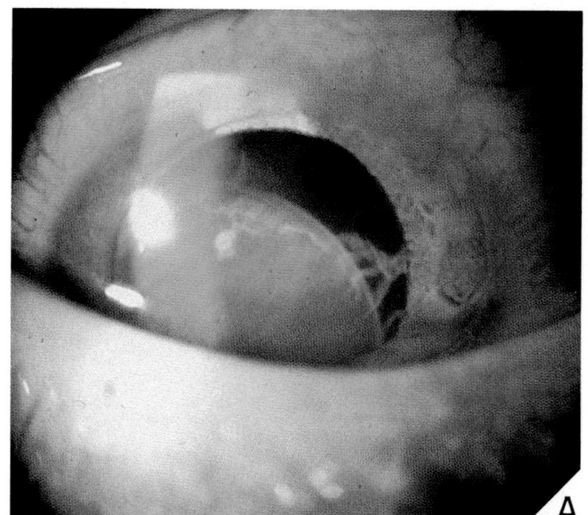

Figure 10.19 Homocystinuria. A A fringe of white zonular remnants is present at the equator of the lens. These remnants tend to undulate slowly when the eye moves. The lens is subluxated inferonasally, the usual location in homocystinuria (in Marfan syndrome it usually is subluxated superotemporally). **B** A histologic section of another case shows a thrombus in the greater arterial circle of the ciliary body. Patients who have homocystinuria are prone to thrombotic episodes, especially during or after general anesthesia. **C** A characteristic thick mantle of abnormal zonular material covers the pars plana of the ciliary body. (**A**, reported in Ramsey MS, et al, 1975; **C**, PAS stain.)

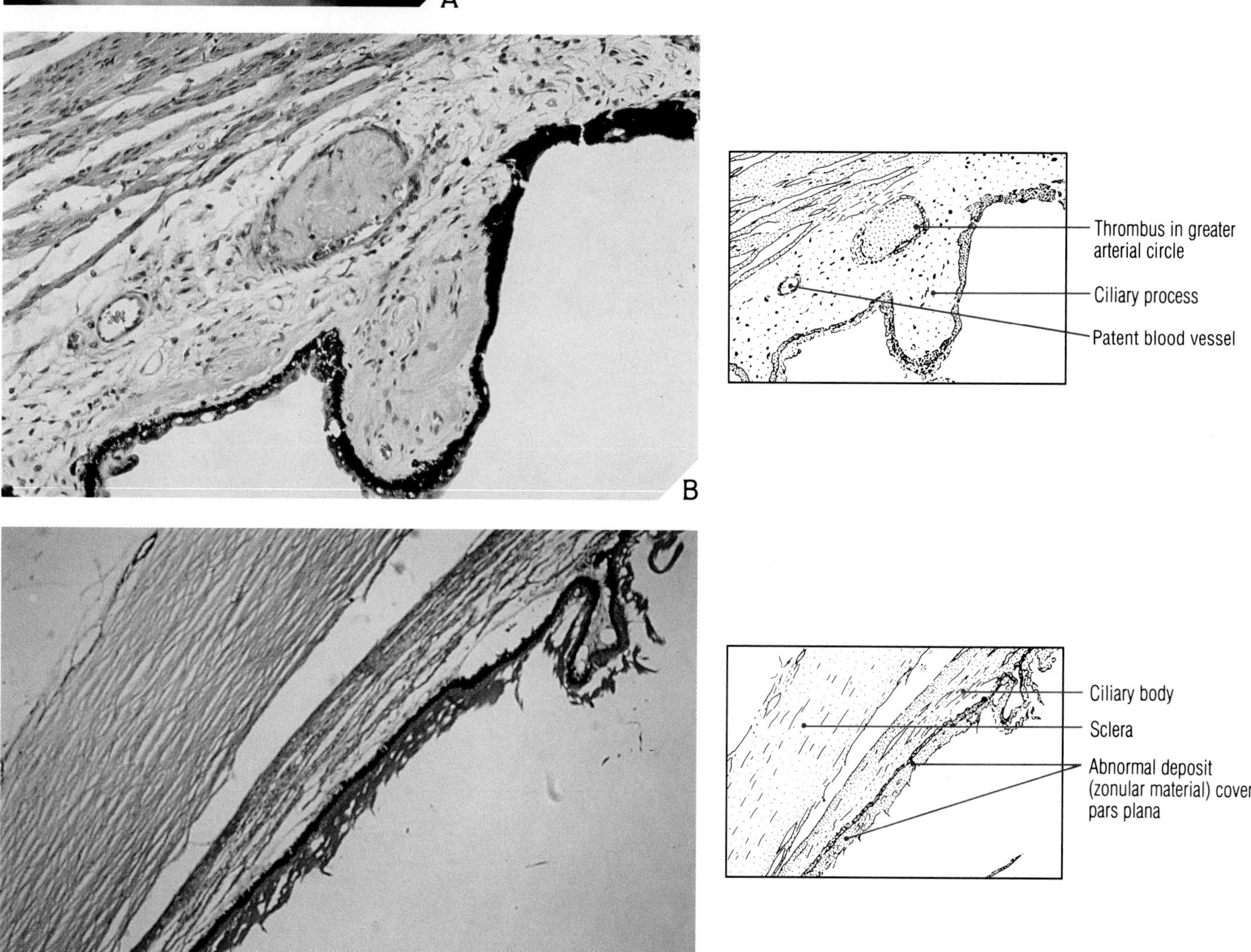

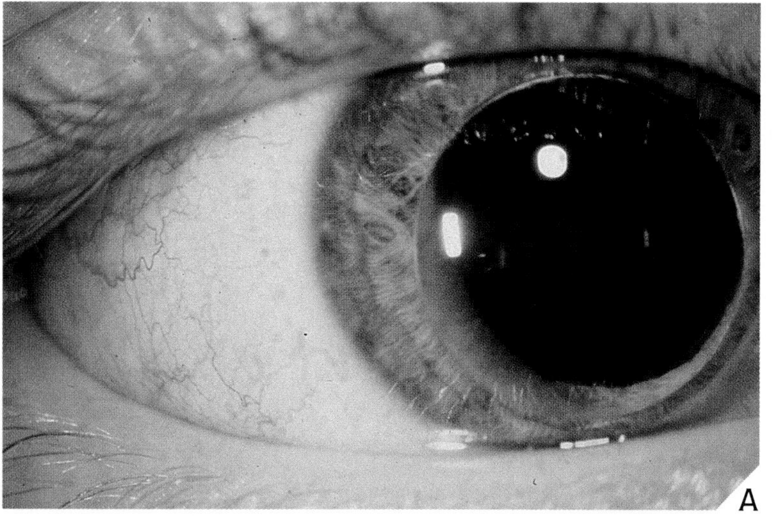

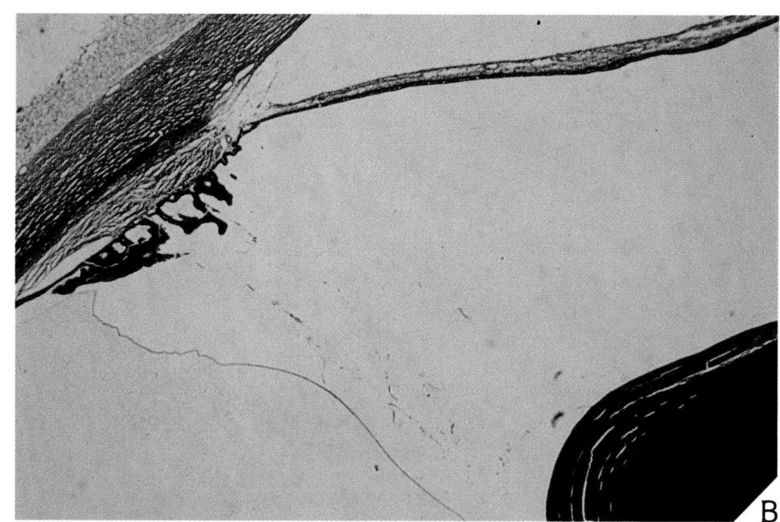

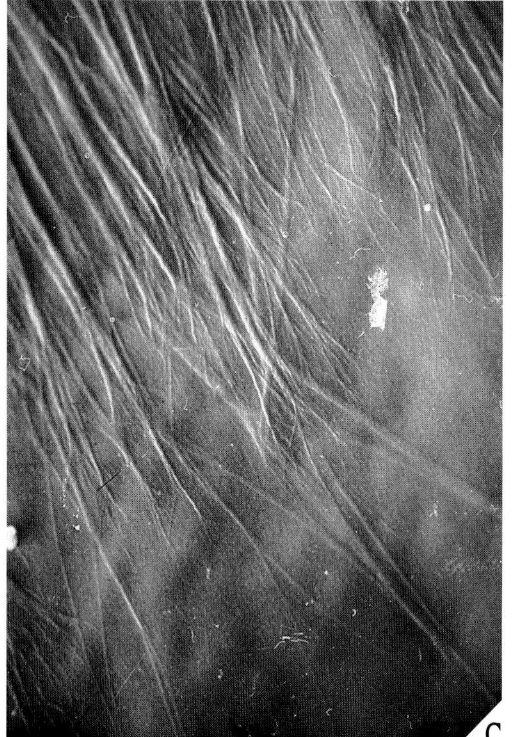

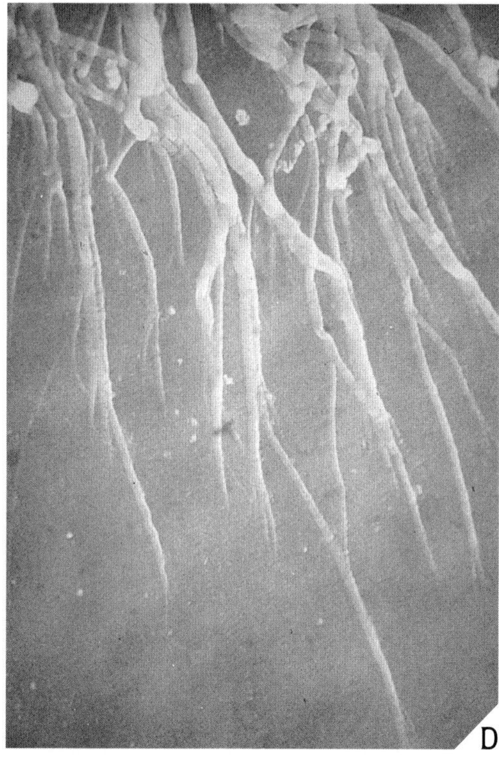

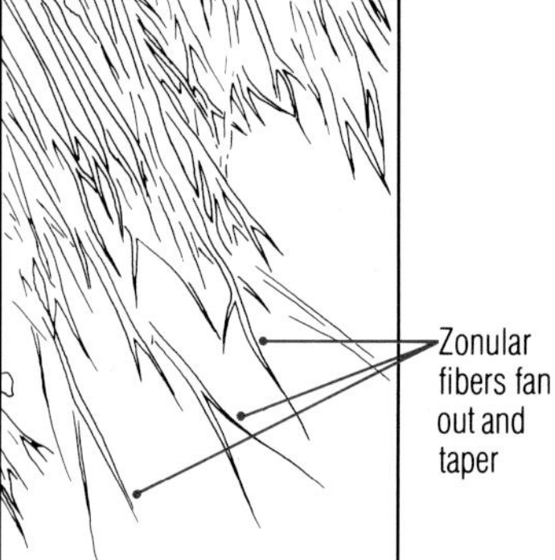

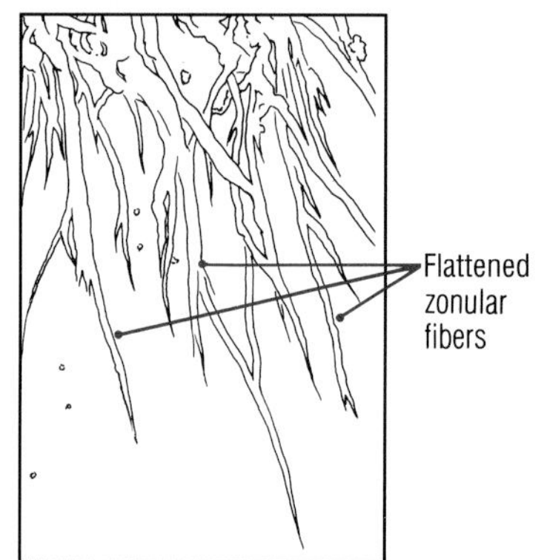

FIGURE 10.20 MARFAN SYNDROME. A The lens has dislocated into the anterior chamber (although in Marfan syndrome the lens usually subluxates superotemporally in the posterior chamber). Anterior dislocation is more common in homocystinuria. **B** A histologic section from an infant shows a relatively normal anterior segment. **C** Electron microscope examination of a normal lens shows the zonular fibers spread out over the anterior lens capsule. Note the fanning out and the tapering of the fibers. **D** The zonular fibers intruding into the anterior capsule of a patient with Marfan syndrome show a flattening and a rapid attenuation of the fibers, along with a lack of wide separation, probably representing a weakened attachment site. (**A**, courtesy of Dr. AC Wulc; **B**, reticulum stain; **C, D**, scanning electron micrographs; **D**, reported in Ramsey MS, et al., 1972.)

Bibliography

Brooks AMV, Grant G, Gillies WE: Comparison of specular microscopy and examination of aspirate in phacolytic glaucoma. Ophthalmology 97:85, 1990.

Cashwell LF, et al: Idiopathic true exfoliation of the lens capsule. Ophthalmology 96:348, 1989.

Flach AJ, Peterson JS, Dolan BJ: Anterior subcapsular cataracts: a review of potential etiologies. Ann Ophthalmol 17:78, 1985.

Goldberg MF: Clinical manifestations of ectopia lentis et pupillae in 16 patients. Trans Am Ophthalmol Soc 86:158, 1988.

Henkind P, Prose P: Anterior polar cataract: electron microscopic evidence of collagen. Am J Ophthalmol 63:768, 1967.

Hu T-S, et al: Age-related cataract in the Tibet eye study. Arch Ophthalmol 107:666, 1989.

Kozart, DM, Yanoff M: Intraocular pressure status in 100 consecutive patients with exfoliation syndrome. Ophthalmology 89:214, 1982.

Leske MC, Chylack LT, Wu S-Y: The lens opacities case-control study. Risk factors for cataract. Arch Ophthalmol 109:244, 1991.

Ramsey MS, Daitz LD, Beaton JW: Lens fringe in homocystinuria. Arch Ophthalmol 93:318, 1975.

Ramsey MS, et al: The Marfan syndrome. A histopathologic study of ocular findings. Am J Ophthalmol 76:102, 1973.

Ramsey MS, Fine BS, Yanoff M: The ocular histopathology of homocystinuria. A light and electron microscopic study. Am J Ophthalmol 74:377, 1972.

Schlötzer-Schrehardt U, Küchle M, Naumann GOH: Electron-microscopic identification of pseudoexfoliation material in extrabulbar tissue. Arch Ophthalmol 109:565, 1991.

Smith ME, Zimmerman LE: Contusive angle recession in phacolytic glaucoma. Arch Ophthalmol 74:799, 1965.

Streeten BW, Eshaghian J: Human posterior subcapsular cataract. A gross and flat preparation study. Arch Ophthalmol 96:1653, 1978.

Streeten BW, et al: Pseudoexfoliation fibrillopathy in the skin of patients with ocular pseudoexfoliation. Am J Ophthalmol 110:490, 1990.

Vrensen G, Willekens B: Biomicroscopy and electron microscopy of early opacities in the aging human lens. Invest Ophthalmol Vis Sci 31:1582, 1990.

Yanoff M, Fine BS: *Ocular Pathology: A Text and Atlas*, 2nd ed. Philadelphia, JB Lippincott, 1982.

Retina

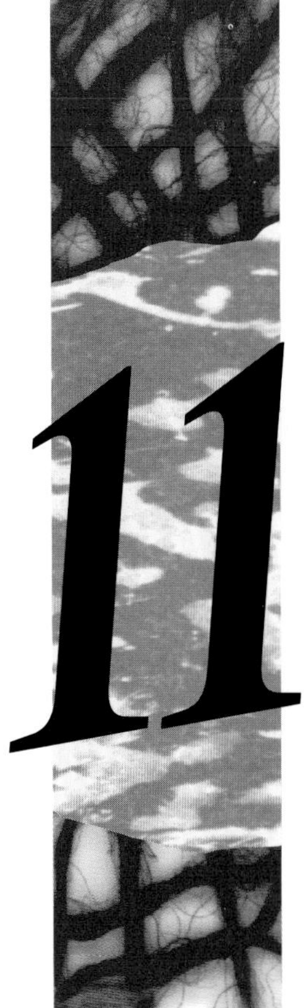

The retina is a highly specialized nervous tissue, in reality a part of the brain that has become exteriorized. It has the equivalent of both white matter (retinal plexiform and nerve fiber layers) and gray matter (retinal nuclear and ganglion cell layers). The glial cells are represented mostly by large all-pervasive specialized Müller cells and, less noticeably, by smaller astrocytes (and possible oligodendrocytes) of the inner retinal layers. As in the brain, a vasculature is present in which the endothelial cells possess tight junctions, producing a blood-retinal barrier. The retina, therefore, is susceptible to many diseases of the central nervous system, as well as to diseases affecting tissues in general. Additionally, the highly specialized photoreceptor cells are subject to their own particular disorders.

Numerous congenital anomalies may involve the retina. These range from common disorders such as albinism to rare disorders such as Oguchi disease. Another common anomaly is the presence of myelinated nerve fibers; this generally occurs contiguous with the optic nerve head in the nerve fiber layer, but also may appear as an isolated retinal lesion. A Lange fold is seen routinely in histological sections of infant eyes, but is a fixation artifact not present in vivo.

Vascular diseases often involve the retina, one of the few places in the body where blood vessels can be viewed directly. Signs of diseases such as diabetes mellitus (see Chapter 15) thus may be viewed directly and detected in their early stages. Retinal ischemia is caused by anything that obstructs the passage of blood through the arteries and arterioles. Hemorrhagic retinopathy, on the other hand, is caused by a partial or complete occlusion of blood leaving the retina via the venules and veins. Arteriolarsclerosis and hypertension leave distinctive signs on the retinal arterioles. Clinical examination of the retina, therefore, may give some clues as to the status of lipid deposition as well as an indication of the magnitude and chronicity of systemic blood pressure in the arterioles and arteries.

Symptoms of systemic diseases, such as sickle-cell anemia and disseminated intravascular coagulation, can be detected in the retina, as can unique ocular entities such as Eales disease or retinopathy due to prematurity (see Chapter 18).

Inflammations of all types may involve the retina. The pathology of such inflammations is similar to that of inflammations in general, covered in Chapters 3 and 4. Injuries have been discussed in Chapter 5.

Degenerations commonly involve the retina. Many (such as microcystoid and "paving stone" degenerations), although quite common, are of little or no clinical significance. Other degenerations (for example, drusen) may lead to very serious abnormalities like macular degeneration. Degenerations may occur in highly myopic eyes, or following ingestion of certain drugs such as chloroquine (toxic retinopathy), or after radiotherapy near the eye (postradiation retinopathy). Degenerations may result from previous injuries or as a consequence of exposure to various noxious agents.

Dystrophies, on the other hand, are primary afflictions of the retina. In general, dystrophies tend to be rare, tend to run in families, and tend to be bilaterally symmetrical. The pathology of many dystrophies has not been described. Some dystrophies, e.g., Stargardt disease and fundus flavimaculatus, have only recently been characterized. The pathology of retinitis pigmentosa, conversely, has been known for a long time, but its cause is unknown.

The retina may be involved secondarily in hereditary disease. Angioid streaks may be found in pseudoxanthoma elasticum, fibrodysplasia hyperelastica (Ehlers-Danlos syndrome), osteitis deformans (Paget disease), sickle-cell anemia, acromegaly, epilepsy, idiopathic thrombocytopenia purpura, trauma, hyperphosphatemia, choriocapillaris atrophy involving posterior eyegrounds, and numerous other entities. Streaks also may be idiopathic. The mucolipidoses (e.g., fucosidosis) mostly involve the anterior part of the eye, especially the cornea, but also may involve the retina. The sphingolipidoses (e.g., Tay-Sachs disease) usually involve the retina, accentuating the normal foveal ("macular") cherry-red spot.

Systemic diseases may affect the retina. The most common of these, diabetes mellitus, is discussed in Chapter 15. Tumors may arise from the retinal pigment epithelium (see Chapter 17), from the neurons (retinoblastoma, see Chapter 18), congenitally (phakomatoses, see Chapter 2), or from the glial elements. The glial cells may proliferate, as in "cellophane maculopathy," where the cells grow out of the retina onto its internal surface to form an epiretinal membrane. Benign neoplasms may develop, such as a benign astrocytoma. Malignant retinal neoplasms almost never occur, except in the rare instance of metastases to the retina.

Retinal detachment, a separation of the neural retina from the retinal pigment epithelium, has many causes. In general, the detachment may be caused by an abnormality of the choroid, causing fluid to collect under the retina, by vitreous membranes that through traction pull the neural retina away from the pigment epithelium, or by a retinal tear (a rhegmatogenous retinal detachment). Following a retinal detachment due to any cause, the outer layers of the retina, removed from their choriocapillaris blood supply, subsequently degenerate.

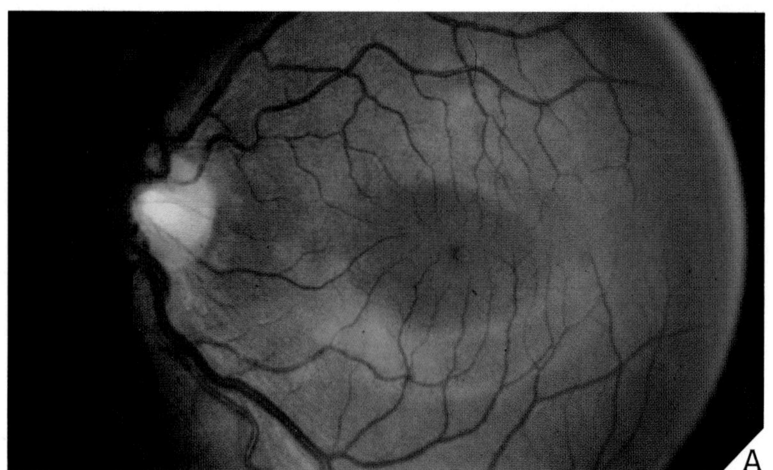

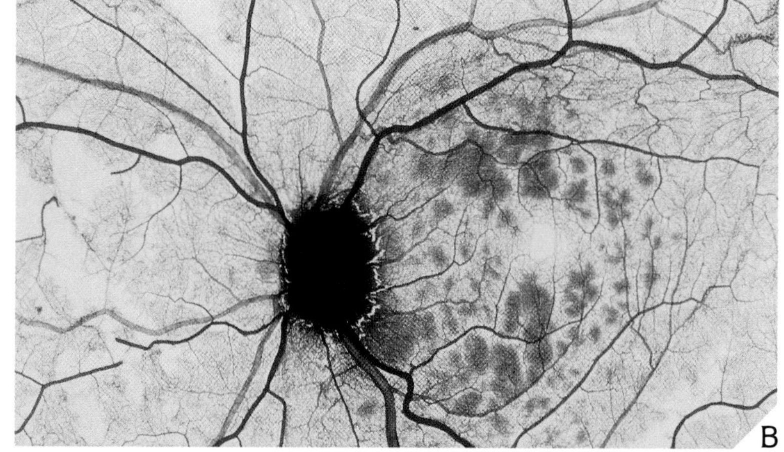

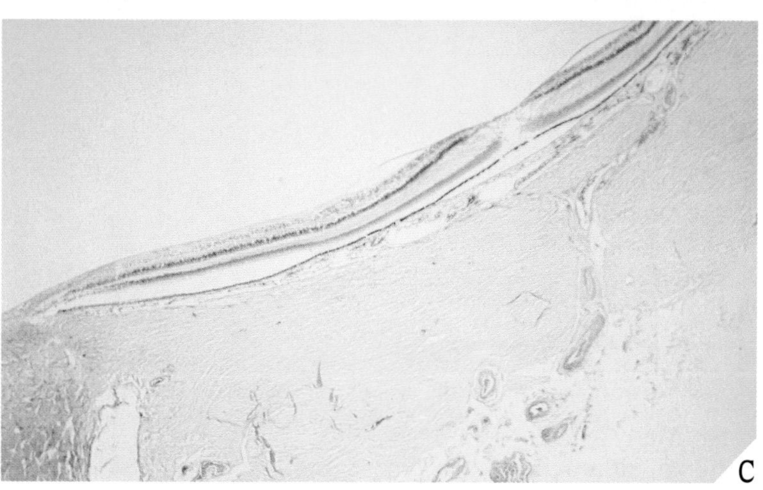

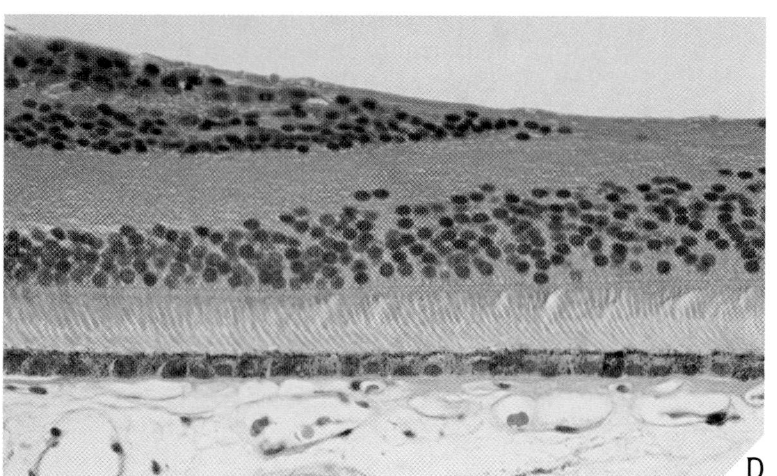

FIGURE 11.1 NORMAL RETINA. A The anatomic fovea (retinal pit, fovea centralis, clinical macula) is about the same size as the optic nerve head and is seen clearly in this child's eye as a central, horizontally oval ring reflex. **B** A retinal trypsin-digesting preparation shows the dark optic nerve head, the arterioles (which have a small surrounding capillary-free zone and are narrower and darker than the venules), the retinal capillaries, the venules, and the avascular area in the central fovea. **C** The ring reflex of the anatomic fovea, as seen in **A**, is caused by a change in the light reflex as the retina changes abruptly from its normal thickness to the thinner central fovea. **D** Increased magnification of the anatomic central foveola (clinical fovea) shows the loss of all layers of the neural (sensory) retina except for the photoreceptors, the external limiting membrane, the outer nuclear layer, the outer-most portion of the outer plexiform layer, and the internal limiting membrane. (**D**, courtesy of Dr. RC Eagle Jr.)

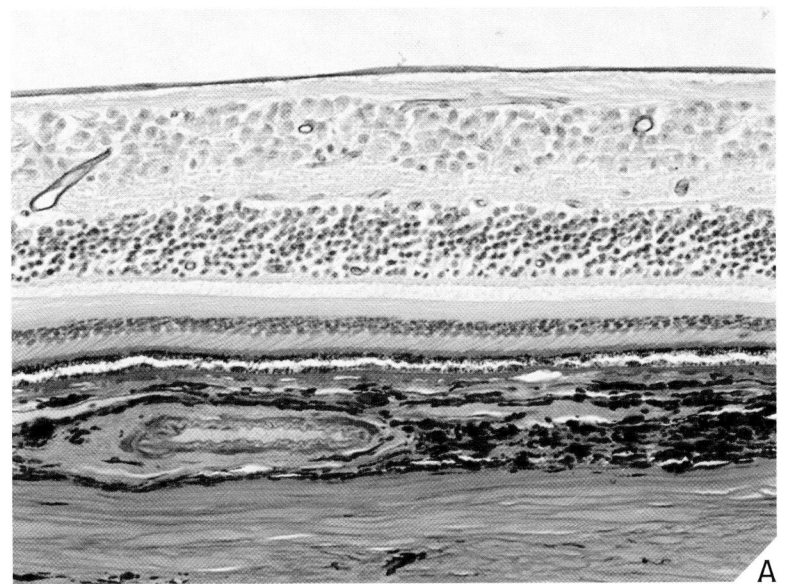

FIGURE 11.2 NORMAL RETINA. A The anatomic macula (posterior pole) is recognized by the multilayered ganglion cell layer, present between the inferior and superior retinal vascular arcades, and from the optic nerve temporally for a distance of about four disc diameters (approx. 6.0 mm). This PAS stain clearly shows the internal limiting membrane. **B** The retina consists of two major parts, the retinal pigment epithelium and the neural (sensory) retina. The latter can be divided into nine layers: 1) photoreceptors (rods and cones); 2) external limiting membrane (terminal bar [zonulae adherentes] attachment sites of adjacent photoreceptors and Müller cells); 3) outer nuclear layer (nuclei of photoreceptors); 4) outer plexiform layer (axonal extensions of photoreceptors), which contains the middle limiting membrane (desmosome-like attachments of photoreceptor synaptic expansions); 5) inner nuclear layer (nuclei of bipolar, Müller, horizontal, and amacrine cells); 6) inner plexiform layer (mostly synapses of bipolar and ganglion cells); 7) ganglion cell layer (here a single layer of continuous cells, signifying a region outside of the macula); 8) nerve fiber layers (axons of ganglion cells); and 9) internal limiting membrane (basement membrane of Müller cells). **C** Increased magnification of the photoreceptors shows that the cones are indeed cone-shaped and the rods rod-shaped. (**B**, modified from Fine BS, Yanoff M, 1979; **C**, courtesy of Dr. RC Eagle Jr.)

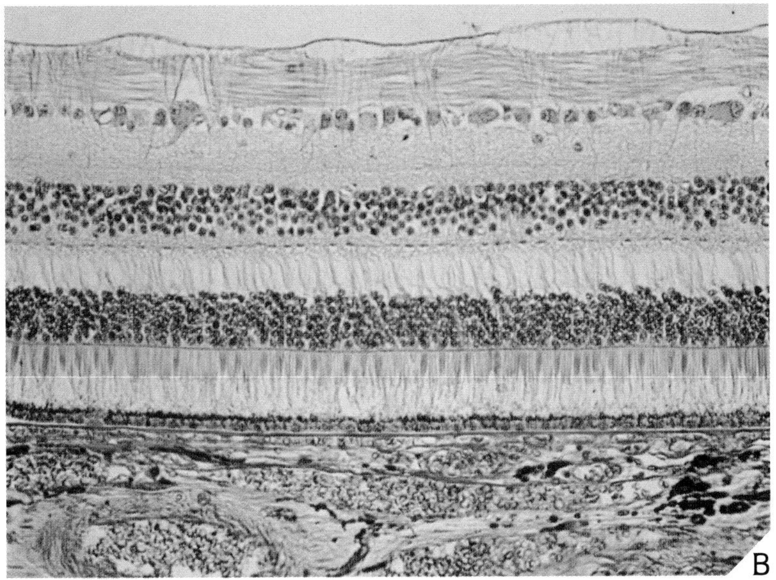

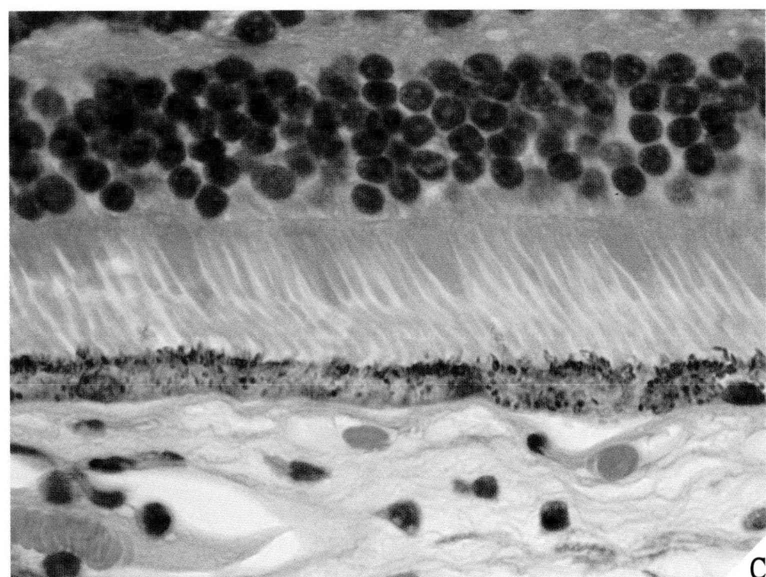

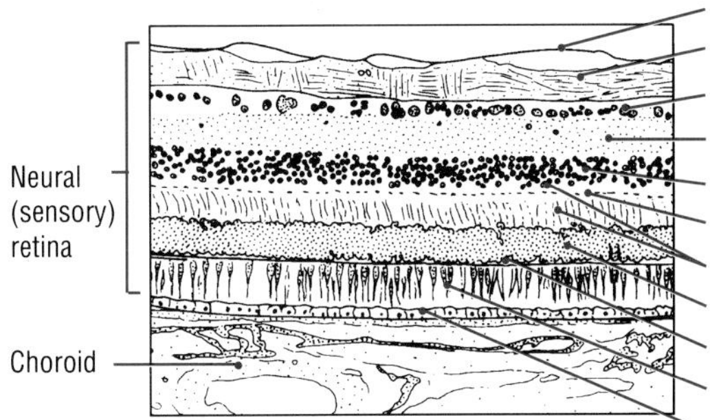

CONGENITAL ANOMALIES OF THE RETINA

- Albinism
- Grouped pigmentation
- Coloboma
- Retinal dysplasia
- Lange fold
- Nonattachment
- Retinal cysts
- Myelination
- Oguchi disease
- Foveomacular anomalies

FIGURE 11.3

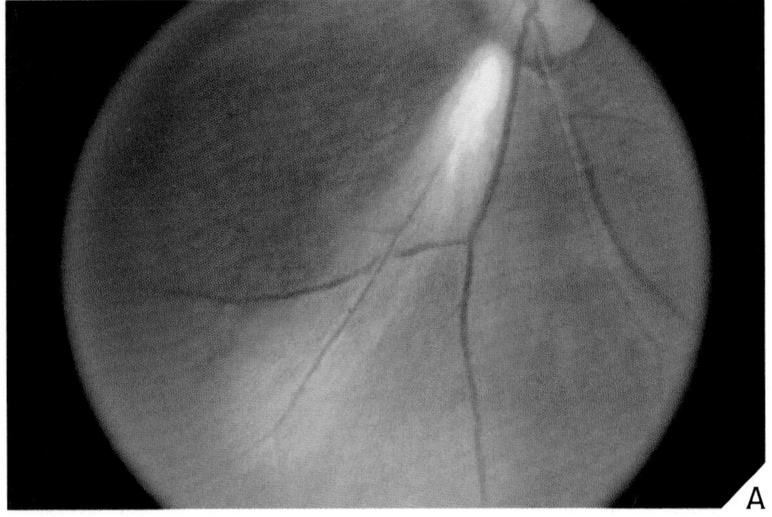

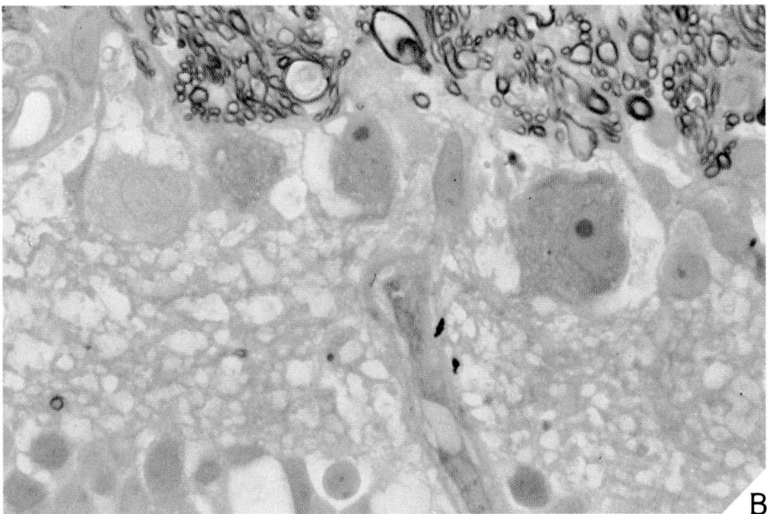

FIGURE 11.4 MYELINATED NERVE FIBERS. A The myelinated nerve fibers fan out from the vicinity of the optic disc. The edges tend to be "feathered." **B** A histologic section shows that the nerve fiber layer, just anterior to the ganglion cell layer, is thickened by heavy myelination. (**B**, PD stain.)

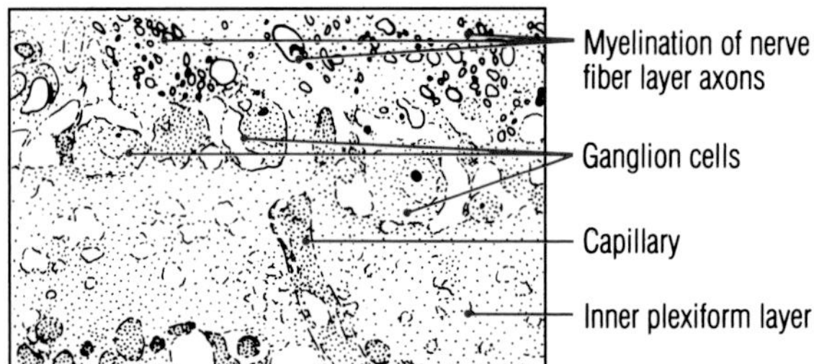

VASCULAR DISEASES OF THE RETINA

Retinal ischemia
Hemorrhagic infarction
Hypertensive retinopathy
Arteriolarsclerotic retinopathy
Diabetes mellitus (see Chapter 15)
Coats (Leber) disease (see Chapter 18)
Familial retinal telangiectasia
Retinal arteriolar macroaneurysms
Sickle-cell disease
Eales disease
Retinopathy of prematurity (see Chapter 18)
Hemangioma (capillary, cavernous)
Rendu-Osler-Weber disease (hereditary hemorrhagic telangiectasia)

FIGURE 11.5

RETINAL ISCHEMIA HISTOLOGY

Early

Coagulative necrosis of inner retinal layers
Cotton-wool spots

Late

Outer half of retina preserved
Inner half shows "homogenized scar"

FIGURE 11.6

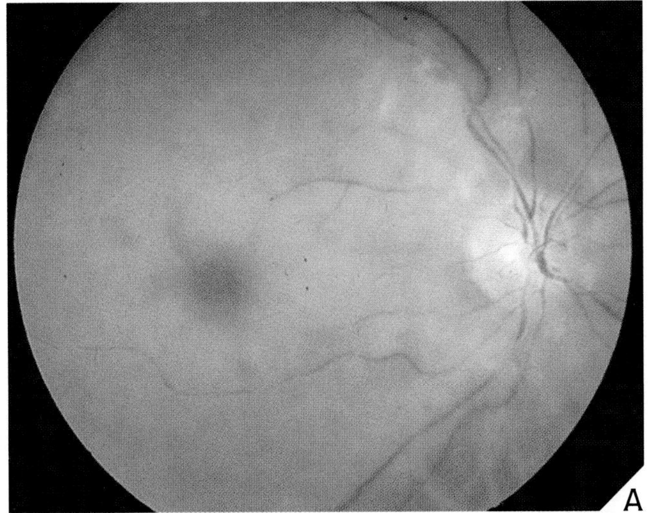

FIGURE 11.7 CENTRAL RETINAL ARTERY OCCLUSION. A The choriocapillaris shows through the central fovea (the thinnest area of the retina) as a red spot. The surrounding thickened edematous retina accentuates the normal red spot (also called a "cherry-red spot"). The retinal arteries are attenuated. **B** The central retinal artery (on the left within the optic nerve) contains an organized thrombus. **C** The early stage of retinal ischemia shows edema of the inner retinal layers and pyknosis of ganglion cell nuclei. **D** The late stage of retinal occlusion (after healing) shows a diffuse homogeneous acellular scar replacing the inner plexiform, ganglion cell, and nerve fiber layers. (**A**, from Yanoff M, Fine BS, *Ocular Pathology*, 2nd ed.; **B**, trichrome stain.)

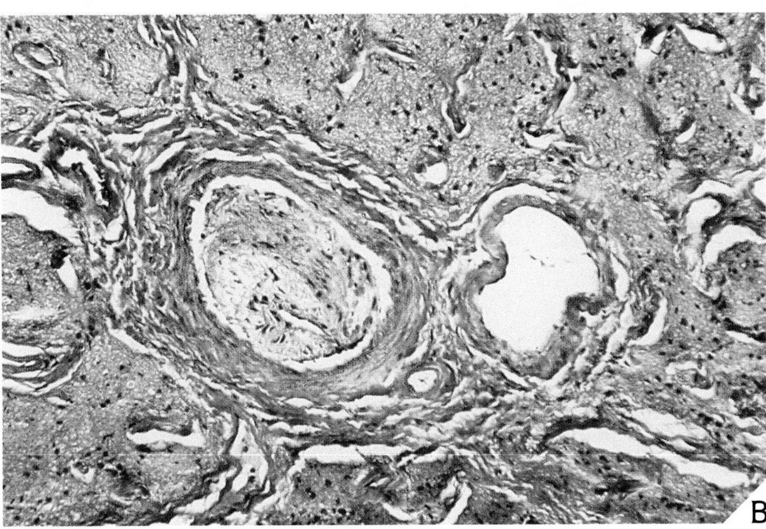

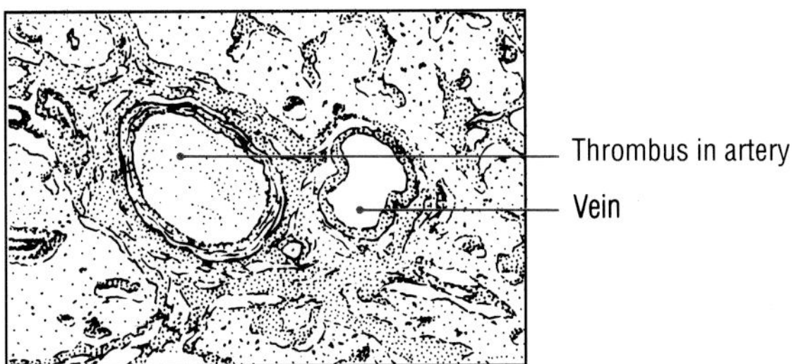

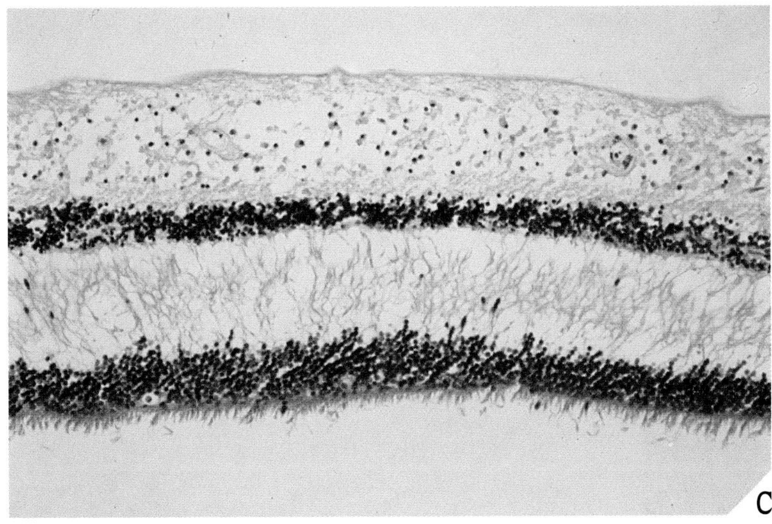

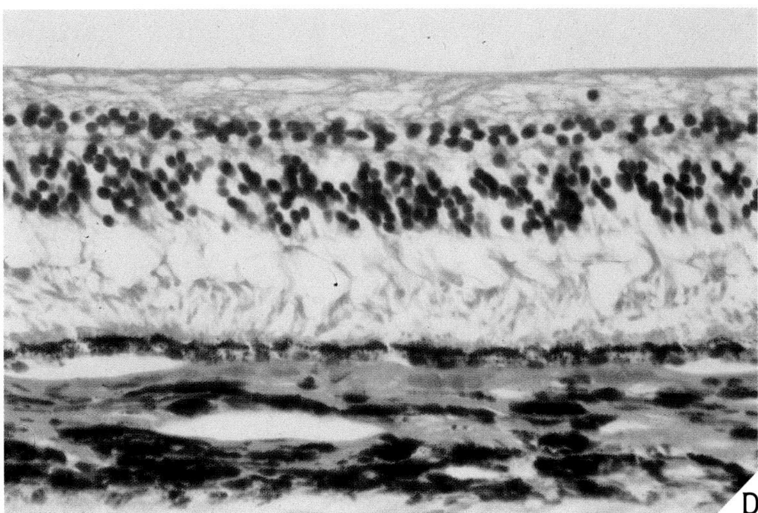

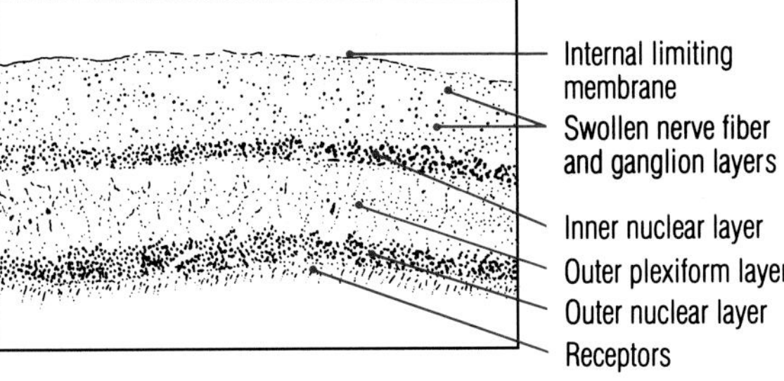

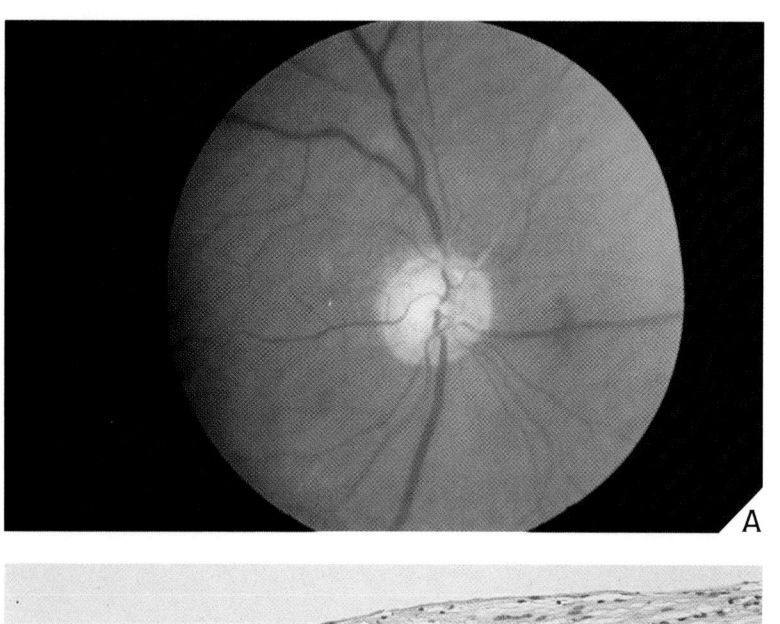

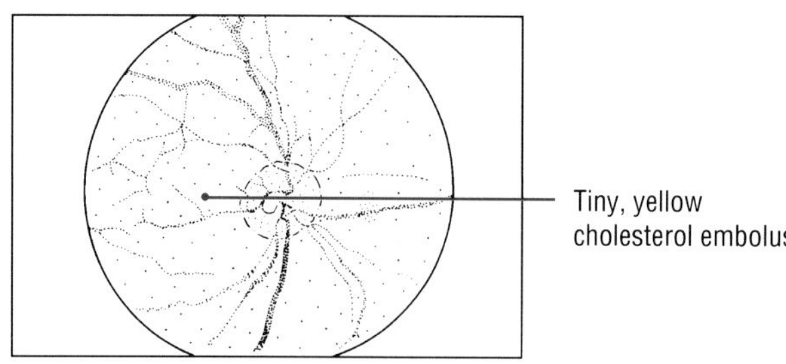

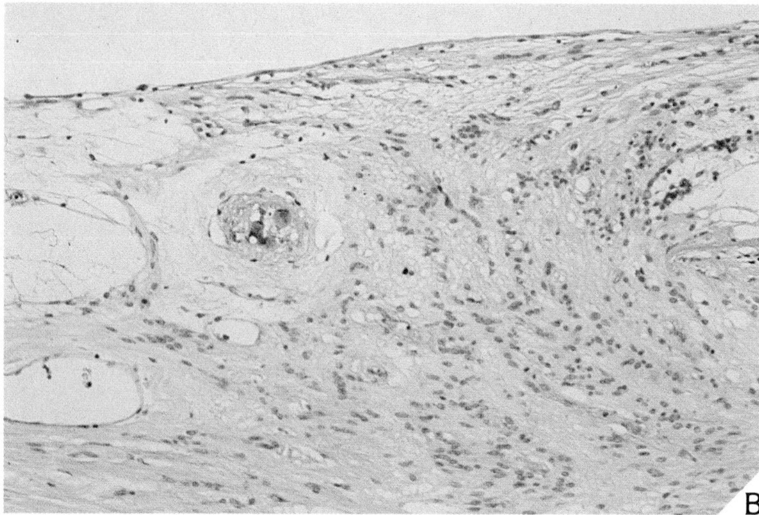

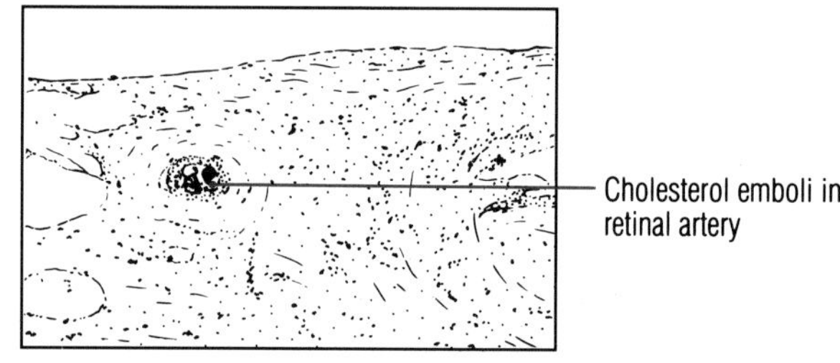

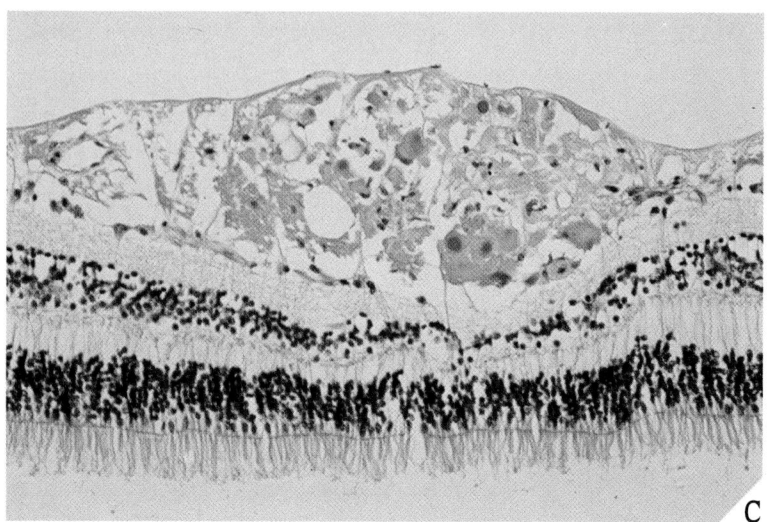

FIGURE 11.8 EMBOLI. A A cholesterol embolus is seen in a tiny vessel just temporal to the optic disc. Scattered "cotton-wool" spots also are present. **B** A histologic section of the same eye shows an intra-arterial embolus within the retinal portion of the optic nerve composed of cholesterol crystals and surrounded by foreign body giant cells. **C** A histologic section of a cotton-wool spot from another case shows a microinfarct of the nerve fiber layer. The individual nerve fibers are swollen and seen as round pink areas, each of which contains a central dark spot (the altered swollen end bulb of the axon). These structures resemble cells and hence are called cytoid bodies.

Central retinal vein occlusion

Primary open-angle glaucoma is present in 8%–20% of cases

Iris neovascularization is seen in 55%–65% of cases within the first six weeks to six months after an ischemic type of occlusion of the central retinal vein

Branch retinal vein occlusion

Neovascularization of the disc or retina may develop, especially if extensive capillary nonperfusion (ischemia) is present in the area of the occlusion

Histology

Early

- Hemorrhages are present throughout the retinal layers
- Normal retinal architecture is disrupted

Late

- Healing occurs by proliferation of glial cells and further disruption of the architectural pattern
- Special stains show iron distributed widely throughout the retina (hemosiderosis)

FIGURE 11.9

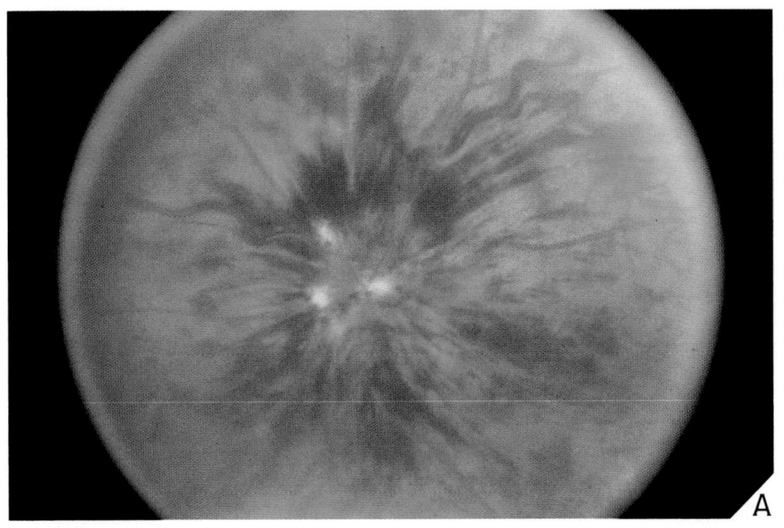

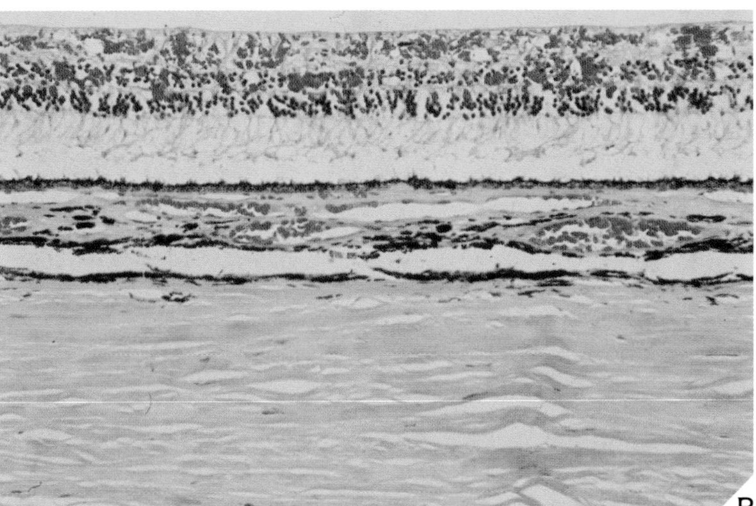

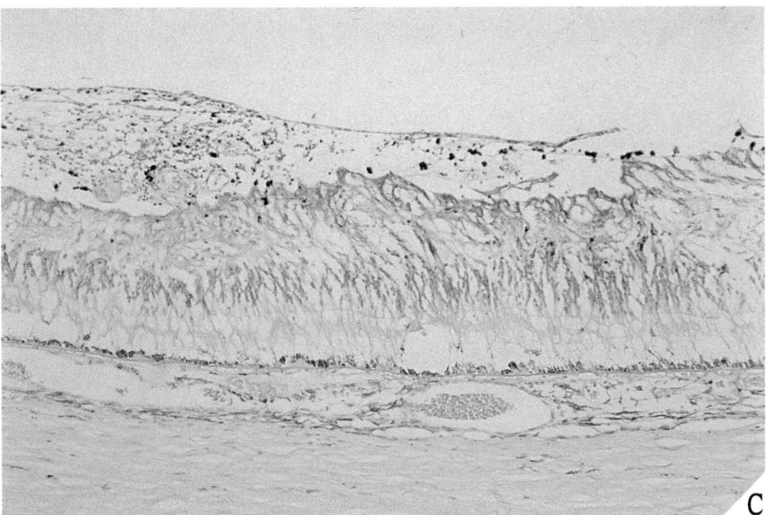

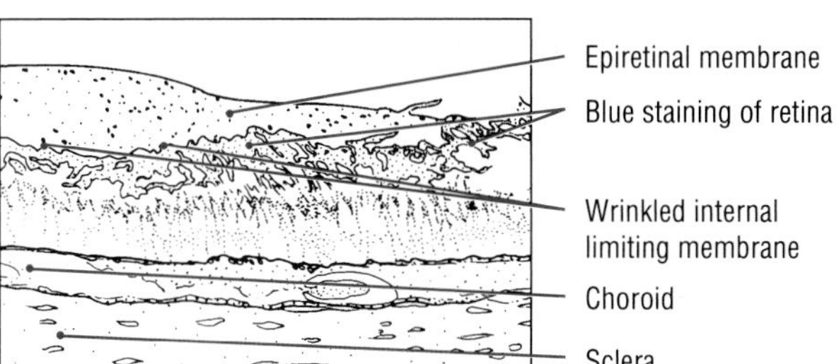

FIGURE 11.10 CENTRAL RETINAL VEIN OCCLUSION. A Typically, widespread hemorrhages and sheets of blood are seen in the fundus. **B** A histologic section shows blood throughout all layers of the retina. **C** With healing, a glial scar is formed. A special stain for iron (Perl stain) is positive (blue) throughout the retina. (**A**, courtesy of Dr. AJ Brucker.)

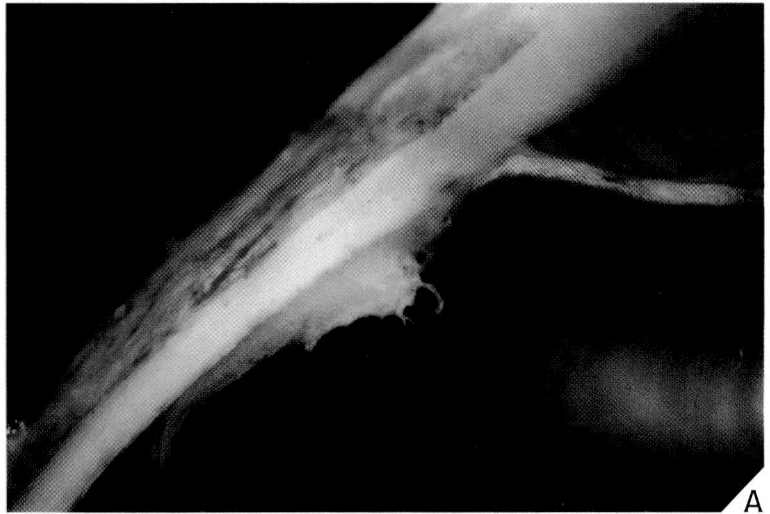

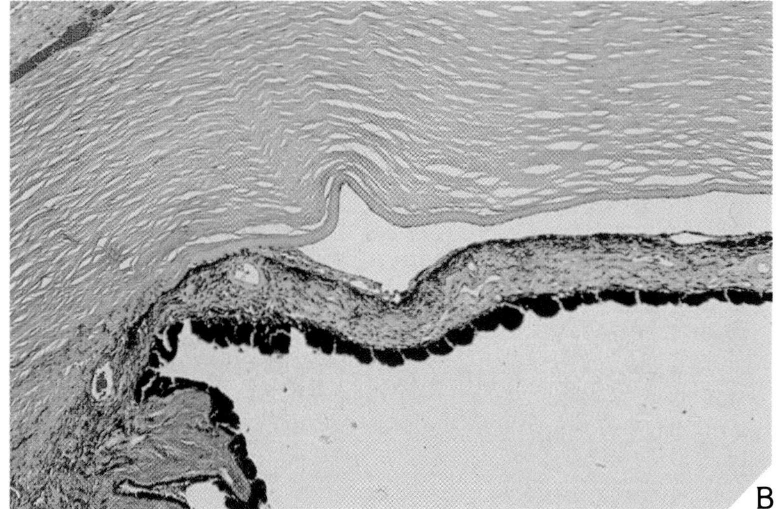

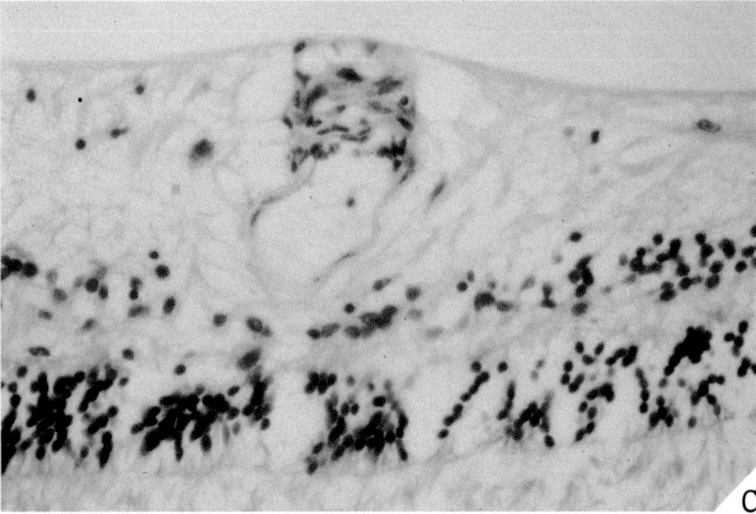

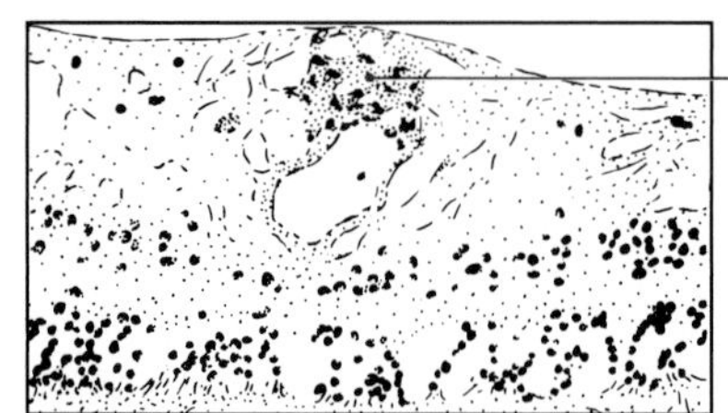

FIGURE 11.11 COMPLICATIONS OF CENTRAL RETINAL VEIN OCCLUSION. **A** A gross specimen shows neovascularization of the iris that has resulted in a peripheral anterior synechia. **B** A histologic section shows tissue present above the anterior border layer of the iris and between the peripheral iris and the cornea. The tissue is neovascular (fibrous tissue and blood vessels). **C** New blood vessels are shown budding off from a retinal venule in this example of early retinal neovascularization.

OCULAR FINDINGS IN SICKLE-CELL ANEMIA

- Peripheral vessel disease, especially occlusion of arterioles
- Peripheral whitening of retina
- Retinitis proliferans ("sea fans")
- Vitreous hemorrhage
- Retinal detachment
- Preretinal hemorrhages ("salmon patches")
- Pigmented chorioretinal lesions ("black sunburst sign")

FIGURE 11.12

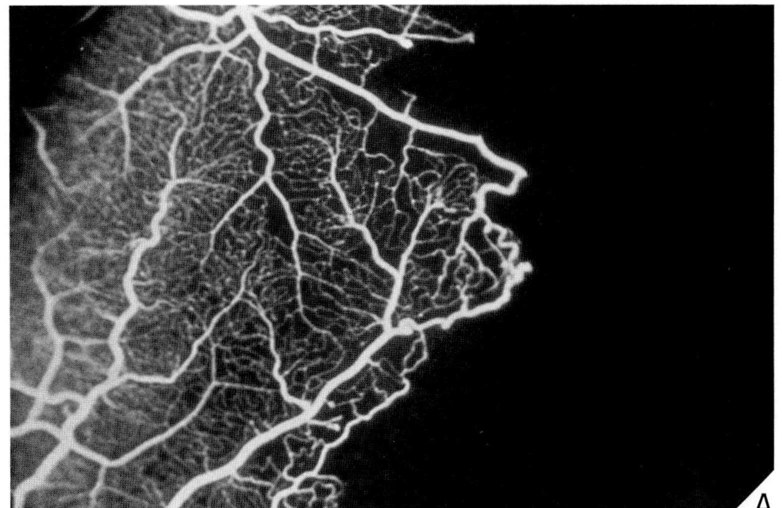

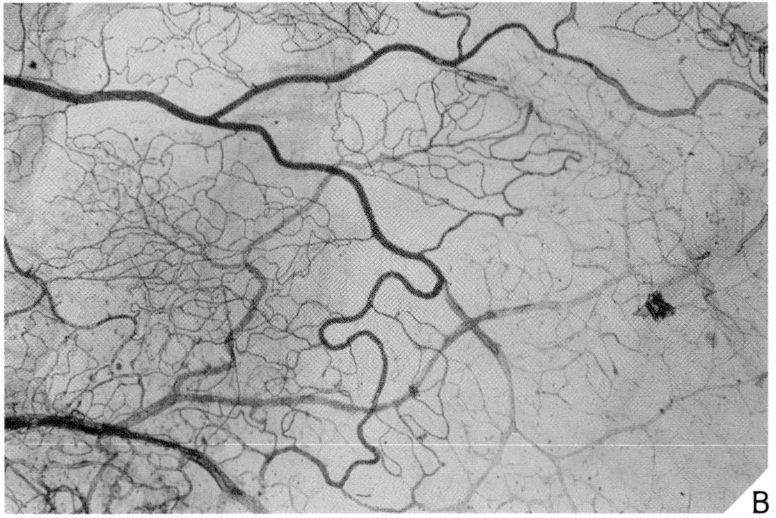

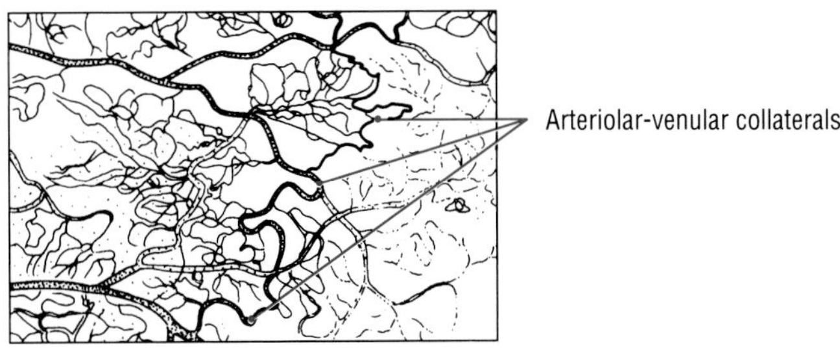

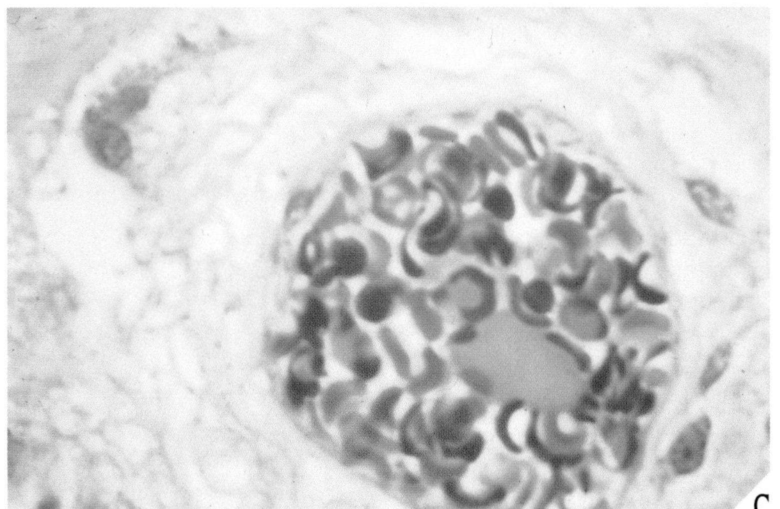

FIGURE 11.13 SICKLE-CELL HEMOGLOBIN C DISEASE. A The perfusion of the retina stops abruptly at the equator, resulting in nonperfusion of the peripheral retina. **B** Trypsin digestion of the equatorial region of the retina (in this case, of sickle cell hemoglobin C disease) shows that peripheral blood vessels are devoid of cells and are nonviable. Arteriolar-venular collaterals are noted in the equatorial region. **C** A peripheral arteriole is occluded by sickled red blood cells. (**B**, PAS stain; **C**, MB stain; case reported by Eagle RC, et al., 1974.)

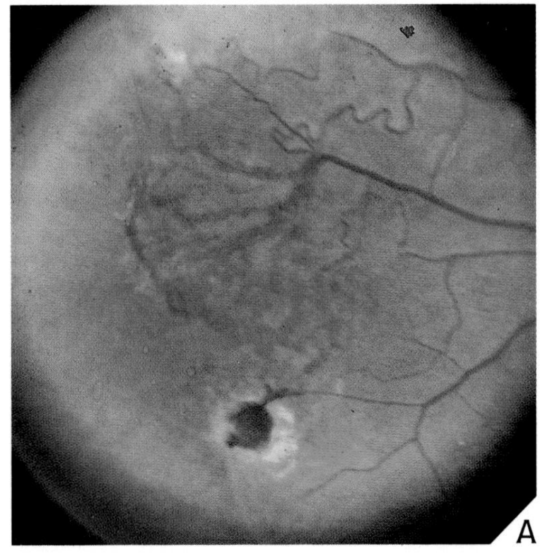

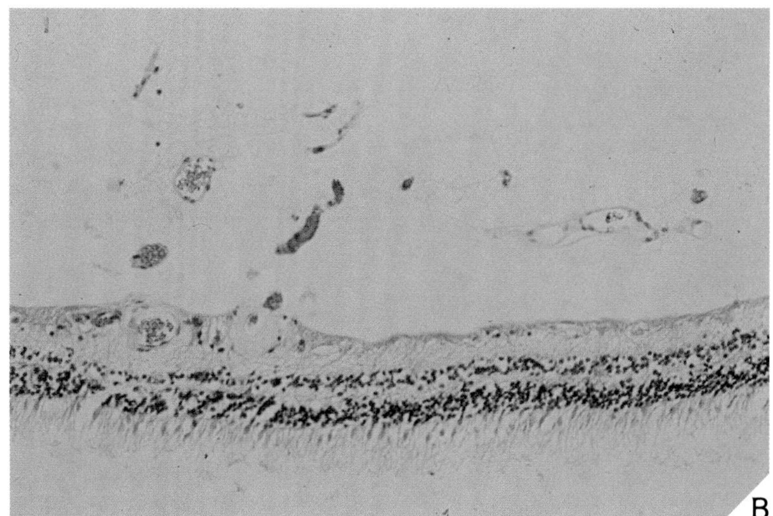

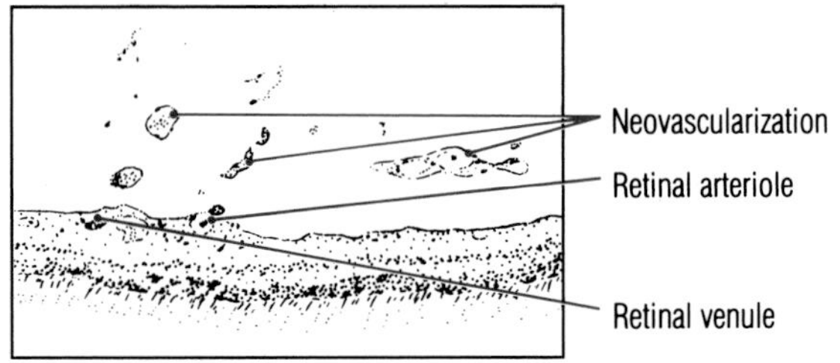

FIGURE 11.14 SICKLE-CELL HEMOGLOBIN C DISEASE. A A sea fan is present at the equator and a sunburst is seen below the sea fan. **B** A histologic section shows that the sea fan lies between the internal surface of the retina and the vitreous body. The neovascularization proceeds from a retinal arteriole into the subvitreal space and then back into a retinal venule. (**A**, courtesy of Dr. MF Rabb.)

DEGENERATIONS

Microcystoid	Drusen	Toxic
Primary retinoschisis	Albinotic spots	Postirradiation
Secondary retinoschisis	Myopic	Traumatic
Paving stone	Macular	

FIGURE 11.15

TYPICAL MICROCYSTOID DEGENERATION AND RETINOSCHISIS

Typical microcystoid degeneration

- Consists of an intraretinal space less than one disc diameter in size
- A universal finding with age
- Bilateral, superior temporal
- Starts at ora serrata and extends posteriorly and circumferentially
- Contains hyaluronic acid within intraretinal spaces
- Pathology involves the middle retinal layers

Typical (senile adult) retinoschisis

- Consists of an intraretinal space greater than one disc diameter in size
- Present in 4% of patients and bilateral in 80%
- Rare under 20 years of age
- Inferior temporal, 70% of cases; superior temporal, 25% of cases
- Small holes in the inner wall, larger outer wall holes
- Tends not to progress posteriorly
- Contains hyaluronic acid within intraretinal spaces
- Pathology involves the middle retinal layers

FIGURE 11.16

RETICULAR MICROCYSTOID DEGENERATION AND RETINOSCHISIS

Reticular microcystoid degeneration

Present in 13% of autopsy eyes and in every decade of life
Bilateral in 41% of patients
Inferior and superior temporal areas involved
It starts posterior to typical microcystoid degeneration
Contains hyaluronic acid within intraretinal spaces
Pathology involves the inner retinal layers (quite similar to that seen in juvenile retinoschisis)

Reticular retinoschisis

Present in 2% of autopsies and rare under 30 years of age
Bilateral in 16% of patients
Inferior temporal quadrant most common
Round or oval holes in the inner layer; rare outer layer holes
Pathology involves the inner retinal layers (quite similar to that seen in juvenile retinoschisis)

FIGURE 11.17

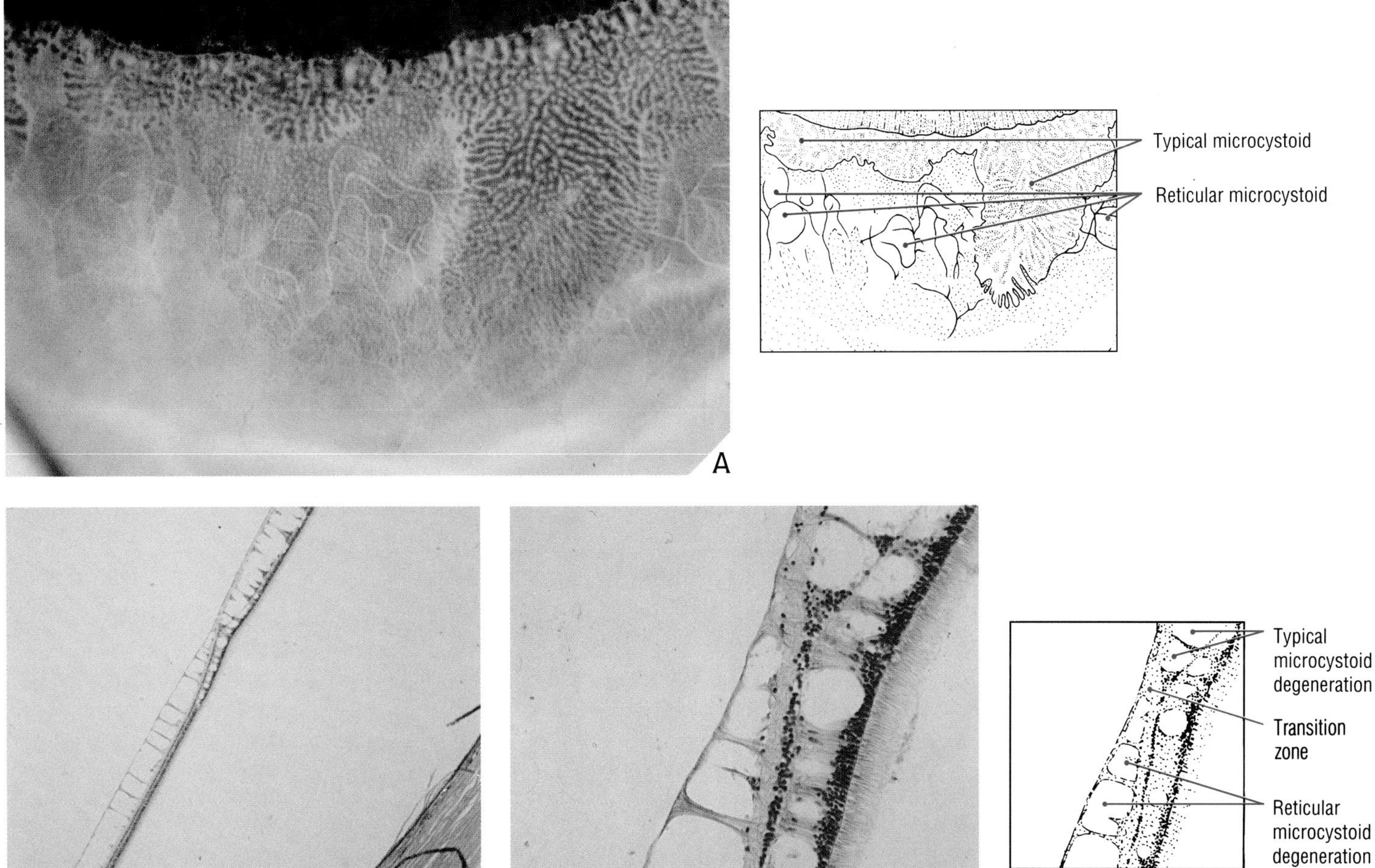

FIGURE 11.18 TYPICAL AND RETICULAR MICROCYSTOID DEGENERATION. **A** Typical microcystoid degeneration starts just posterior to the ora serrata. Reticular cystoid degeneration is present just posterior to the typical microcystoid degeneration. **B** A transitional zone from typical (middle retinal layers) to reticular (inner retinal layers) cystoid degeneration is seen. The typical microcystoid degeneration is to the right (shown under increased magnification in **C**). (**B**, **C**, courtesy of Dr. RY Foos.)

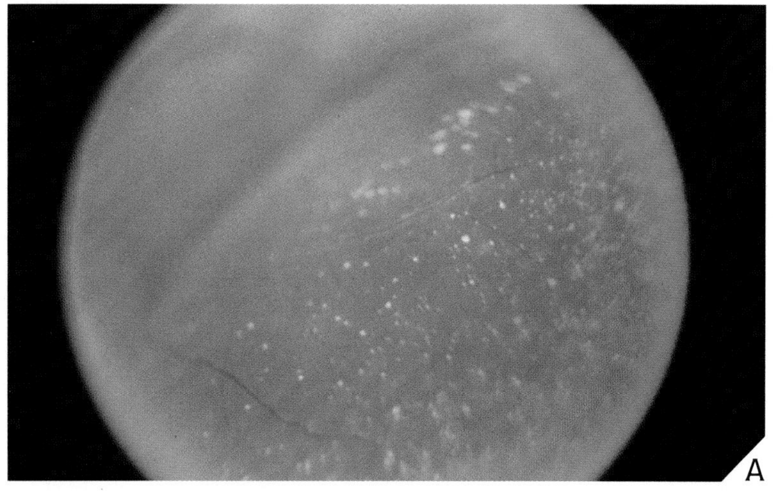

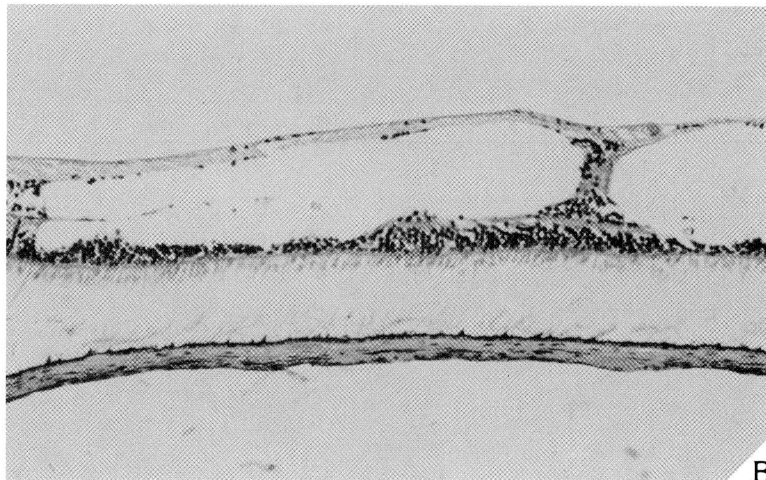

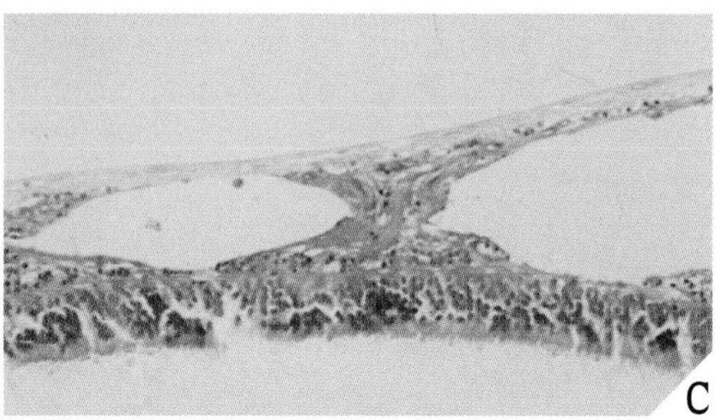

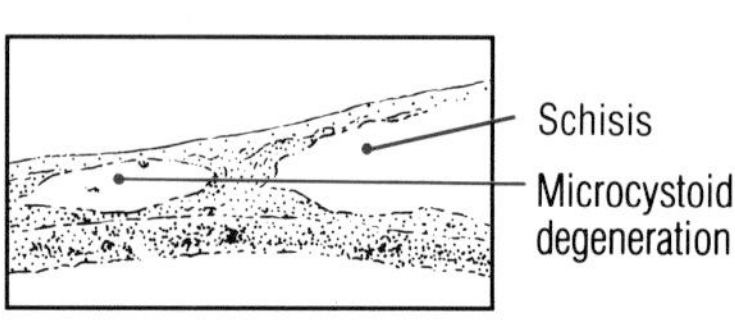

FIGURE 11.19 TYPICAL AND RETICULAR RETINOSCHISIS. A A large dome-shaped retinoschisis is present. Glistening yellow-white dots are seen on its surface. **B** A histologic section shows typical retinoschisis. In order to determine whether retinoschisis is typical or reticular, the beginning part of the lesion (to the left) needs to be examined. Here the lesion seems to start in the middle retinal layers. **C** A histologic section of reticular retinoschisis shows that the lesion starts in the inner retinal layers.

PAVING STONE DEGENERATION

Incidence: 22%–40% of patients
Involves inferior and temporal quadrants
Degeneration of outermost retinal layers
Does not make the eye more susceptible to retinal detachment

FIGURE 11.20

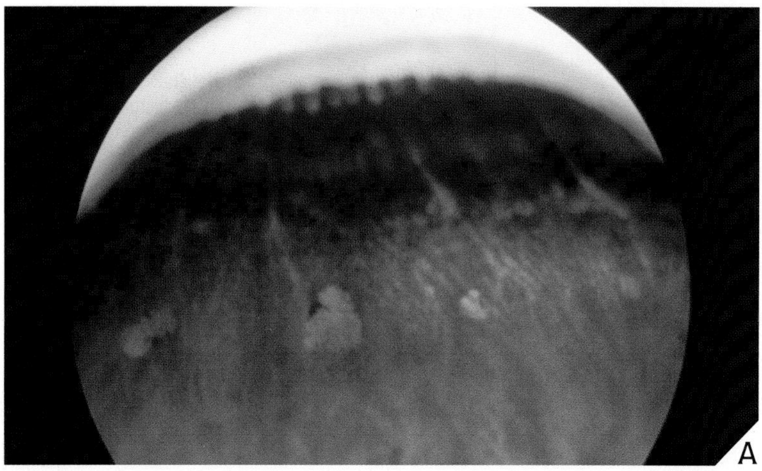

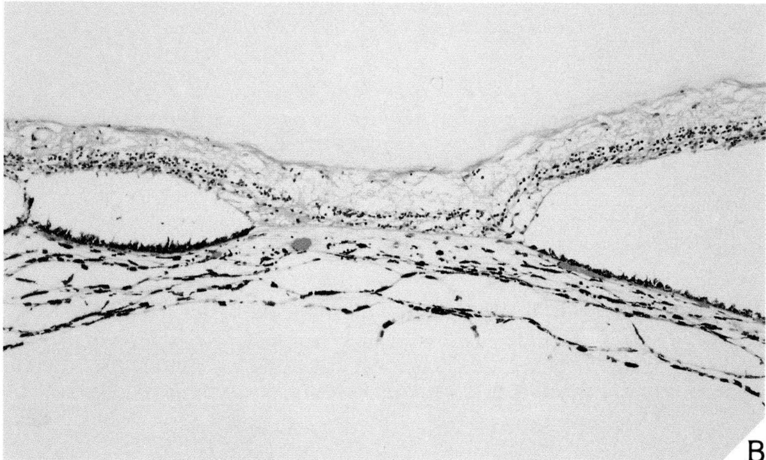

FIGURE 11.21 PAVING STONE DEGENERATION. A Examination of the gross specimen shows nonelevated, sharply demarcated yellow-white lesions which are present between the ora serrata and the equator. These lesions may extend and become confluent. **B** The retinal pigment epithelium ends abruptly in the area of degeneration. The Bruch membrane remains intact, but the overlying retina and the underlying choroid are atrophic.

IDIOPATHIC MACULAR DEGENERATION

Precursors

Central serous chorioretinopathy
Detachment of the retinal pigment epithelium
Drusen maculopathy

Types

"Dry" (atrophic)—no subretinal neovascularization (SRN)
"Wet" (exudative, disciform)—SRN present

FIGURE 11.22

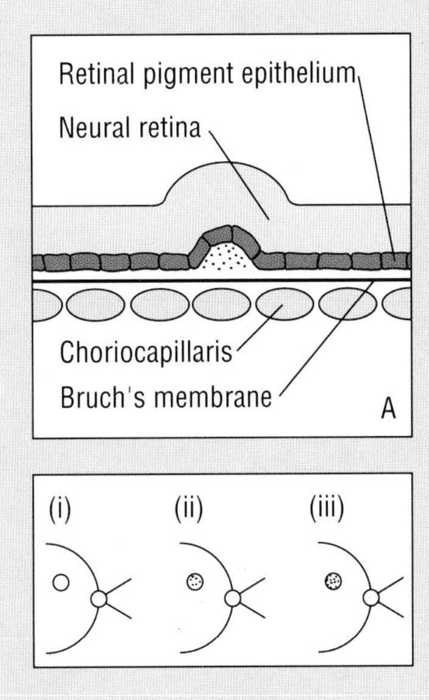

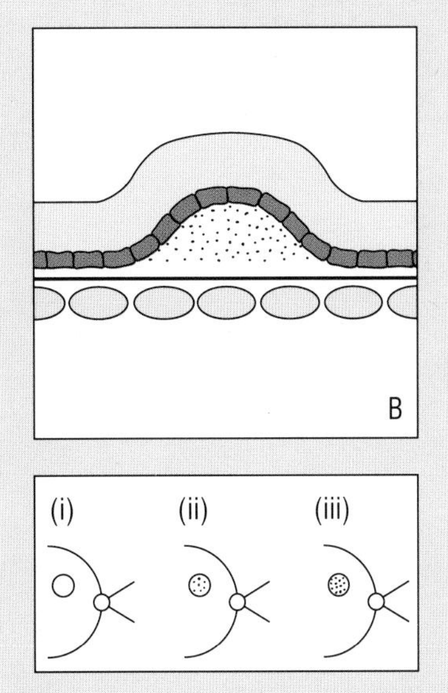

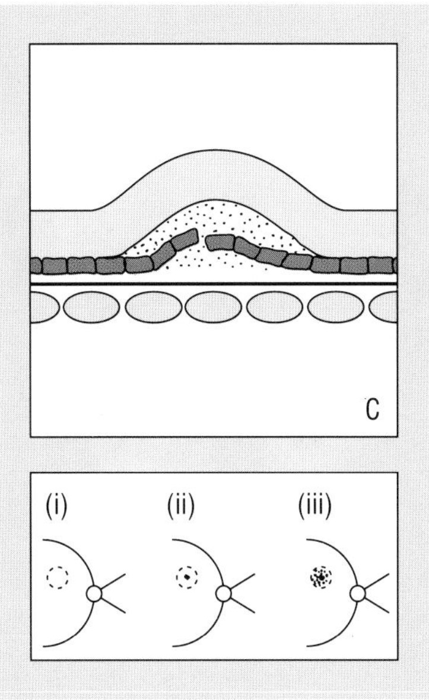

FIGURE 11.23 DETACHMENTS OF THE RETINAL PIGMENT EPITHELIUM AND NEURAL RETINA. The schematic histology drawings in the upper panels correspond with the schematic drawings of the fundus pictures in the lower panels. **A** A small, simple retinal pigment epithelium (RPE) detachment. **B** A large RPE detachment. **C** A small RPE detachment with an overlying neural retina (NR) serous detachment. The triple drawings of the fundus represent (i) before fluorescein injection, (ii) the early fluorescein stage, and (iii) the late fluorescein stage. Note that the RPE detachments are sharply demarcated and fill with fluorescein completely in the late stage, whereas the NR serous detachment has fuzzy borders and does not fill completely in the late stage. (Adapted from Figure 11.39 from Yanoff M, Fine BS, *Ocular Pathology*, 2nd ed.)

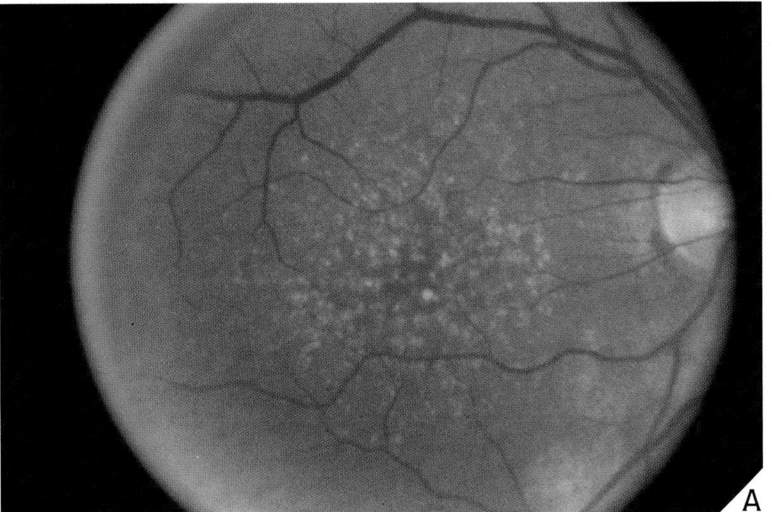

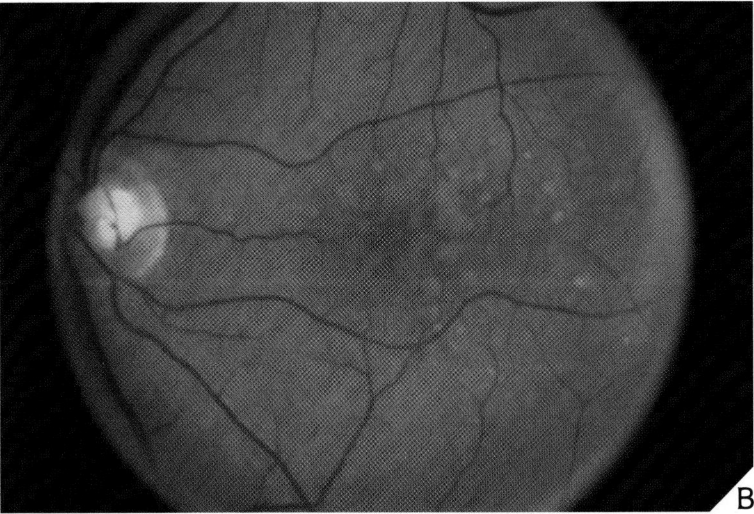

FIGURE 11.24 DRUSEN. A The fundus picture shows small "hard" drusen. Hard drusen apparently predispose the eye to geographic atrophy of the RPE ("dry" macular degeneration). **B** Large "soft" drusen are present. Soft drusen apparently result from large amounts of abnormal basement membrane material that accumulate between the RPE and the Bruch membrane. Soft drusen seem to predispose the eye to subretinal neovascularization ("wet" macular degeneration). (**A**, courtesy of Dr. RC Eagle Jr.)

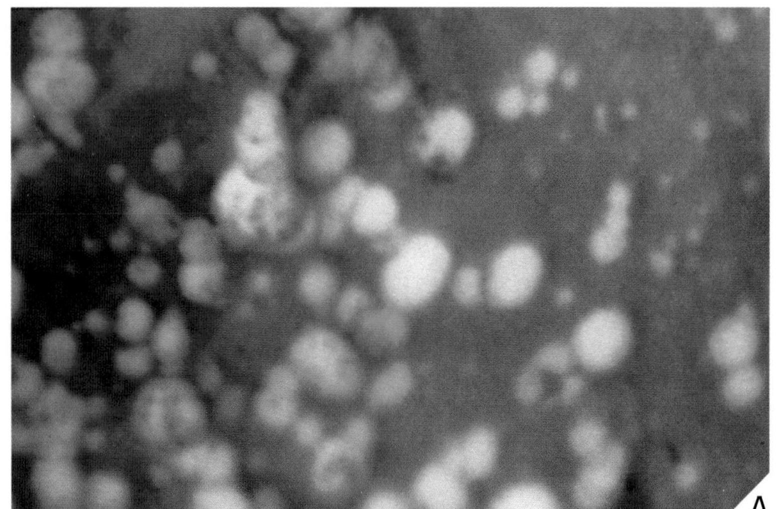

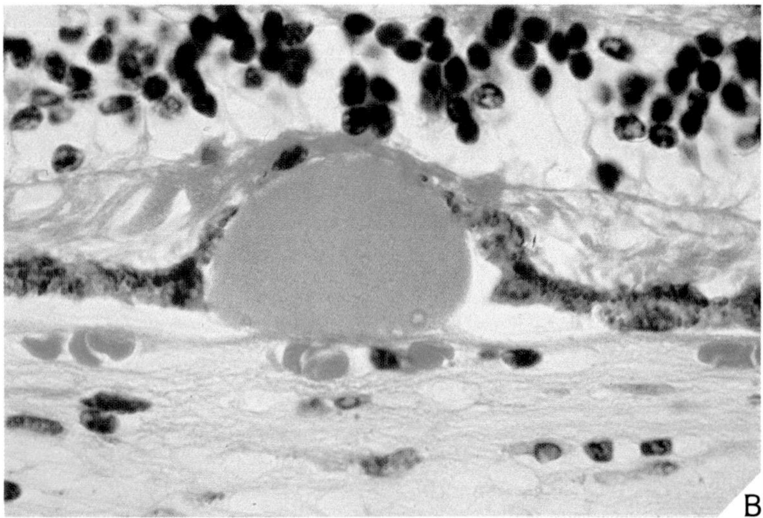

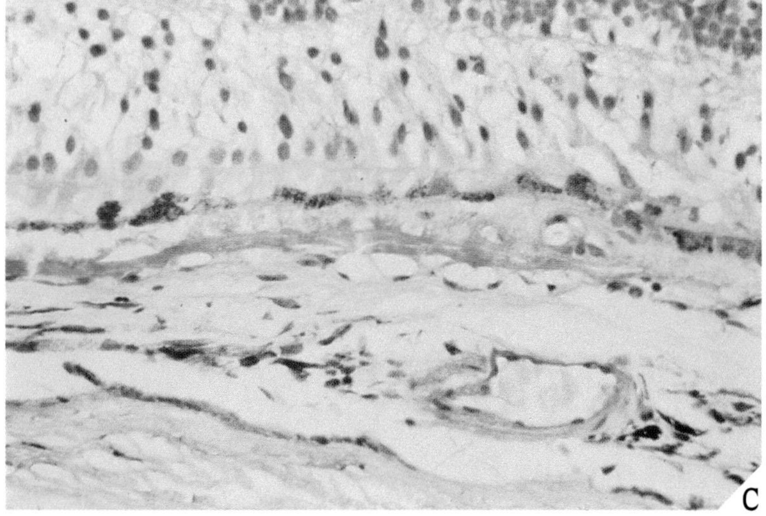

FIGURE 11.25 DRUSEN. A In this gross specimen, the neural retina has been removed. The drusen protrude from the choroid and RPE. **B** A hard druse appears as a collection of basement membrane material between the attenuated RPE and the Bruch membrane. **C** In this example, confluent drusen are present, analogous to the soft drusen seen clinically. Small blood vessels are present within the drusen. (**B**, courtesy of Dr. RC Eagle Jr.)

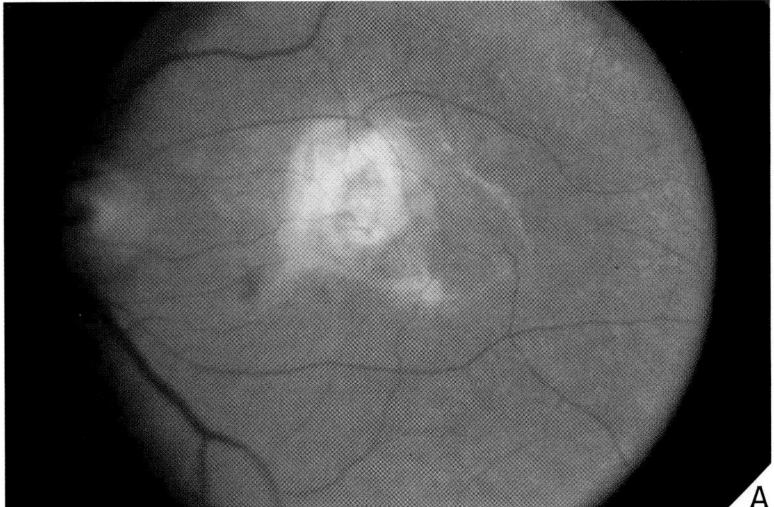

Figure 11.26 Disciform (Wet) Macular Degeneration. A The patient had subretinal neovascularization followed by numerous episodes of hemorrhage, resulting in an organized scar. **B** A small vessel has grown through the Bruch membrane into the sub-RPE space, resulting in hemorrhage and fibroplasia. **C** The end stage of the process shows a thick fibrous scar between the choroid and the outer retinal layers (trichrome stain). Note the good preservation of the retina, except for the complete degeneration of the receptors. (**B**, reported in Frayer WC, 1955.)

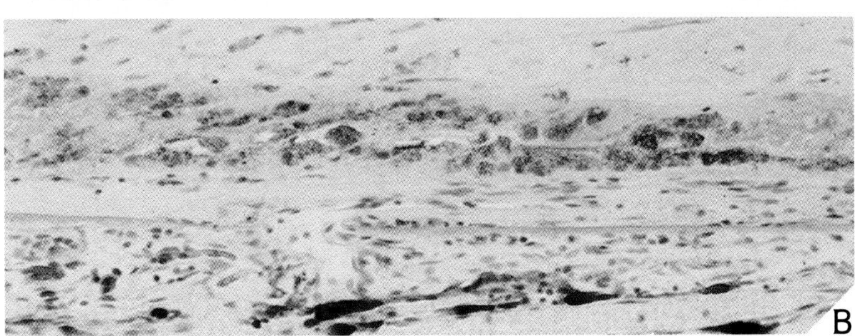

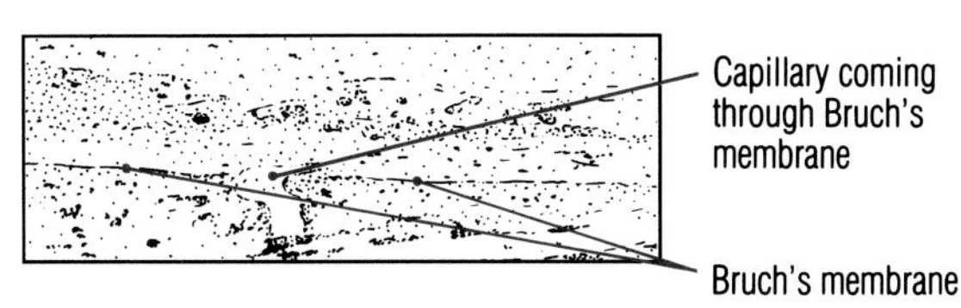

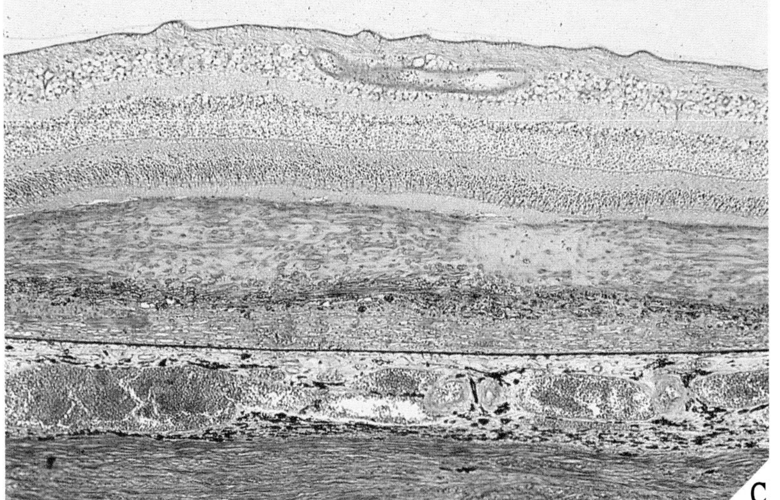

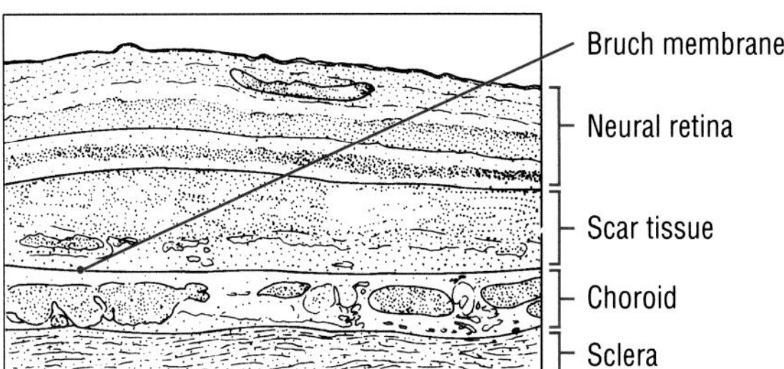

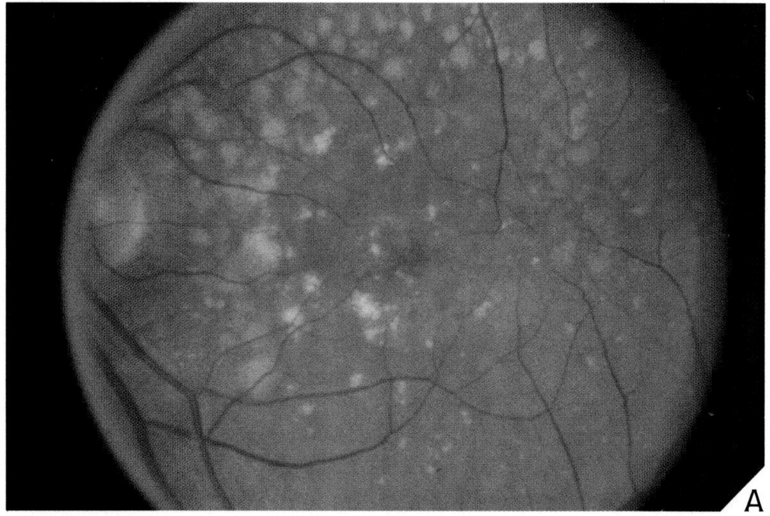

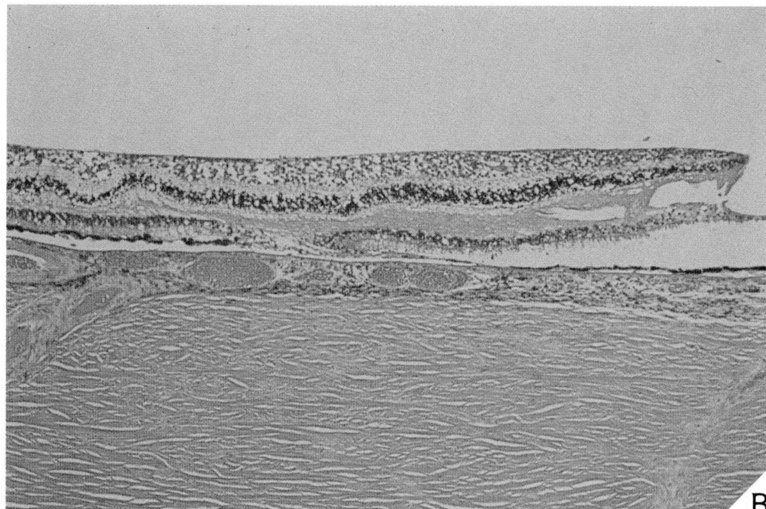

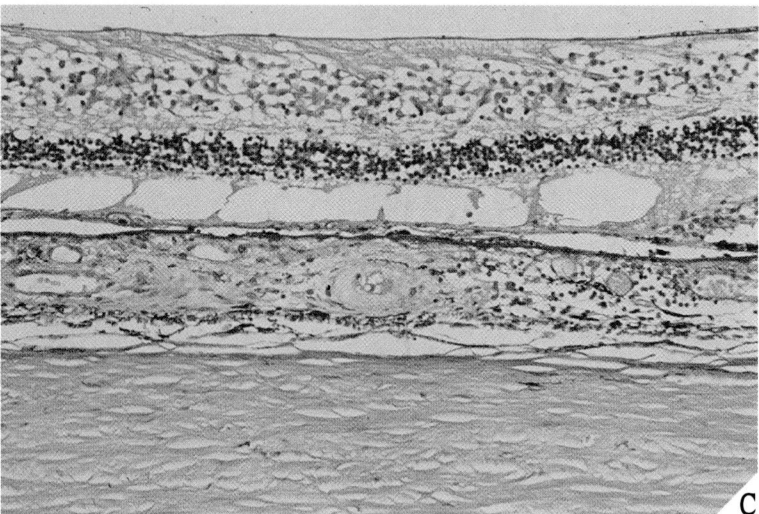

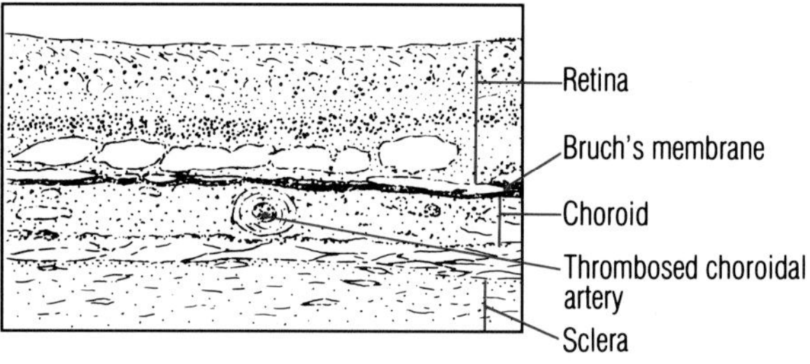

FIGURE 11.27 ATROPHIC (DRY) MACULAR DEGENERATION. A The patient showed drusen and other abnormalities of the RPE in the form of increased translucency, pigment mottling, and pigment loss. No subretinal neovascularization (SRN) was present in this eye. However, SRN was present in the other eye. **B** A histologic section of another eye shows irregular degeneration of the RPE and the outer retinal layers, as well as cystic changes in the outer plexiform layer. **C** Another level of the same eye shows similar retinal changes along with a thrombus in a choroidal artery. Whether the choroidal thrombosis is related to the retinal changes in atrophic macular degeneration is not known. (**C**, from Yanoff M, Fine BS, *Ocular Pathology*, 2nd ed.)

HEREDITARY PRIMARY RETINAL DYSTROPHIES

- Juvenile retinoschisis
- Choroidal (choriocapillaris, gyrate, central areolar, serpiginous)
- Stargardt disease and fundus flavimaculatus
- Retinitis pigmentosa (RP), peripheral and central
- Retinitis punctata albescens (may be a form of RP)
- Dominant drusen
- Dominant cystoid macular dystrophy
- Fenestrated sheen macular dystrophy
- Vitelliform (Best syndrome)
- Dominant progressive foveal dystrophy
- Progressive cone dystrophy
- Crystalline retinopathy
- Macular pattern (reticular, spider, butterfly)
- Pseudoinflammatory dystrophy
- Pigment epithelial dystrophy
- Central areolar pigment epithelial dystrophy

FIGURE 11.28

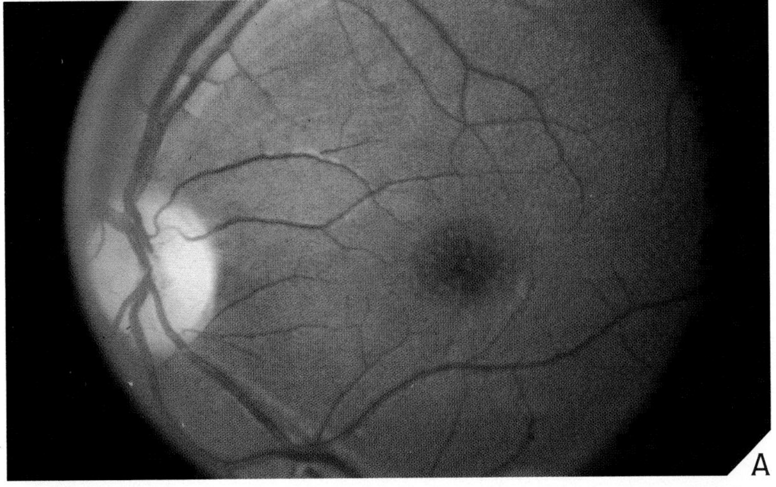

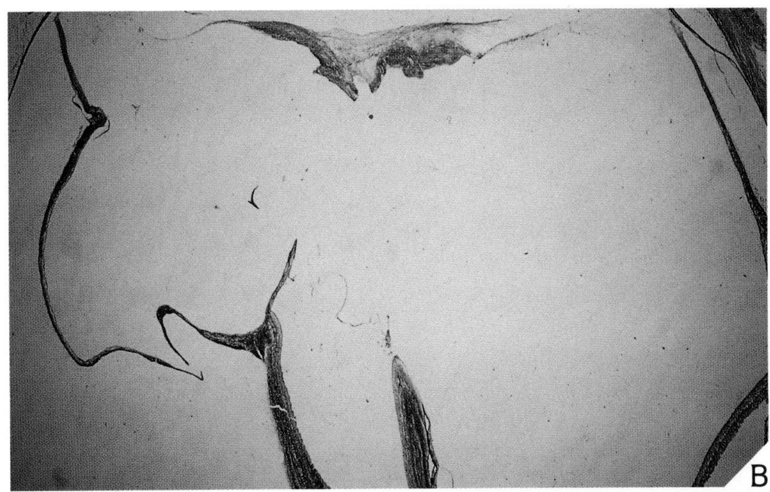

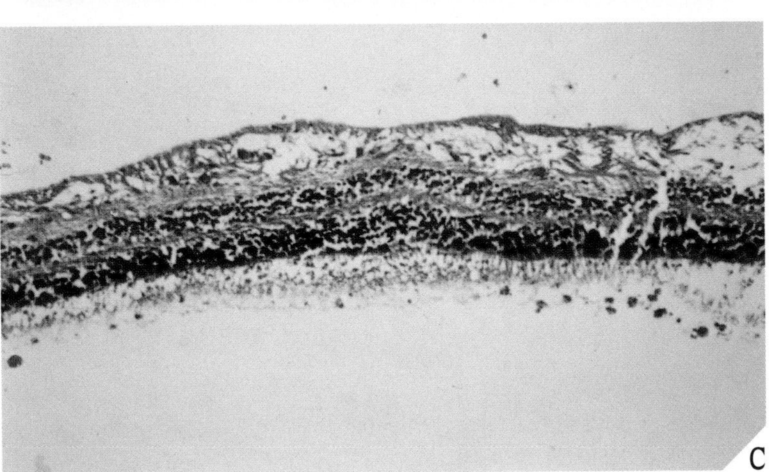

FIGURE 11.29 JUVENILE RETINOSCHISIS. A The characteristic foveal lesion, resembling a polycystic fovea, is shown. Typically, no leakage is present when fluorescein angiography is performed. **B** A histologic section of another eye shows a large temporal peripheral retinoschisis cavity. **C** A histologic section of another area of the same eye shows a splitting in the ganglion and nerve fiber layers of the retina, the earliest finding in juvenile retinoschisis. The area of pathology is the same as that seen in reticular microcystoid degeneration and retinoschisis. (**A**, courtesy of Dr. AJ Brucker; **B**, **C**, case reported by Yanoff M, et al., 1968.)

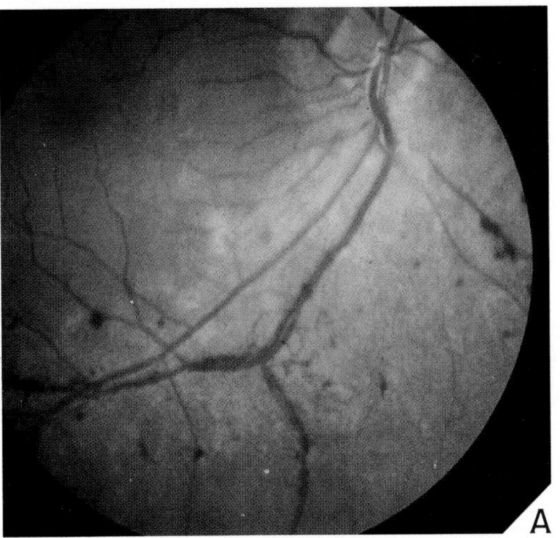

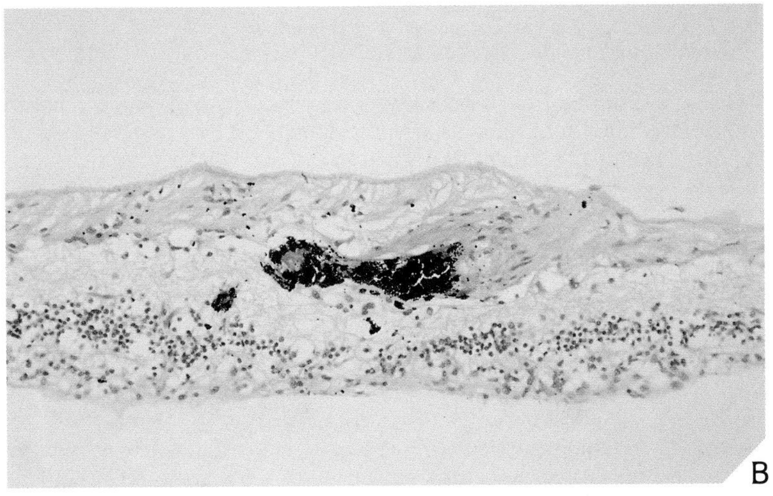

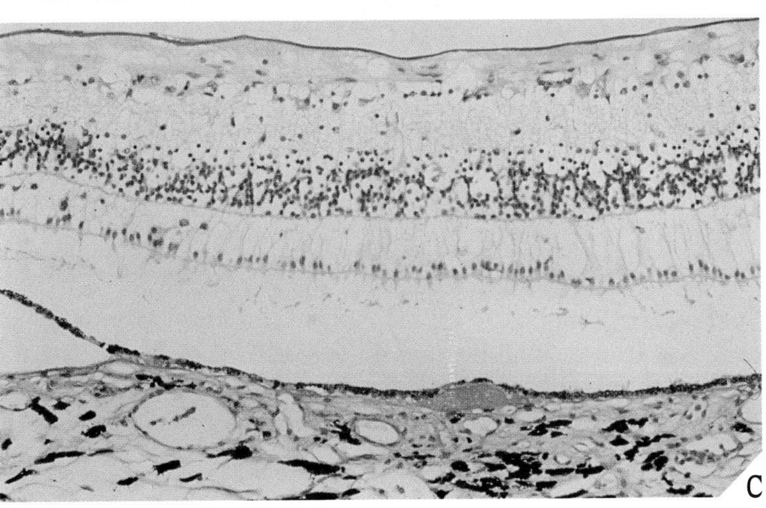

FIGURE 11.30 RETINITIS PIGMENTOSA. A The fundus picture shows a characteristic sharp demarcation from the relatively normal posterior pole to the "moth-eaten" appearance of the retina that extends out to the equator. Bone-corpuscular retinal pigmentation is present. **B** A histologic section of another case shows melanin-filled macrophages and RPE cells within the neural retina, mainly around blood vessels, resulting in the clinically seen bone-corpuscular retinal pigmentation. **C** A histologic section of the posterior pole shows loss of photoreceptors and atrophy of the choriocapillaris. (See Fig. 10.11B for picture of cataract in retinitis pigmentosa.)

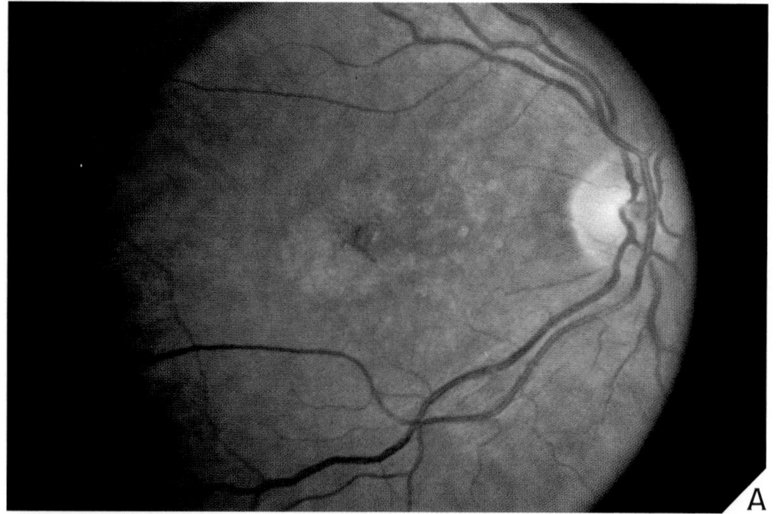

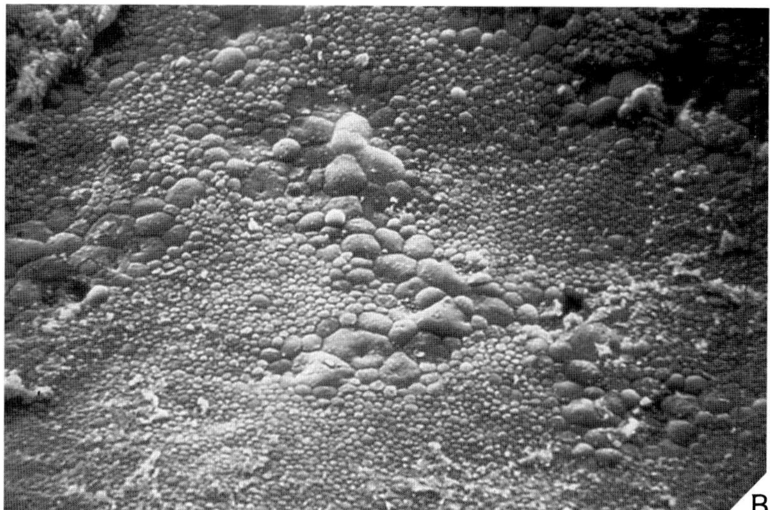

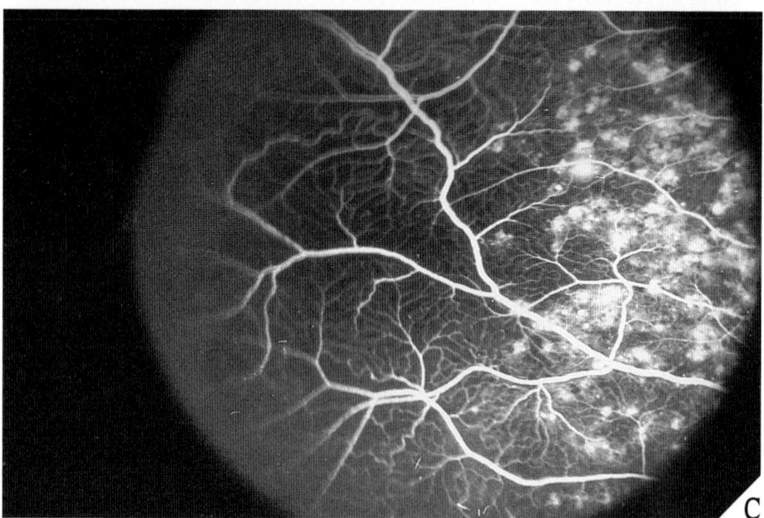

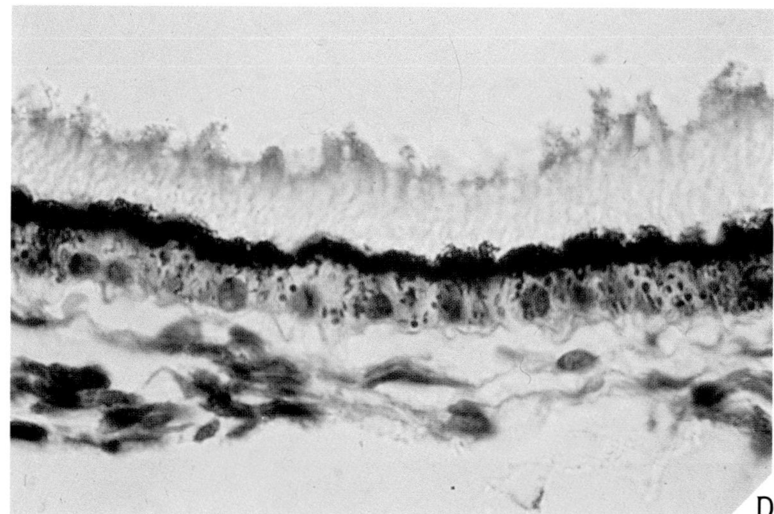

FIGURE 11.31 STARGARDT DISEASE (FUNDUS FLAVIMACULATUS). A Characteristic yellow-white flecks and an annular zone of foveal retinal pigment epithelial atrophy ("bull's-eye" maculopathy) are present. **B** A scanning electron micrograph of an enucleated eye from the brother of the woman whose eye is shown in **A** demonstrates that the yellow-white flecks are caused by irregular pisciform aggregates of enormous RPE cells, surrounded by a mosaic of smaller, relatively normal RPE cells. **C** Fluorescein angiography performed on the patient shown in **A** reveals a characteristic damping out of the background choroidal fluorescence (dark fundus). **D** A histologic section of the eye of the patient in **B** shows that the fluorescein effect is caused by enlarged lipofuscin-containing RPE cells, which act as a fluorescence filter. (**B**, **D**, case reported by Eagle RC Jr, et al., 1980.)

CAUSES OF BULL'S-EYE MACULOPATHY

- Age-related macular degeneration ("dry" type)
- Benign concentric annular macular dystrophy
- Chloroquine retinopathy
- Cone dystrophy
- Dominant slowly progressive macular dystrophy
- Fenestrated sheen macular dystrophy
- Fucosidosis
- Hallervorden-Spatz disease
- Neuronal ceroid lipofuscinosis (Batten disease)
- Olivopontocerebellar atrophy
- Retinitis pigmentosa
- Sjögren-Larsson syndrome
- Stargardt disease

FIGURE 11.32

HEREDITARY SECONDARY RETINAL DYSTROPHIES

- Angioid streaks
- Sjögren-Larsson syndrome
- Mucopolysaccharidoses
- Mucolipidoses
- Sphingolipidoses
- Other lipidoses
- Disorders of carbohydrate metabolism
- Osteopetrosis
- Homocystinuria

FIGURE 11.33

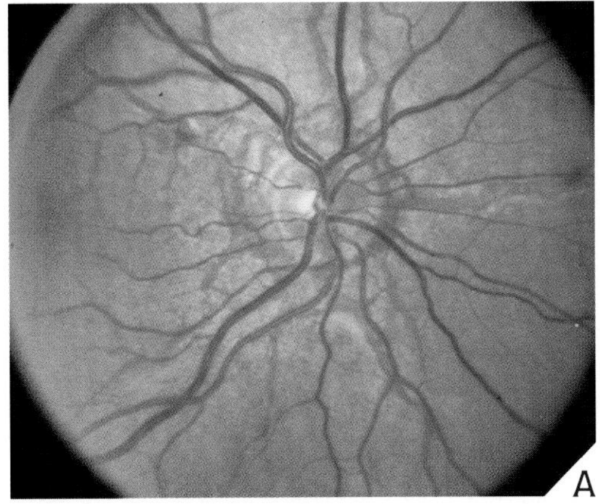

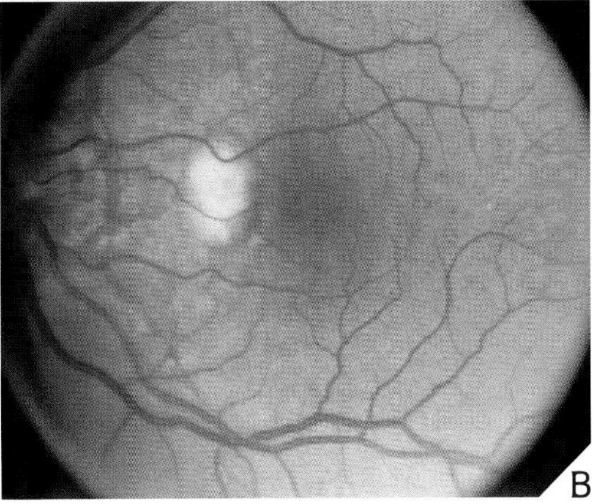

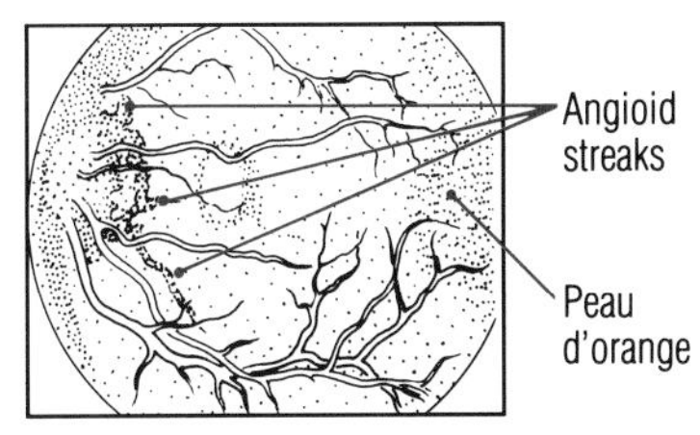

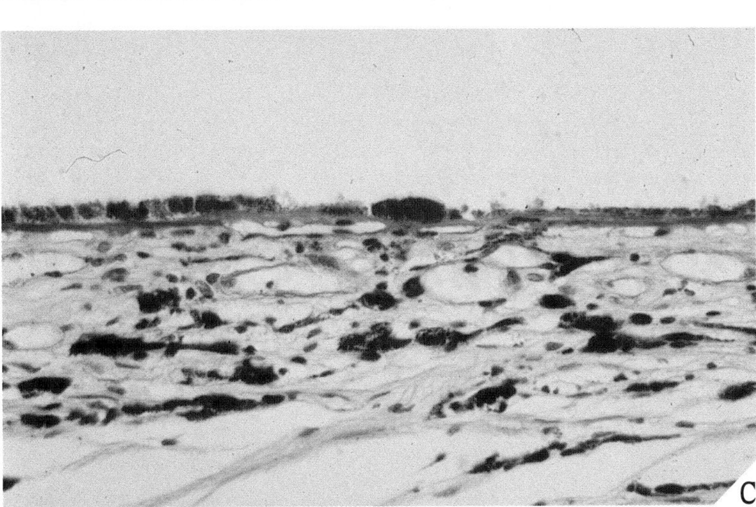

FIGURE 11.34 ANGIOID STREAKS. A This patient with angioid streaks also had pseudoxanthoma elasticum. The breaks in the Bruch membrane around the optic nerve resulted in angioid streaks. **B** Similar breaks away from the optic nerve have resulted in "peau d'orange" appearance. The yellow area just temporal to the optic nerve represents subretinal neovascularization. **C** A histologic section of another case, from a patient with Paget disease, also shows streaks caused by an interruption (break) in the Bruch membrane. Other causes of angioid streaks include acromegaly, Bassen-Kornzweig syndrome, chromophobe adenoma, diffuse lipomatosis, dwarfism, Ehlers-Danlos syndrome, epilepsy, facial angiomatosis, hemoglobinopathies, hyperphosphatemia, idiopathic thrombocytopenic purpura, lead poisoning, neurofibromatosis, and trauma. About half of angioid streak cases are idiopathic.

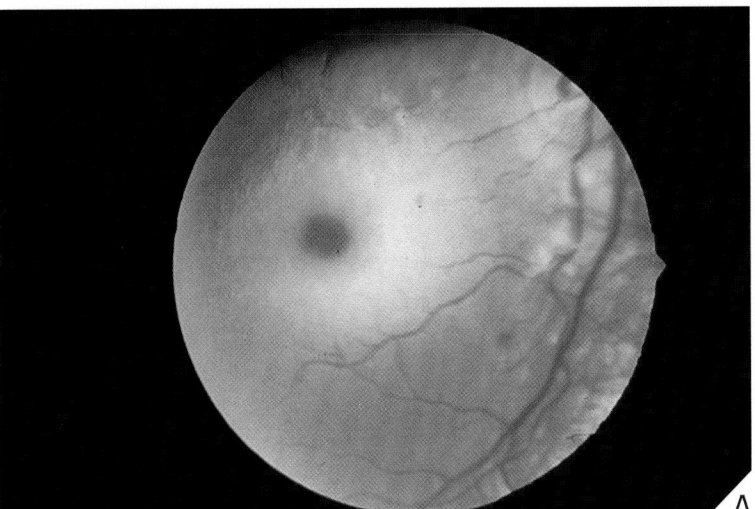

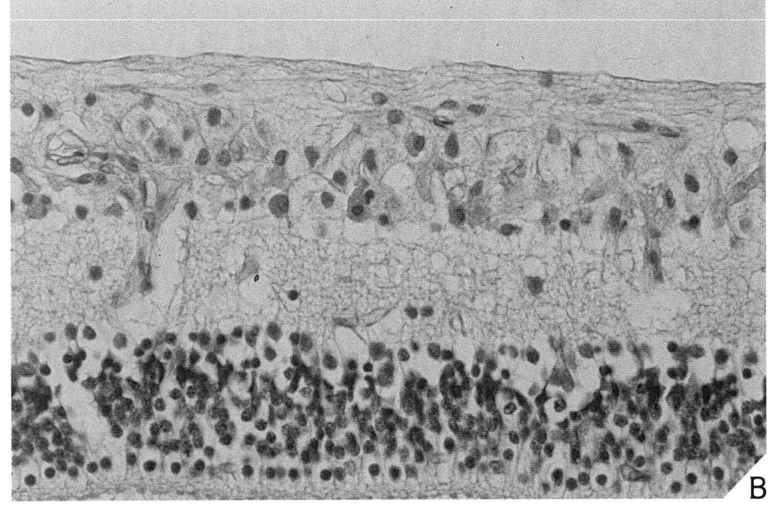

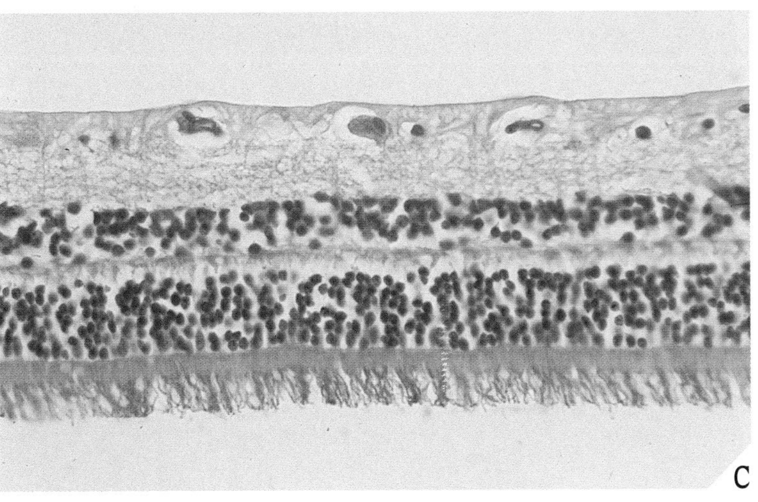

FIGURE 11.35 TAY-SACHS DISEASE. A A characteristic cherry-red spot is present in the central macula. **B** A histologic section shows a normal macular retina, except for ganglion cells that are swollen by PAS-positive material (sphingolipid). **C** The peripheral retina also shows ganglion cells whose cytoplasm is swollen by PAS-positive material. (**B**,**C**, PAS stain.)

SYSTEMIC DISEASES INVOLVING THE RETINA

Hereditary secondary retinal dystrophies
Diabetes mellitus (see Chapter 15)
Hypertension and arteriolarsclerosis
Collagen diseases
Blood dyscrasias
Demyelinating diseases (see Chapter 13)

FIGURE 11.36

TUMORS OF THE RETINA

Glial (usual glial scar and massive gliosis)
Phakomatosis (see Chapter 2)
Retinal pigment epithelium (see Chapter 17)
Retinoblastoma (see Chapter 18)
Pseudogliomas (see Chapter 18)

FIGURE 11.37

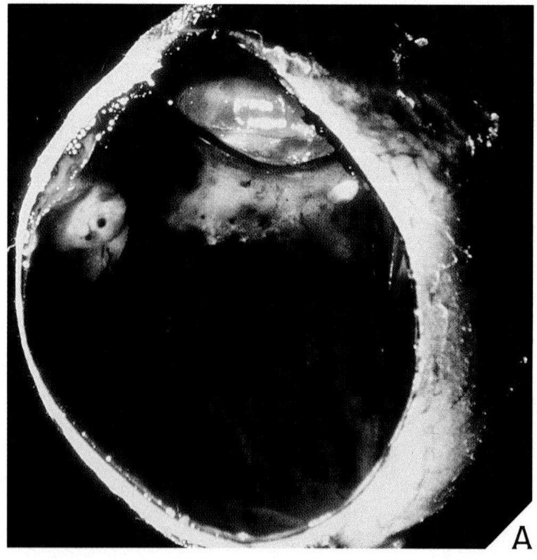

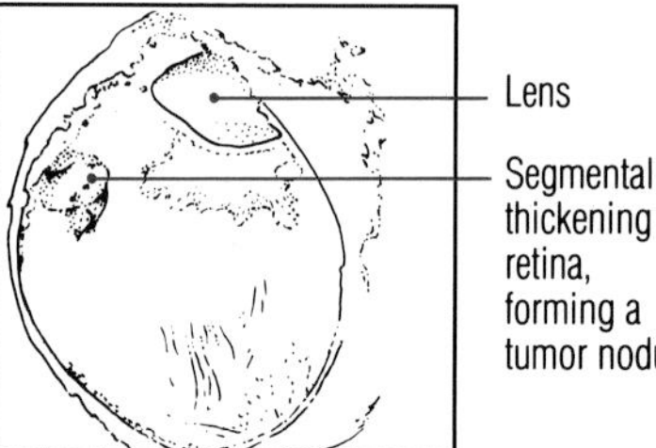

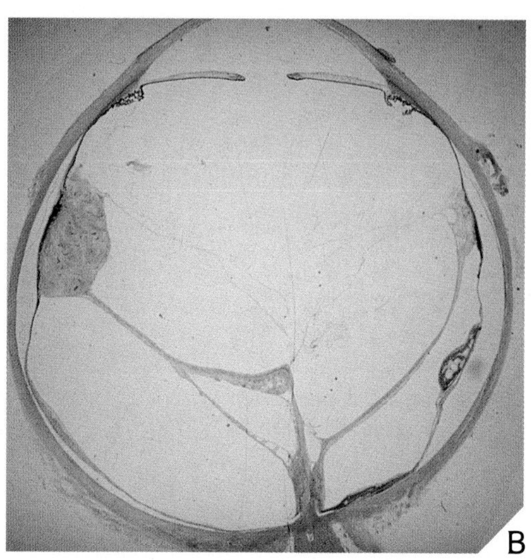

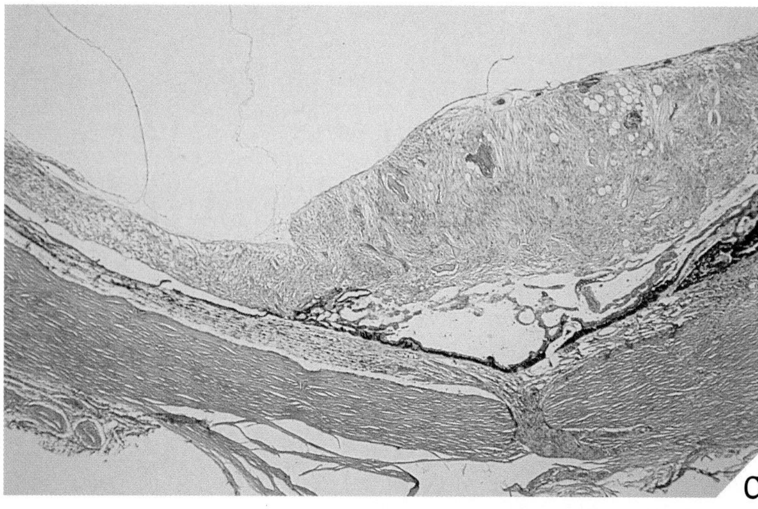

FIGURE 11.38 MASSIVE GLIOSIS. A Segmental thickening of the retina is seen in this gross specimen. The lesion was mistaken for a malignant melanoma and the eye was enucleated. **B** A histologic section of another case shows a sudden transition peripherally from a retina of normal thickness to a thickened, abnormal one. **C** Massive gliosis is characterized histologically by total replacement and thickening of the retina by glial tissue and abnormal blood vessels. Frequently, calcium and even inflammatory round cells are present within the tumor. (**A–C**, cases reported by Yanoff M, et al., 1971.)

MAJOR CAUSES OF RETINAL DETACHMENT

Fluid under intact sensory retina
Harada disease
Coats disease
Malignant hypertension
Eclampsia of pregnancy

Traction bands in vitreous
Post-traumatic
Diabetes

Fluid under broken sensory retina
Rhegmatogenous retinal detachment

FIGURE 11.39

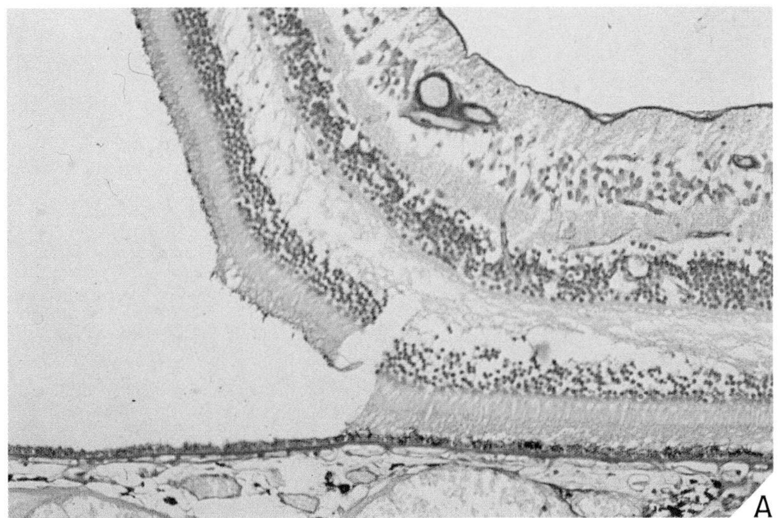

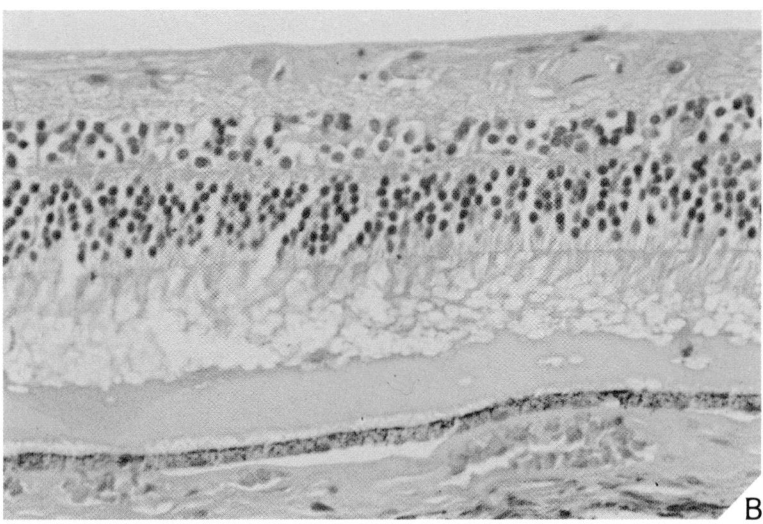

FIGURE 11.40 RETINAL DETACHMENT. A An artifactitious retinal detachment (RD) shows no fluid in the subneural retinal space, pigment adherent to the tips of the photoreceptors, and good preservation of the normal retinal architecture in all layers. **B** A true RD shows material in the subneural retinal space and degeneration of the outer retinal layers.

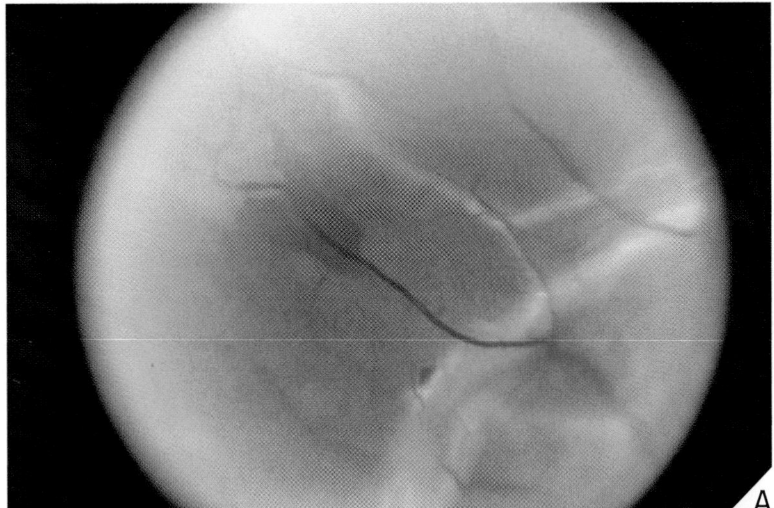

FIGURE 11.41 HORSESHOE RETINAL TEAR. A The horseshoe retinal tear is more easily seen with red-free (green) light than with ordinary light (**B**). **C** A histologic section shows the characteristic adherence of the vitreous to the anterior (uplifted) lip of the retinal tear and nonadherence to the posterior lip of the tear. (**B**, from Yanoff M, Fine BS, *Ocular Pathology*, 2nd ed.)

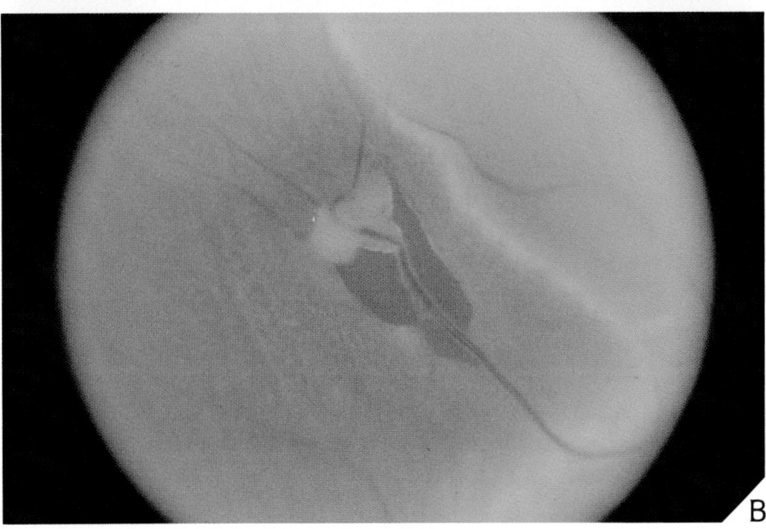

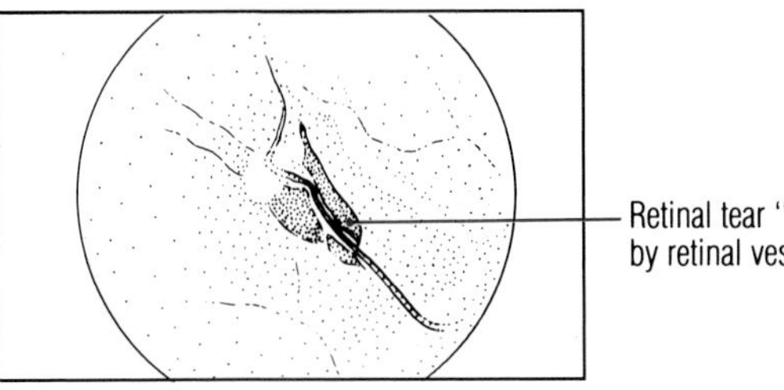

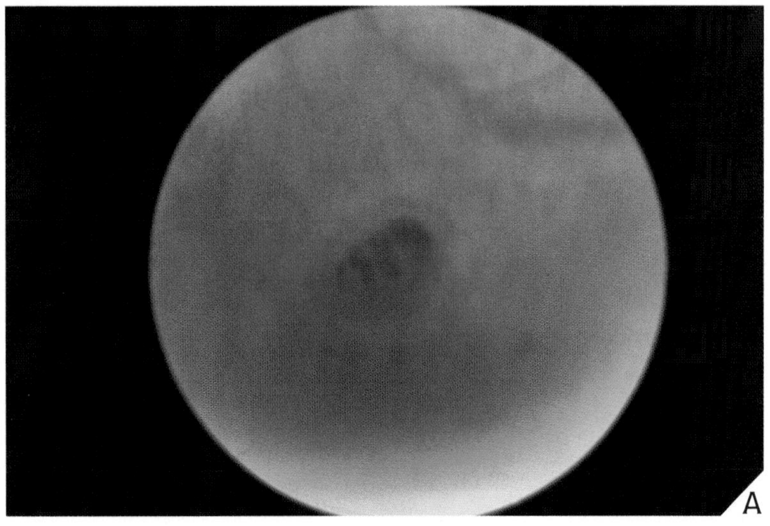

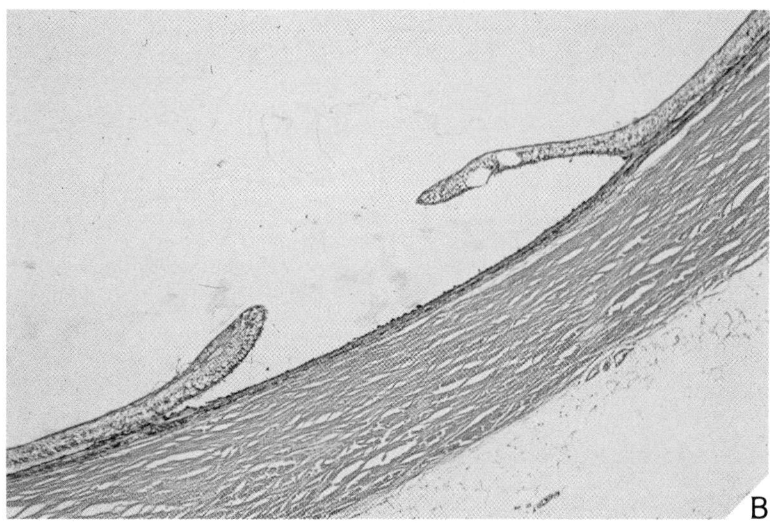

FIGURE 11.42 ROUND RETINAL TEAR. A A round retinal tear is surrounded by a small retinal detachment in the inferior retina. **B** A histologic section shows that, in a round retinal tear, vitreous is not adherent to the edge of the tear. Note the round smooth edges of the tear. An artifactitious retinal tear has sharp edges. (**B**, courtesy of Dr. WR Green.)

PREDISPOSING FACTORS TO RETINAL DETACHMENT (RD)

Juvenile and senile retinoschisis

Lattice retinal degeneration
- Cause of RD in 20%–30% of patients with retinal detachment
- Fewer than 1% of retinas with lattice become detached

Retinal pits

Vitreoretinal adhesions

Trauma (surgical and nonsurgical)

Myopia

Diabetes mellitus

FIGURE 11.43

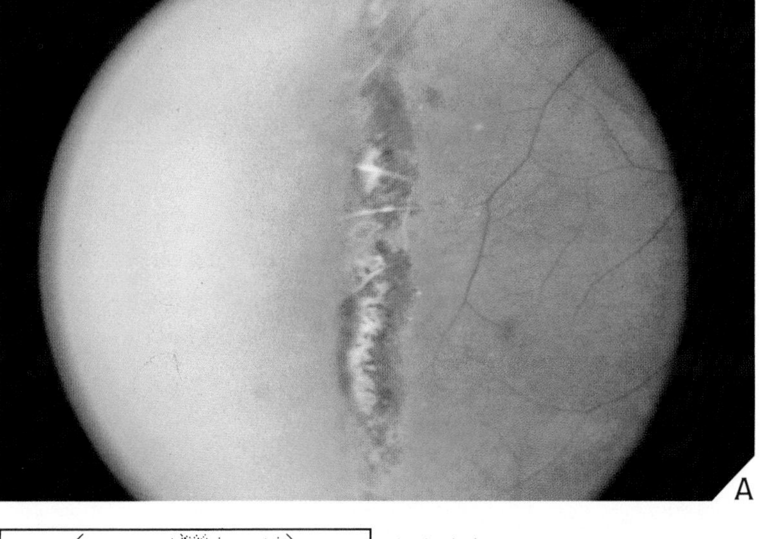

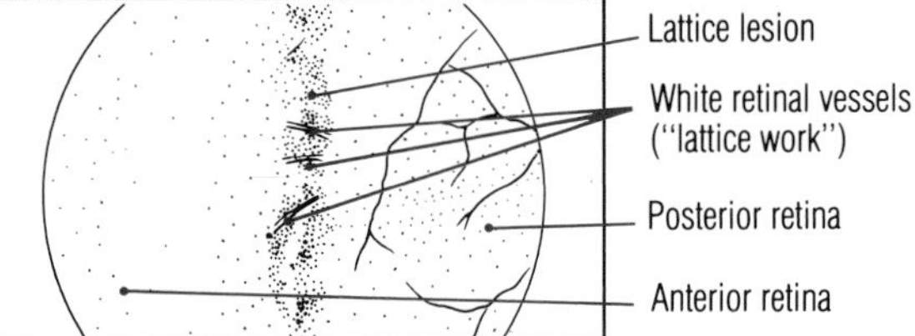

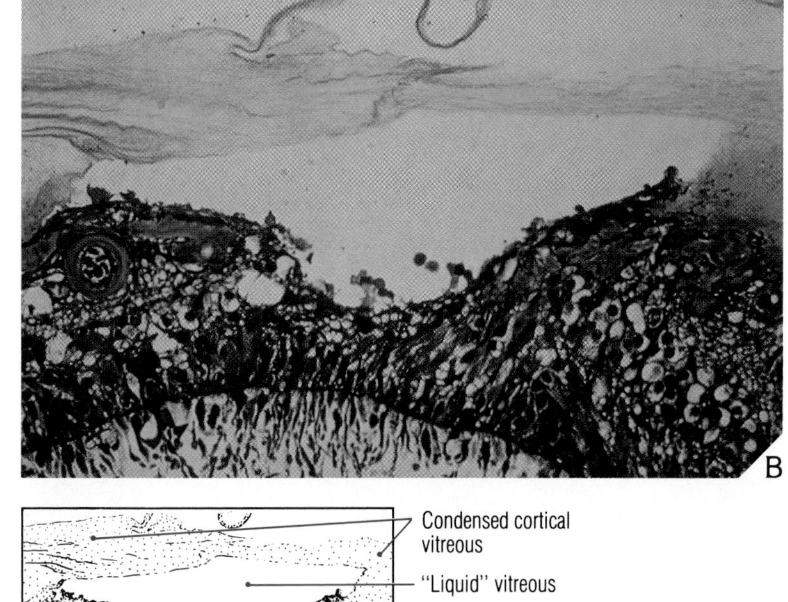

FIGURE 11.44 LATTICE RETINAL DEGENERATION. A Heavy pigmentation and thinning of the retina are present circumferentially in an oval area. **B** The internal layers of the retina, including the internal limiting membrane, are not present. The overlying formed vitreous is split (vitreoschisis) or separated from the retina by fluid.

PATHOLOGIC CHANGES FOLLOWING RETINAL DETACHMENT

Retinal atrophy

Subsensory retinal collections

Glial or RPE membrane growth
Fixed folds
Demarcation lines
Ringschwiele

Intraretinal cysts

Calcium oxalate crystals

FIGURE 11.45

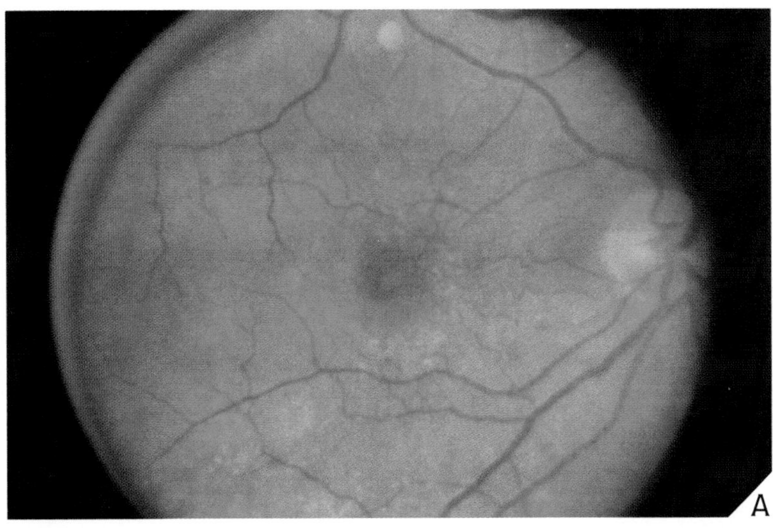

FIGURE 11.46 EPIRETINAL (FLAT) GLIOSIS. A The fundus shows characteristic crinkling or "cellophane" appearance of the retina in the posterior pole. **B** A histologic section of another case shows a fine glial membrane on the internal surface of the retina. **C** A histologic section of a more advanced case shows that contraction of the glial membrane produced many folds of the internal surface of the retina.

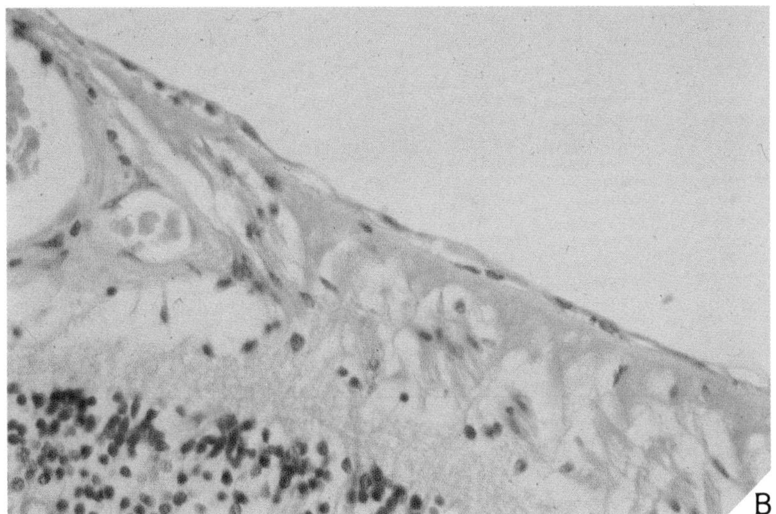

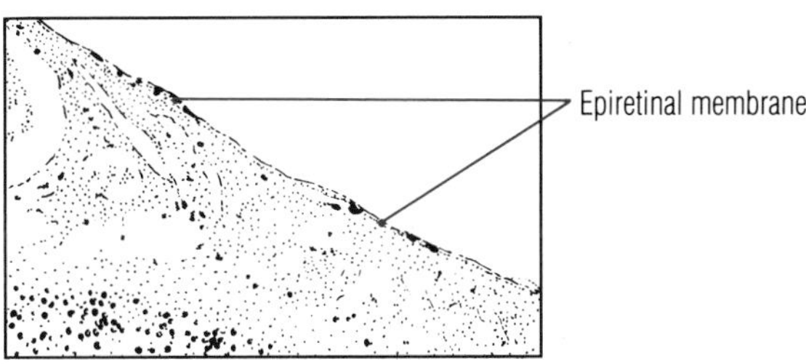

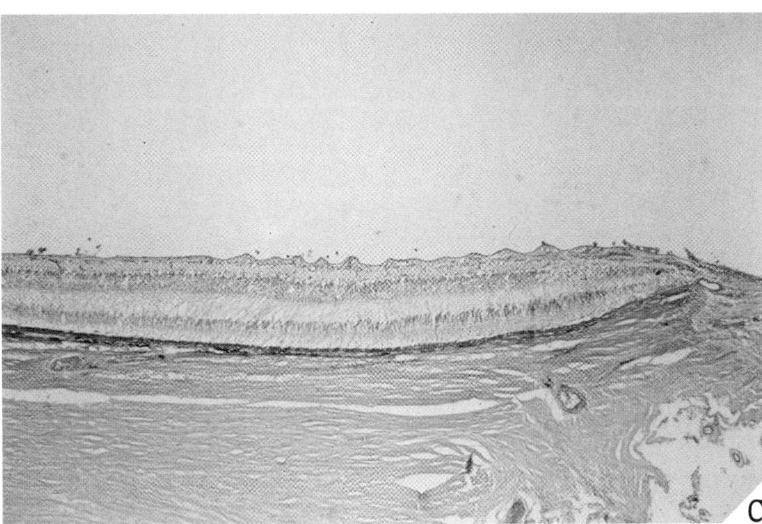

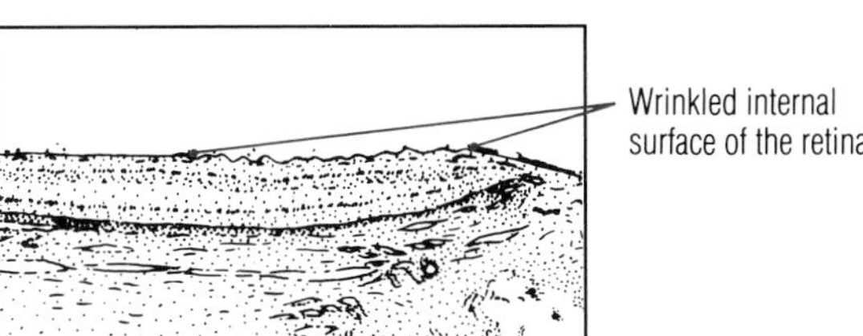

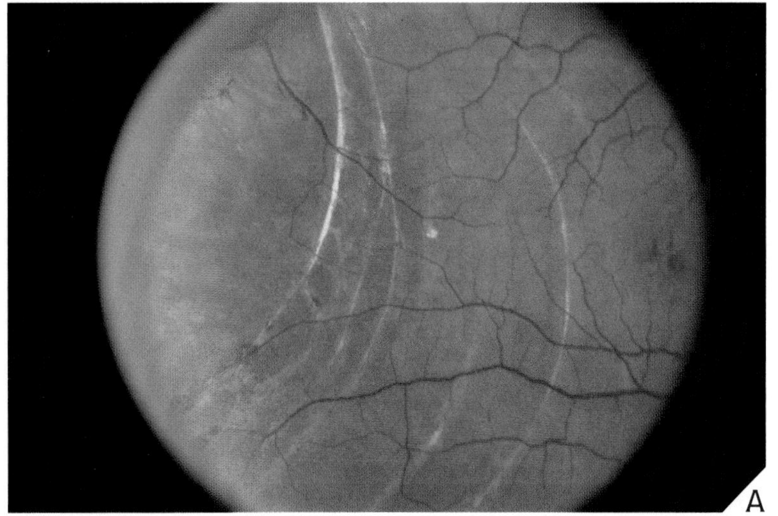

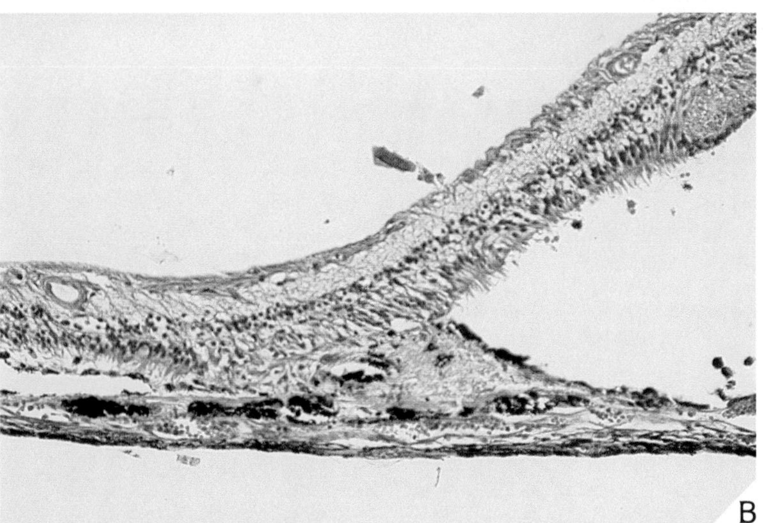

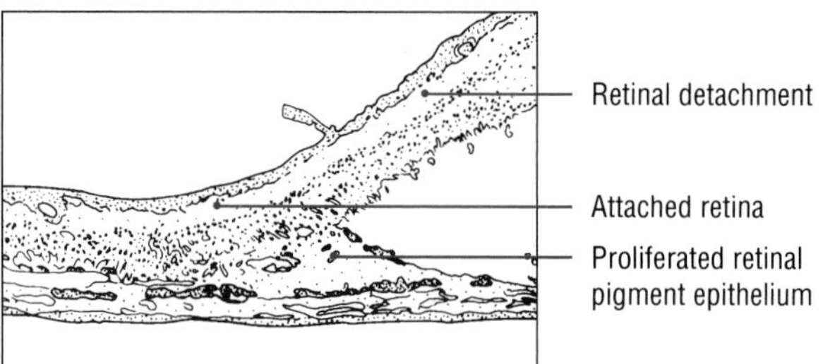

FIGURE 11.47 DEMARCATION LINE. A Concentric yellow-white lines are present at the edge of a retinal detachment. Some pigment also is present. **B** A histologic section shows the region of transition between retinal detachment and attachment. The RPE has undergone proliferation and the thickness of the basement membrane has increased. The yellow-white appearance of the demarcation lines presumably is due to the basement membrane material. When the RPE cells are sufficiently pigmented, the demarcation lines also will be pigmented. (**B**, courtesy Dr. WR Green.)

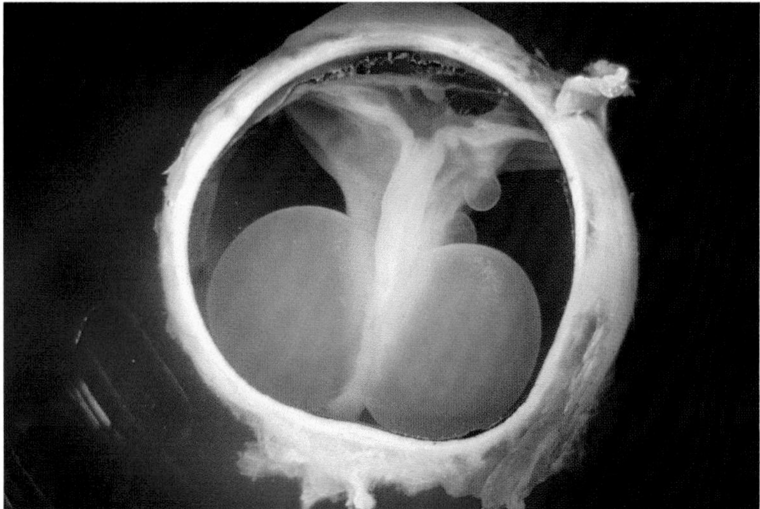

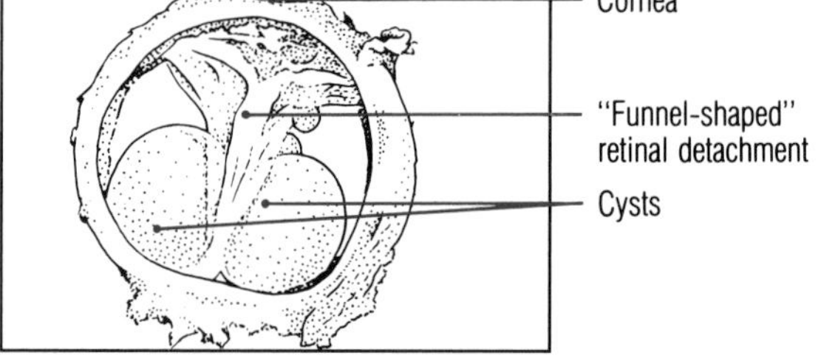

FIGURE 11.48 RETINAL CYSTS. This gross specimen shows numerous large retinal cysts from a case of longstanding retinal detachment.

Bibliography

Aaby AA, Kushner BJ: Acquired and progressive myelinated nerve fibers. Arch Ophthalmol 103:542, 1985.

Aessopos A, et al: Angioid streaks in homozygous B thalassemia. Am J Ophthalmol 107:356, 1989.

Bressler SB, et al: Relationship of drusen and abnormalities of the retinal pigment epithelium to the prognosis of neovascular macular degeneration. Arch Ophthalmol 109:1442, 1990.

Byer NE: The natural history of asymptomatic retinal breaks. Ophthalmology 89:1033, 1982.

Byer NE: Long-term natural history of lattice degeneration of the retina. Ophthalmology 96:1396, 1989.

Duker JS, et al: A prospective study of acute central retinal artery obstruction. The incidence of secondary ocular neovascularization. Arch Ophthalmol 109:339, 1991.

Eagle RC Jr: Mechanisms of maculopathy. Ophthalmology 91:613, 1984.

Eagle RC Jr, et al: Retinal pigment epithelial abnormalities in fundus flavimaculatus. A light and electronic microscopic study. Ophthalmology 7:1189, 1980.

Eagle RC Jr, Yanoff M, Fine BS: Hemoglobin SC retinopathy and fat emboli to the eye. A light and electron microscopical study. Arch Ophthalmol 92:28, 1974.

Fine BS, Yanoff M: Ocular Histology: A Text and Atlas, 2nd ed. Hagerstown, Harper & Row, 1979.

Foos RY, Feman SS: Reticular cystoid degeneration of the peripheral retina. Am J Ophthalmol 69:392, 1970.

Foos RY, Simons KB: Vitreous in lattice degeneration of the retina. Ophthalmology 91:452, 1984.

Frayer WC: Elevated lesions of the macular area. A histopathologic study emphasizing lesions similar to disciform degeneration of the macula. Arch Ophthalmol 53:82, 1955.

Greven CM, Moreno RJ, Tasman W: Unusual manifestations of X-linked retinoschisis. Trans Am Ophthalmol Soc 88:211, 1990.

Lopez PF, et al: Autosomal-dominant fundus flavimaculatus. Clinicopathologic correlation. Ophthalmology 97:798, 1990.

Miyake Y, et al: Bull's-eye maculopathy and negative electroretinogram. Retina 9:210, 1989.

Pagon RA: Retinitis pigmentosa. Surv Ophthalmol 33:137, 1988.

Pauleikhoff D, et al: Drusen as risk factors in age-related macular disease. Am J Ophthalmol 109:38, 1990.

Pauleikhoff D, Harper CA, Marshall J: Aging changes in Bruch's membrane. A histochemical and morphologic study. Ophthalmology 97:171, 1990.

Quinlan PM, et al: The natural course of central retinal vein occlusion. Am J Ophthalmol 110:118, 1990.

Rabb MF, Gagliano DA, Teske MP: Retinal arterial macro aneurysms. Surv Ophthalmol 33:73, 1988.

Vinores SA, Campochiaro PA, Conway BP: Ultrastructural and electron-immunocytochemical characterization of cells in epiretinal membranes. Invest Ophthalmol Vis Sci 31:14, 1990.

West SK, et al: Exposure to sunlight and other risk factors for age-related macular degeneration. Arch Ophthalmol 107:875, 1989.

Yanoff M, Rahn EK, Zimmerman LE: Histopathology of juvenile retinoschisis. Arch Ophthalmol 79:49, 1968.

Yanoff M, Zimmerman LE, Davis R: Massive gliosis of the retina. A continuous spectrum of glial proliferation. Int Ophthalmol Clin 11:211, 1971.

Vitreous

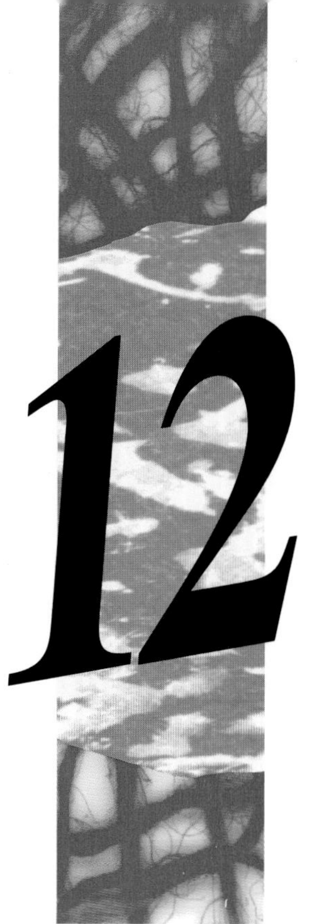

The vitreous body is one of the most delicate and transparent connective tissues. It occupies the posterior or largest compartment of the eye, filling the globe between the retina and the lens. The structure is composed of a framework of extremely delicate or embryonic collagen filaments closely associated with a large quantity of water-binding hyaluronic acid.

Embryologically, the developing avascular secondary vitreous surrounds and compresses the vascularized primary vitreous into a canal that extends from the optic disc to the back of the lens, forming the hyaloid canal (canal of Cloquet) through which passes the hyaloid vessel. With embryonic maturation, the hyaloid vessel atrophies, disappearing before birth. Persisting remnants of the primary vitreous or hyaloid vessel produce congenital anomalies, the most common being retention of fragments on the back of the lens (Mittendorf dot; see Chapter 10), retention of tissue on the optic disc (Bergmeister papilla), and persistent hyperplastic primary vitreous (see Chapter 18), which often encroaches on the posterior lens.

Inflammatory diseases may involve the vitreous primarily or secondarily. The inflammations are quite similar to those already discussed in Chapters 3 and 4.

Vitreous adhesions, membranes, and opacities may form secondary to a variety of causes. They may be congenital, may follow trauma or inflammation, may be secondary to systemic or familial diseases, or may be idiopathic. Hemorrhage into the vitreous is a common cause of vision loss. Most frequently, hemorrhage occurs in a diabetic patient and is secondary to the presence of abnormal, easily ruptured vessels (see Chapter 15). Vitreous hemorrhage also may be secondary to trauma, retinal tears, vitreoretinal separation, hypertensive or sickle-cell retinopathy, Eales disease, retinal vascularization from any cause, age-related macular degeneration ("wet" type), blood dyscrasias, uveitis, malignant melanoma, retinoblastoma, metastatic intraocular tumors, Terson syndrome (subarachnoid hemorrhage plus vitreous hemorrhage), retinal angiomas, juvenile retinoschisis, or choroidal hemorrhage with extension. Hemorrhage into the vitreous compartment between the vitreous body and the internal surface of the retina generally resorbs rapidly (within a few weeks to a few months). Hemorrhage into the vitreous body may be spontaneously reabsorbed (although it usually takes three months or more), or it may organize and form fibrous membranes. The membranes shrink and cause traction on the retina, which may then produce a retinal detachment (see Chapter 11). Glaucoma, in the form of hemolytic glaucoma (see Chapter 16), also may be a complication of an intravitreal hemorrhage.

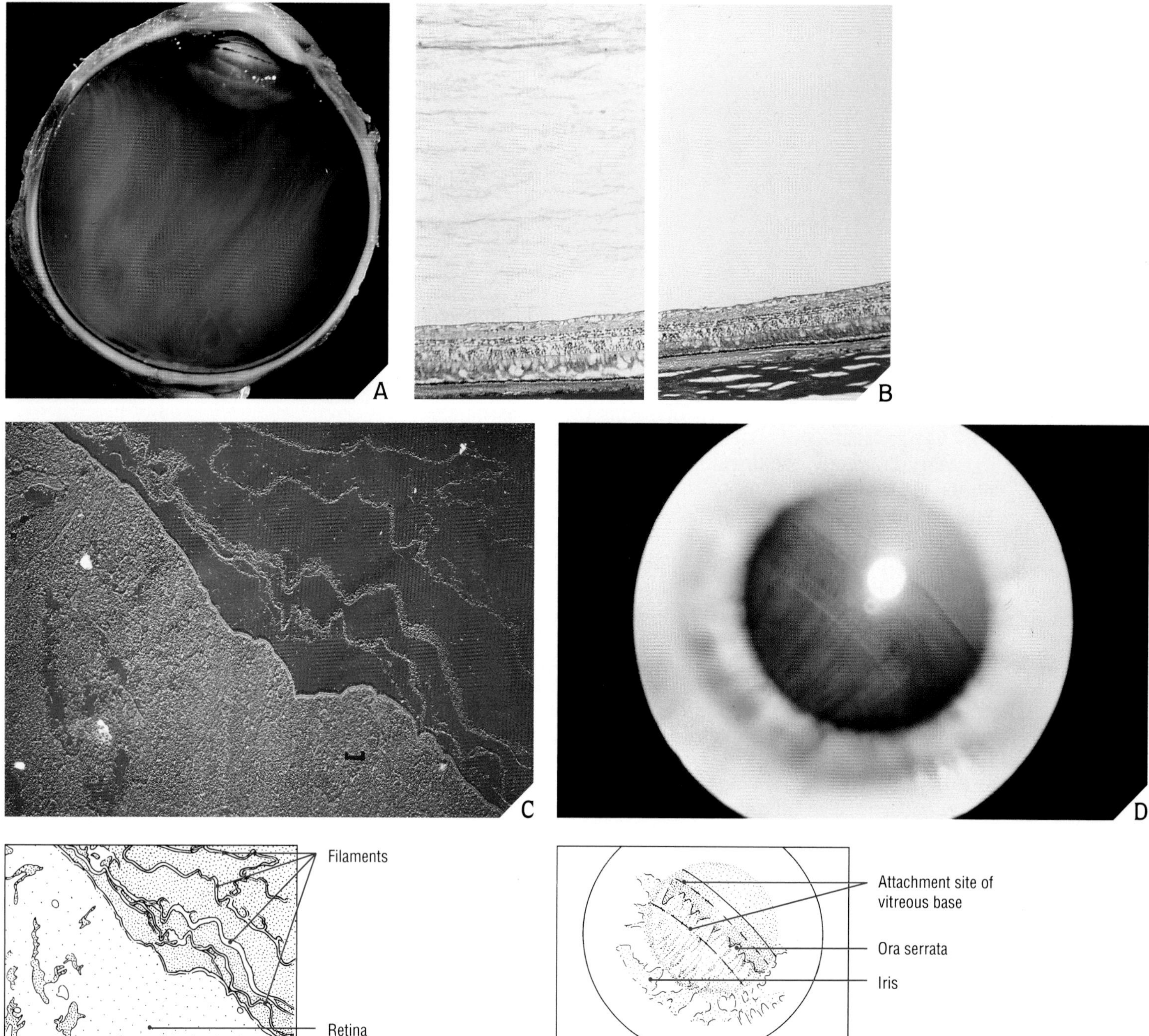

FIGURE 12.1 NORMAL VITREOUS. A The vitreous compartment is filled completely by the vitreous body. The major components of the vitreous are hyaluronic acid and delicate, collagenous filaments. **B** On the left is a vitreous body stained with colloidal iron so that it appears blue. On the right the tissue was first treated with hyaluronidase and no staining occurred, indicating that the blue-staining material on the left is hyaluronic acid. **C** The other major component, the collagenous delicate vitreous filaments, are well demonstrated by this electron micrograph of a shadow-cast preparation. The retina occupies the diagonal lower left side and the filaments the diagonal upper right side. **D** A ciliary body melanoma has elevated the ora serrata region so that it is seen clearly. Note the attachment site of the vitreous base appears as two white lines, one easily seen just anterior to the ora serrata and the other less easily seen just posterior to the ora serrata. This is the strongest attachment site of the vitreous body. The next strongest attachment site surrounds the optic nerve head, followed by a ring within the clivus of the anatomic fovea centralis. (**B**, **C**, modified from Fine BS, Yanoff M, 1979.)

CONGENITAL ANOMALIES

Persistent primary vitreous

Anterior remnants: lenticular portion of hyaloid; Mittendorf dot

Posterior remnants: vascular loops; Bergmeister papilla; congenital cysts

Anterior persistent hyperplastic primary vitreous (see Chapter 18)

Posterior persistent hyperplastic primary vitreous

FIGURE 12.2

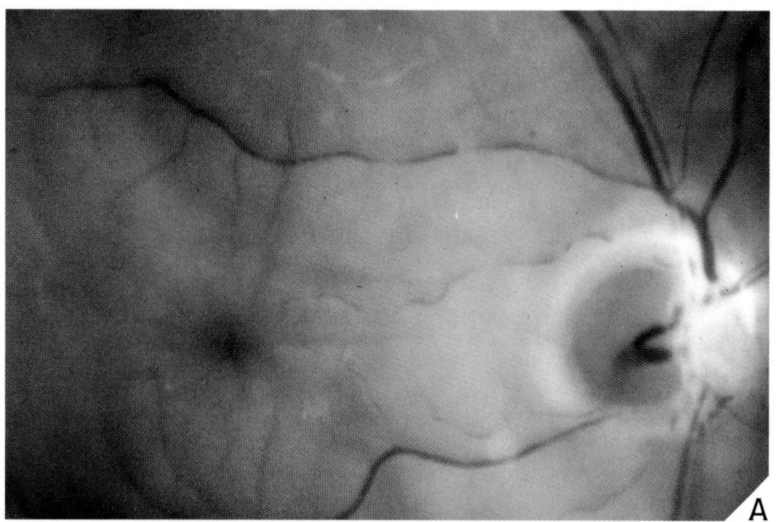

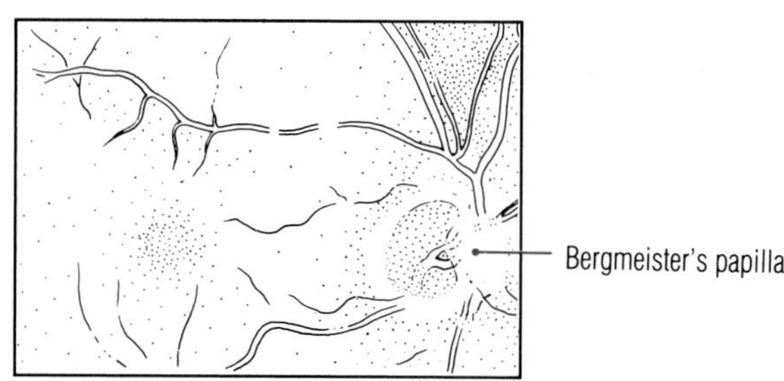

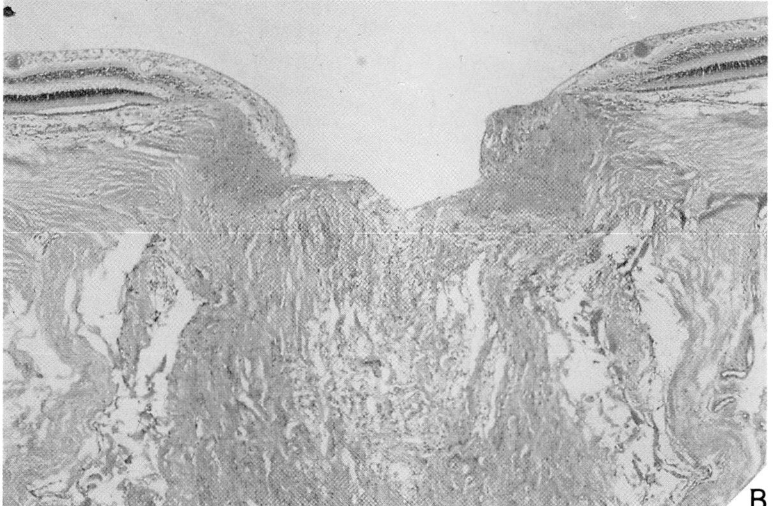

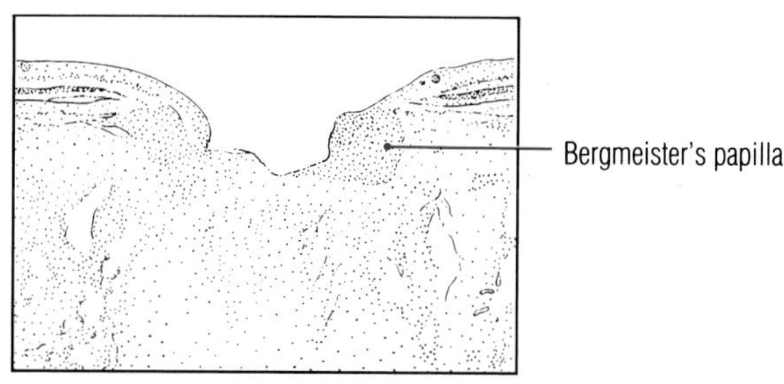

FIGURE 12.3 BERGMEISTER PAPILLA. A The enucleated eye shows posterior remnants of the hyaloid system over the nasal portion of the optic nerve head. **B** Histologic section shows a Bergmeister papilla in the form of a glial remnant of the hyaloid system.

VITREOUS

Inflammation (see Chapters 3 and 4)

Acute

Chronic

FIGURE 12.4

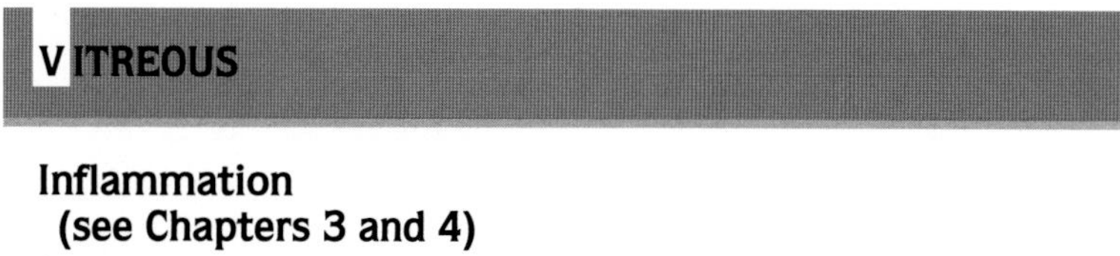

POSTTRAUMATIC AND SURGICAL VITREOUS ADHESIONS

Vitreocorneal
Corneal "touch" syndrome

Iridovitreal
Posterior synechiae
- Total synechiae leads to seclusion of pupil and iris bombé

Pupillary membrane leads to occlusion of pupil

Vitreoretinal
Irvine-Gass syndrome
"Cellophane" retina
Postinflammation
Idiopathic

FIGURE 12.5

VITREOUS OPACITIES

Hyaloid vessel remnants

Acquired vitreous floaters
Posterior vitreous detachment
- Present in more than 50% of patients over 50 years of age
- Present in 65% of patients over 65 years of age

Proteinaceous deposits

Inflammatory cells

Red blood cells

Iridescent particles
Asteroid hyalosis—calcium soaps
Synchysis scintillans—cholesterol (see Figs. 5.26 and 5.27)

Tumor cells

Pigment dust

Cysts

Retinal fragments

Traumatic avulsion of vitreous base

Anterior vitreous detachment

Autosomal dominantly inherited vitreoretinal disorders
Autosomal dominant neovascular inflammatory vitreoretinopathy (ADNIV)
Autosomal dominant vitreoretinochoroidopathy (ADVIRC)
Autosomal dominant cystoid macular edema
Familial exudative vitreoretinopathy
Snowflake degeneration
Wagner-Stickler syndrome

Amyloid
Primary familial
- Sheet-like vitreous veils
- Deposits in lids, orbit, nerves, and ganglia
- Widespread systemic deposits
- Histology shows pale, amorphous material that is Congo-red-positive, metachromatic, dichroic, and birefringent

FIGURE 12.6

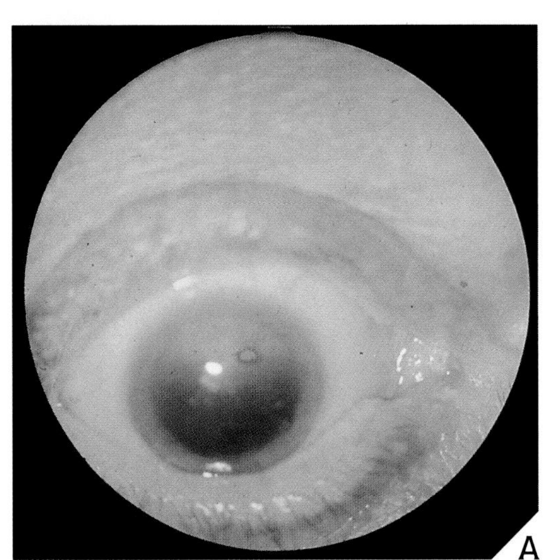

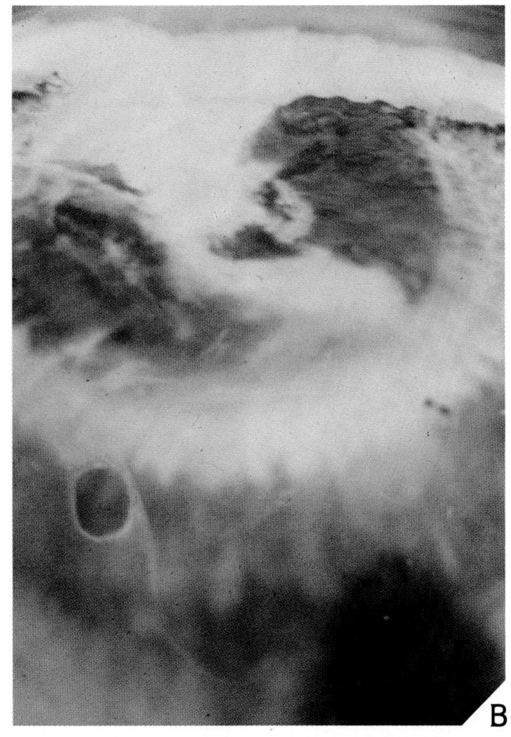

FIGURE 12.7 POSTERIOR VITREOUS DETACHMENT. A The fundus reflex shows the characteristic "donut" or "peep-hole" of posterior vitreous detachment (PVD). **B** An enucleated eye shows the previous attachment site of the vitreous around the optic nerve head, now floating freely in the central vitreous compartment as a round fibrous band. **C** Another enucleated eye shows that the vitreous is detached posteriorly everywhere except around the optic nerve head. **D** The vitreous is detached posteriorly, except around the optic nerve head where it is attached to the edges of the nerve.

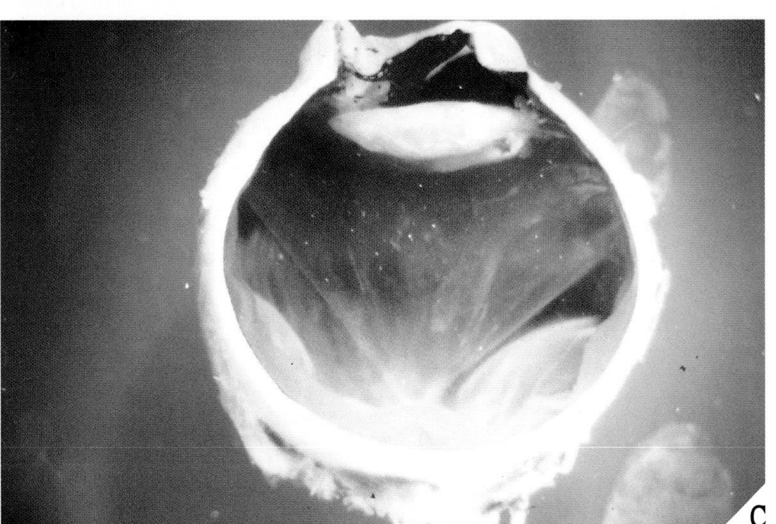

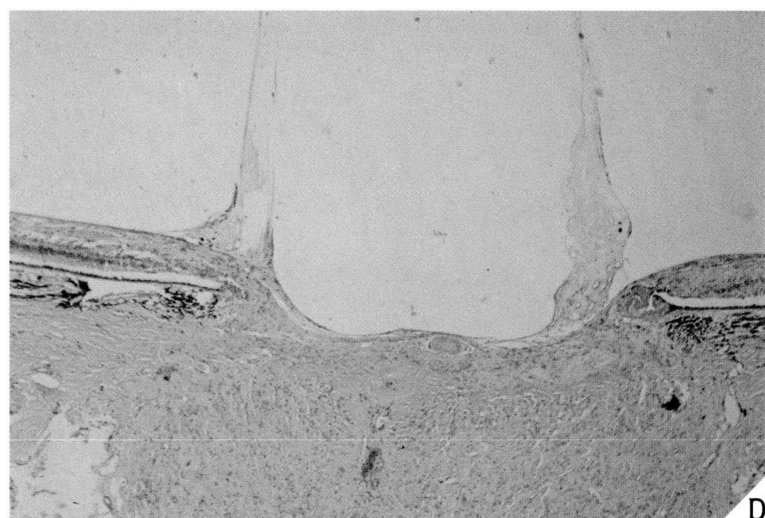

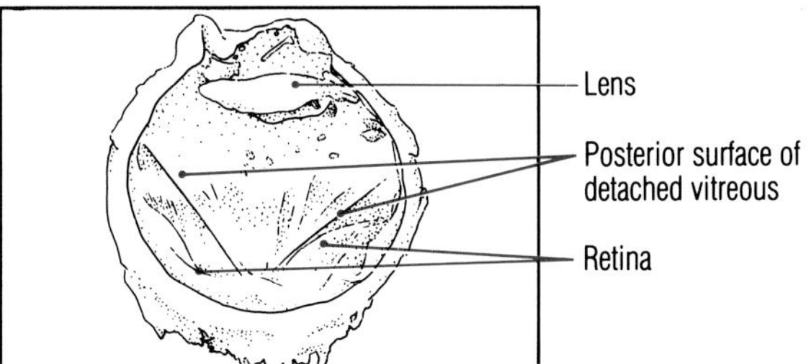

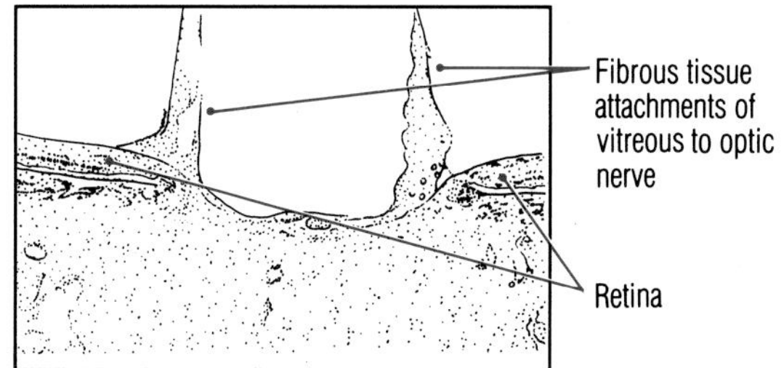

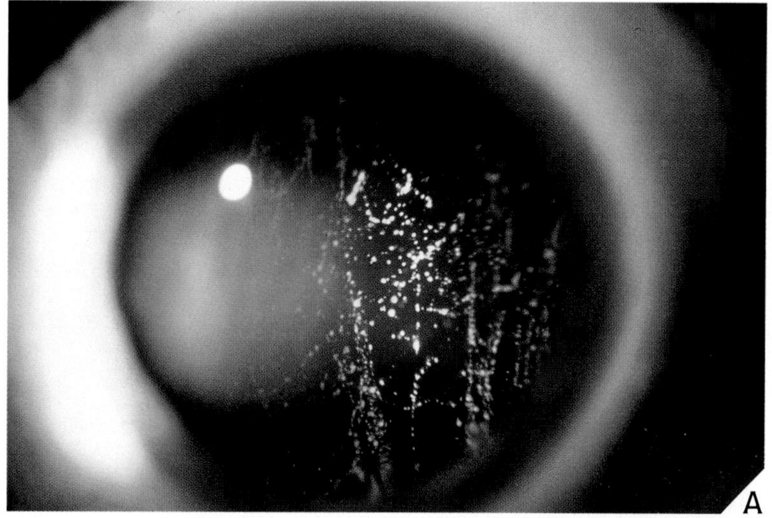

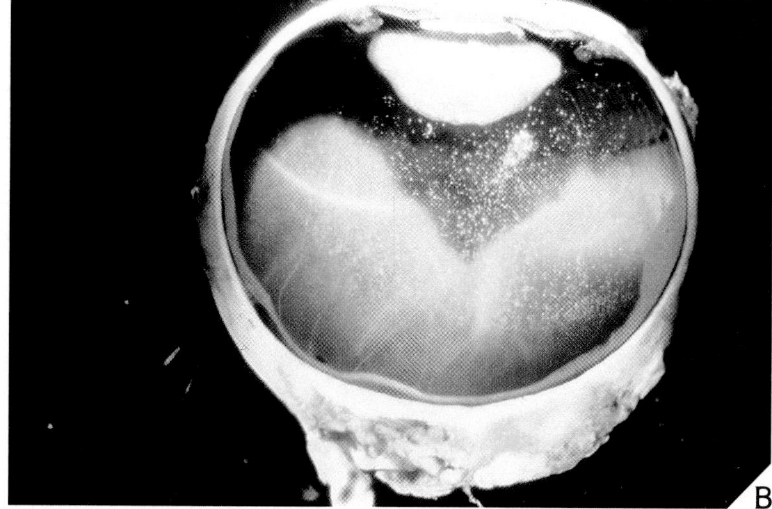

FIGURE 12.8 ASTEROID HYALOSIS. **A** The fundus reflex shows tiny gold-colored balls in the anterior vitreous. **B** The enucleated globe shows multiple tiny white spherules suspended throughout the vitreous body. **C** A histologic section shows that the spherules are birefringent in polarized light.

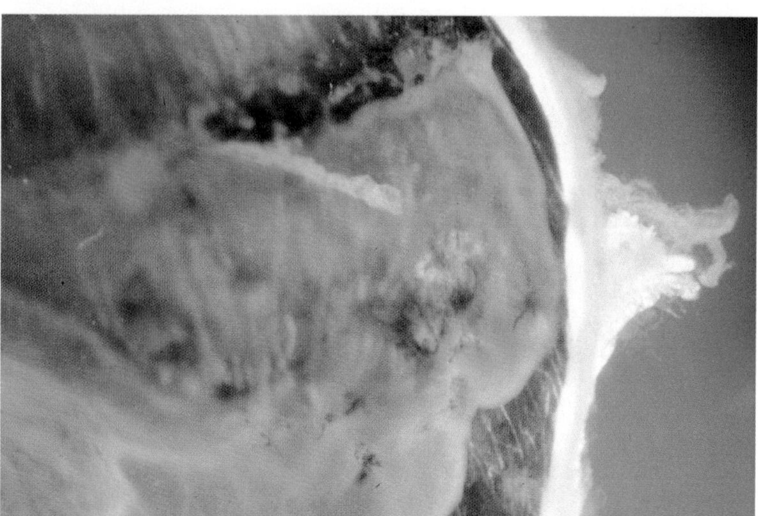

FIGURE 12.9 AVULSION OF THE VITREOUS BASE. The vitreous base is seen to be partially avulsed. The patient had blunt injury to this eye.

VITREOUS HEMORRHAGE

Definitions

Intravitreal—within the vitreous

Subvitreal—between the vitreous body and the internal surface of the retina

Subhyaloid—confusing term: a clinical subhyaloid hemorrhage usually is actually within the retina between the internal limiting membrane (ILM) and the nerve fiber layer (submembranous, intraretinal)

Causes

Retinal tears
Vitreoretinal separations
Trauma
Diabetic retinopathy
Hypertensive retinopathy
Sickle-cell retinopathy
Eales disease
Retinal neovascularization
Age-related macular degeneration
Choroidal hematoma
Juvenile retinoschisis
Blood dyscrasias
Uveitis
Malignant melanoma
Retinoblastoma
Metastatic tumor
Retinal angiomas
Subarachnoid hemorrhage (Terson syndrome)

FIGURE 12.10

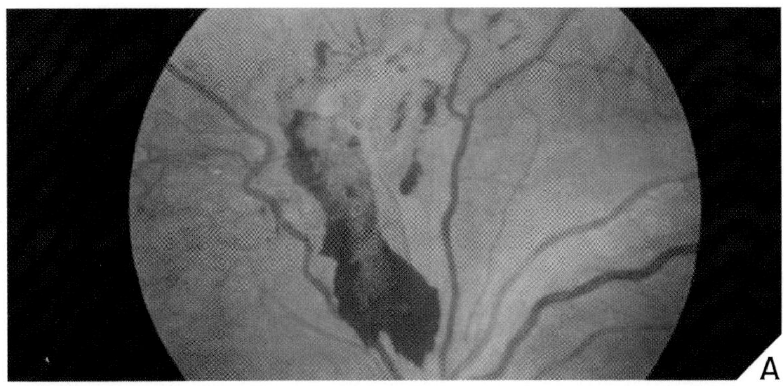

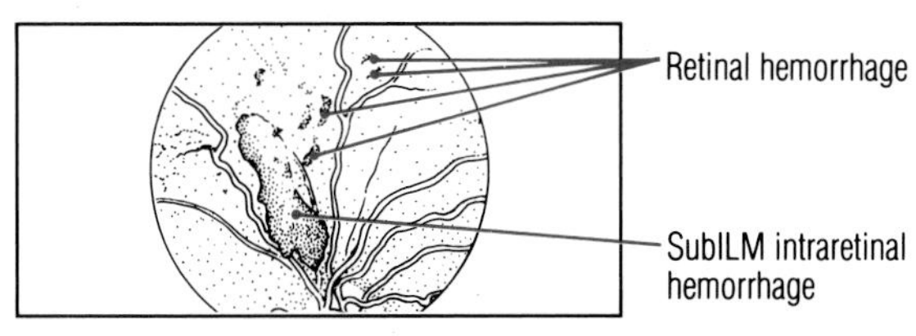

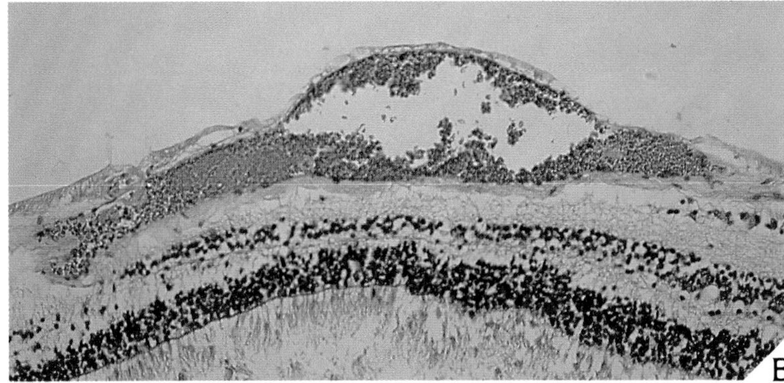

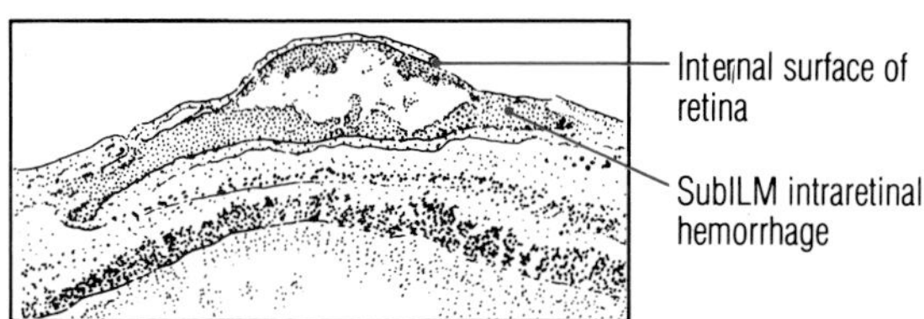

FIGURE 12.11 SUBMEMBRANOUS INTRARETINAL HEMORRHAGE. A A hemorrhage is seen between the internal limiting membrane (ILM) and the nerve fiber layer of the retina. This is often mistakenly called a subhyaloid hemorrhage. **B** A histologic section of another case shows that the hemorrhage lies entirely within the retina, separated from the vitreous compartment by a thick basement membrane (ILM).

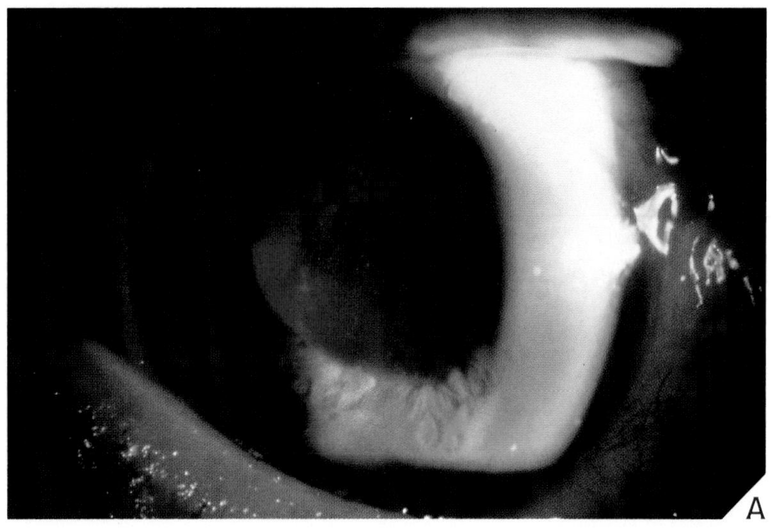

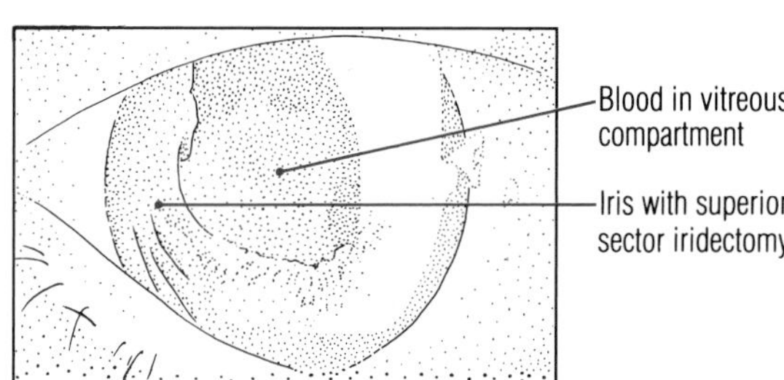

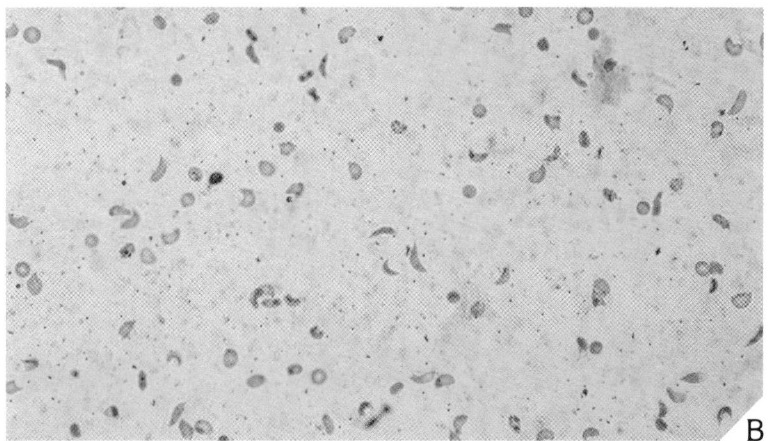

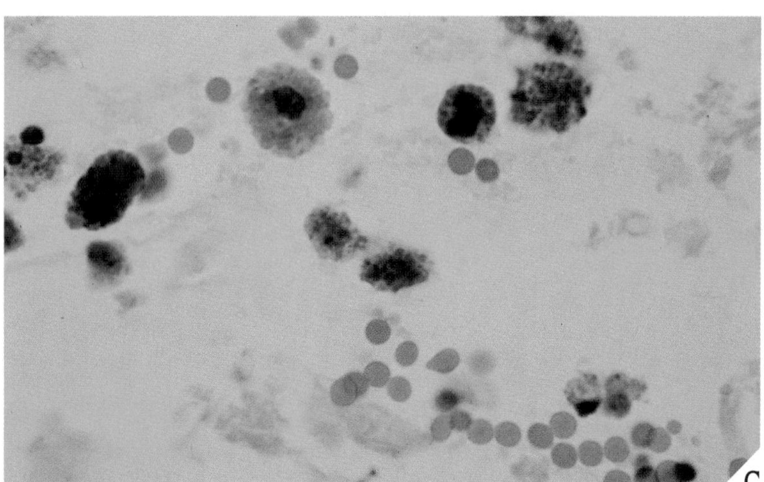

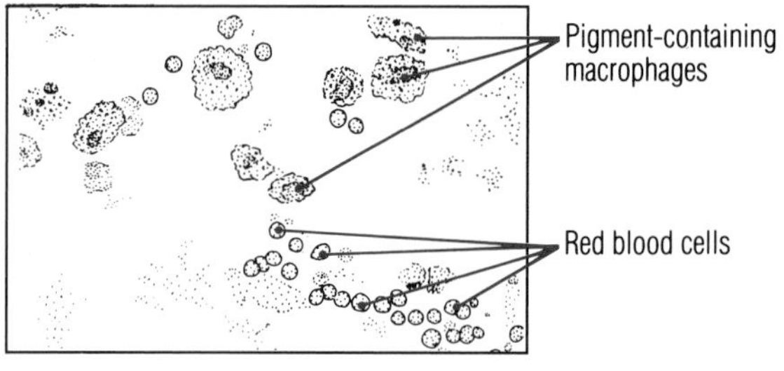

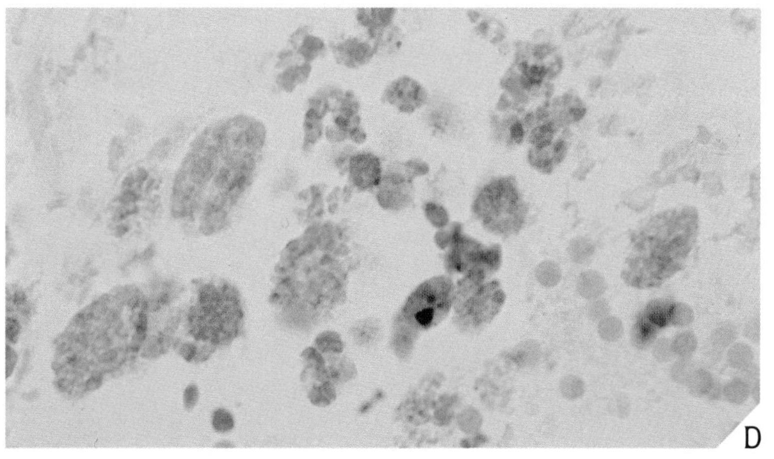

FIGURE 12.12 INTRAVITREAL HEMORRHAGE. A A hemorrhage is seen within the vitreous body. **B** In this vitrectomy specimen of an intravitreal hemorrhage from a 67-year-old black man, the red blood cells were noted to have a sickle configuration; a diagnosis of sickle-cell trait was made. The diagnosis had not been made previously. **C** Another vitrectomy specimen shows red blood cells and pigment-containing macrophages. **D** A special stain for iron (Perl stain) shows that the pigment in some of the macrophages stains positively (blue), signifying hemosiderin; the pigment in other macrophages does not stain, and presumably represents melanin or hemoglobin not yet oxidized to hemosiderin. (**A**, courtesy of Dr. SH Sinclair; **B**, **C**, **D**, courtesy of Dr. RC Eagle Jr.)

Bibliography

Bergren RL, Brown GC, Duker JS: Prevalence and association of asteroid hyalosis with systemic diseases. Am J Ophthalmol 111:289, 1991.

Eagle RC Jr, Yanoff M: Cholesterolosis of anterior chamber. Albrecht von Graefes Arch Klin Ophthalmol 193:121, 1975.

Fine BS, Yanoff M: *Ocular Histology: A Text and Atlas,* 2nd ed. Hagerstown, Harper & Row, 1979.

Fishman GA: Discussion of Bennett SR, Folk JC, Kimura AE, et al: Autosomal-dominant neovascular inflammatory vitreoretinopathy. Ophthalmology 97:1135, 1991.

Foos RY: Posterior vitreous detachment. Trans Am Acad Ophthalmol Otolaryngol 76:480, 1972.

Forrester JV, Lee WR, Williamson J: The pathology of vitreous hemorrhage. I. Gross and histological appearances. Arch Ophthalmol 96:703, 1978.

Goldberg MF, et al: Histopathologic study of autosomal-dominant vitreoretinochoroidopathy. Peripheral annular pigmentary dystrophy. Ophthalmology 96:1736, 1989.

Jerdan JA, et al: Proliferative vitreoretinopathy membranes. An immunohistochemical study. Ophthalmology 96:801, 1989.

Miller H, et al: Asteroid bodies—an ultrastructural study. Invest Ophthalmol Vis Sci 24:133, 1983.

Orellana J, et al: Pigmented free-floating vitreous cysts in two young adults. Electron microscopic observations. Ophthalmology 92:297, 1985.

Optic Nerve

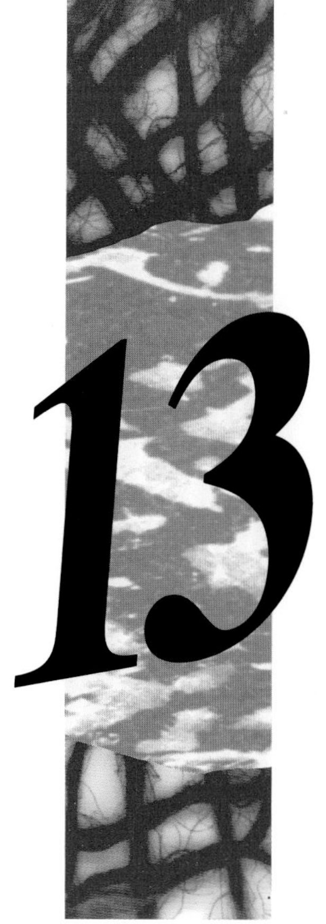

The optic nerve is made up of a number of components. White matter, in the form of glial supporting elements and axons from the retinal ganglion cells, is the major constituent. All the meningeal sheaths (dura, arachnoid, and pia) are present, along with an intrinsic and extrinsic blood supply. The optic nerve is continuous at one end with the retina and at the other end with the brain, making it vulnerable to a variety of ocular and central nervous system diseases.

Numerous anatomic variations and congenital defects may involve the optic nerve. These range from complete absence of the optic nerve (aplasia) to minor abnormalities such as differences in the size and shape of the optic nerve head. An optic pit may be seen within the optic nerve head, usually in the inferotemporal quadrant. The pit may be associated with a serous detachment of the central (macular) retina.

Swelling of the optic nerve, manifested as optic disc edema, may have a local cause within the eye, may be an extension of an intracranial disorder, or may be part of a systemic abnormality such as malignant hypertension. The optic nerve may become inflamed, which results in a condition called optic neuritis. The inflammation may be caused by a local phenomenon such as uveitis or may be part of a generalized condition such as multiple sclerosis. Atrophy of the optic nerve may result from many diverse conditions, but whatever the cause, histologic findings in optic atrophy inevitably reflect a loss of parenchyma (myelinated neurites) and a compensatory increase in glial cell mass—an increase, however, insufficient to compensate for the parenchymal loss.

The optic nerve may give rise to primary tumors, as in juvenile pilocytic astrocytoma (glioma) and meningioma, or may be the site of secondary tumors, due for example to invasion by retinoblastoma or to leukemic involvement. Tumors can cause secondary effects, such as optic disc edema or optic atrophy.

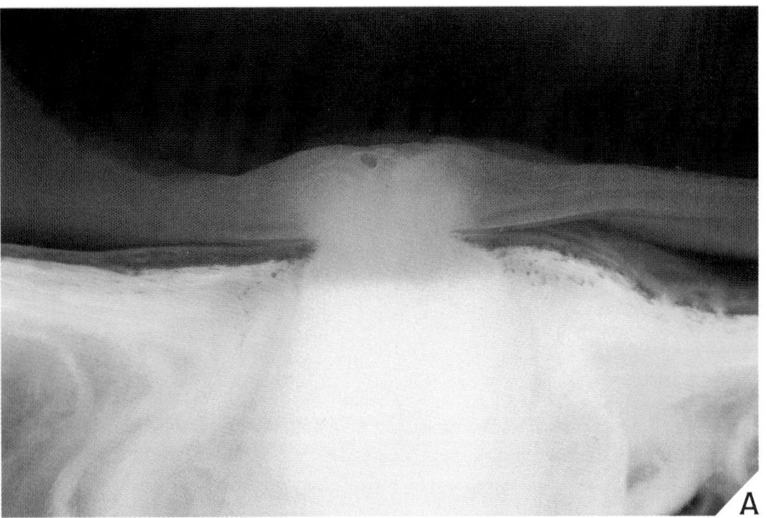

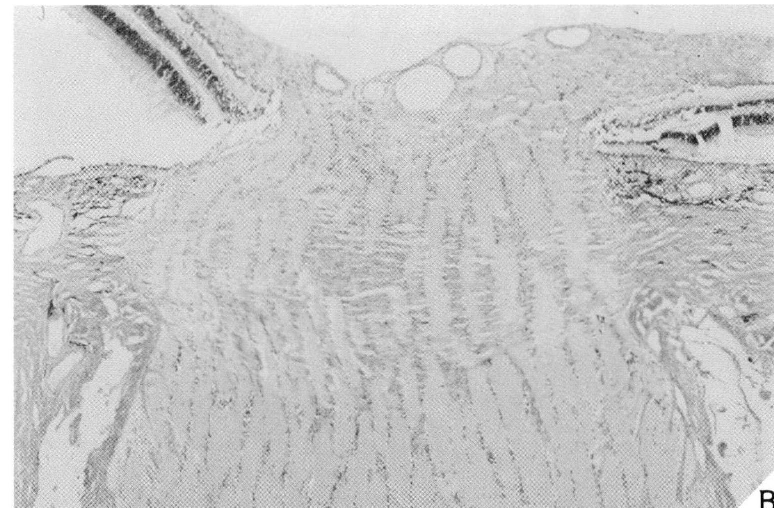

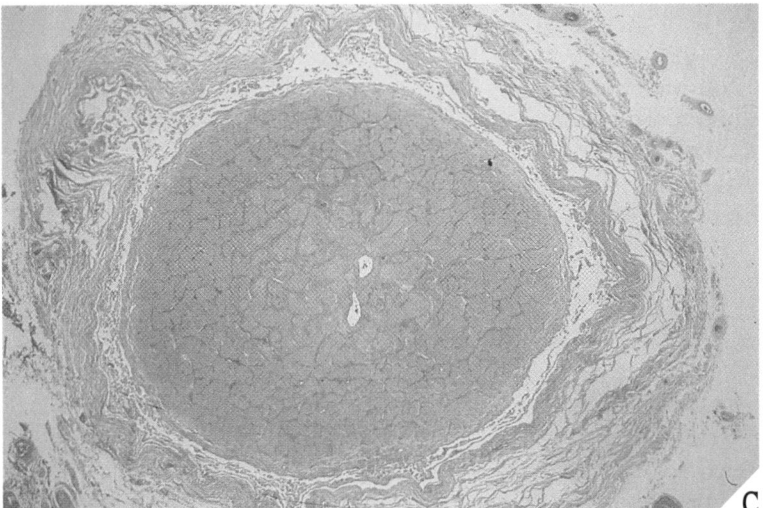

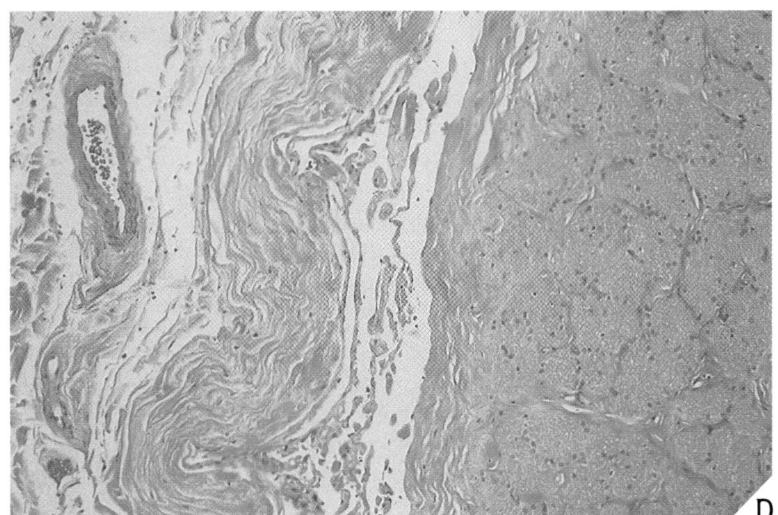

FIGURE 13.1 NORMAL OPTIC NERVE. A and **B** Longitudinal sections (gross and microscopic, respectively) of the optic nerve (ON) shows the intraocular (within the scleral canal) and retrobulbar portions of the ON. The intraocular portion is divided into three parts or layers: the inner retinal layer anteriorly; the middle choroidal layer where white mylination of the ON begins (**A**); and the outer scleral layer posteriorly. The anterior surface of the retinal layer (the optic disc or ON head) measures about 1.5 mm; as the ON exits the scleral canal posteriorly to form the retrobulbar portion, it measures 3 to 4 mm; the increased width mainly is caused by the addition of myelin (seen as white within the ON in **A**). **C** and **D** Cross sections (low and medium magnification, respectively) of the ON shows the central parenchyma that contains axons, central retinal artery and vein, other blood vessels, astrocytes, oligodendrocytes, and pial septa. This is surrounded by pia mater, subarachnoid "space", arachnoid mater, subdural "space', and dura. (**A**, courtesy of Dr. RC Eagle Jr; **C**, **D**, courtesy of Dr. MG Farber.)

CONGENITAL DEFECTS AND ANATOMIC VARIATIONS

- Aplasia
- Hypoplasia
- Dysplasia
- Anomalous shape of optic disc and optic cup
- Congenital crescent or conus
- Congenital optic atrophy
- Coloboma
  - Optic pit
  - Morning glory syndrome
- Myopia

FIGURE 13.2

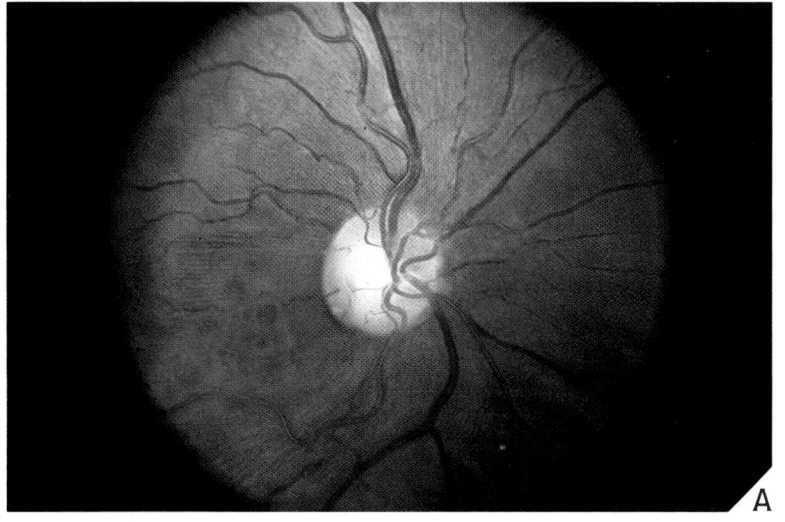

A

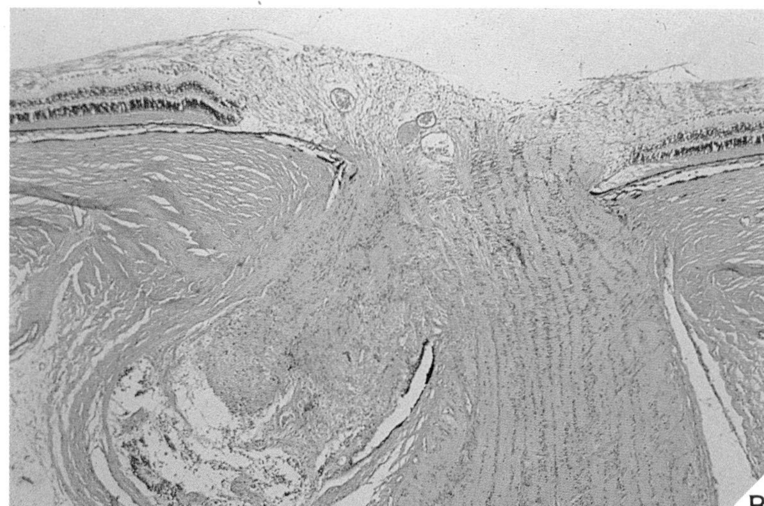

B

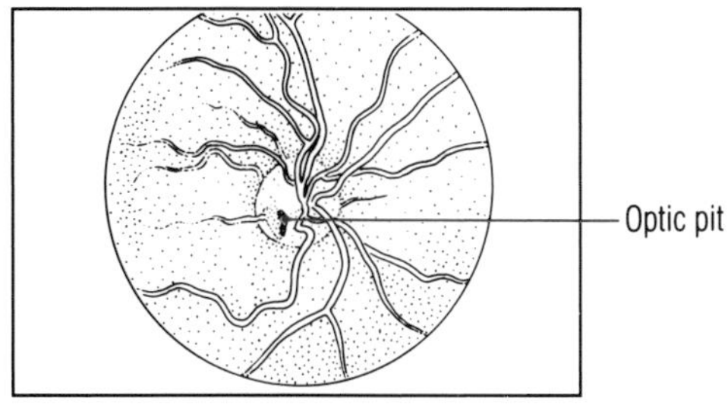

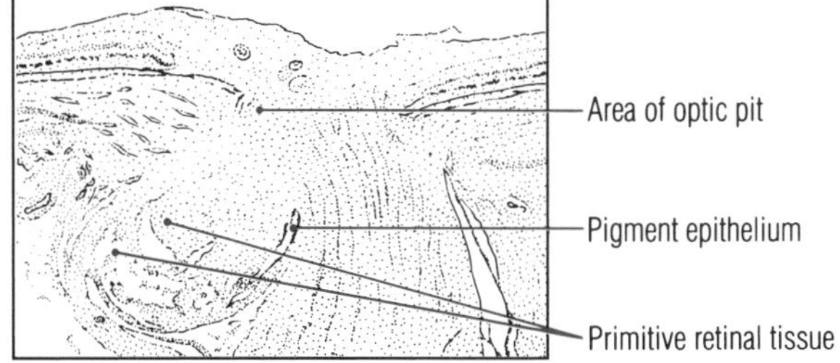

FIGURE 13.3 COLOBOMA OF THE OPTIC NERVE. A An optic pit, a form of optic nerve coloboma, is present as a small angular depression in the inferotemporal quadrant of the disc. This is the usual location for a pit. The patient had an associated detachment of the macular retina. **B** A histologic section of another case shows the herniation of retinal tissue through the enlarged scleral opening along one side of the optic nerve. **C** The enlarged, deeply excavated optic disc resembles a morning glory flower, hence the name "morning glory syndrome," another form of optic nerve coloboma. (**B**, courtesy of Dr. JB Crawford, from Irvine AR, et al., 1986; **C**, courtesy of Dr. GR Diamond.)

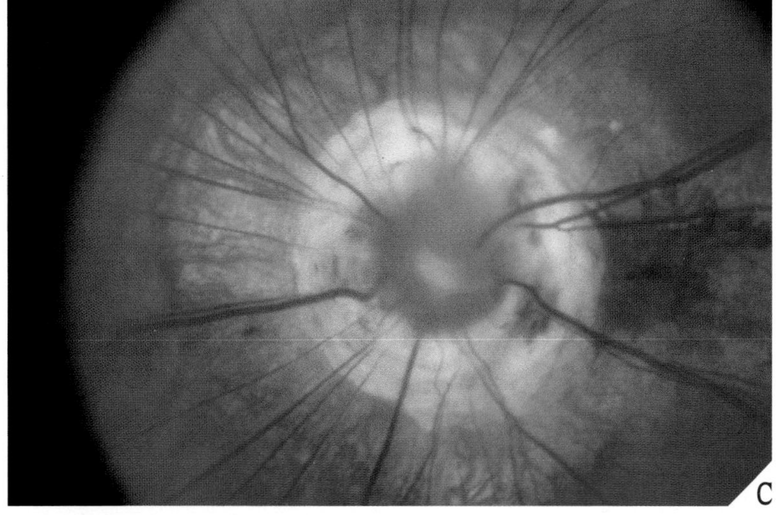

C

OPTIC DISC EDEMA

Causes

Increased venous pressure at or posterior to the lamina cribrosa
- Acute glaucoma
- Brain tumors

Increased venous pressure at or anterior to the lamina cribrosa
- Ocular hypotony
- Central retinal vein occlusion

Local phenomena
- Irvine-Gass syndrome
- Iron deficiency anemia

Histology

Acute
- Edema, blockage of axoplasmic flow, vascular congestion, increased volume of tissue, hemorrhages, and narrowing of phsyiologic cup
- Displacement of sensory retina away from the optic disc and the peripapillary retinal and choroidal folds
- Peripapillary retinal detachment

Chronic
- Degeneration of nerve fibers
- Gliosis and optic atrophy

FIGURE 13.4

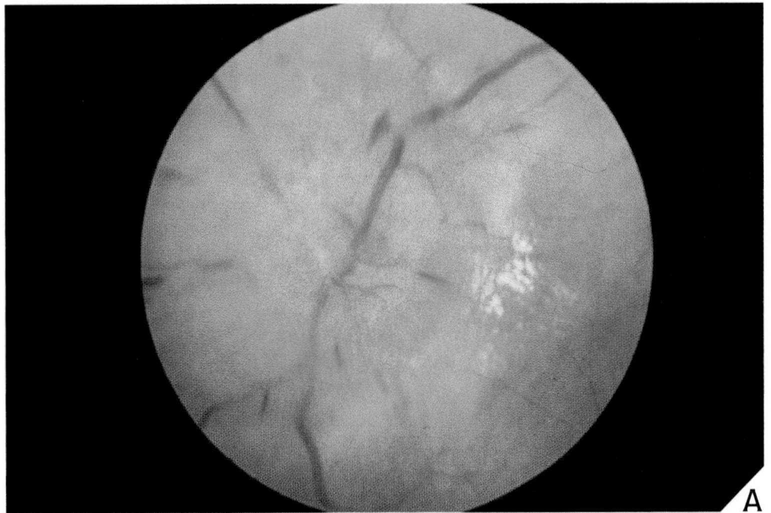

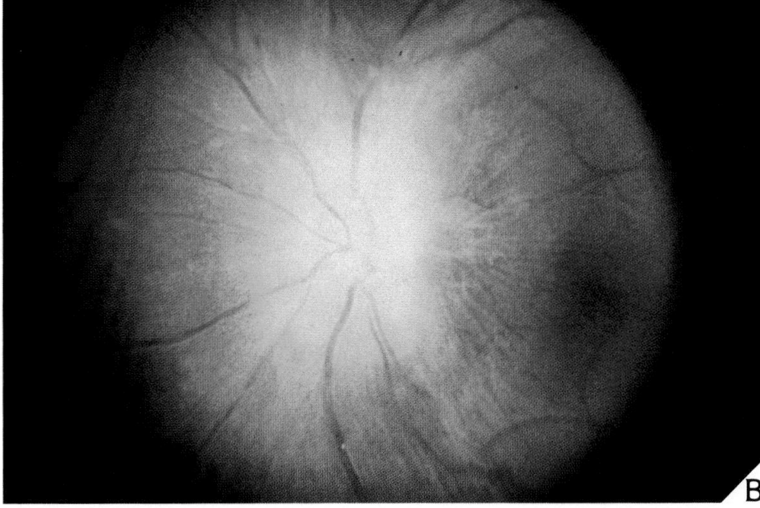

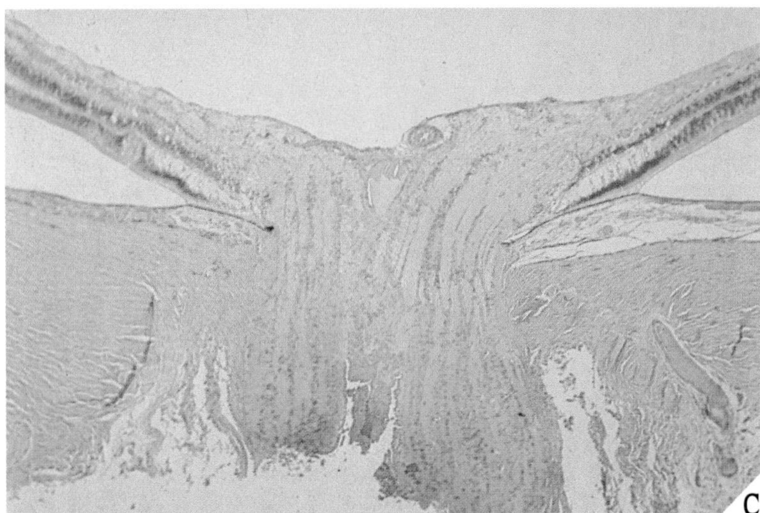

FIGURE 13.5 OPTIC DISC EDEMA. A The acutely swollen optic nerve head is surrounded by concentric retinal folds. Note the flame-shaped retinal hemorrhages and exudates. The patient had severe hypertension. **B** This patient had chronic bilateral optic disc edema, secondary to orbital pseudotumor. **C** A histologic section of another case of acute optic disc edema shows the characteristic findings. Increased mass is caused by axonal swelling, tissue edema, and vascular congestion. The photoreceptors are displaced laterally from the Bruch membrane, which terminates in a ring at the optic nerve. (**C**, from Yanoff M, Fine BS, *Ocular Pathology*, 3rd ed.)

PSEUDOPAPILLEDEMA

Hypermetropic optic disc
Drusen of optic nerve head
Congenital developmental abnormalities
Optic neuritis and perineuritis
Myelinated (medullated) nerve fibers

FIGURE 13.6

CAUSES OF OPTIC NEURITIS

Secondary to ocular disease
- Keratitis
- Uveitis
- Endophthalmitis

Secondary to orbital disease
- Cellulitis
- Thrombophlebitis
- Arteritis

Secondary to intracranial disease
- Meningitis

Secondary to vascular disease
- Temporal arteritis

Secondary to demyelinating disease

Secondary to spread of distant infection

Secondary to nutritional, toxic, or metabolic processes
- Tobacco-alcohol amblyopia

Secondary to hereditary conditions

Secondary to idiopathic causes

FIGURE 13.7

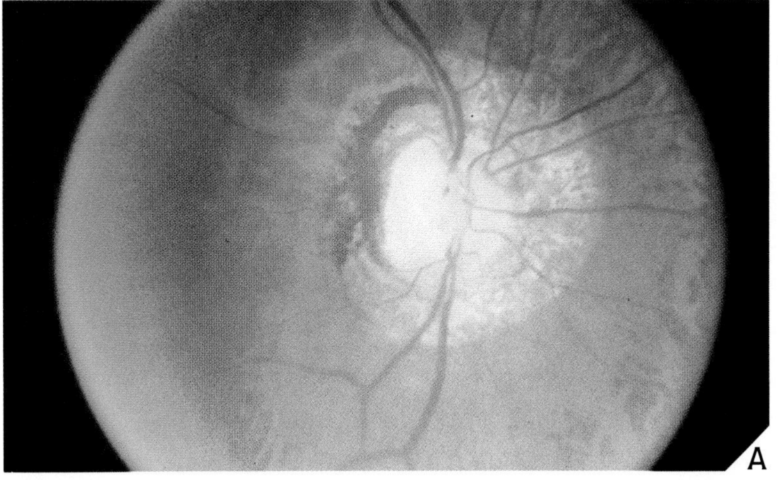

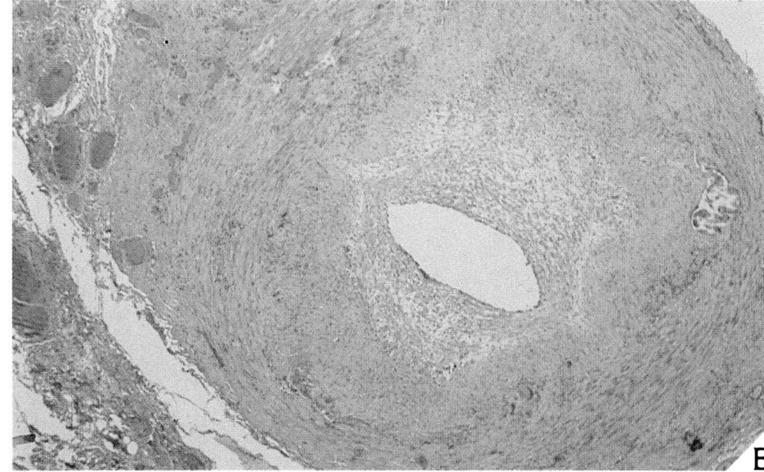

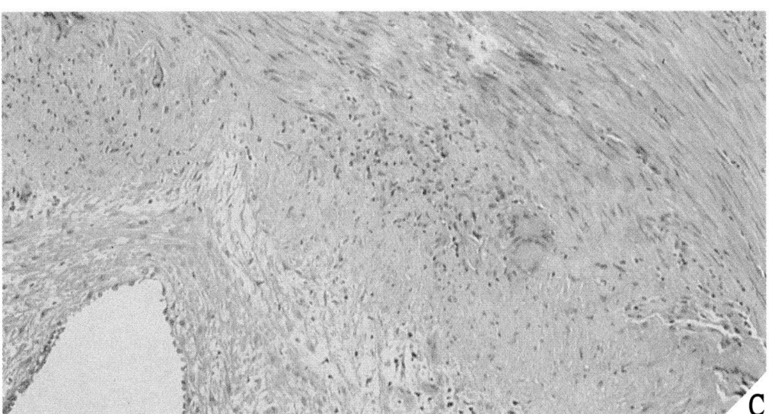

FIGURE 13.8 TEMPORAL ARTERITIS. A The patient had a gradual decrease in vision in his left eye, along with generalized weakness and a 11.4 kg weight loss. The fundus shows an atrophic optic nerve head as a result of temporal arteritis. **B** A histologic section of the temporal artery from this case shows a granulomatous giant cell reaction in the inflamed wall of the artery. The internal elastic lamina of the artery is fragmented. **C** Increased magnification shows the giant cells and granulomatous inflammation.

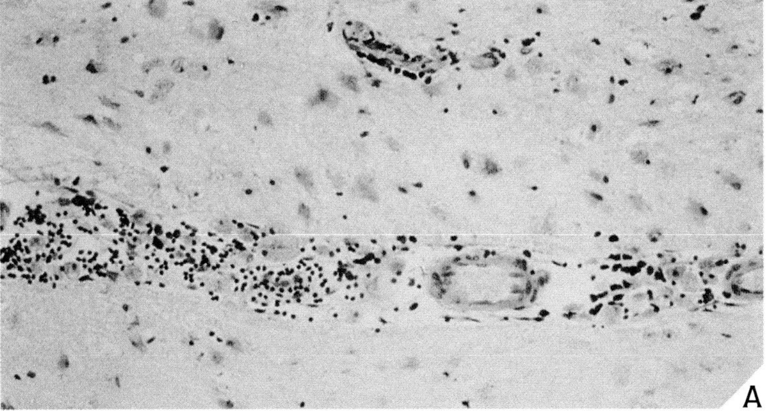

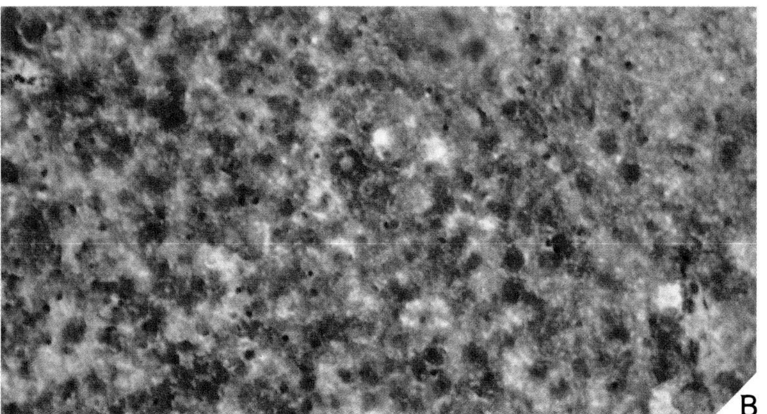

FIGURE 13.9 DEMYELINATING DISEASE. A A histologic section of the occipital lobe from a patient who had Schilder disease shows a marked perivascular inflammatory reaction, which consists mainly of lymphocytes and some plasma cells. The surrounding brain parenchyma demonstrates a reactive gliosis and contains a proliferation of astrocytes. **B** Special stains for fat (oil red-O) show considerable amounts of lipid present in the tissue.

CAUSES OF OPTIC ATROPHY

Ascending

Primary lesion in retina or optic disc (e.g., glaucoma) and secondary effects on the optic nerve and brain

Descending

Primary lesion in the optic nerve or brain (e.g., tabes dorsalis, hydrocephalus)

Inherited

Leber optic atrophy
Behr optic atrophy
Friedreich ataxia

FIGURE 13.10

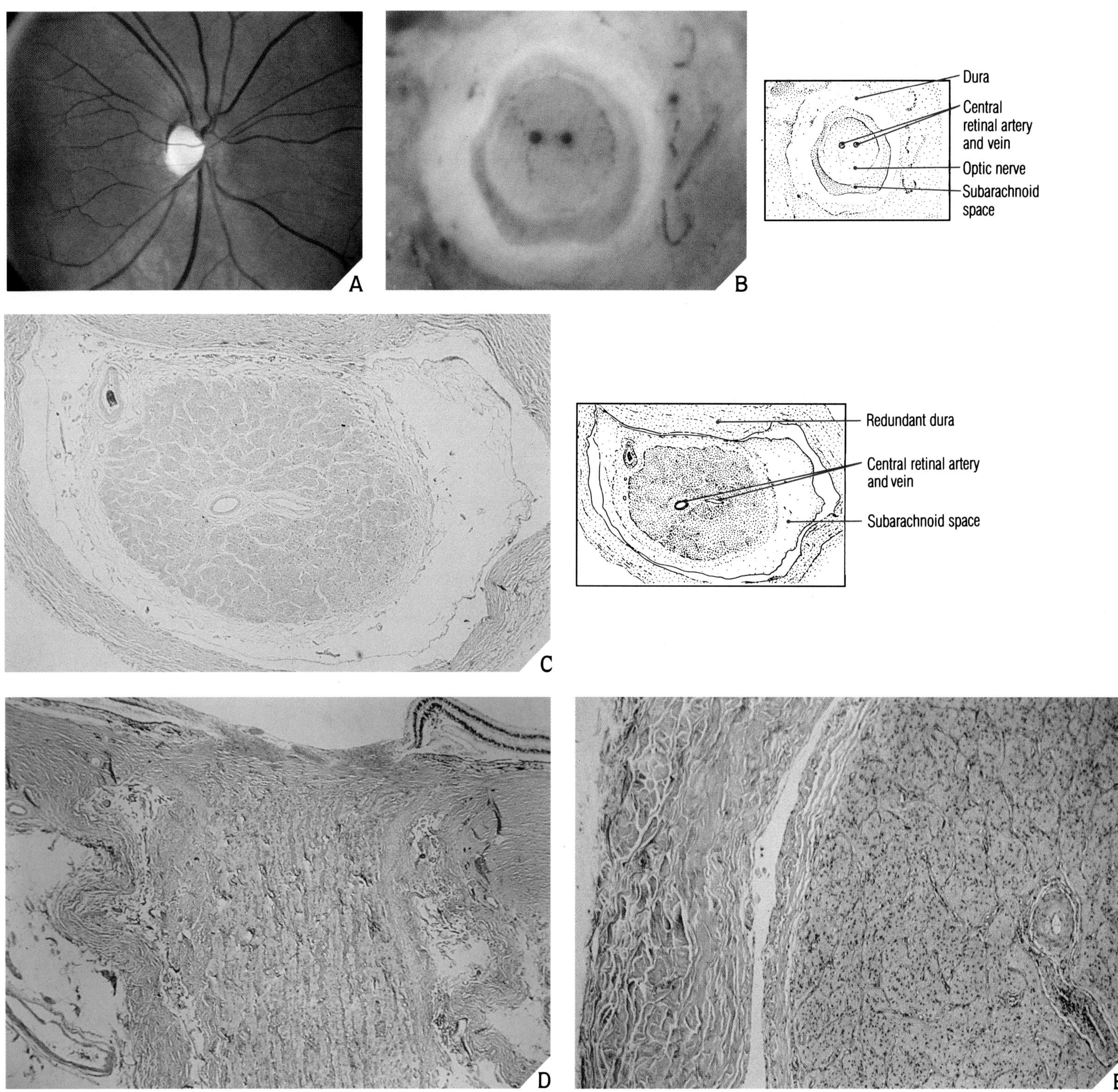

FIGURE 13.11 OPTIC ATROPHY. A The patient had retrobulbar neuritis in this eye, leaving him with optic atrophy of the temporal half of the optic nerve head. **B** Gross examination of an enucleated eye in another case shows marked atrophy of the parenchyma of the optic nerve, which has resulted in a widened subarachnoid space. **C** A histologic cross-section shows the optic nerve to be atrophic and shrunken, resulting in an increased size of the subarachnoid space, a redundancy of the dura, a widening of the pial septa, and gliosis. **D** A longitudinal histologic section shows that the optic nerve is of the same diameter where it enters the eye as it is when posterior to the sclera. Normally, the optic nerve doubles in diameter behind the sclera because of the accumulation of myelin. The narrowness of the optic nerve is due to atrophy. The subarachnoid space is widened and the dura is redundant. **E** Increased magnification of another case shows the marked cellularity of the atrophic nerve caused by proliferation of astrocytes.

Juvenile pilocytic astrocytoma ("glioma")
Oligodendrocytoma
Malignant astrocytoma
Meningioma
Melanocytoma (see Chapter 17)
Hemangioma
Medulloepithelioma (see Chapter 17)
Giant drusen (see Chapter 2)
Ordinary drusen
Juxtapapillary retinal pigment epithelial drusen
Corpora amylacea
Corpora arenacea

FIGURE 13.12

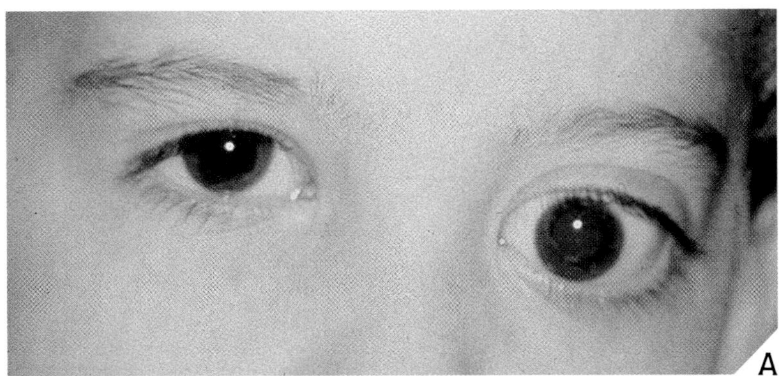

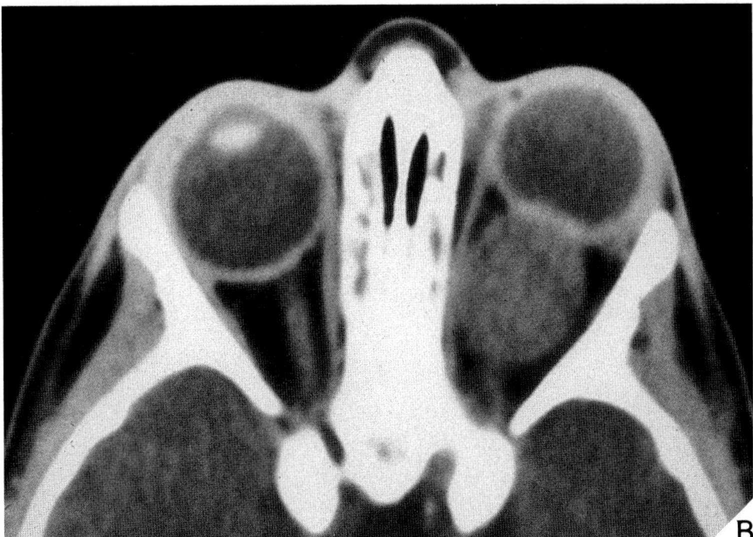

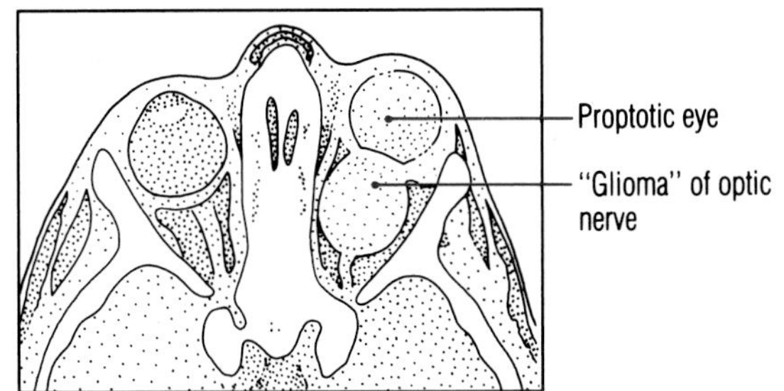

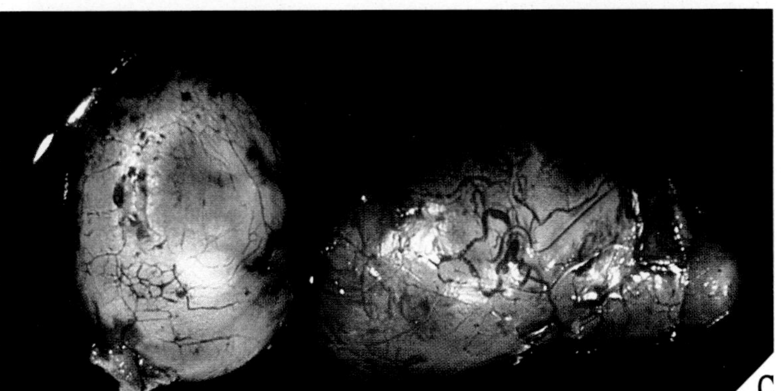

FIGURE 13.13 OPTIC NERVE "GLIOMA". A The patient has proptosis of the left eye caused by a glioma of the optic nerve. Most of the time the proptosis is in a downward and outward direction. **B** The CT scan of this case shows the glioma enlarging the retrobulbar optic nerve. **C** This gross specimen from another case shows the optic nerve thickened by tumor, starting just behind the globe. (**A**, **B**, case presented by Dr. JA Shields to the Armed Forces Institute of Pathology Alumni, 1987; **C**, courtesy of Dr. WC Frayer, from Yanoff M, Fine BS, *Ocular Pathology*, 3rd ed.)

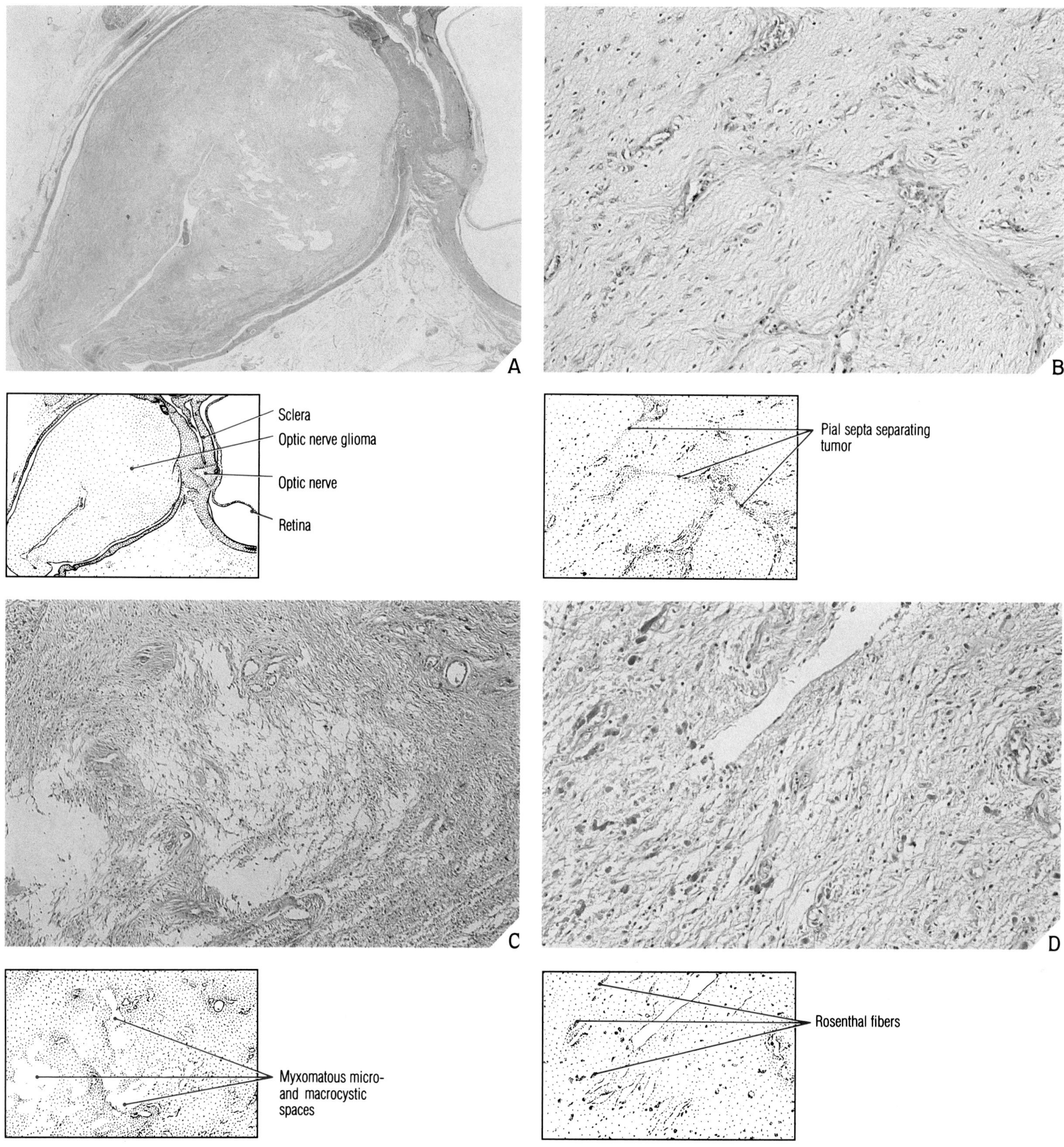

FIGURE 13.14 OPTIC NERVE "GLIOMA". A A large tumor involves and thickens the optic nerve. **B** Increased magnification shows enlarged neural bundles between the spread-out pial septa. The neural bundles contain expanded, disordered glial cells and a few axons. **C** An area of necrosis within the tumor shows myxomatous microcystoid and macrocystoid spaces. **D** Many astrocytes contain intracytoplasmic eosinophilic structures, called Rosenthal fibers. (**A**, from Yanoff M, Fine BS, *Ocular Pathology*, 3rd ed.)

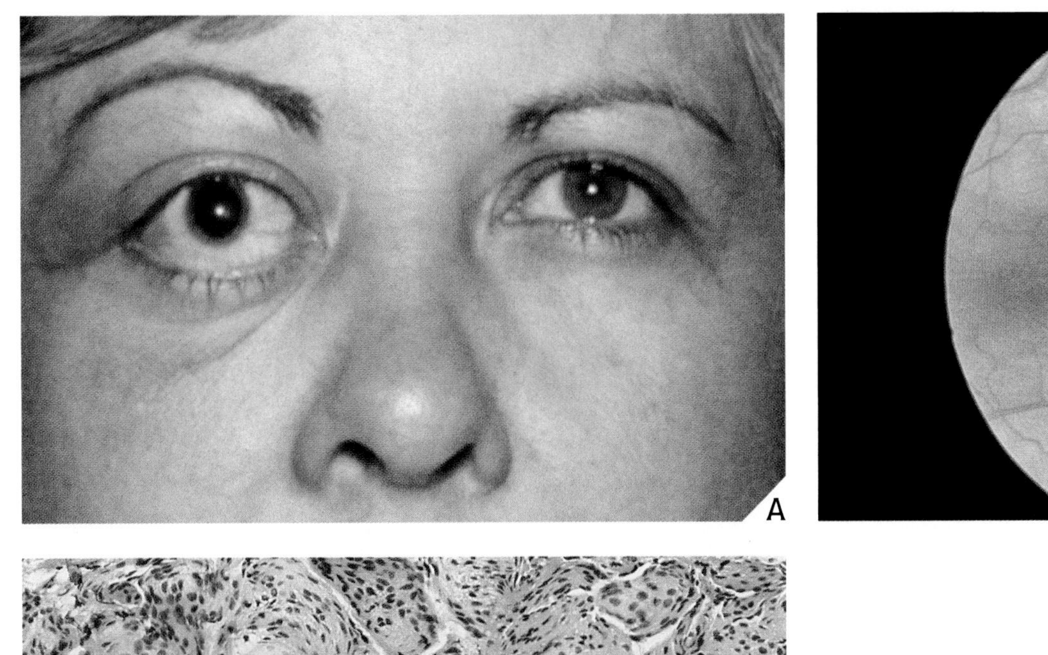

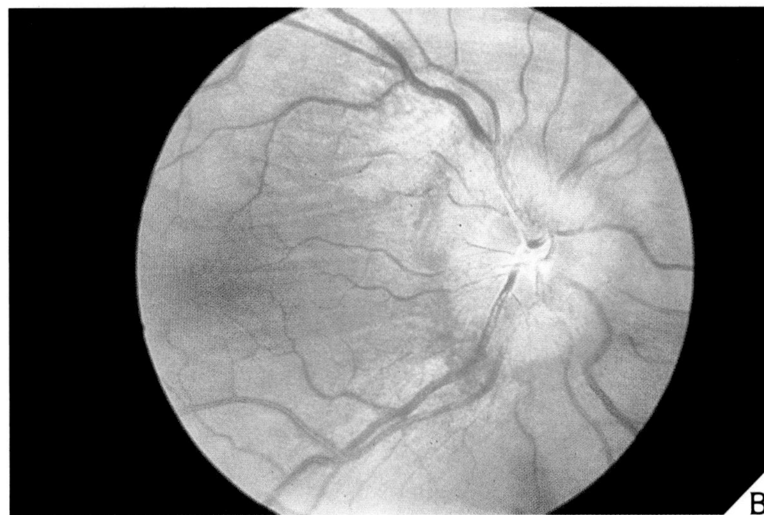

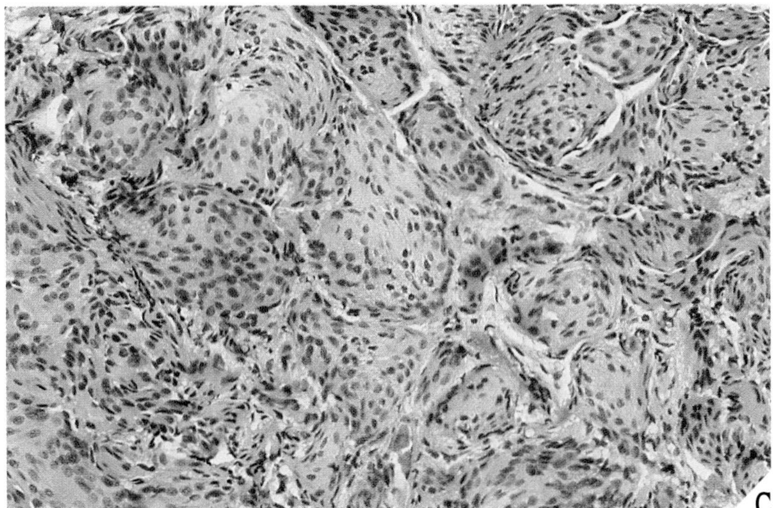

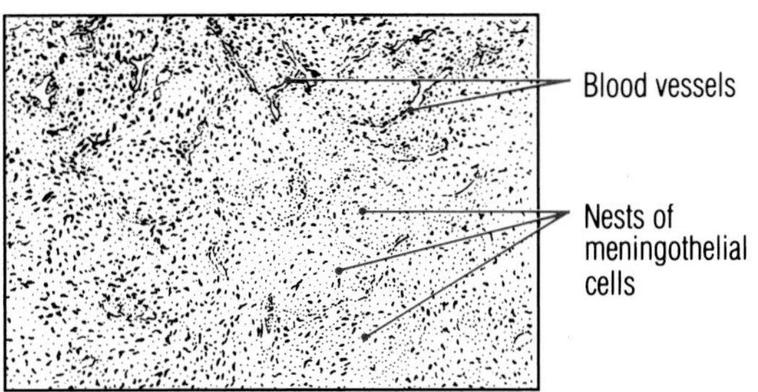

FIGURE 13.15 MENINGIOMA. A A meningioma of the orbital portion of the optic nerve has caused proptosis of the right eye, **B** Fundus examination shows optic disc edema of long-term duration. **C** A biopsy of another case shows a proliferation of meningothelial cells. As is often the case, no psammoma bodies are present. (**A**, **B**, courtesy of Dr. WC Frayer.)

SECONDARY OPTIC NERVE TUMORS

Retinoblastoma (see Chapter 18)
Malignant melanoma (see Chapter 17)
Hamartoma of retinal pigment epithelium (see Chapter 17)
Metastatic carcinoma
Leukemia and lymphoma
Glioblastoma multiforme
Myelin artifact

FIGURE 13.16

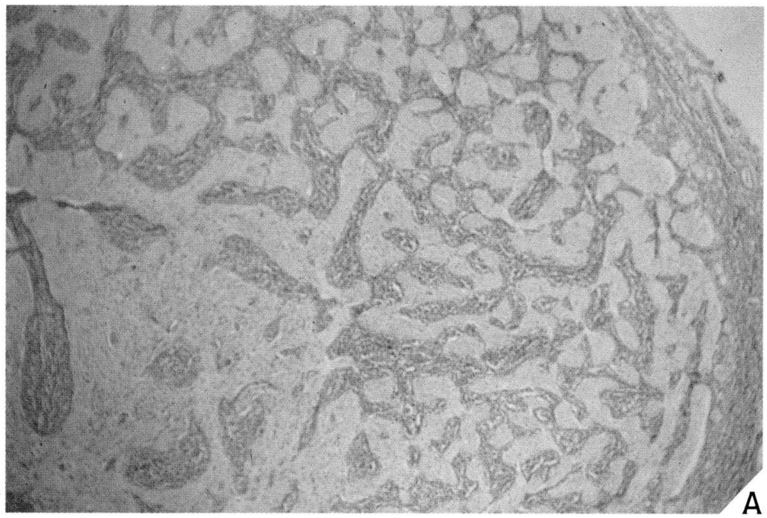

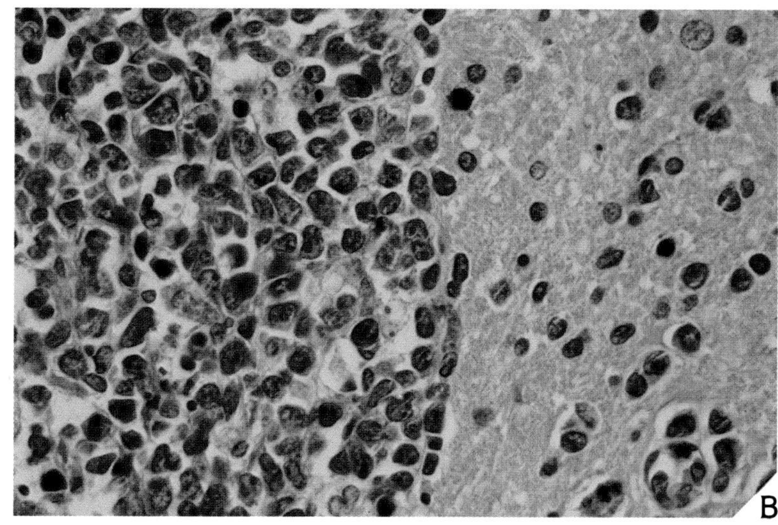

Figure 13.17 Leukemic Infiltrate. A The pial septa of the optic nerve are markedly thickened. The subarachnoid space contains a cellular infiltrate. **B** Increased magnification shows that the pial septa are thickened by blastic leukemic cells.

Bibliography

Brodsky MC, et al: Optic nerve hypoplasia. Identification by magnetic resonance imaging. Arch Ophthalmol 108:1562, 1990.

Coons SW, Davis JR, Way DL: Correlation of DNA content and histology in prognosis of astrocytomas. Am J Clin Pathol 90:289, 1988 .

Imes RK, et al: Evolution of optociliary veins in optic nerve sheath meningiomas. Arch Ophthalmol 103:59, 1985.

Irvine AR, Crawford JB, Sullivan JH: The pathogenesis of retinal detachment with morning glory disc and optic pit. Retina 6:146, 1986.

Kincaid MC, Green WR: Ocular and orbital involvement in leukemia (Review). Surv Ophthalmol 27:211, 1983.

Quigley HA, Miller NR, Green WR: The pattern of optic nerve fiber loss in anterior ischemic optic neuropathy. Am J Ophthalmol 100:769, 1985

Rizzo JF, Lessell S: Risk of developing multiple sclerosis after uncomplicated optic neuritis: a long-term prospective study. Neurology 38:185, 1988.

Sadun AA, Bassi CJ: Optic nerve damage in Alzheimer's disease. Ophthalmology 97:9, 1990.

Sibony PA, et al: Optic nerve sheath meningiomas. Clinical manifestations. Ophthalmology 91:1313, 1984.

Slusher MM, et al: The spectrum of cavitary optic disc anomalies in a family. Ophthalmology 96:342, 1989.

Sobol WM, et al: Long-term visual outcome in patients with optic nerve pit and serous retinal detachment of the macula. Ophthalmology 97:1539, 1990.

Stone EM, et al: *Mae* III positively detects the mitochondrial mutation associated with type I Leber's hereditary optic neuropathy. Arch Ophthalmol 108:1417, 1990.

Wells KK, et al: Temporal artery biopsies. Correlation of light microscopy and immunofluorescence microscopy. Ophthalmology 96:1058, 1989.

Yanoff M, Davis R, Zimmerman LE: Juvenile pilocytic astrocytoma ("glioma") of optic nerve: clinicopathologic study of 63 cases. In: Jakobiec FA (ed): *Ocular and Adnexal Tumors.* Birmingham, Aesculapius Publishing, 1978, pp 685–707.

Zimmerman CF, Schatz NJ, Glaser JS: Magnetic resonance imaging of optic nerve meningiomas. Enhancement with gadolinium-DTPA. Ophthalmology 97:585, 1990.

Orbit

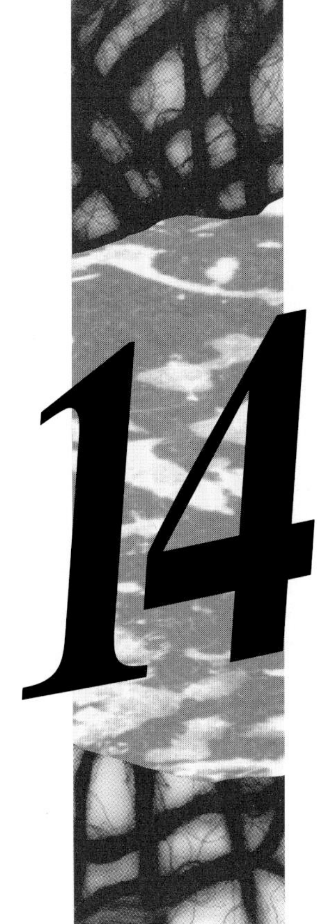

In addition to the eye and the optic nerve, the orbit contains many soft tissue structures such as fat, muscle (striated and nonstriated), cartilage, bone, fibrous tissue, nerves, and blood vessels. Orbital disease, whatever its cause, tends to increase the bulk of the orbit, so the main presenting sign is exophthalmos. Other than the epithelia in the eye, the lacrimal gland is the only epithelial structure within the orbit. All orbital structures may be involved in disease processes. Many congenital anomalies may affect both the bony structure of the orbit and the soft tissues within the orbit. Inflammatory diseases of all types may affect the orbit. Inflammation has been already discussed in general in Chapters 3 and 4.

Many systemic diseases may involve the orbit. The most important of these is Graves disease, which is one of the most common causes of exophthalmos.

Orbital tumors may arise initially in the orbit, extend into the orbit from contiguous structures, or secondarily affect the orbit from distant sites (metastatic). Congenital tumors that contain tissue normally present (e.g., blood vessels) are called hamartomas. Congenital tumors that contain tissue not normally present (e.g., hair follicles) are called choristomas. Many mesenchymal tumors may arise from orbital soft tissues. The most important of these are fibrous histiocytoma and rhabdomyosarcoma. Numerous neural tumors involve the orbit. Neurofibroma has been described in Chapter 2. Glioma of the optic nerve and meningioma have been described in Chapter 13. Neurilemmoma is illustrated in this chapter.

The major epithelial tumors found in the orbit arise from the lacrimal gland. The most common benign lacrimal gland tumor is the benign mixed tumor. The most common malignant tumor is adenoid cystic carcinoma. Lymphoid lesions, both benign and malignant, and leukemias often involve the orbit. In fact, lymphoid lesions and Graves disease are the most common causes of exophthalmos. Other diseases, such as fibrous dysplasia and Langerhans granulomatoses (histiocytosis X), also may affect the orbit. The most common entity involving the orbit in the group of Langerhans granulomatoses is eosinophilic granuloma.

DEVELOPMENTAL ABNORMALITIES

Developmental abnormalities of bony orbit
Microphthalmos with cyst
Cephaloceles
Congenital alacrima

FIGURE 14.1

ORBITAL INFLAMMATION (SEE CHAPTERS 3 AND 4)

Acute
Nonsuppurative
Suppurative
Purulent infection
Phycomycosis (mucormycosis)

Chronic
Nongranulomatous
Granulomatous

FIGURE 14.2

INJURIES (SEE CHAPTER 5)

Penetrating wounds
Nonpenetrating wounds

FIGURE 14.3

VASCULAR DISEASE

Primary
Varix
Cavernous sinus thrombosis

Part of systemic disease
Collagen disease
Wegener granulomatosis
Allergic vasculitis
Temporal arteritis (see Chapter 13)

FIGURE 14.4

OCULAR MUSCLE INVOLVEMENT IN SYSTEMIC DISEASES

Graves disease
Myasthenia gravis
Myotonia dystrophica
Collagen diseases
Sarcoidosis
Trichinosis
Primary amyloidosis

FIGURE 14.5

GRAVES DISEASE

Mild
Onset early in adult life
Affects predominantly women
Bilateral (initially may be unilateral)
Ocular proptosis nil to mild to moderate (lid retraction often simulates exophthalmos)
Prognosis for vision good

Severe
Onset in middle age (average: 50 years)
Affects both sexes equally (except post-thyroidectomy, when men predominate 4:1)
Bilateral (initially may be unilateral)
Severe proptosis
Poor visual prognosis
The patient may be hypothyroid, hyperthyroid, or euthyroid

FIGURE 14.6

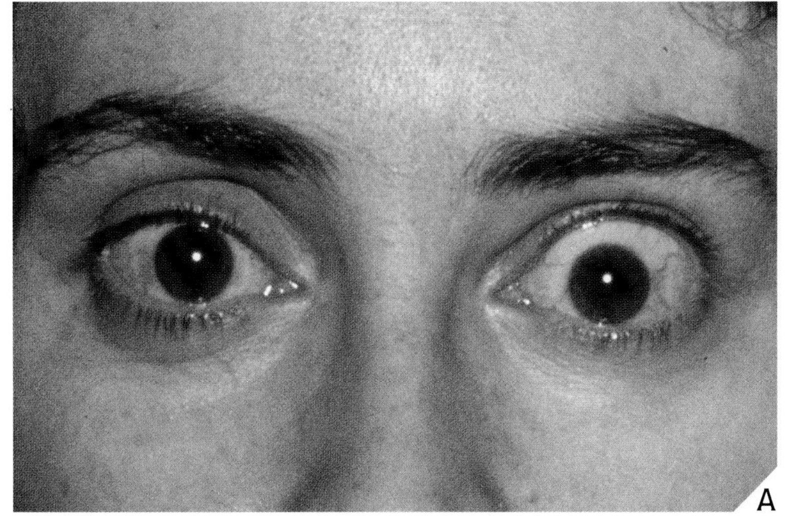

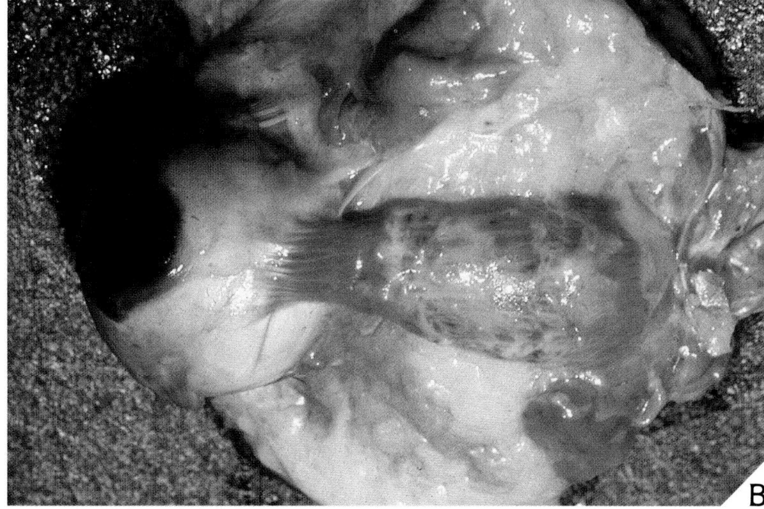

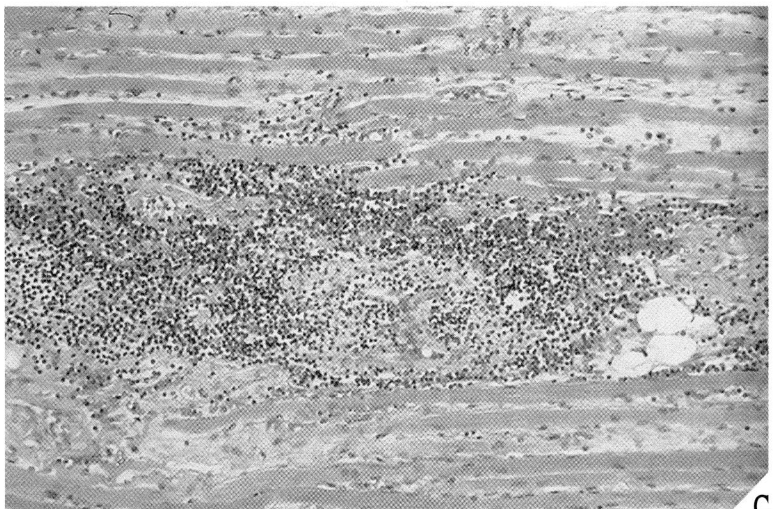

FIGURE 14.7 GRAVES DISEASE. A In Graves disease, exophthalmos often looks more pronounced than it actually is because of the extreme lid retraction that may occur. This patient, for instance, had minimal proptosis of the left eye but marked lid retraction. **B** The orbital contents obtained postmortem from a patient with Graves disease. Note the enormously thickened extraocular muscle. **C** A histologic section shows both fluid and inflammatory cells separating the muscle bundles. The inflammatory cells are predominantly lymphocytes plus plasma cells. (**A**, courtesy of Dr. HG Scheie; **B, C**, courtesy of Dr. RC Eagle Jr, from Hufnagel TJ, et al., 1984.)

CLASSIFICATION OF ORBITAL TUMORS

Primary in orbit
Choristomas
Hamartomas
Mesenchymal
Neural
Lymphoid and inflammatory
Epithelial (lacrimal gland)

Direct extension

Metastatic from distant sites

FIGURE 14.8

CHORISTOMAS

Dermoid
Epidermoid
Teratoma
Ectopic lacrimal gland

FIGURE 14.9

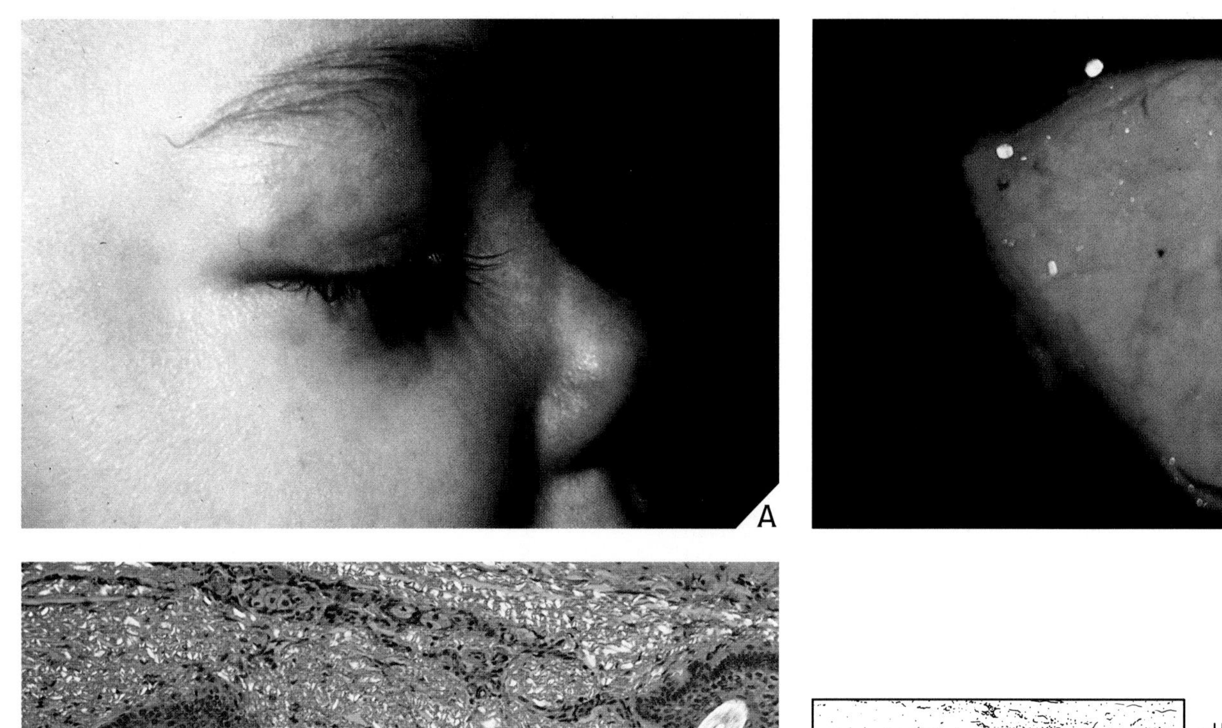

FIGURE 14.10 DERMOID. A A dermoid tumor is present in its most common location, the superior temporal portion of the orbit. **B** Gross examination of the cut surface of the tumor shows a cyst filled with "cheesy" material. **C** A histologic section, viewed using polarized light, shows a cyst lined by stratified squamous epithelium. Hair follicles (which contain birefringent hair shafts) and other epidermal appendages are contained in the wall of the cyst. The cyst itself contains keratin debris and hair shafts which are birefringent in the polarized light. (**A**, courtesy of Dr. JA Katowitz; **B**, from Yanoff M, Fine BS, *Ocular Pathology*, 3rd ed.)

HAMARTOMAS

- Lymphangioma
- Hemangioma
- Hemangiosarcoma
- Hemangiopericytoma
- Kaposi sarcoma (especially associated with AIDS)
- Phacomatoses (see Chapter 2)

FIGURE 14.11

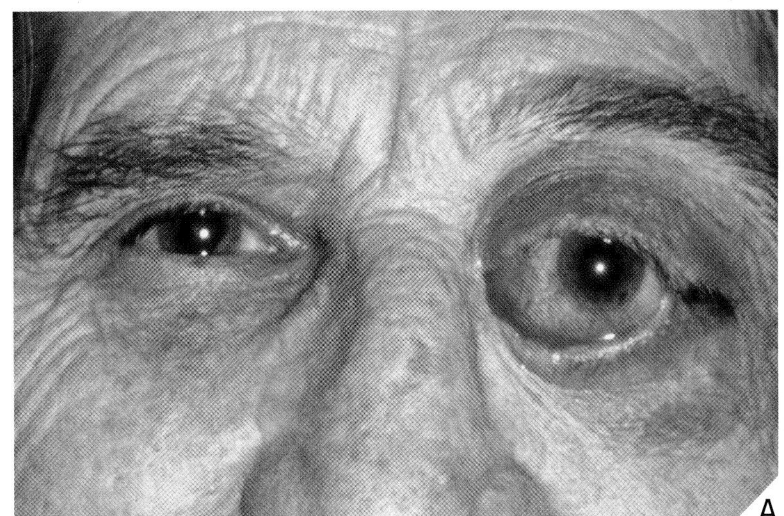

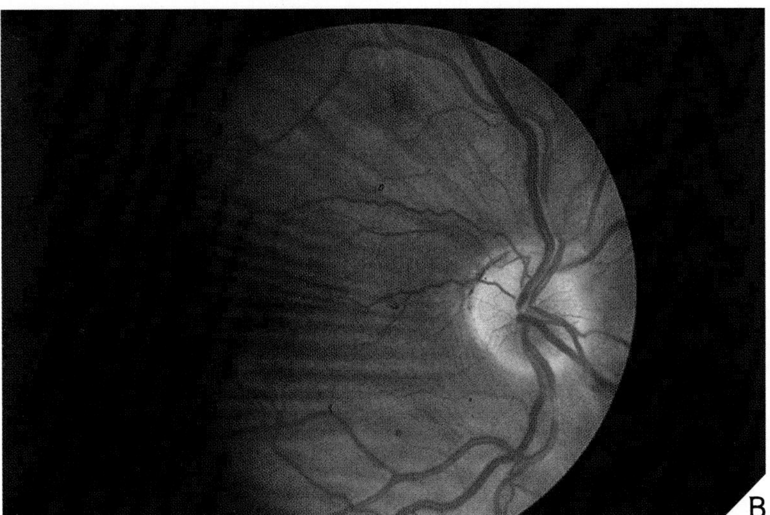

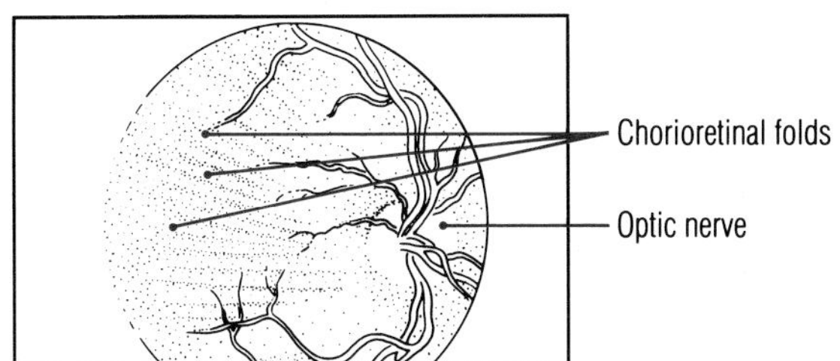

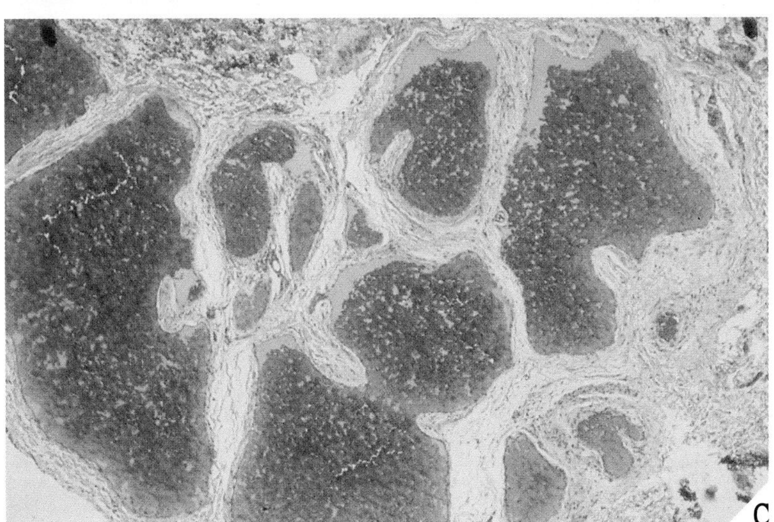

Figure 14.12 Hemangioma. A The patient had increasing proptosis of the left eye. Even though a hemangioma is a congenital tumor, the increase in size often does not occur until adult life because of hemorrhage into the tumor or inflammatory changes. **B** Another case shows that the orbital hemangioma has caused chorioretinal folds. **C** A histologic section shows large blood-filled spaces, lined by endothelium. The septa between the blood channels are of differing thicknesses. (**A, B**, courtesy of Dr. HG Scheie.)

Mesenchymal Tumors

Lipoma*, liposarcoma*
Fibroma*, fibrosarcoma*
Fibrous histiocytoma

Chondroma*, chondrosarcoma*
Osteoma*, osteosarcoma*

Leiomyoma*, leiomyosarcoma*
Rhabdomyoma*, rhabdomyosarcoma

*Rare except following radiation therapy

Figure 14.13

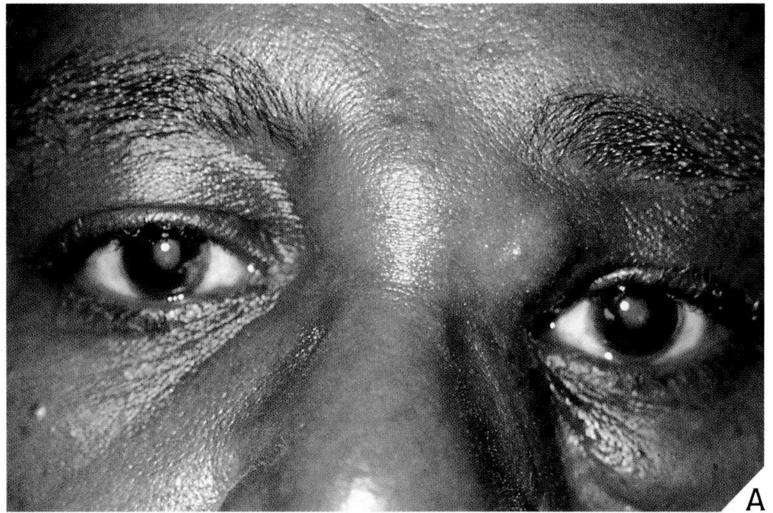

FIGURE 14.14 FIBROUS HISTIOCYTOMA. A This is the fourth recurrence of an orbital tumor that first had been excised 10 years previously. The histology of the primary lesion and of the four recurrences all appear identical. **B** A histologic section shows the diphasic pattern consisting of a histiocytic component and a fibrous component. **C** Increased magnification shows that the fibrous component forms a storiform or matted pattern. Controversy exists as to whether the tumor arises from histiocytes or fibroblasts (most of the evidence points toward a primitive mesenchymal cell origin). (Case reported by Jones WD III, et al., 1979.)

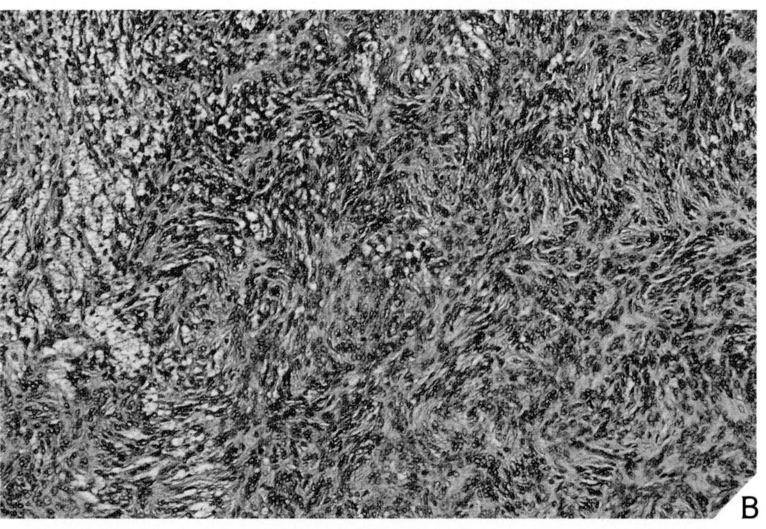

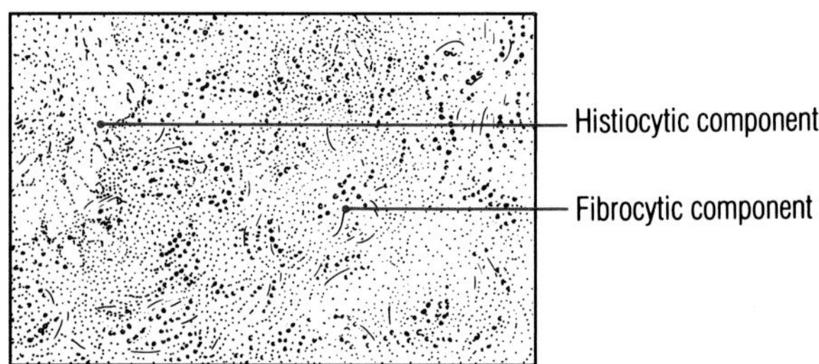

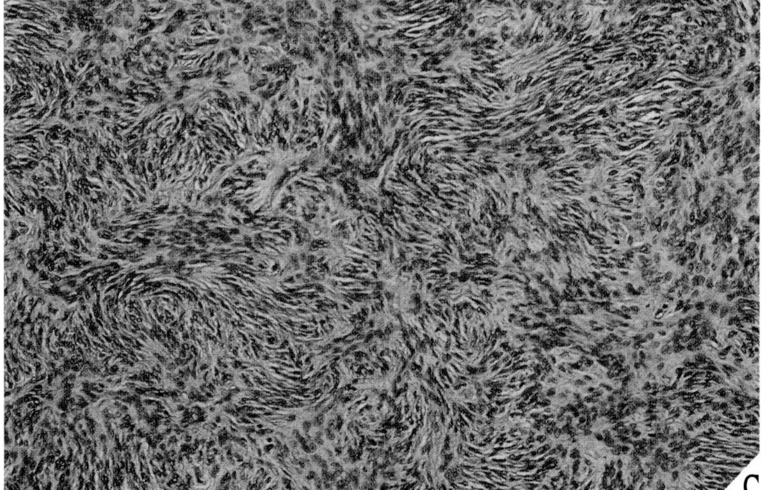

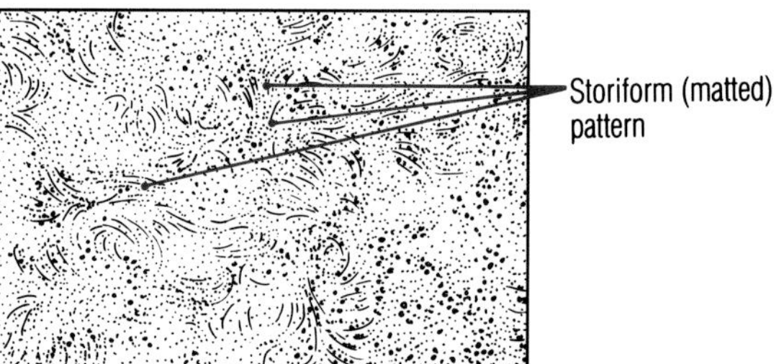

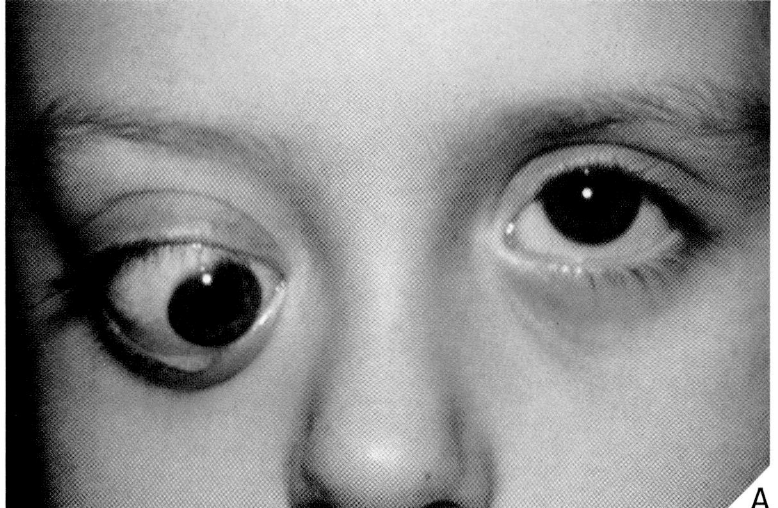

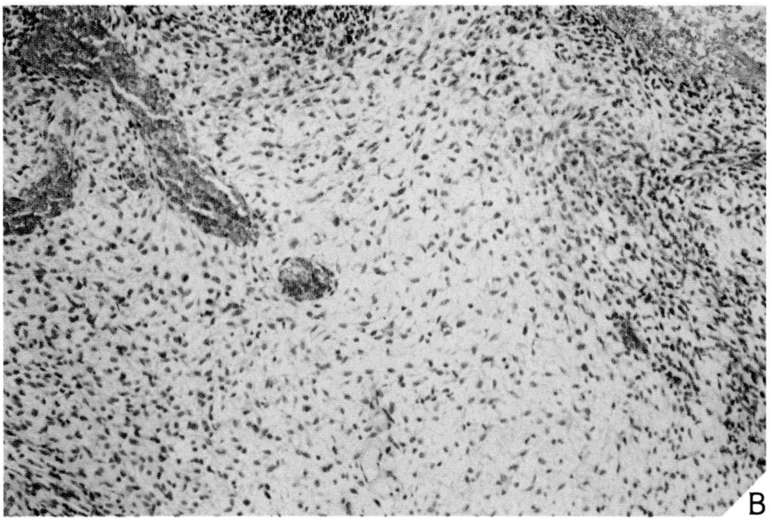

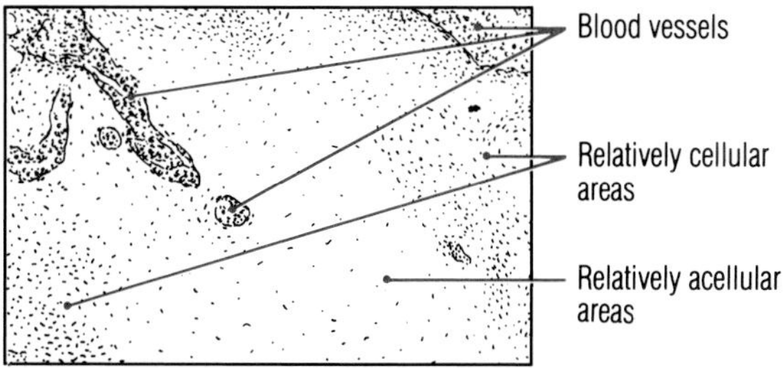

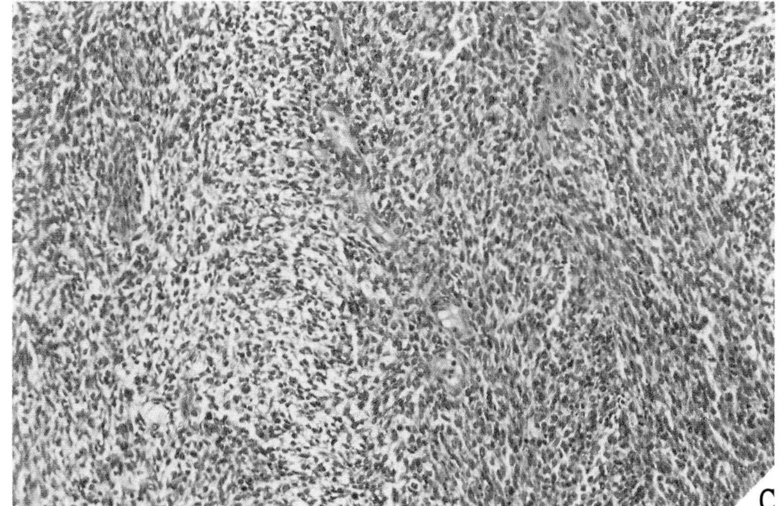

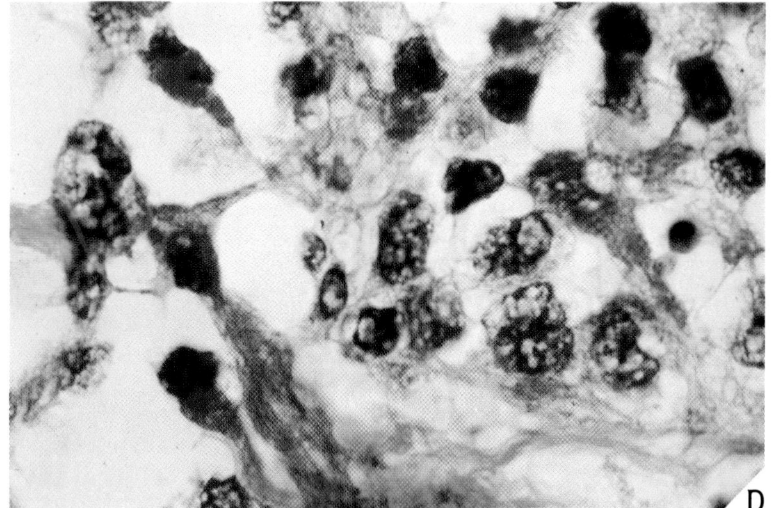

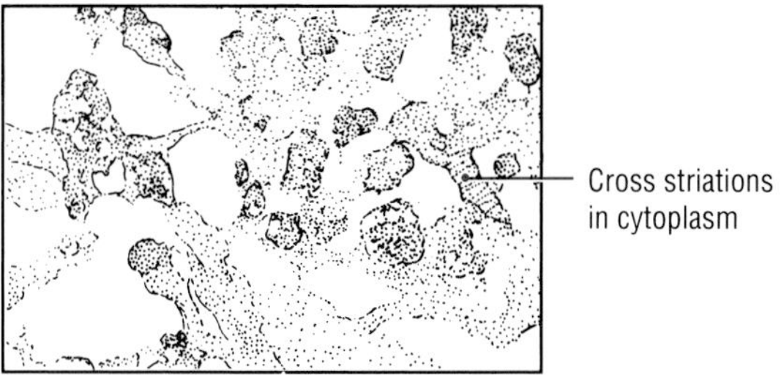

FIGURE 14.15 RHABDOMYOSARCOMA. A The patient has a unilateral proptosis of very recent onset. Often, rhabdomyosarcoma presents rapidly, causes lid redness, and is mistaken for orbital inflammation. **B** A histologic section shows a marked embryonic cellular pattern, hence the term embryonal rhabdomyosarcoma. **C** Increased magnification shows the primitive nature of the rhabdomyoblasts; these tend to cluster in groups, separated by relatively acellular areas. **D** A trichrome stain shows characteristic cross-striations in the cytoplasm of some of the rhabdomyoblasts. Cross-striations, although not abundant in embryonal rhabdomyosarcoma, can be seen in sections stained with hematoxylin and eosin but are easier to see with special stains.

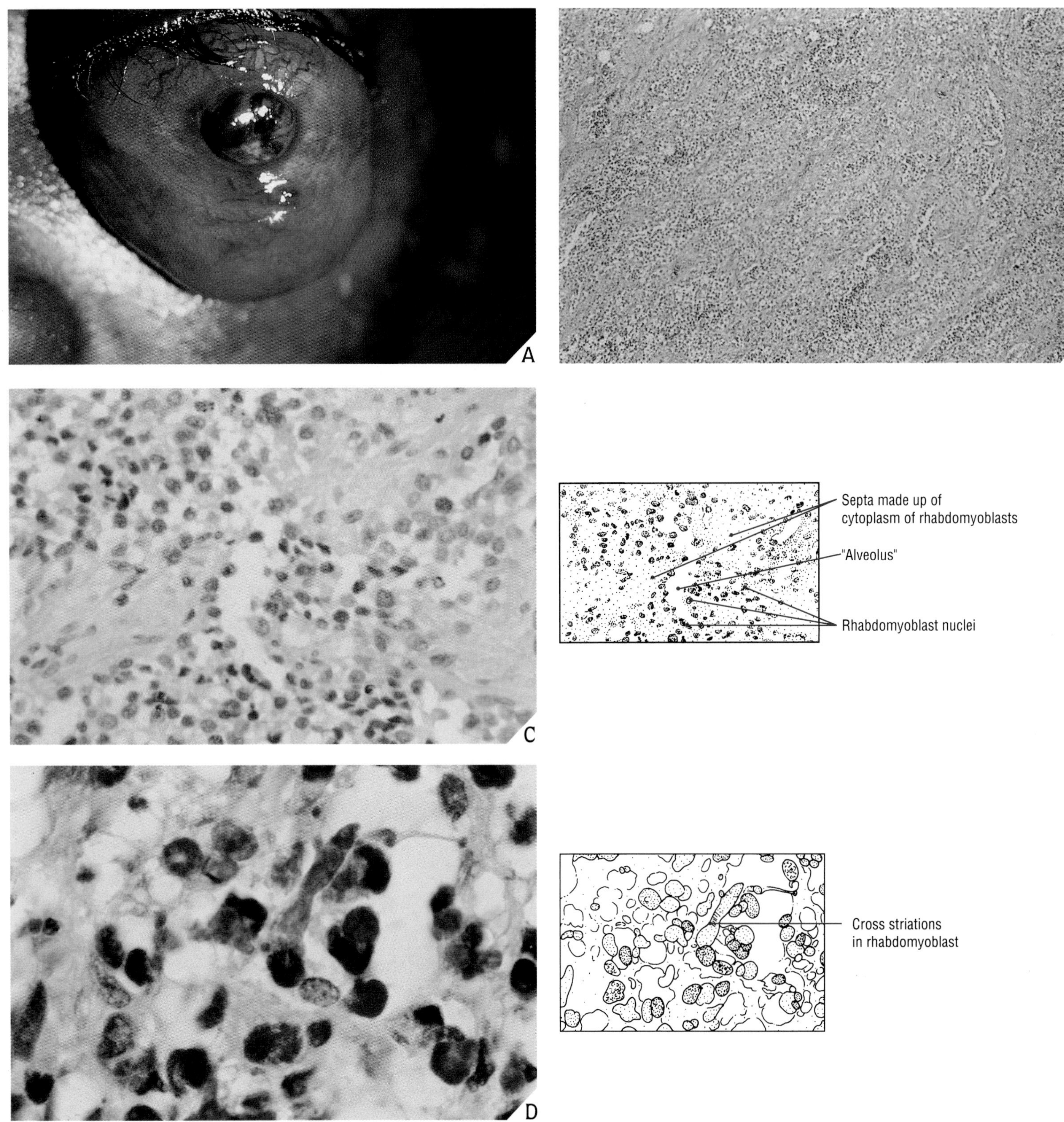

FIGURE 14.16 RHABDOMYOSARCOMA. A This 21-year-old man presented with proptosis of his left eye. **B** A reticulin stain shows delicate septa, which give the tumor an alveolated appearance (hence the term alveolar rhabdomyosarcoma). **C** Increased magnification shows that the cytoplasm of the rhabdomyoblasts makes up part of the septa. **D** A trichrome stain shows typical cross-striations. Cross-striations are least abundant and hardest to find in alveolar rhabdomyosarcoma. In the third type of rhabdomyosarcoma (differentiated), unlike in embryonal and alveolar types, most of the cells are differentiated, and cross-striations are easy to find.

NEURAL TUMORS

Amputation neuroma
Neurofibroma (see Chapter 2)
Neurilemmoma (schwannoma)
Juvenile pilocytic astrocytoma (glioma) of optic nerve (see Chapter 13)
Meningioma (see Chapter 13)
Nonchromaffin paraganglioma (carotid body tumor)
Granular cell tumor
Alveolar soft-part sarcoma

FIGURE 14.17

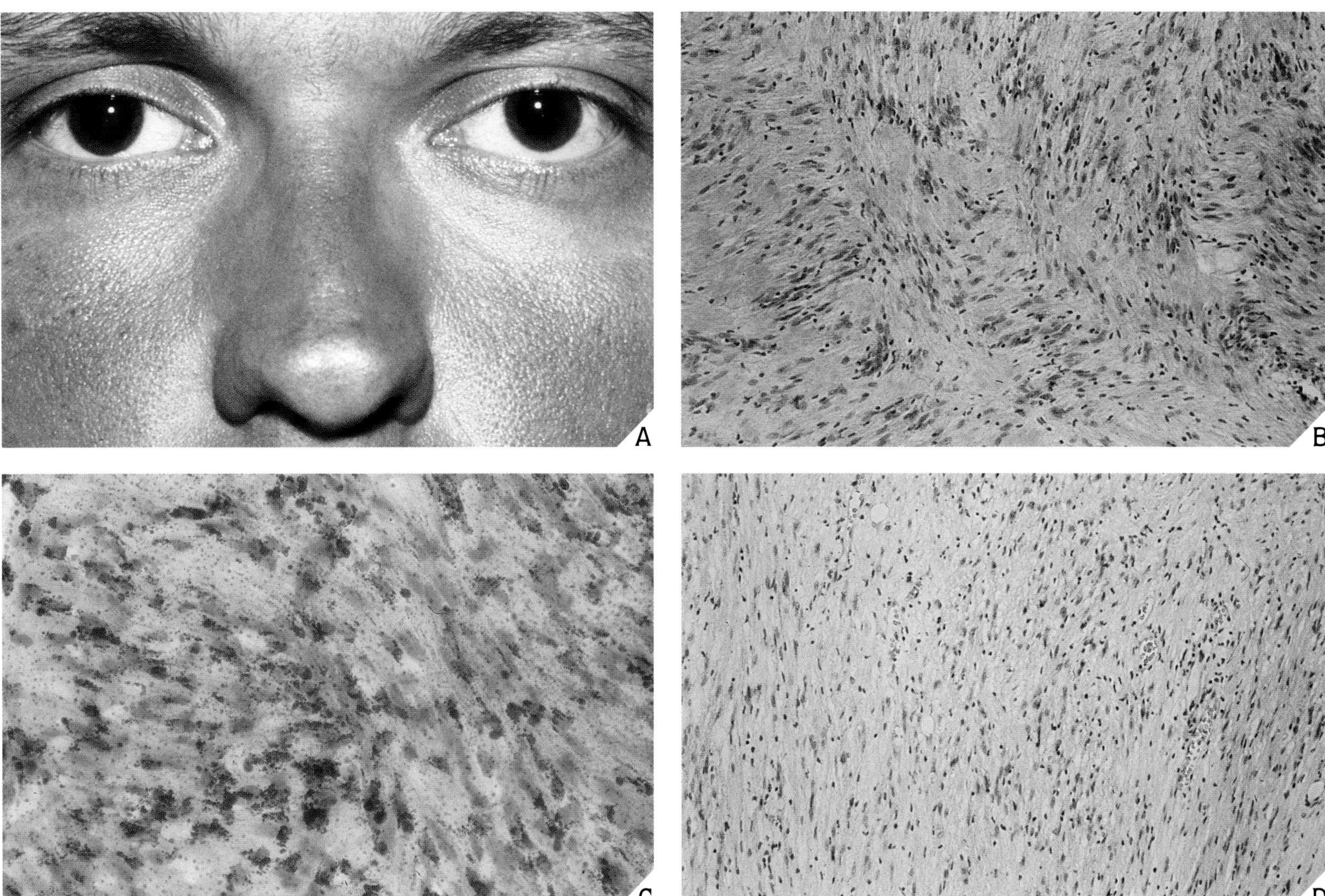

FIGURE 14.18 NEURILEMMOMA. A Proptosis of the patient's left eye had been present for many months and was increasing in size. An orbital tumor was removed. **B** A histologic section shows ribbons of spindle Schwann cell nuclei, which show a tendency toward palisading. Areas of relative acellularity, mimicking tactile corpuscles, are called Verocay bodies. This pattern is called the Antoni type A pattern. **C** Oil red-O stain shows the cytoplasm of the tumor cells is clearly lipid positive. **D** In this area of necrosis, inflammatory cells and microcystoid degeneration are present, a pattern called the Antoni type B pattern.

EPITHELIAL TUMORS OF THE LACRIMAL GLAND

Benign (about 50%)	**Malignant (about 50%)**
Benign mixed tumor	Adenoid cystic carcinoma (most frequent malignant tumor)
	Malignant mixed tumor
	Mucinous adenocarcinoma
	Mucoepidermoid carcinoma

FIGURE 14.19

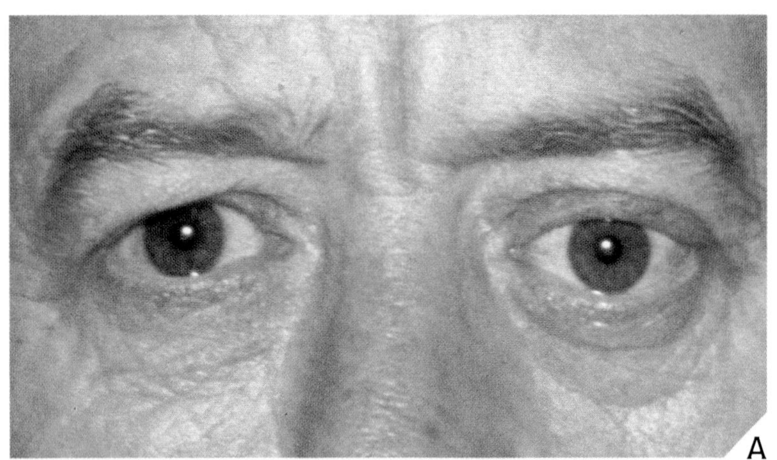

FIGURE 14.20 BENIGN MIXED TUMOR. A The patient had proptosis of the left eye for quite some time. It had gradually increased in severity. **B** A histologic section shows the characteristic diphasic pattern, consisting of a pale background that has a myxomatous stroma and a relatively amorphous appearance, contiguous with quite cellular areas that contain mainly epithelial cells. **C** Increased magnification shows the characteristic epithelial ductal structures lined by two layers of epithelium. The outer layer often undergoes myxoid and even cartilaginous metaplasia, whereas the inner layer may secrete mucus or may undergo squamous metaplasia, both of which are present here. (**A**, from Yanoff M, Fine BS: *Ocular Pathology*, 3rd ed.)

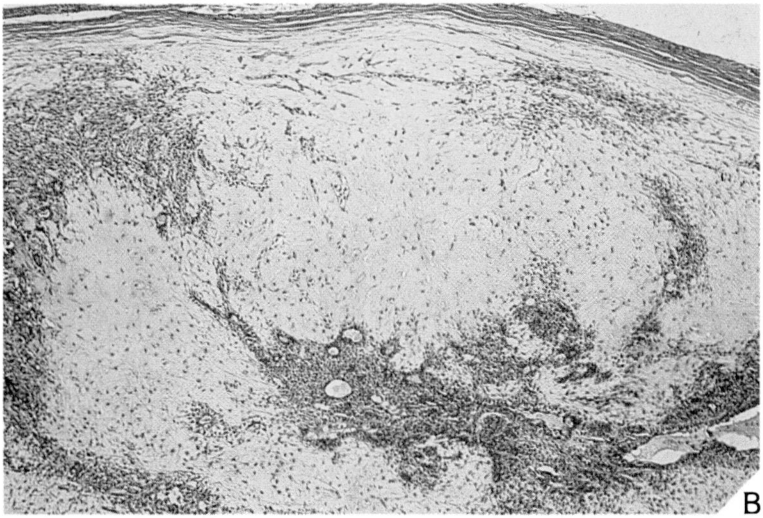

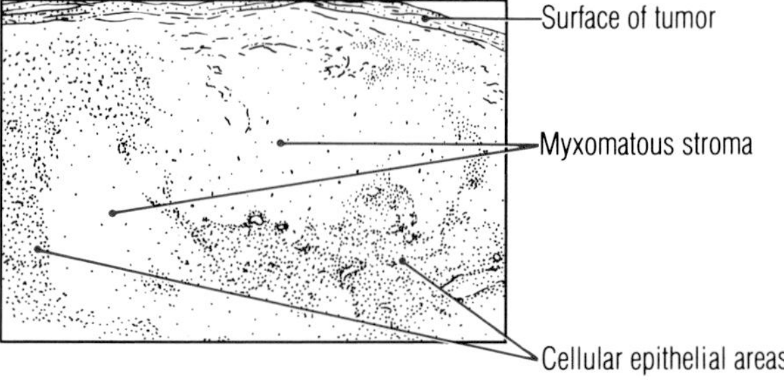

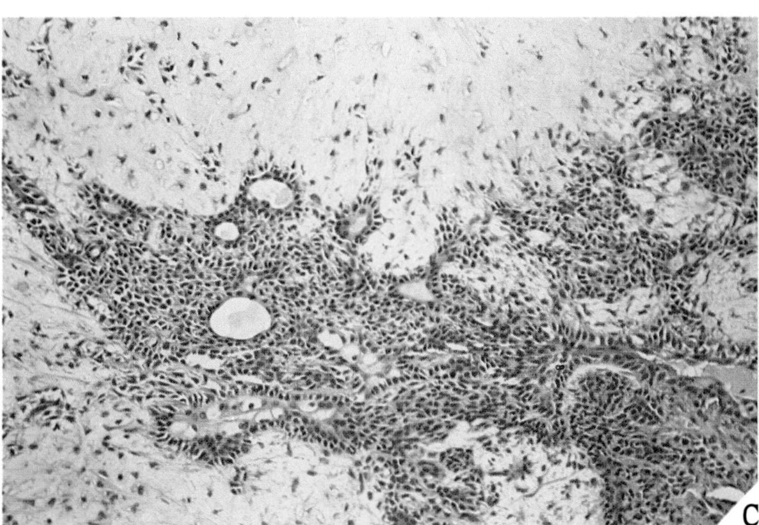

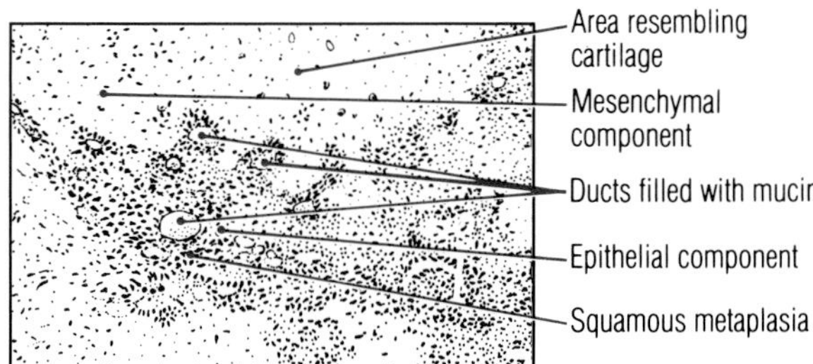

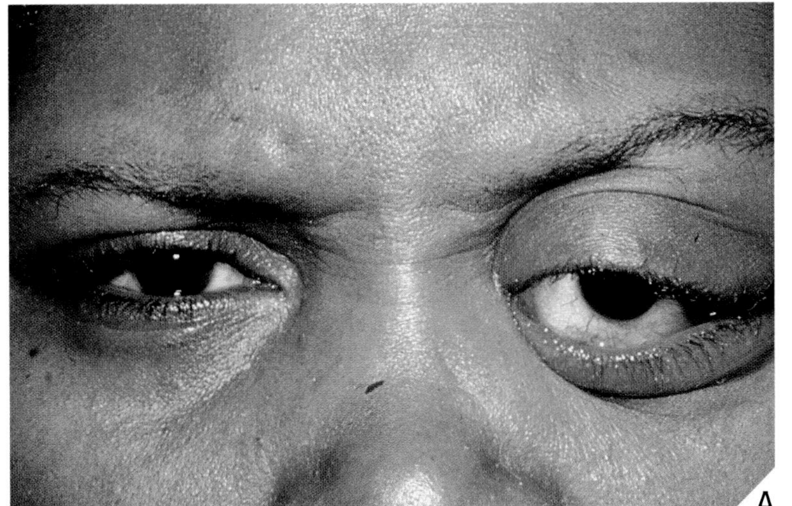

FIGURE 14.21 ADENOID CYSTIC CARCINOMA. A The patient had a rapidly progressing proptosis of the left eye. **B** A histologic section shows the characteristic "swiss cheese" pattern of adenoid cystic carcinoma. The "swiss cheese" tumor also is present in the perineural sheath around a ciliary nerve. Adenoid cystic carcinoma is noted for its rapid invasion of ciliary nerves. **C** The tumor may superficially resemble a basal cell carcinoma, but it tends to have a relatively acellular hyalin-like stroma between the islands of poorly differentiated, tightly packed, small dark epithelial cells. A basal cell carcinoma tends to have a very cellular desmoplastic stroma between the nests of malignant basal cells. **D** In this area, a more solid pattern (basaloid pattern) is seen. This type of pattern is present in about 50% of tumors. If no basaloid pattern is present, the 5-year survival rate is 70%; with a basaloid pattern, the 5-year survival rate is 20%. (**A, B**, from Yanoff M, Fine BS: *Ocular Pathology*, 3rd ed.)

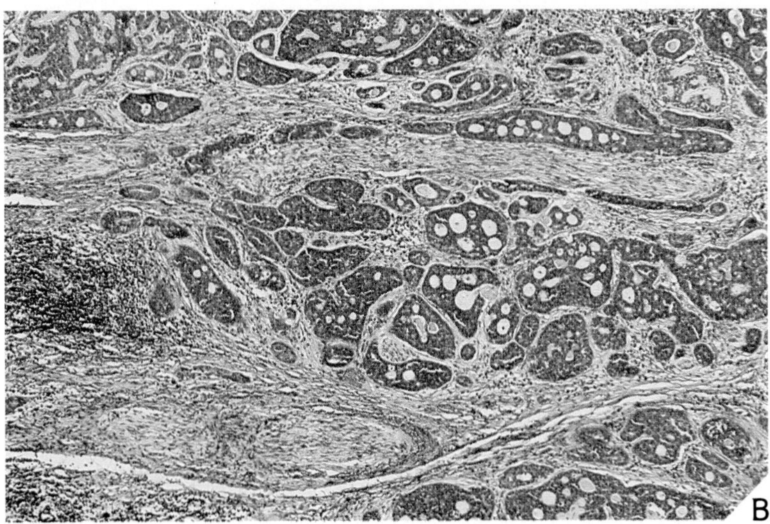

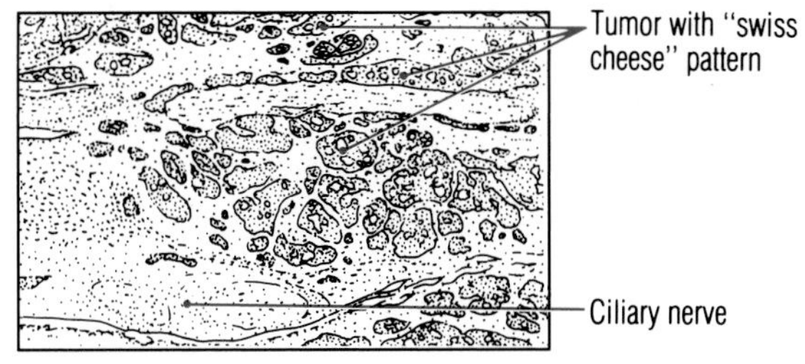

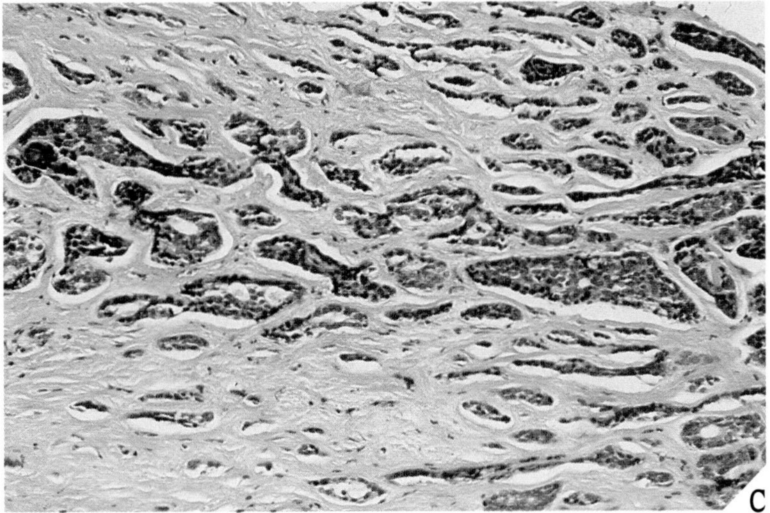

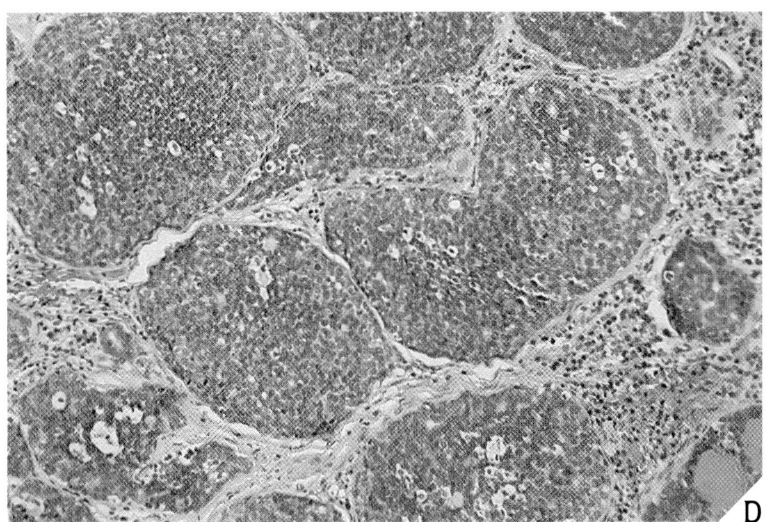

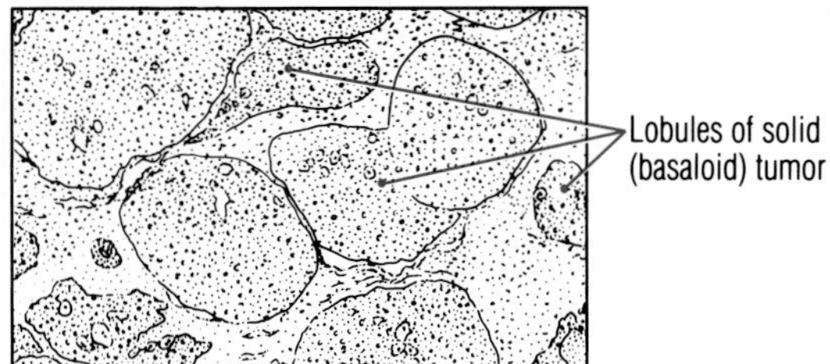

LESIONS OF THE IMMUNE SYSTEM

Inflammatory pseudotumor
Benign lymphoid hyperplasia
Malignant lymphoma and leukemia
Sinus histiocytosis

FIGURE 14.22

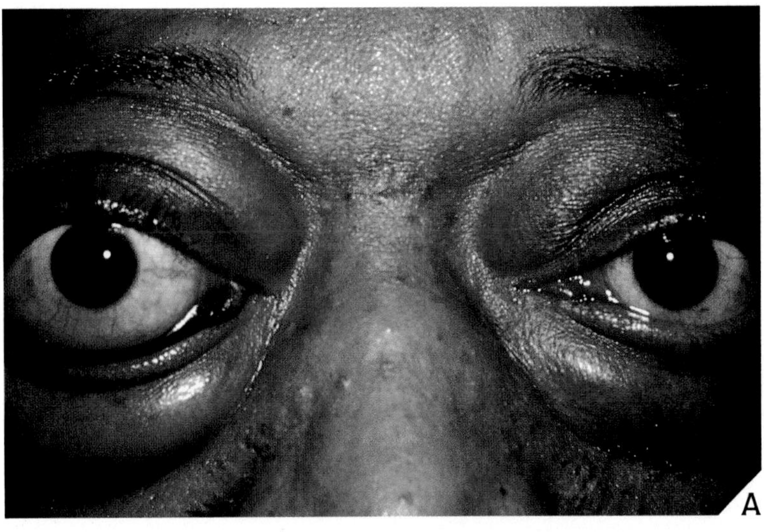

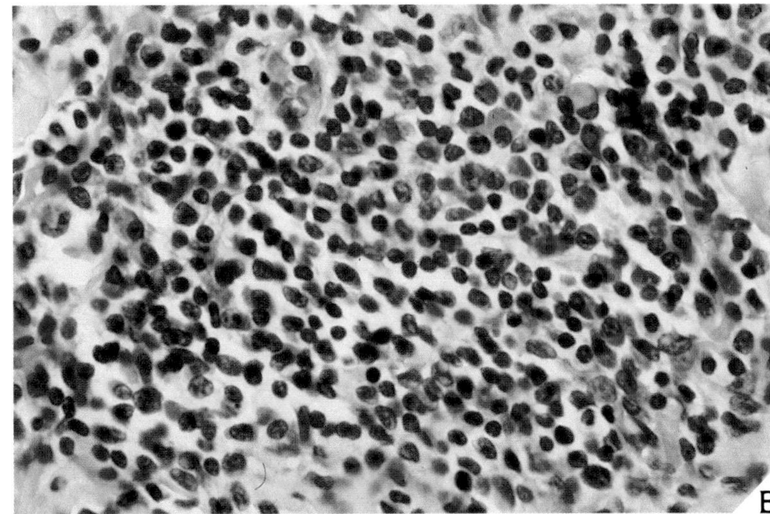

FIGURE 14.23 INFLAMMATORY PSEUDOTUMOR. A A 45-year-old man has bilateral exophthalmos that is much worse in the right eye. **B** A biopsy of the right orbital tumor shows a mixed inflammatory infiltrate of lymphocytes, plasma cells, and histiocytes. Other sections showed lymphoid follicles which contained germinal centers and young budding capillaries. This pattern is characteristic of an inflammatory pseudotumor. Histologically, cases like this are easy to diagnose as inflammatory. (**A**, from Yanoff M, Fine BS: *Ocular Pathology*, 3rd ed.)

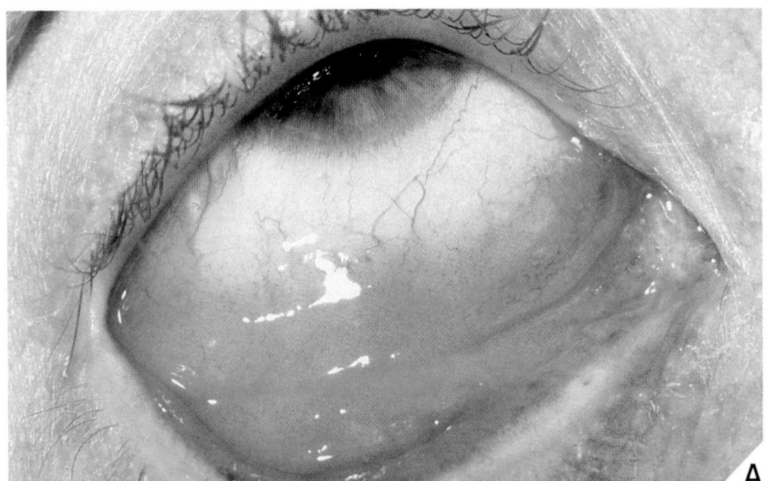

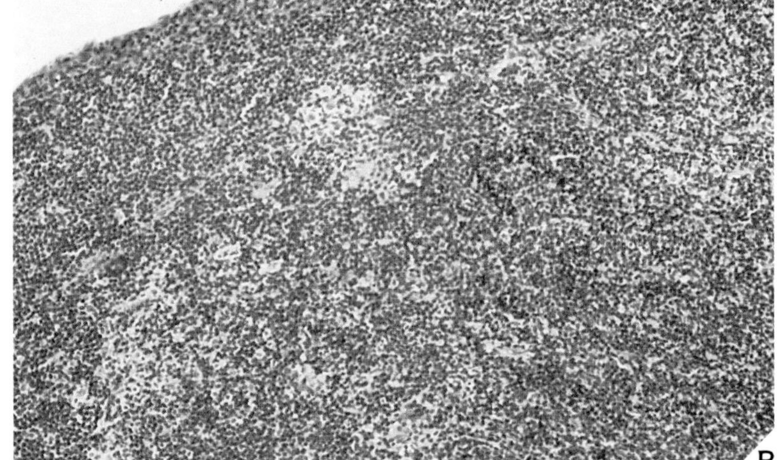

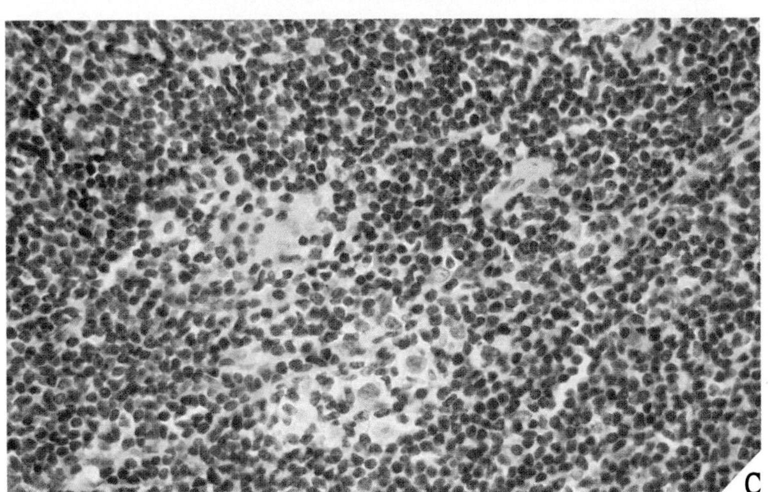

FIGURE 14.24 BENIGN LYMPHOID HYPERPLASIA. A The patient noted a fullness of the lower right lid. Large thickened redundant folds of conjunctiva in the inferior cul de sac are seen. The conjunctival lesion has a characteristic "fish-flesh" appearance and contains few blood vessels. The clinical differential diagnosis here is between a lymphoid lesion and amyloidosis. **B** A histologic section shows a lymphoid infiltrate. **C** Increased magnification shows that the lymphocytes are mature, quite small, and uniform; occasional plasma cells and large histiocytes are seen. The uniformity of the lymphocytes makes it difficult to differentiate this benign lesion from a well differentiated lymphosarcoma. The very mature appearance of the cells and the absence of atypical cells, along with the presence of plasma cells, helps to make the diagnosis of a benign lesion. In such cases, testing using monoclonal antibodies may be quite helpful. If the population is a mixed population of B- and T- cells, chances are the tumor is benign. If it is predominantly of one cell type or the other, it probably is malignant. (**A**, from Yanoff M, Fine BS: *Ocular Pathology*, 3rd ed.)

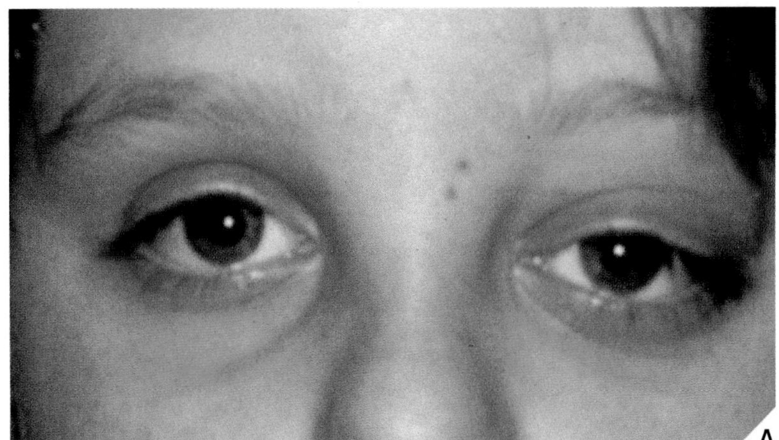

FIGURE 14.25 LEUKEMIA. A A 9-year-old boy presented with a drooping left upper lid and proptosis of the left eye. A painless left orbital mass was found. The work-up, including a complete blood count, showed normal results. He had no other signs or symptoms. An orbital biopsy was performed. **B** A histologic section shows a diffuse cellular infiltrate of primitive granulocytic leukemic cells. **C** Because of the findings in the orbital biopsy, a bone marrow aspirate was obtained. The smear shows blast cells. In most malignant lymphomas and leukemias, the atypical cell types make the diagnosis of malignancy relatively easy. (**A**, from Yanoff M, Fine BS: *Ocular Pathology*, 3rd ed.)

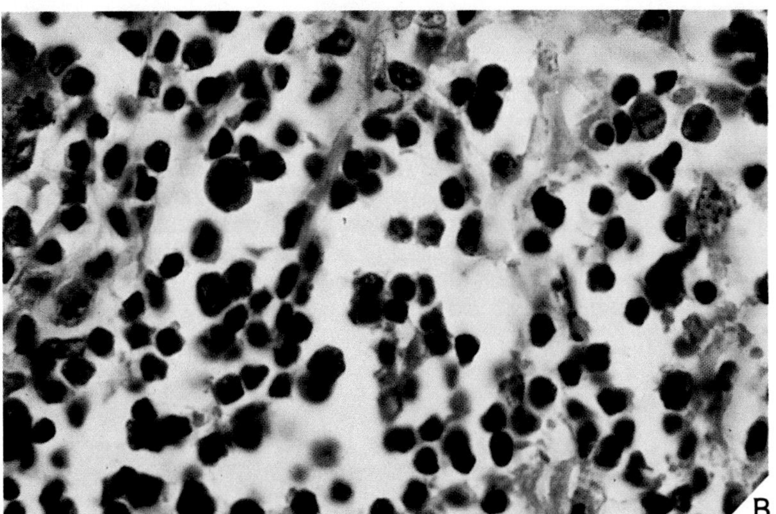

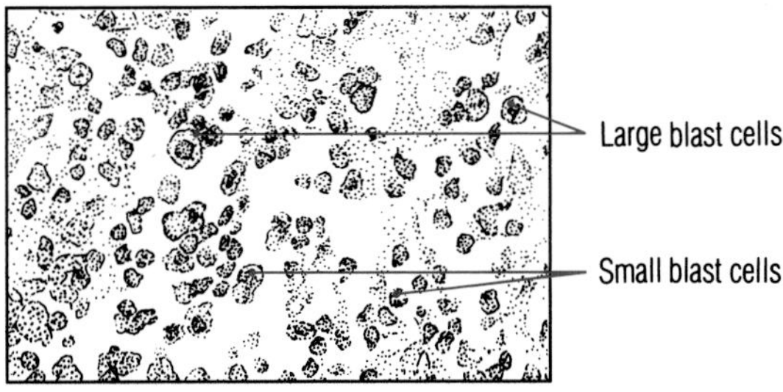

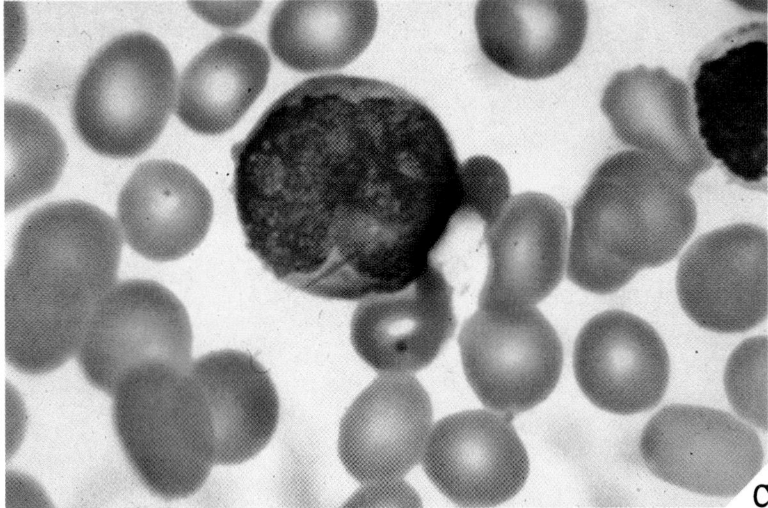

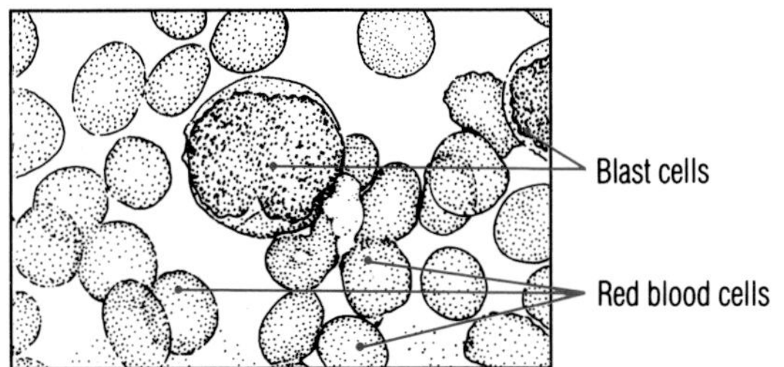

ORBITAL TUMORS RELATED TO SYSTEMIC DISEASE

Langerhans cell granulomatosis (histiocytosis X)
Juvenile fibromatosis
Fibrous dysplasia

FIGURE 14.26

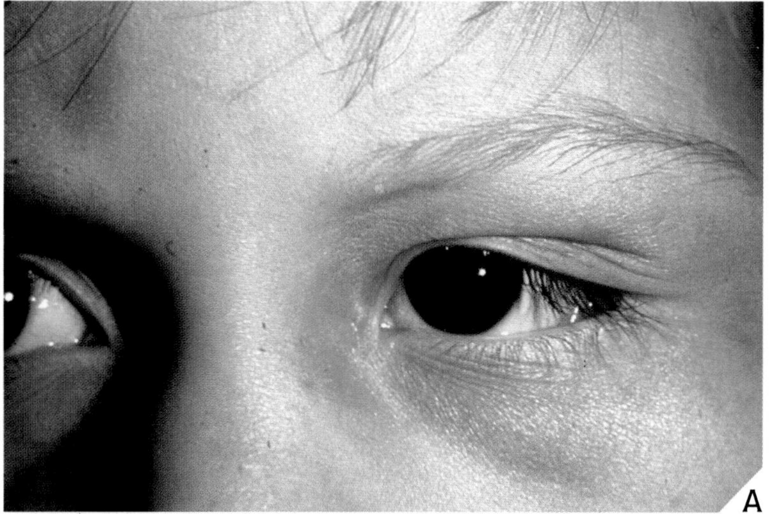

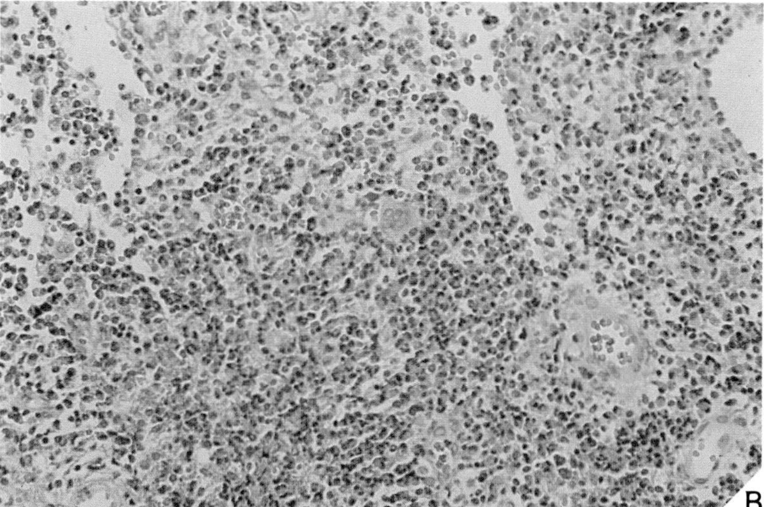

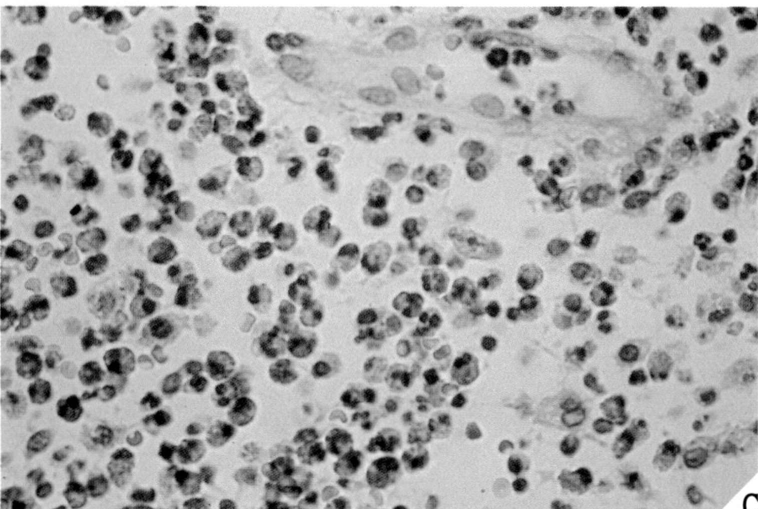

FIGURE 14.27 EOSINOPHILIC GRANULOMA. A This 4-year-old boy presented with a rapid onset of erythema and swelling over the lateral edge of his orbit. Osteomyelitis or rhabdomyosarcoma were diagnosed. A biopsy was performed. **B** A histologic section shows numerous large abnormal histiocytes and many eosinophils. **C** Increased magnification shows the abnormal histiocytes, which contain pale cytoplasm and large vesicular nuclei along with many eosinophils. Eosinophilic granuloma is classified within the group of Langerhans cell granulomatosis (histiocytosis X). (**A**, from Yanoff M, Fine BS: *Ocular Pathology*, 3rd ed.)

SECONDARY ORBITAL TUMORS

Direct extension

Malignant melanoma of uvea, conjunctiva, or lid
Retinoblastoma
Squamous cell carcinoma of conjunctiva
Basal cell carcinoma of lid
Sebaceous gland carcinoma of lid
Tumors of the upper respiratory tract
Tumors of the nasolacrimal apparatus
Meningioma

Metastatic from distant sites

Breast
Lung
Adrenal (neuroblastoma)
Pancreas
Other sites

FIGURE 14.28

Bibliography

Bullock JD, Goldberg SH, Connelly PJ: Orbital varix thrombosis. Ophthalmology 97:251, 1990.

Capps DH, et al: Orbital intramuscular schwannoma. Am J Ophthalmol 110:535, 1990.

Fajardo LF: The complexity of endothelial cells. A review. Am J Clin Pathol 92:241, 1989.

Font RL, Hidayat AA: Fibrous histiocytoma of the orbit. A clinicopathologic study of 150 cases. Hum Pathol 13:199, 1982.

Greiner TC, Robinson RA, Maves MD: Adenoid cystic carcinoma. A clinicopathologic study with flow cytometry analysis. Am J Clin Pathol 92:711, 1989.

Grossniklaus HE, Abbuhl MF, McLean IW: Immunohistologic properties of benign and malignant mixed tumor of the lacrimal gland. Am J Ophthalmol 110:540, 1990.

Guterman C, Abboud E, Mets MB: Microphthalmos with cyst and Edward's syndrome. Am J Ophthalmol 109:228, 1990.

Harris GJ, et al: An analysis of thirty cases of orbital lymphangioma. Pathophysiologic consideration and management recommendations. Ophthalmology 97:1583, 1990.

Henderson JW, Farrow GM, Garrity JA: Clinical course of an incompletely removed cavernous hemangioma of the orbit. Ophthalmology 97:625, 1990.

Hufnagel TJ, et al: Immunohistochemical and ultrastructural studies on the exenterated orbital tissues of a patient with Graves' disease. Ophthalmology 91:1411, 1984.

Jakobiec FA, Knowles DM: An overview of ocular adnexal lymphoid tumors. Trans Am Ophthalmol Soc 87:443, 1989.

Jones WD III, Yanoff M, Katowitz JA: Recurrent facial fibrous histiocytoma. Br J Plast Surg 32:46, 1979.

Raikow RB, et al: Immunohistochemical evidence for IgE involvement in Graves' orbitopathy. Ophthalmology 97:629, 1990.

Schachat AP, et al: Ophthalmic manifestations of leukemia. Arch Ophthalmol 107:697, 1989.

Shields CL, et al: Clinicopathologic review of 142 cases of lacrimal gland lesions. Ophthalmology 96:431, 1989.

van Veen S, et al: Granulocytic sarcoma (chloroma). Presentation of an unusual case. Am J Clin Pathol 95:567, 1991.

Yanoff M, Fine BS: Ocular Pathology: A Text and Atlas, 3rd ed. Philadelphia, JB Lippincott, 1989.

Yasunaga C, et al: Heterogeneous expression of endothelial cell markers in infantile hemangioendothelioma. Immunohistochemical study of two solitary cases and one multiple one. Am J Clin Pathol 91:673, 1989.

Diabetes Mellitus

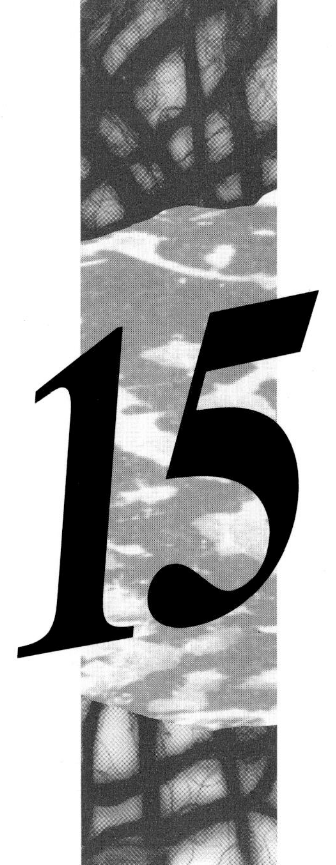

Diabetic retinopathy currently is the leading cause of blindness in adults under the age of 65. In addition, diabetic retinopathy is the second leading cause of new blindness each year. Approximately 70% of those who have had diabetes mellitus for more than ten years will develop retinopathy. In fewer than 10% of these cases, however, will the retinopathy progress to blindness.

Diabetes affects many ocular structures. Major effects may be seen, clinically and histologically, in the retina as diabetic retinopathy and in the iris as neovascularization of the stroma and vacuolization of the pigment epithelium. Other significant changes may be seen histologically in the ciliary body (thickened basement membrane) and in the choroid (diabetic choroidopathy). It now appears that diabetics show an earlier or an increased incidence of cataract development. The optic nerve may be involved in neovascularization or in ischemic (nonarteritic) optic neuropathy.

FINDINGS IN BACKGROUND DIABETIC RETINOPATHY

Microaneurysms	Exudates
Edema	Hemorrhages

FIGURE 15.1

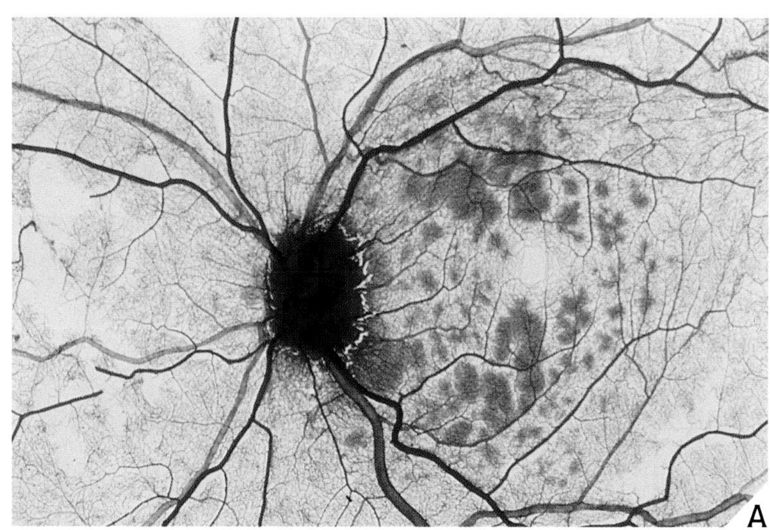

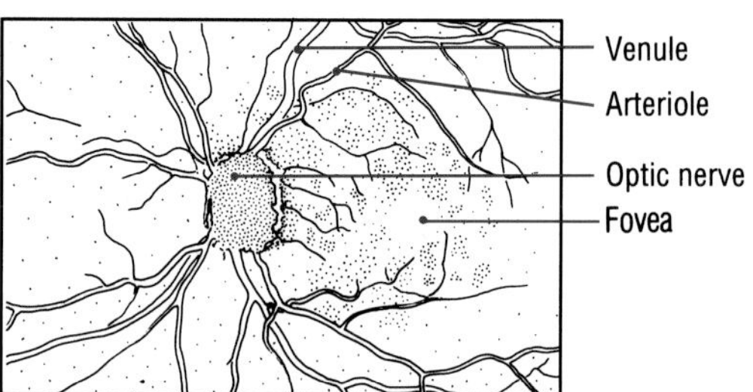

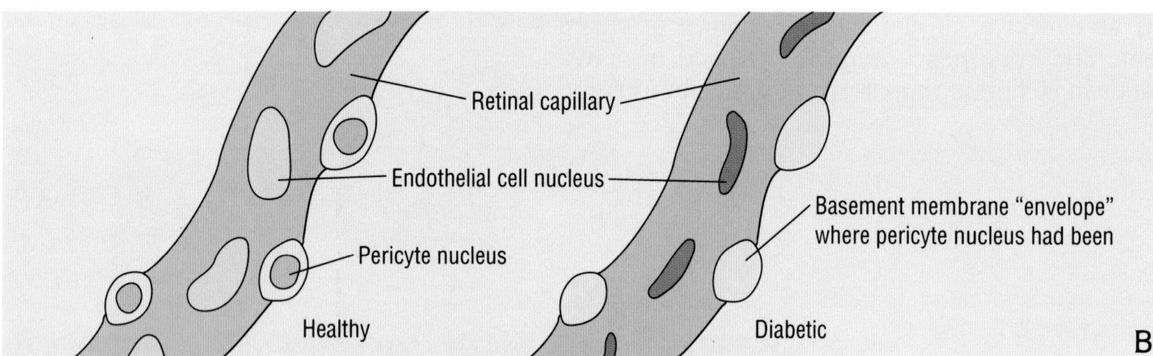

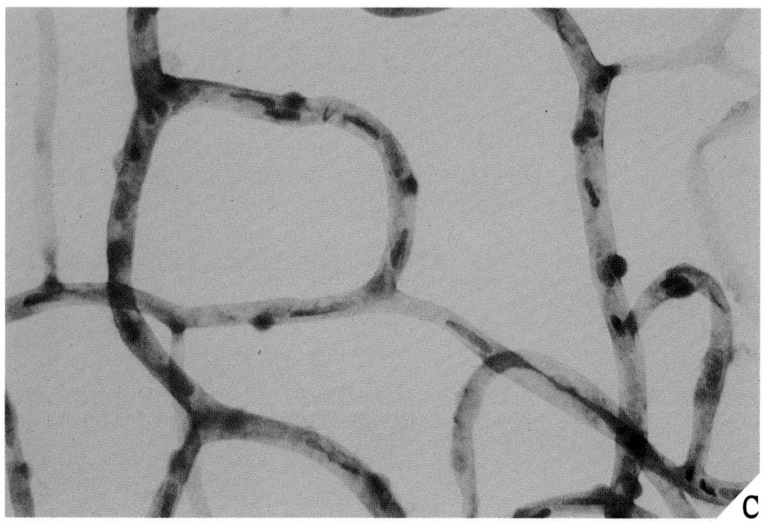

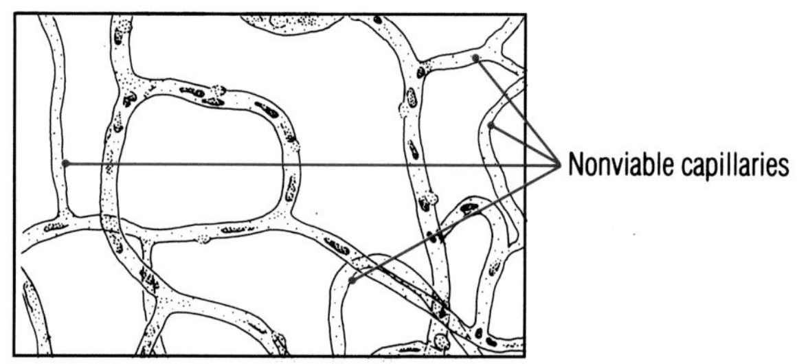

FIGURE 15.2 RETINAL VASCULATURE (NORMAL AND DIABETIC). A A trypsin-digest preparation of the retina, stained with PAS and hematoxylin, shows the optic nerve and the major retinal blood vessels. The capillary-free zone of the fovea is seen clearly. **B** In a retinal capillary of a normal eye the ratio of pericyte nuclei to endothelial cell nuclei is 1:1. In a diabetic, the ratio is decreased due to a loss of pericyte nuclei. Even though the endothelial cells are present in the diabetic, their nuclei appear pyknotic. The normal endothelial cell cytoplasm, covered externally by a basement membrane, makes up the wall of the retinal capillary. The normal pericyte nucleus sits like a button on the surface of the capillary and sends cytoplasmic processes discontinuously around the capillary. The normal pericyte is completely surrounded by a basement membrane envelope. **C** In capillaries of diabetic patients, the basement membrane envelopes no longer contain pericyte nuclei and are themselves thickened by PAS-positive material. The endothelial cells, although somewhat pyknotic, remain in relatively normal numbers.

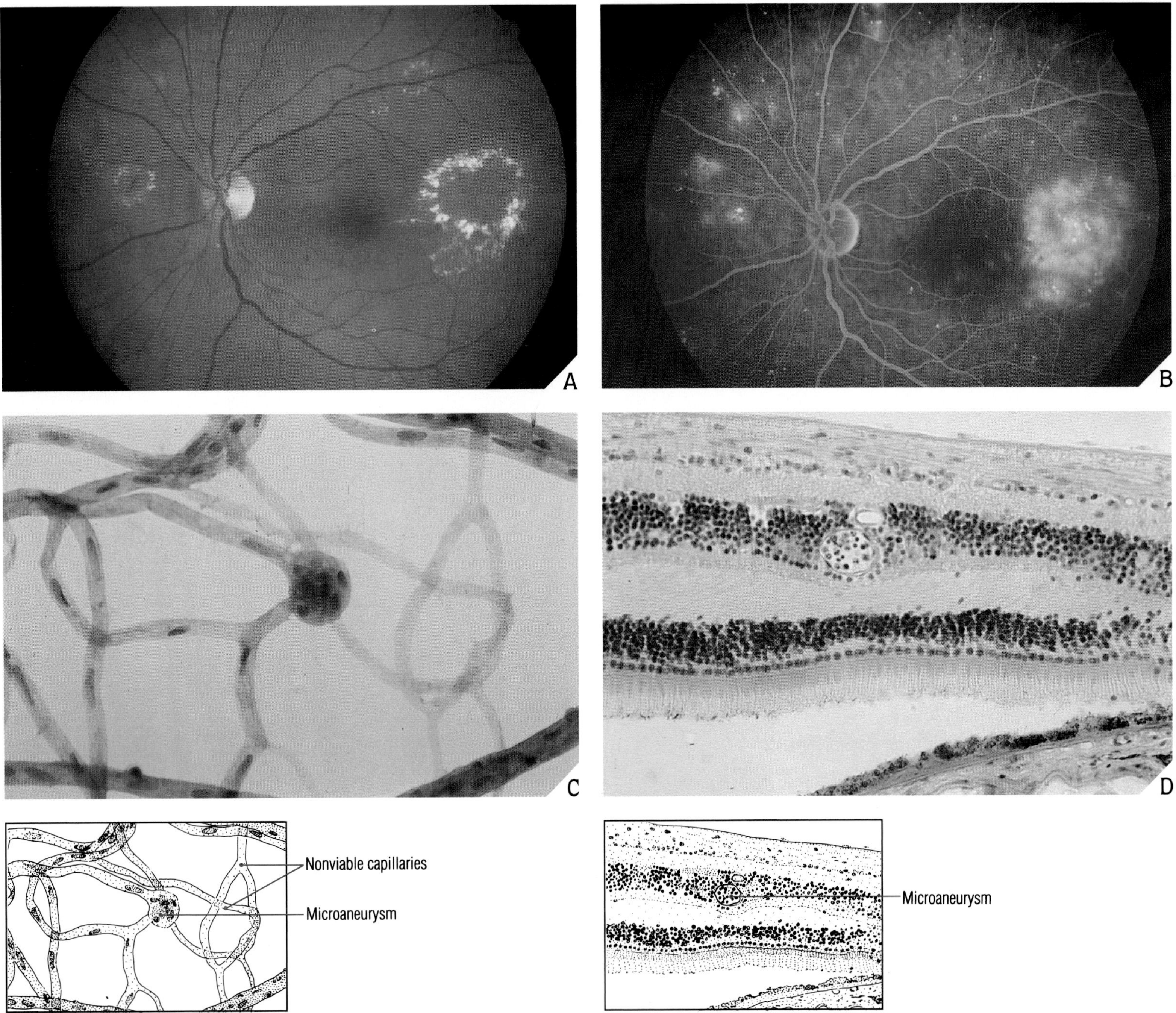

FIGURE 15.3 RETINAL CAPILLARY MICROANEURYSM. A Background diabetic retinopathy consists of retinal capillary microaneurysms (RCMs), hemorrhages, edema, and exudates (here in a circinate pattern). **B** The RCMs are seen more easily with fluorescein. The areas of circinate retinopathy show leakage. (see also Figs. 15.4 and 15.7A) **C** Trypsin digest preparation shows that an RCM consists of a proliferation of endothelial cells. **D** A histologic section shows a large blood-filled space lined by endothelium. The caliber is about that of a venule. Venules, however, do not occur in this location (in the inner nuclear layer), but are found mainly in the nerve fiber layer. By a process of elimination, the "vessel," therefore is identified as a cross-section of an RCM. (**A, B** courtesy of Dr. GE Lang; **D**, from Yanoff M, Fine BS: *Ocular Pathology*, 3rd ed.)

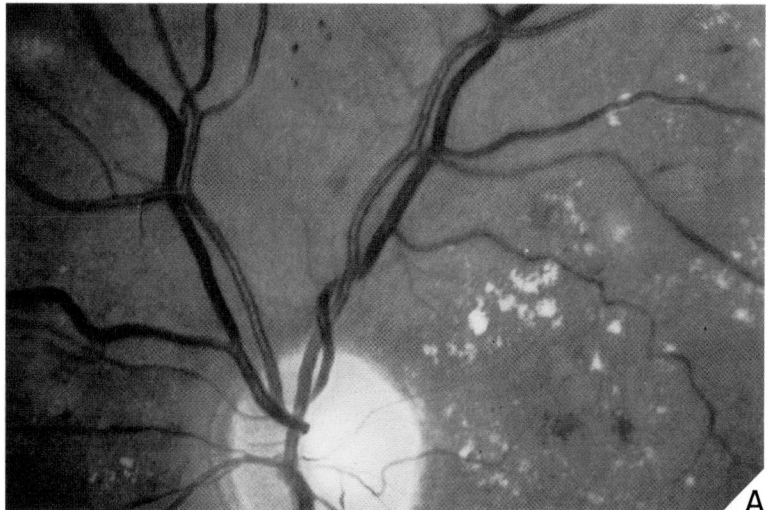

FIGURE 15.4 EXUDATES. A In addition to retinal capillary microaneurysms and retinal hemorrhages, scattered hard waxy exudates are seen. **B** A histologic section of another case shows a collection of eosinophilic material in the outer plexiform layer, the characteristic location of diabetic exudates. The nuclei within the fluid represent histiocytes. **C** A thin section of a plastic-embedded retina shows collections of fluid within the outer plexiform layer. In some areas, the exudate is occupied completely by histiocytes. **D** With oil red-O the material within the exudates stains positive (red) (**A**, from Yanoff M, Fine BS: *Ocular Pathology*, 3rd ed., **B** from Yanoff M, Fine BS: *Ocular Pathology*, 2nd ed.)

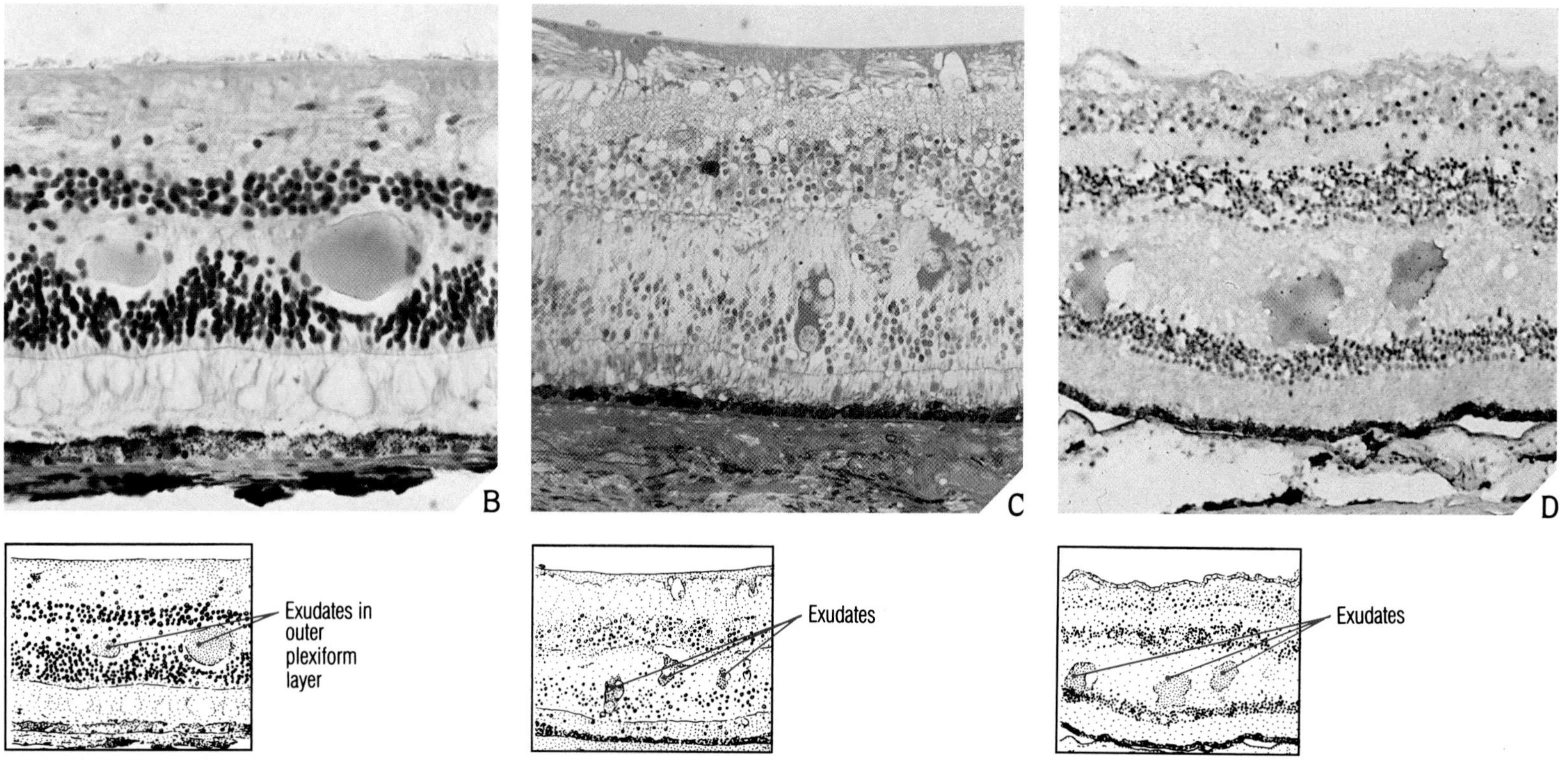

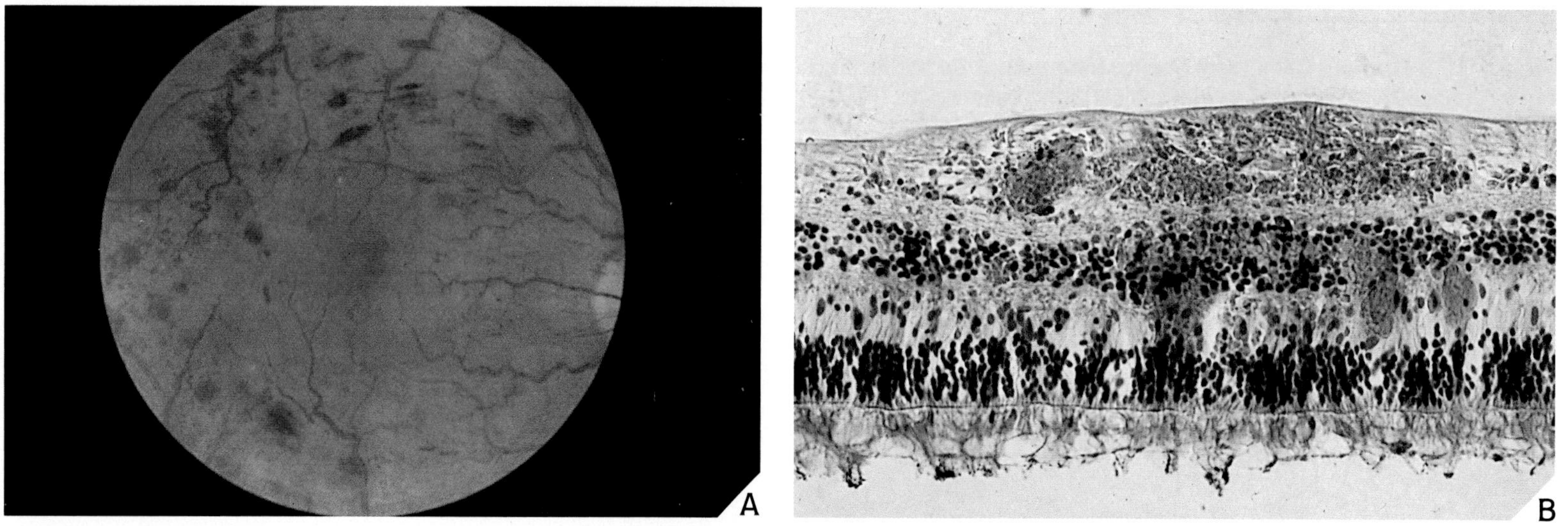

FIGURE 15.5 HEMORRHAGIC RETINOPATHY. A Dot, blot, flame-shaped, and globular hemorrhages are present within the retina. **B** Flame-shaped or splinter hemorrhages consist of small collections of blood in the nerve fiber layer. Dot and blot hemorrhages are caused by small hemorrhagic collections in the inner nuclear and outer plexiform layers. (**A**, from Yanoff M, Fine BS: *Ocular Pathology*, 3rd ed.)

FINDINGS IN PREPROLIFERATIVE RETINOPATHY

Cotton-wool spots
Venous beading
Intraretinal microvascular abnormalities (IRMA)
Increasing retinal hemorrhages

FIGURE 15.6

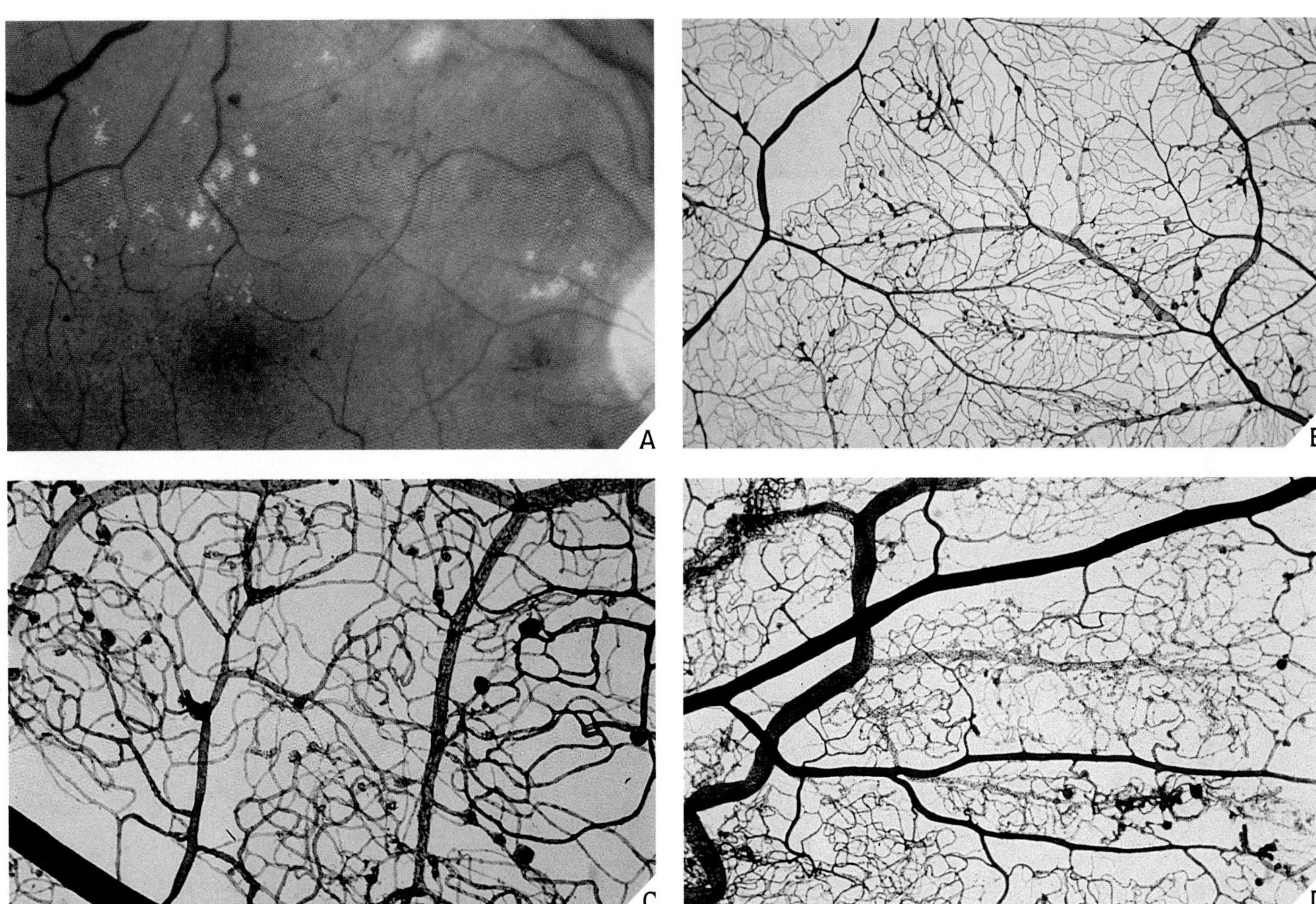

Venule
Arteriolar-venular collateral
Arteriole

FIGURE 15.7 PREPROLIFERATIVE RETINOPATHY. A A cotton-wool spot of recent onset is present just inferior to the superior arcade. Note also retinal "hard" exudates, capillary microaneurysms, and hemorrhages. **B** Trypsin-digest preparation shows sausage-shaped dilated venules. **C** An arteriolar-venular collateral vessel is present. **D** Intraretinal microvascular abnormalities (IRMA) are present in the form of dilated capillaries, capillary buds and loops, and areas of capillary closure.

FINDINGS IN PROLIFERATIVE RETINOPATHY

Pure neovascularization
Fibrovascular membranes
Retinal detachment

FIGURE 15.8

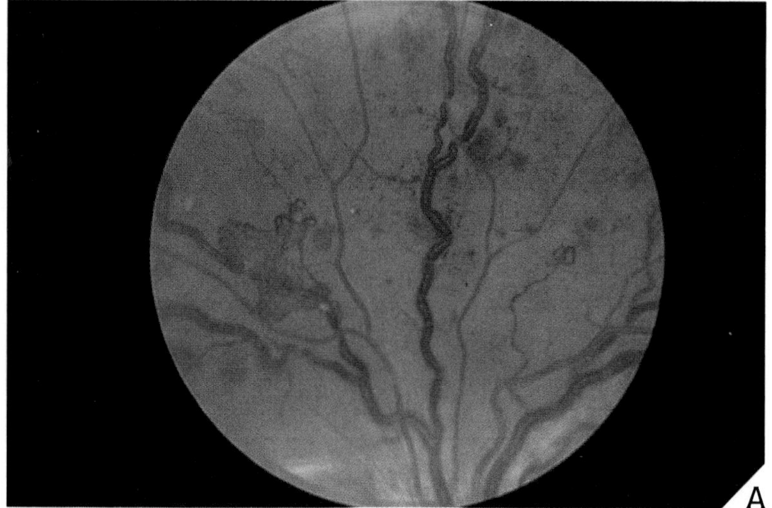

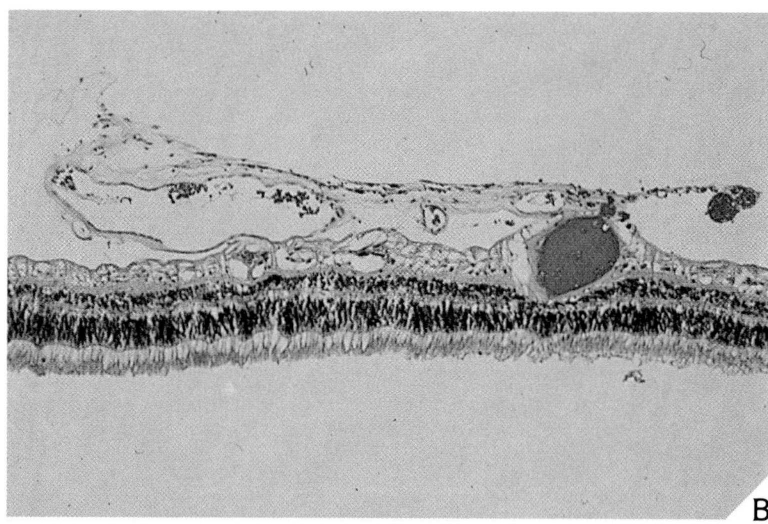

FIGURE 15.9 NEOVASCULARIZATION. A The superior venule is dilated and beaded. Neovascular tufts arise from the venules. **B** A histologic section of another case shows new blood vessels arising from a retinal venule, perforating the internal limiting membrane, and spreading out on the internal surface of the retina between the internal limiting membrane and the vitreous body. In this location, the fragile new abnormal blood vessels may be subject to trauma (e.g., vitreous detachment), resulting in a subvitreal hemorrhage between the retinal internal limiting membrane and the posterior hyaloid of the separated vitreous body. (**A**, from Yanoff M, Fine BS: *Ocular Pathology*, 3rd ed.)

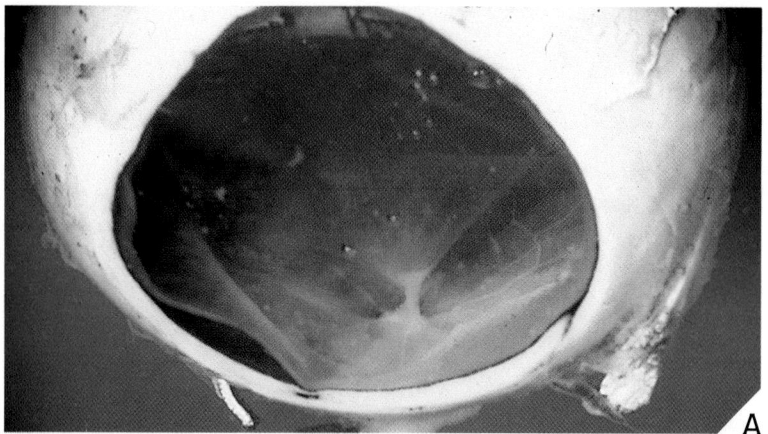

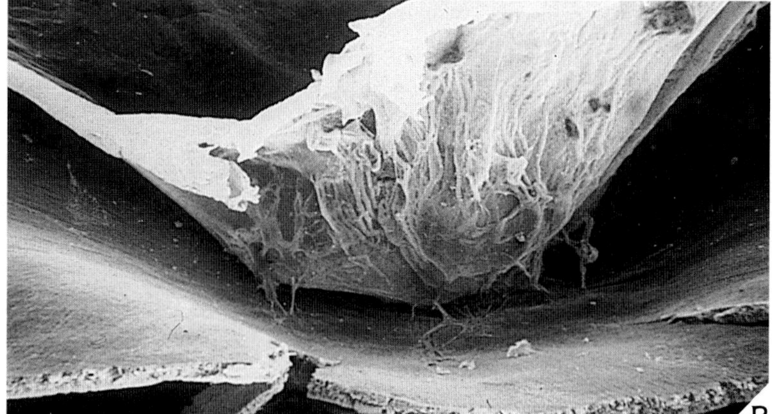

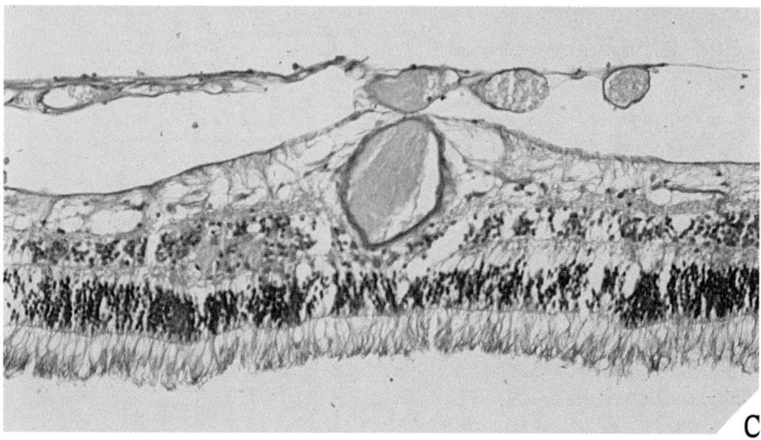

FIGURE 15.10 NEOVASCULARIZATION. A tuft of neovascularization arising from the optic nerve head is attached to the posterior surface of an otherwise detached vitreous body. **B** Scanning electron microscopy shows blood vessels arising from the internal surface of the retina and attaching to the posterior surface of the partially detached vitreous. **C** A PAS-stained histologic section shows blood vessels originating from a retinal venule and attaching to the posterior surface of the vitreous. **D** The gross specimen shows the end stage of diabetic retinopathy. Extensive neovascularization of the retina and the detached vitreous have resulted in a traction retinal detachment. The subretinal space is filled with a gelatinous material. (**B**, courtesy of Dr. RC Eagle Jr; **D**, from Yanoff M, Fine BS: *Ocular Pathology*, 3rd ed.)

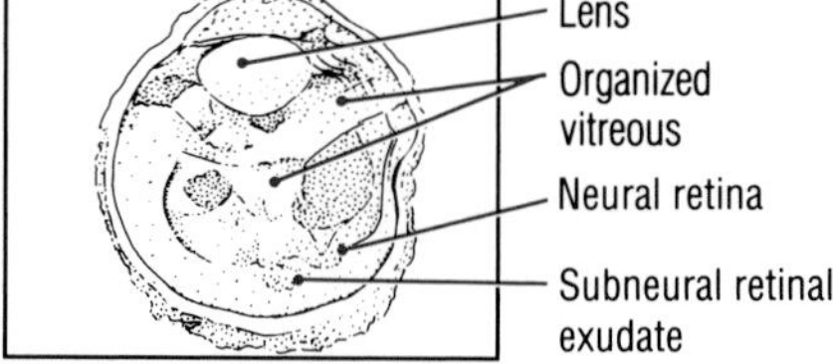

DIABETIC CHANGES IN THE IRIS, CHOROID, AND CILIARY BODY

Diabetic iridopathy
Neovascularization
Lacy vacuolization

Diabetic choroidopathy
Occlusion of the choriocapillaris
Thickening (hyperproduction) of vascular basement membranes
Arteriolarsclerosis

Diabetic changes in the ciliary body
Diffuse thickening of the outer basement membrane of the pars plicata

FIGURE 15.11

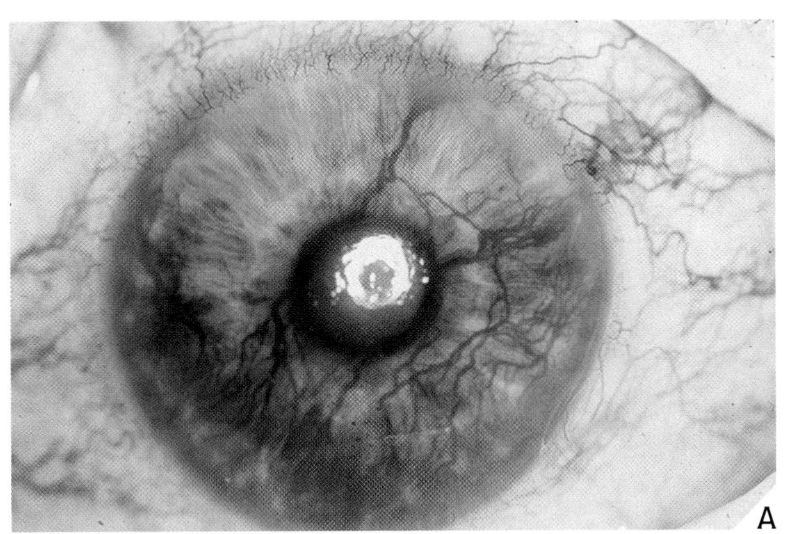

FIGURE 15.12 IRIS NEOVASCULARIZATION. A Clinical appearance of iris neovascularization. The reddish coloration of the iris, caused by the abnormal anterior surface blood vessels, is called rubeosis iridis. **B** A histologic section of another case shows a peripheral anterior synechia and a thick mantle of tissue anterior to the pigmented anterior border layer of the iris. The tissue is fibrovascular tissue. Contraction of the tissue has caused an eversion of the iris pigment epithelium and sphincter muscle. This eversion is called ectropion uveae. Tissue anterior to the normally avascular anterior border layer of the iris usually signifies neovascularization (as in this case), inflammation, or neoplasm. **C** In yet another case, a histologic section shows that the neovascularization has caused adherence between the peripheral iris and the cornea, called peripheral anterior synechia.

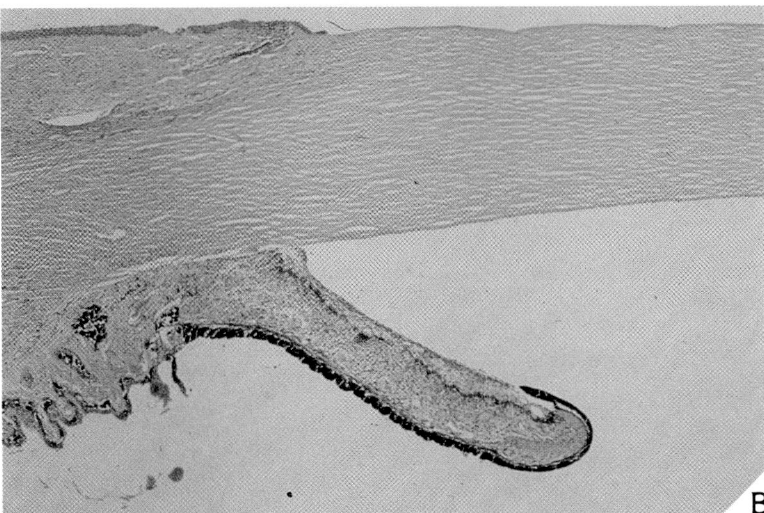

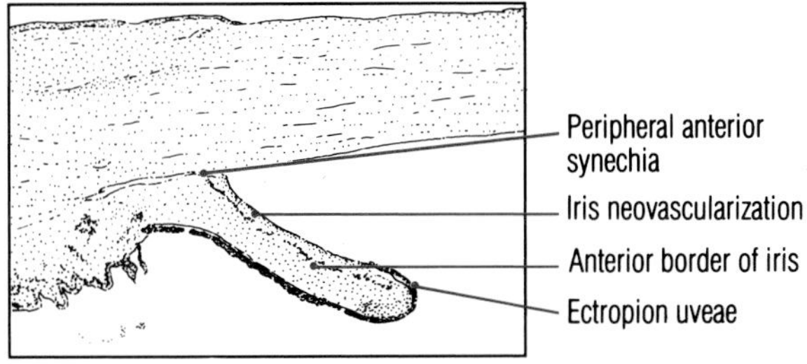

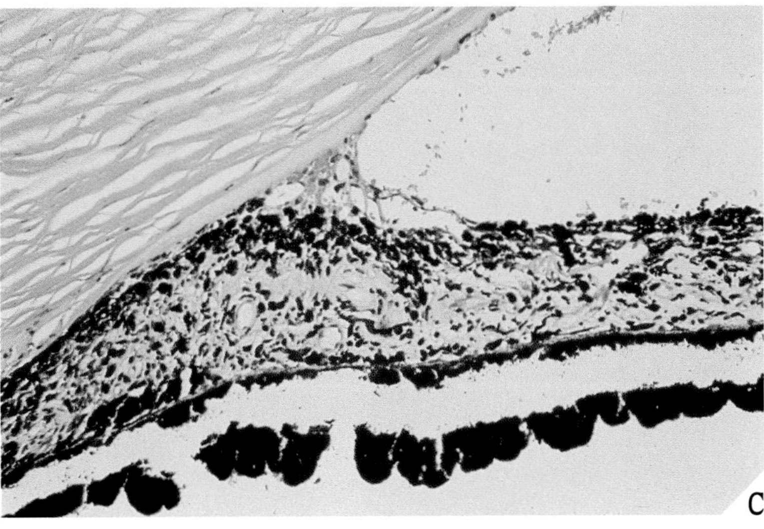

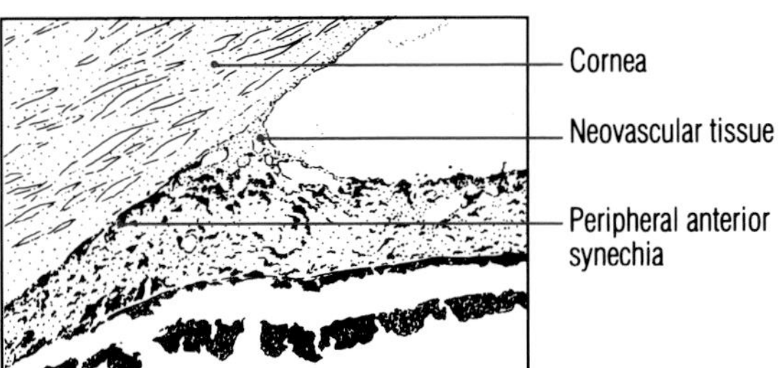

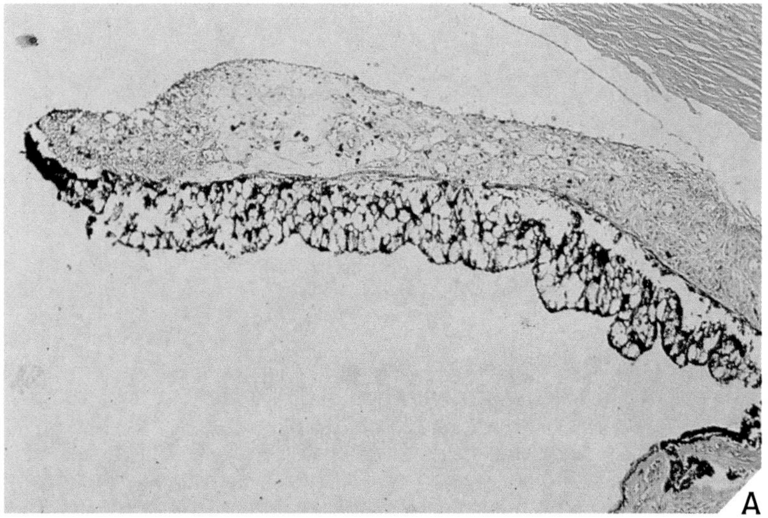

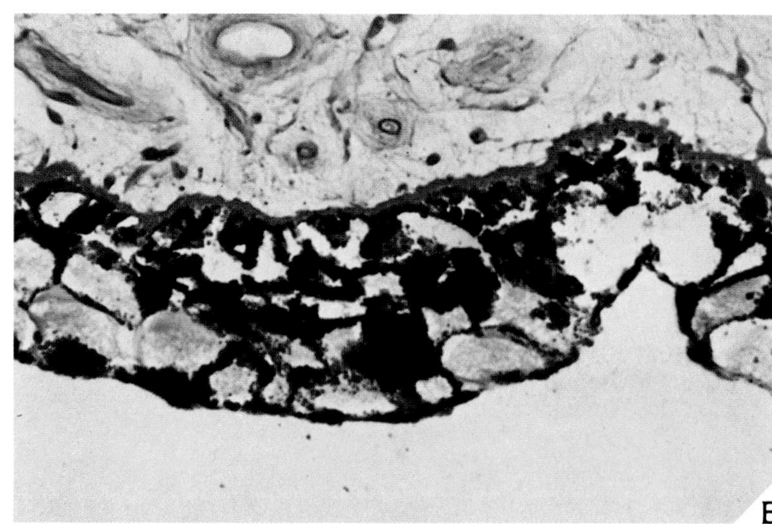

FIGURE 15.13 LACY VACUOLIZATION OF IRIS PIGMENT EPITHELIUM. A Large vacuoles are present in both the anterior and posterior layers of the iris pigment epithelium. The vacuoles appear empty in sections stained with hematoxylin and eosin. **B** PAS stain shows that the vacuoles contain a PAS-positive material. Pretreatment of the sections with diastase eliminates the PAS reaction, signifying that the vacuolar material contains glycogen.

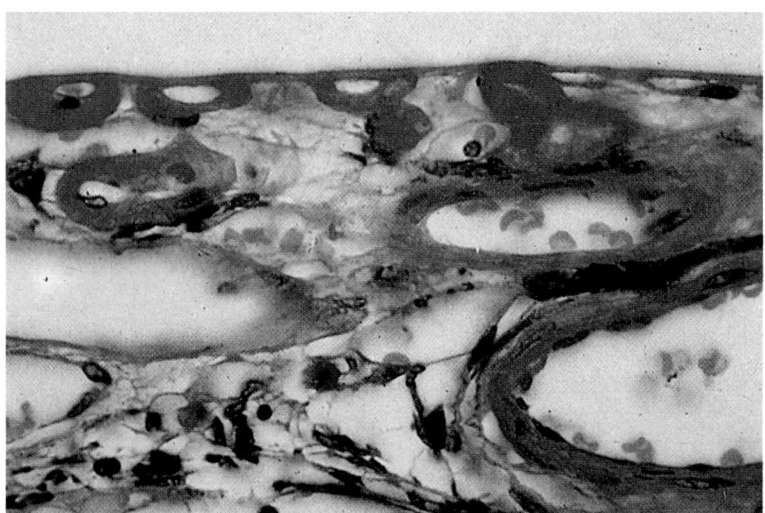

FIGURE 15.14 CHOROIDOPATHY. A A histologic section of the foveomacular region shows diffuse thickening of choroidal vessels by periodic acid-Schiff (PAS) positive material. The choriocapillaris is prominently involved and partially occluded. The retinal pigment epithelium is absent. (Modified from Hidayat AA, Fine BS, 1985.)

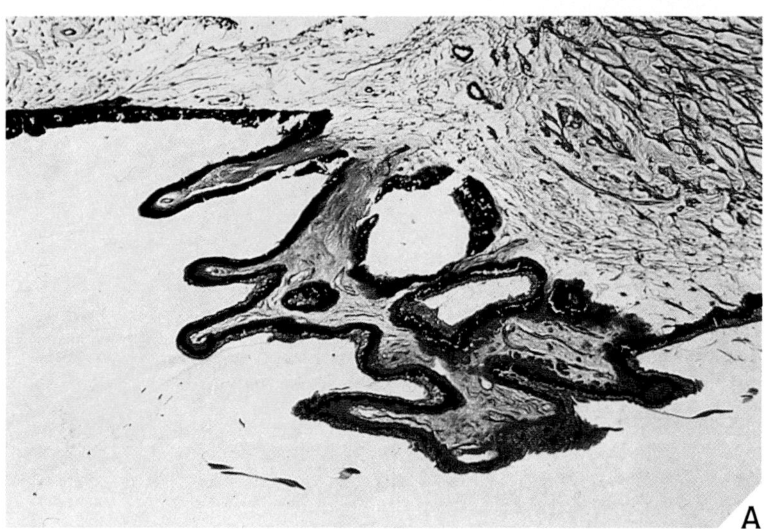

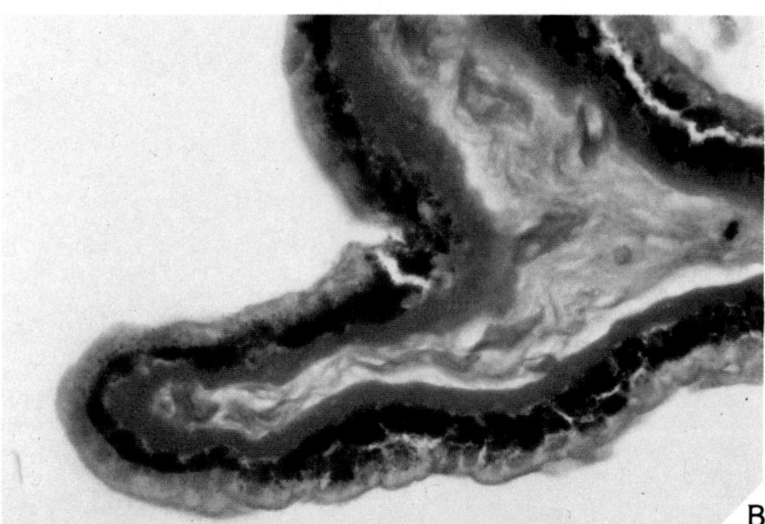

FIGURE 15.15 CILIARY BODY. A PAS stain shows a diffuse thickening of the basement membrane of the pigmented ciliary epithelium in the pars plicata only. **B** Increased magnification of another section shows the thickened basement membrane characteristic of diabetes mellitus.

Bibliography

Bergren RL, Brown GC, Duker JS: Prevalence and association of asteroid hyalosis with systemic diseases. Am J Ophthalmol 111:289, 1991.

Buzney SM, et al: Retinal vascular endothelial cells and pericytes. Differential growth characteristics in vitro. Invest Ophthalmol Vis Sci 24:470, 1983.

Engerman RL: Pathogenesis of diabetic retinopathy. Diabetes 38:1203, 1989.

Hidayat AA, Fine BS: Diabetic choroidopathy—light and electron microscopic observations of seven cases. Ophthalmology 92:512, 1985.

Klein R, et al: The Wisconsin epidemiologic study of diabetic retinopathy. IX. Four-year incidence and progression of diabetic retinopathy when age at diagnosis is less than 30 years. Arch Ophthalmol 107:237, 1989.

Klein R, et al: The Wisconsin epidemiologic study of diabetic retinopathy. X. Four-year incidence and progression of diabetic retinopathy when age at diagnosis is 30 years or more. Arch Ophthalmol 107:244, 1989.

Klein R, et al: The relationship of retinal microaneurysm counts to the 4-year progression of diabetic retinopathy. Arch Ophthalmol 107:1780, 1989.

Klein R, et al: The Wisconsin epidemiologic study of diabetic retinopathy. XI. The incidence of macular edema. Ophthalmology 96:1501, 1989.

Miller H, et al: Diabetic neovascularization: permeability and ultrastructure. Invest Ophthalmol Vis Sci 25:1338, 1984.

Muraoka K, Shimizu K: Intraretinal neovascularization in diabetic retinopathy. Ophthalmology 91:1440, 1984.

Niki T, Muraoka K, Shimizu K: Distribution of capillary nonperfusion in early-stage diabetic retinopathy. Ophthalmology 91:1431, 1984.

Yanoff M: Ocular pathology of diabetes mellitus. Am J Ophthalmol 67:21, 1969.

Yanoff M, Fine BS, Berkow JW: Diabetic lacy vacuolation of iris pigment epithelium. Am J Ophthalmol 69:201, 1970.

Glaucoma

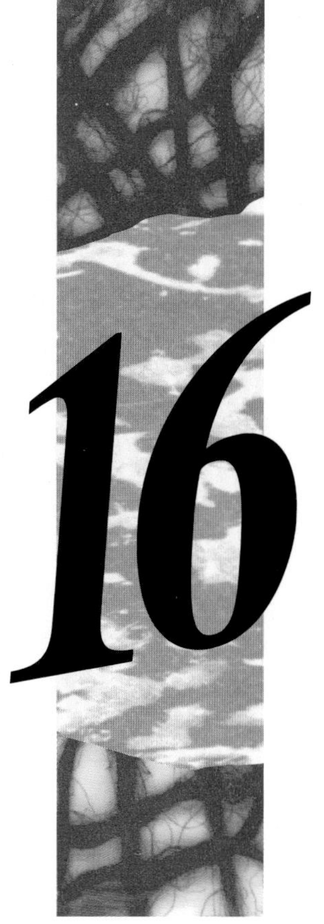

Glaucoma is the leading cause of blindness among the 500,000 people legally classified as blind in the United States. Glaucoma affects:
• 0.5%–1% of the population;
• 2% of people age 35 years or older;
• 3% of people age 65 years or older;
• 14% (1:7) of blind people.

Glaucoma is characterized by an intraocular pressure sufficiently elevated to produce ocular tissue damage, either temporary or permanent. The condition is not a single disease entity; it may be primary or it may develop secondary to a variety of ocular and systemic diseases. Glaucoma, therefore, is a syndrome, not an intraocular pressure reading.

A patient presenting with increased intraocular pressure without detectable ocular tissue damage or visual functional impairment may be said to have ocular hypertension or be a glaucoma-suspect. Ocular hypertension leads to ocular tissue damage, and hence to glaucoma, at an incidence of about 1% per year.

Glaucoma may be divided into two different types. One is extremely rare and is characterized by a normal outflow but a hypersecretion of aqueous. The other is the common type that shows impaired outflow, which can be subdivided as follows:
• congenital glaucoma;
• primary open- and closed-angle glaucomas;
• secondary open- and closed-angle glaucomas.

Primary open-angle glaucoma accounts for about two-thirds of all glaucomas seen in whites, and has a prevalence between 0.5 and 1% of the population. In blacks it occurs at a rate of approximately 1.5% of the population. Primary closed-angle glaucoma occurs in less than 0.5% of the population. This type of glaucoma is much more common in whites than in blacks. However, a high percentage of blacks have the chronic rather than the acute type of closed-angle glaucoma.

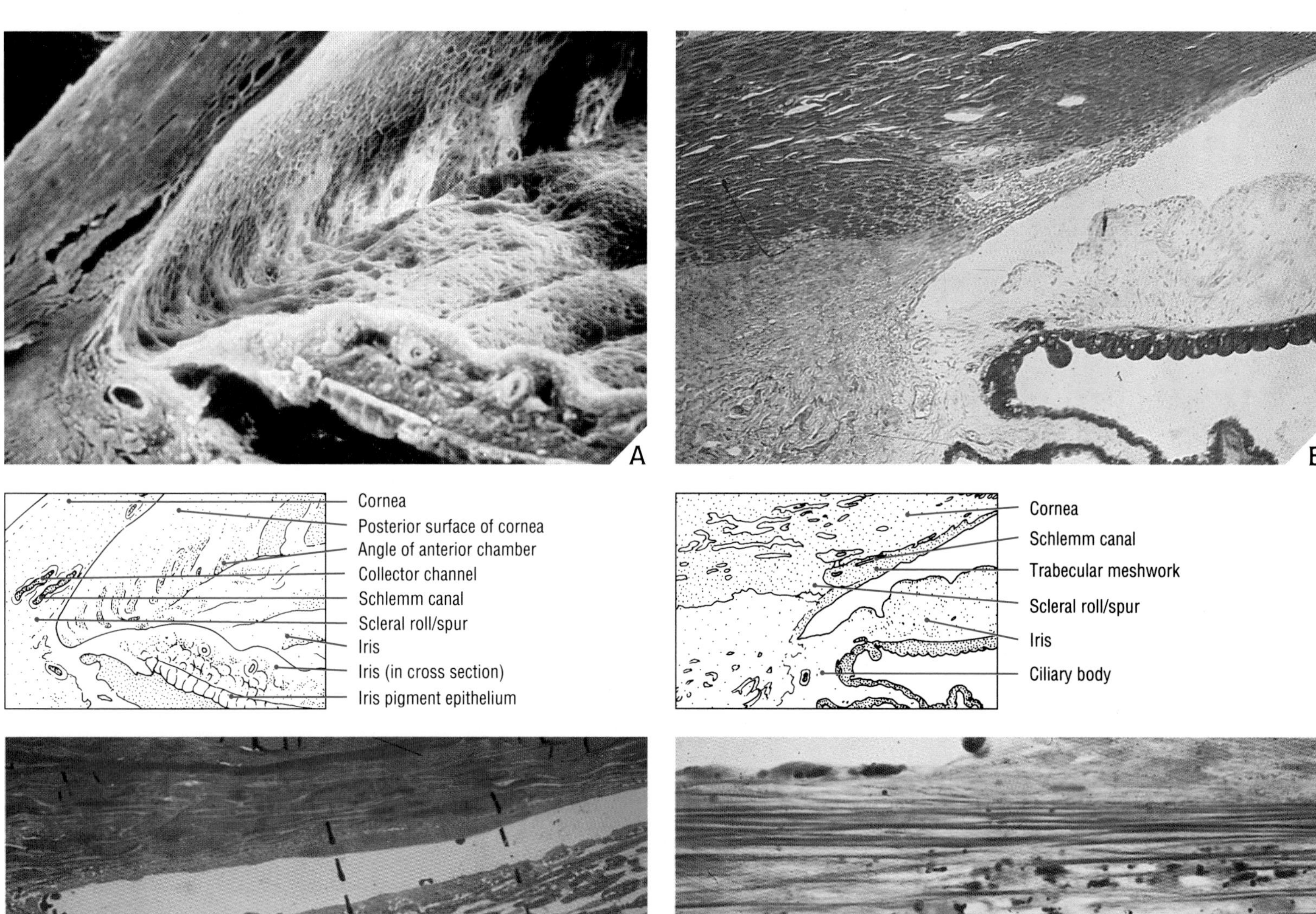

FIGURE 16.1 NORMAL ADULT ANGLE. **A** Scanning electron microscopy shows the main aqueous drainage area, i.e., the angle of the anterior chamber. Aqueous drains through the trabecular meshwork into the canal of Schlemm, the collector channels, and the aqueous veins, as well as into the uveal tract and out via the anterior ciliary and vortex veins. Some aqueous also drains into the iris and out through the iris vessels. **B** In an adult the scleral roll becomes thickened by compacting of the uveal meshwork to form the scleral spur. Between the scleral spur and the cornea lies the corneoscleral trabecular meshwork (TM). Just posterior lies the uveal TM and just anterior, adjacent to the Schlemm canal, lies the juxtacanalicular connective tissue (see Fig. 16.11A). **C** We usually view the transtrabecular and intertrabecular TM spaces meridionally. A section perpendicular to this plane, through the dotted lines, results in an anterior-posterior (coronal or frontal) view of the TM intertrabecular drainage spaces or canals, as seen in **D** (see Fig. 16.11A, C). (**A**, courtesy of Dr. RC Eagle Jr.)

CLINICAL FEATURES OF CONGENITAL GLAUCOMA

Affects 1:5000–1:10,000 live births
Autosomal-recessive
About 65% are male children
About 75% are bilateral

FIGURE 16.2

CONGENITAL GLAUCOMA

Age at onset	Percentage
At birth	40
Birth–6 months	34
6 months–1 year	12
1 year–6 years	11
Over 6 years	2
No information	1

FIGURE 16.3

DISEASES AND SYNDROMES ASSOCIATED WITH CONGENITAL GLAUCOMA

Aniridia	Rubella
Peters anomaly	Marfan syndrome
Phakomatoses	Axenfeld anomaly
Lowe syndrome	Rieger syndrome
Pierre Robin syndrome	

FIGURE 16.4

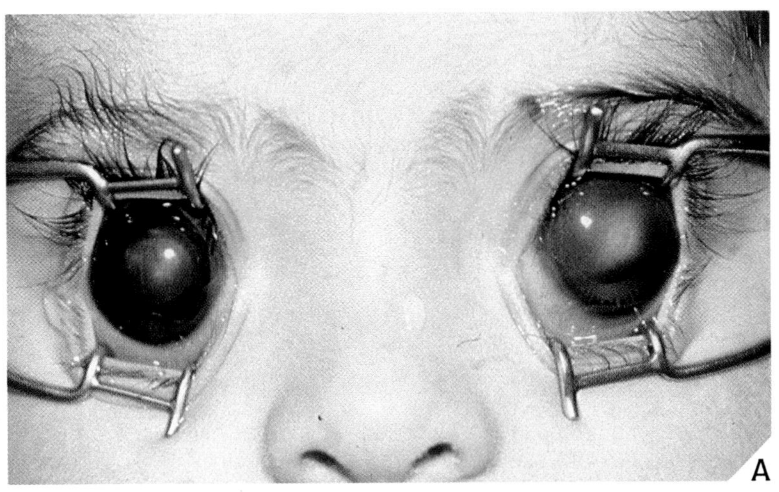

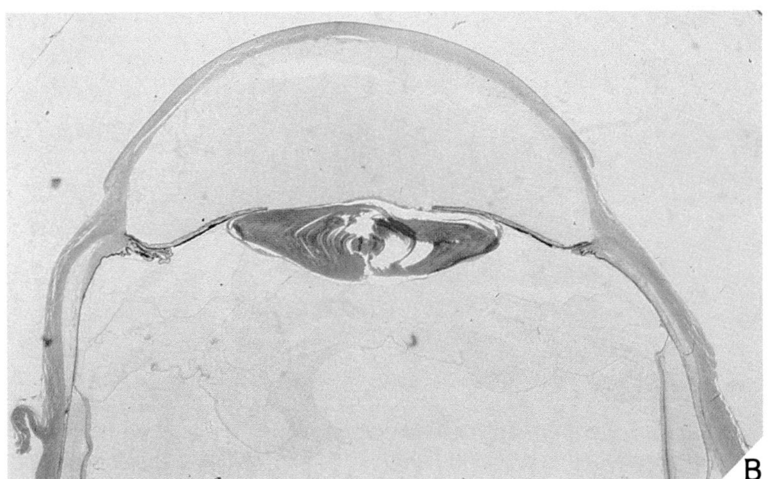

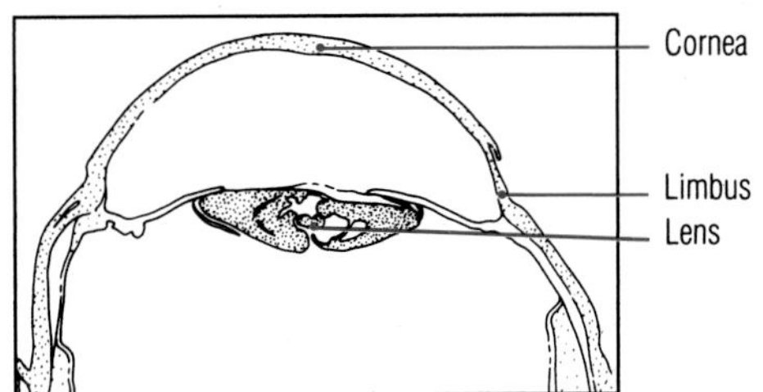

FIGURE 16.5 CONGENITAL GLAUCOMA. A The enlarged corneas are secondary to abnormal intraocular pressure in a patient who has congenital glaucoma, buphthalmos, and aniridia. Congenital glaucoma often presents with symptoms of tearing and photophobia. **B** In buphthalmos, enlargement of the globe is predominantly in the anterior segment and mainly in the limbal region, causing limbal ectasia. If the ectatic limbus is lined by uveal tissue in the form of iris, it is called limbal staphyloma. (**A**, courtesy of Dr. HG Scheie.)

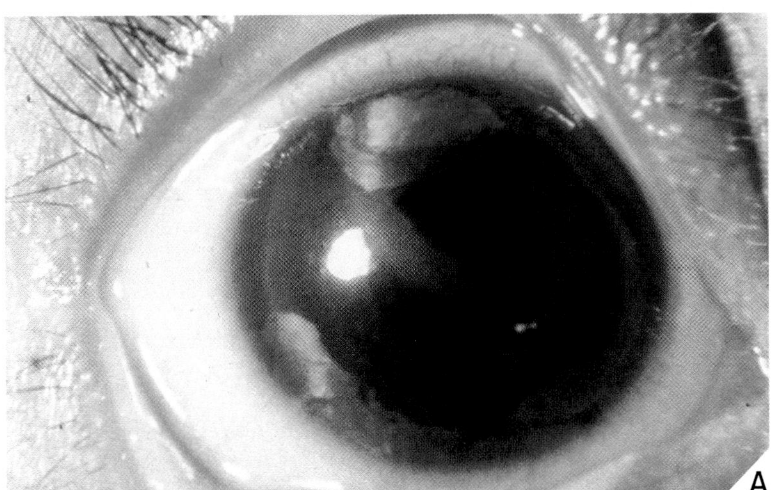

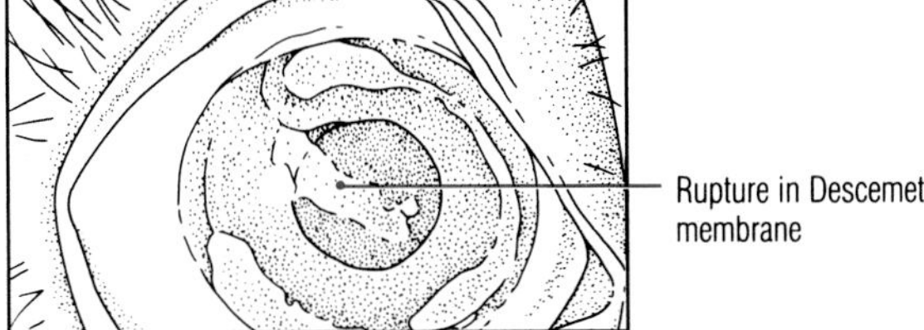

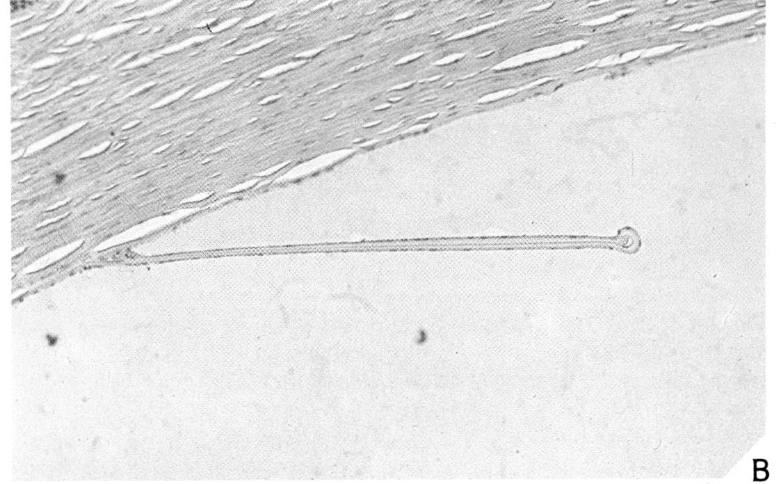

FIGURE 16.6 CONGENITAL GLAUCOMA. A The patient presented with congenital glaucoma, including enlarged corneas and ruptures in the Descemet membrane. **B** The ruptured ends of the Descemet membrane have sealed over. The ends, which extend into the anterior chamber, are scroll-like and covered by endothelium. (**A**, courtesy of Dr. HG Scheie.)

CAUSES OF PRIMARY CLOSED-ANGLE GLAUCOMA

Anatomic predisposition	Precipitating factors
High hypermetropia	Dim light leading to mid-dilatation
	Swelling of cataractous lens

FIGURE 16.7

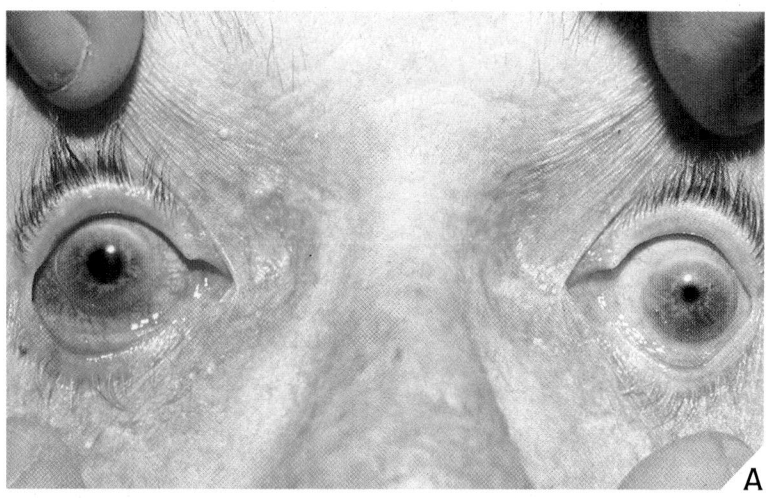

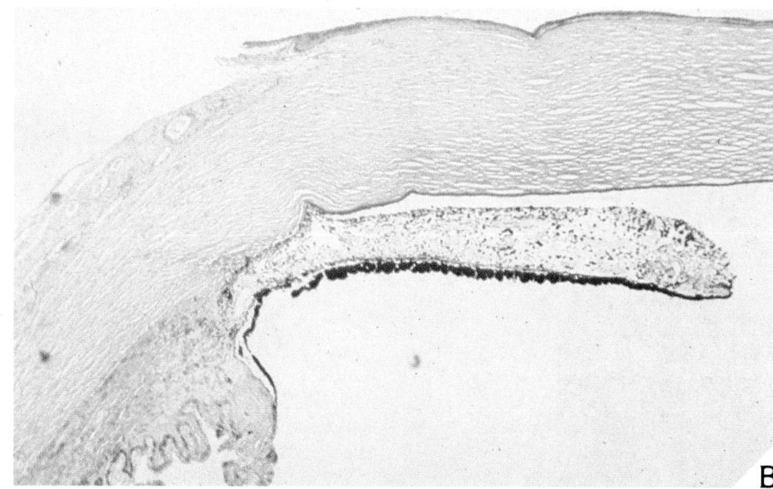

FIGURE 16.8 CLOSED-ANGLE GLAUCOMA. A The patient complained of pain, photophobia, and seeing halos around lights. Note the semidilated pupil and the ciliary injection in the right eye. **B** The eye was removed from another patient who had closed-angle glaucoma. The anterior chamber angle is occluded completely by a peripheral anterior synechia. The iris shows segmental necrosis consisting of stromal atrophy, loss of the dilator muscle, and necrosis of the sphincter muscle. Segmental iris necrosis can be mimicked clinically by *Herpes zoster*. (**B**, PAS stain.)

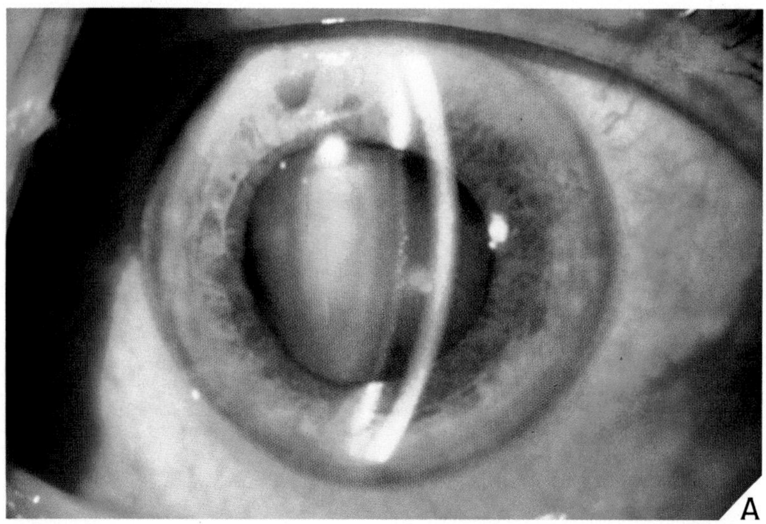

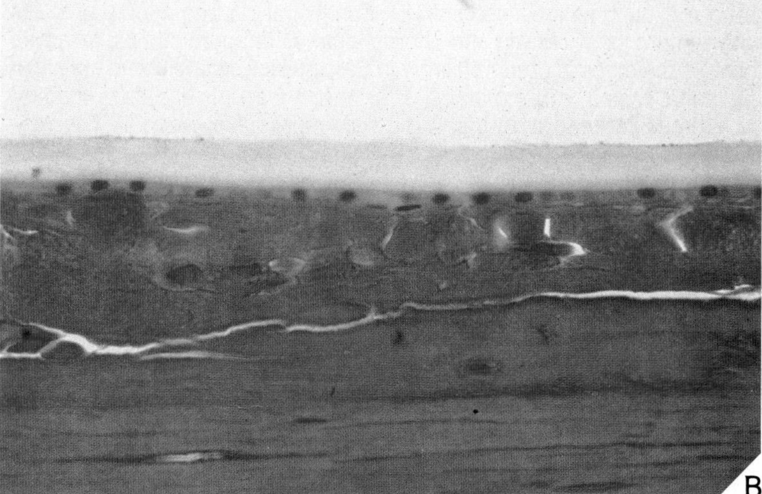

FIGURE 16.9 CLOSED-ANGLE GLAUCOMA. A Lens exhibits presence of glaukomflecken (tiny, white, anterior, subcapsular lens opacities). **B** Histologic section shows small areas of epithelial necrosis in the lens and tiny adjacent areas of subcapsular cortical degeneration. (**A**, courtesy of Dr. DM Kozart.)

CAUSES OF PRIMARY OPEN-ANGLE GLAUCOMA

Causes and pathology unclear but seem related to acceleration of aging process

Autosomal-recessive

FIGURE 16.10

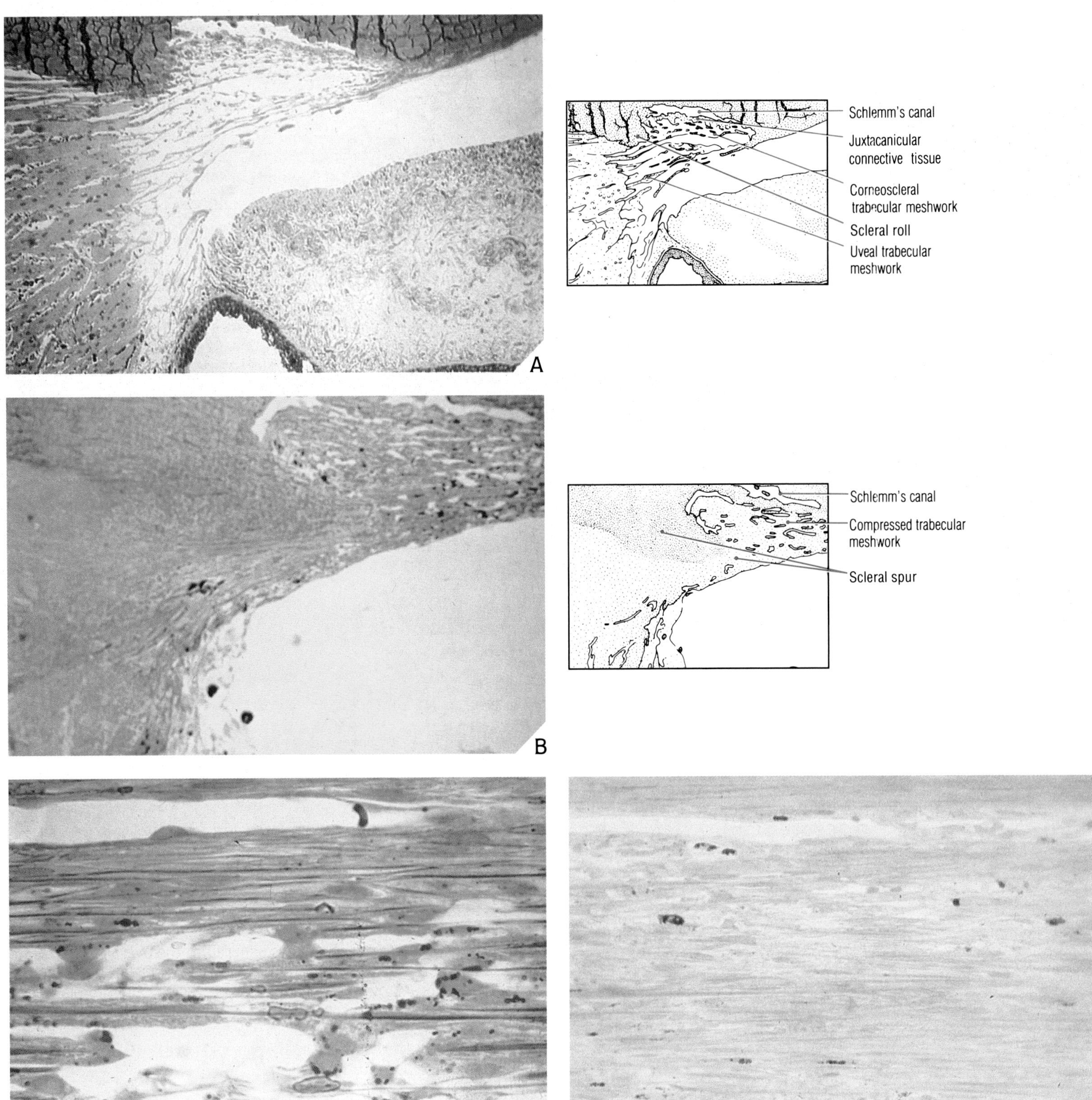

FIGURE 16.11 OPEN-ANGLE GLAUCOMA. A The normal anterior chamber angle shows a loose arrangement of trabecular meshwork in both the corneoscleral and uveal components. The juxtacanalicular connective tissue of the trabecular meshwork is adjacent to the Schlemm canal. **B** An eye removed from a patient who had chronic open-angle glaucoma shows the results of the aging process. The normally loose tissue in the uveal trabecular meshwork and angle recess has compacted, producing a prominent scleral spur. **C** A coronal section taken through normal trabecular meshwork shows that the loose beams of the meshwork form large tubes running in an anterior-posterior direction. **D** Coronal sections through the trabecular meshwork in a patient who had chronic open-angle glaucoma show that the aging process has caused marked compaction of the trabecular meshwork beams, resulting in occlusion of most of the tubes. (**A–D**, PD stain; case reported in Fine BS, et al., 1981; **A**, rhesus monkey.)

CAUSES OF SECONDARY CLOSED-ANGLE GLAUCOMA

Chronic primary closed angle
Phacomorphic lens swelling
Anterior lens dislocation
Post-traumatic flat anterior chamber
Iridocorneal endothelial (ICE) syndrome
Anterior uveitis
Spherophakia
Seclusion of pupil (iris bombé)
Retinopathy of prematurity
Persistent hyperplastic primary vitreous
Endo- or epithelialization
Iris neovascularization
Cysts of iris and ciliary body
Juvenile xanthogranuloma
Uveal melanoma

FIGURE 16.12

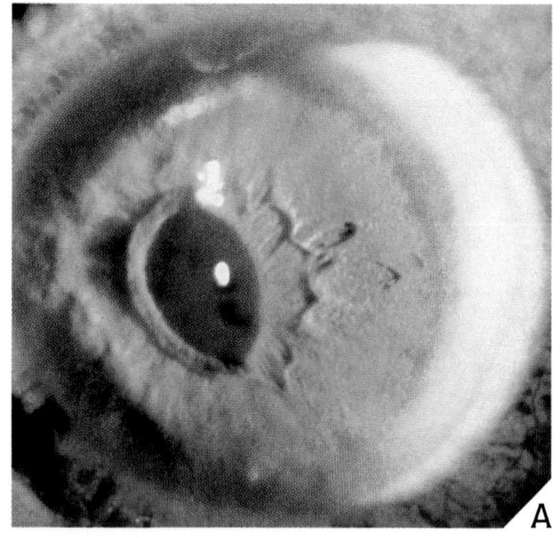

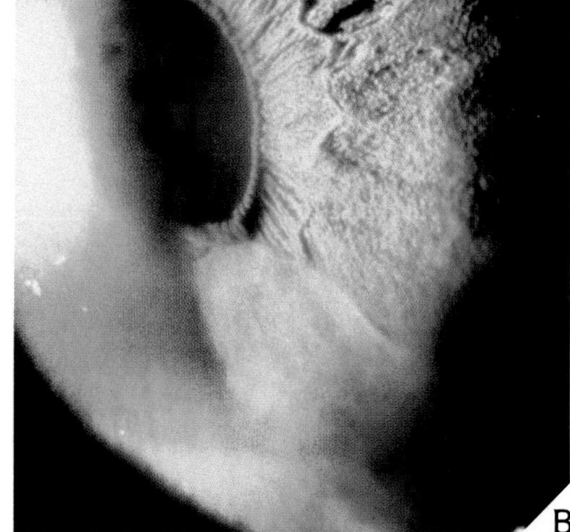

FIGURE 16.13 IRIDOCORNEAL ENDOTHELIAL (ICE) SYNDROME (IRIS NEVUS SYNDROME VARIANT). A Unilateral corneal edema and heterochromia in a patient with ICE syndrome. The temporal half of the iris is relatively normal; the nasal half shows ectropion uvea and effacement of the normal iris pattern by a membrane (probably the Descemet). **B** The inferior temporal transition zone between the normal temporal section of the iris and the membrane is clear. Note the corneal blebs in region of the pupil. (**A**, **B**, courtesy of Dr. DM Kozart, from Yanoff M, Fine BS: *Ocular Pathology,* 3rd ed.)

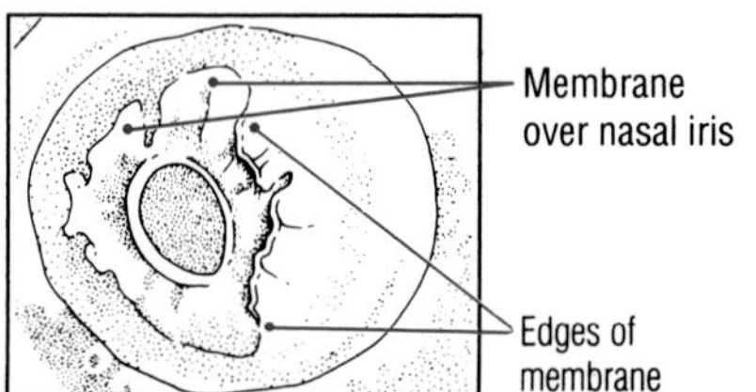

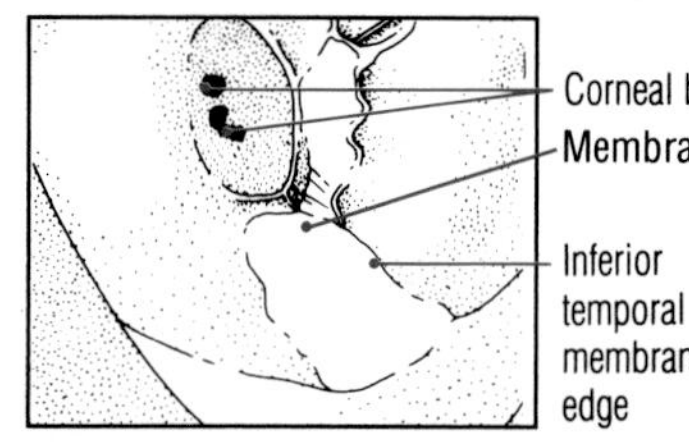

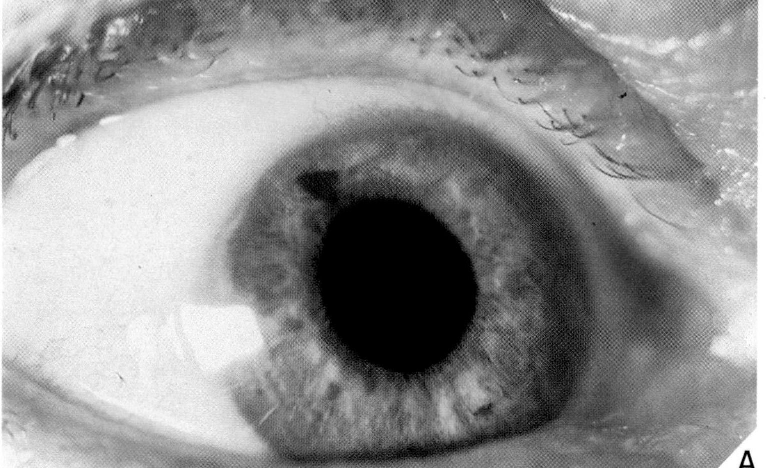

FIGURE 16.14 ICE SYNDROME (IRIS NEVUS SYNDROME VARIANT). A Note the irregularity on the superior aspect of the pupillary margin, the dark iris nevus, and the effacement of the iris stroma superiorly. **B** An excisional biopsy of the superior iris shows deep stromal pigmentation. Bleached sections revealed that the pigmented cells were nevus cells. Traction pulls the pigment epithelium and sphincter forward to form an ectropion uveae. **C** At a different level, the peripheral iris has adhered to the overlying Descemet membrane. Migration and proliferation of corneal endothelium from the Descemet membrane over the stromal bridge onto the anterior surface of the iris has occurred both centrally and peripherally, laying down a new Descemet membrane. The endothelium over the surface of the superior iris probably has contracted and caused the ectropion uveae. (**C**, PAS stain; case reported in Jakobiec FA, et al., 1977.)

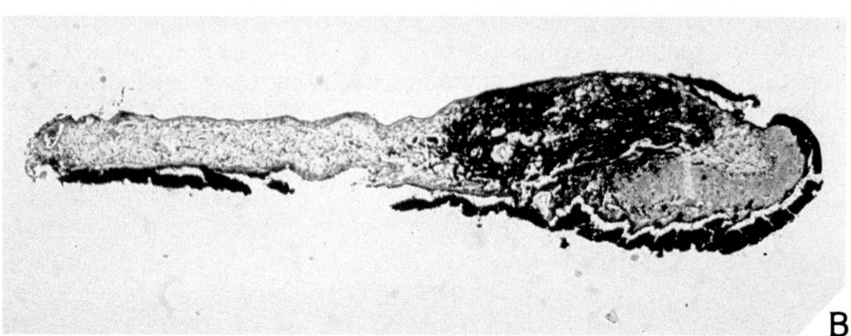

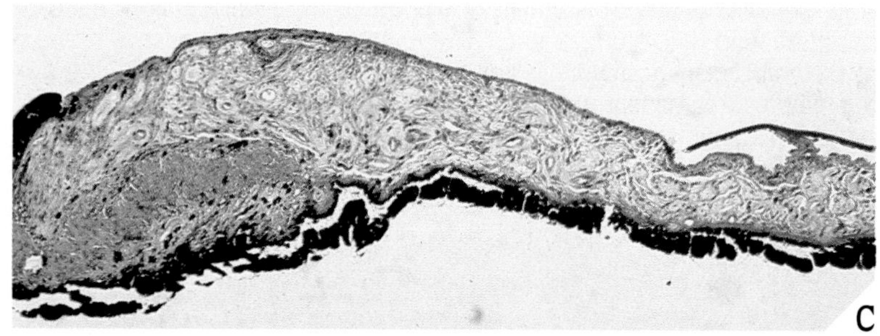

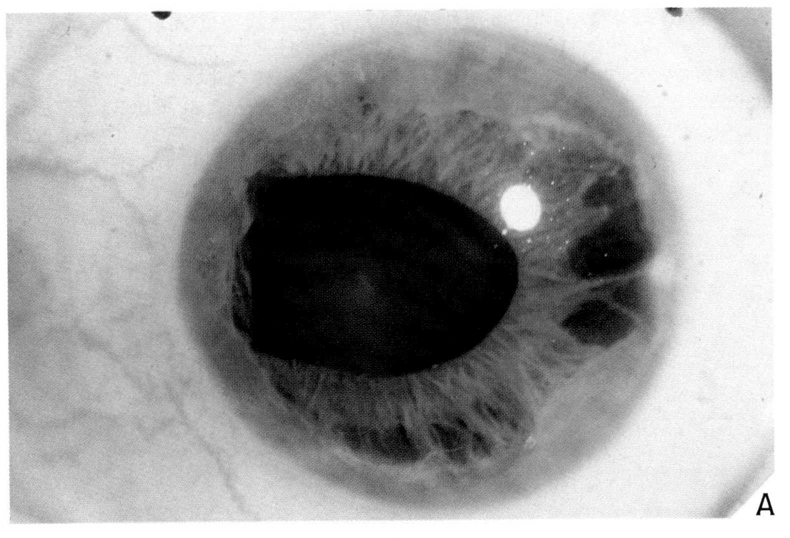

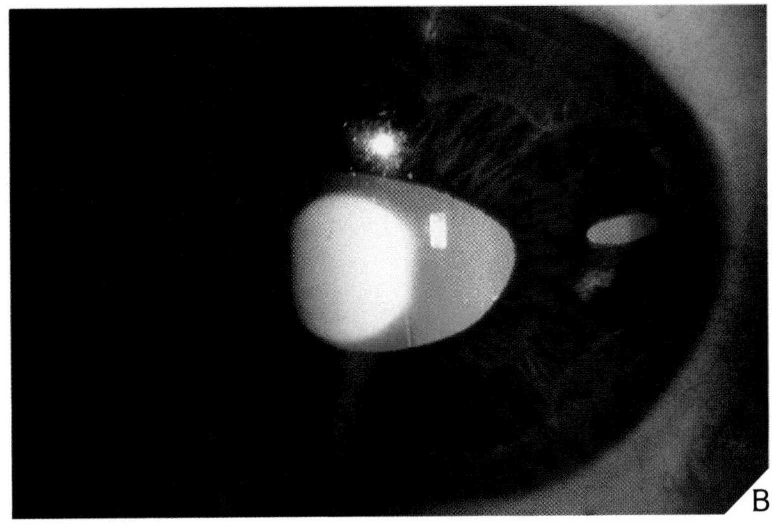

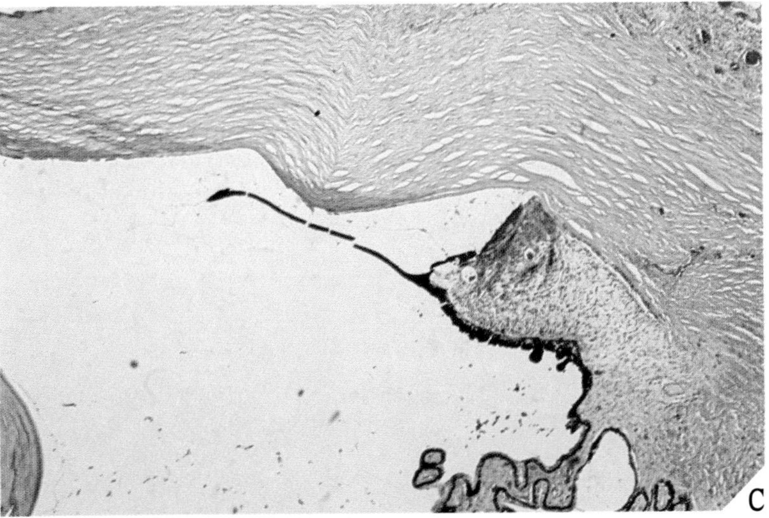

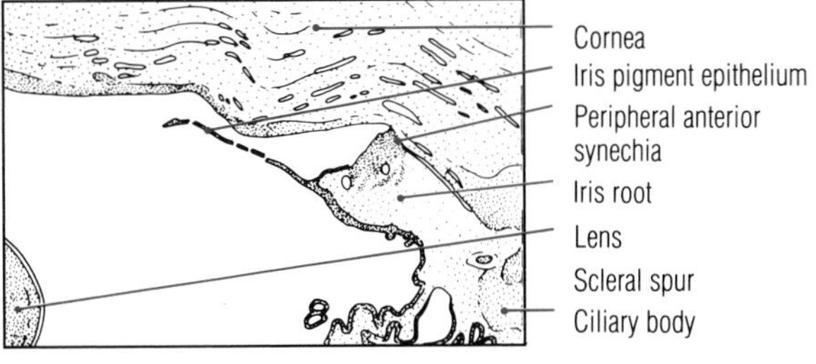

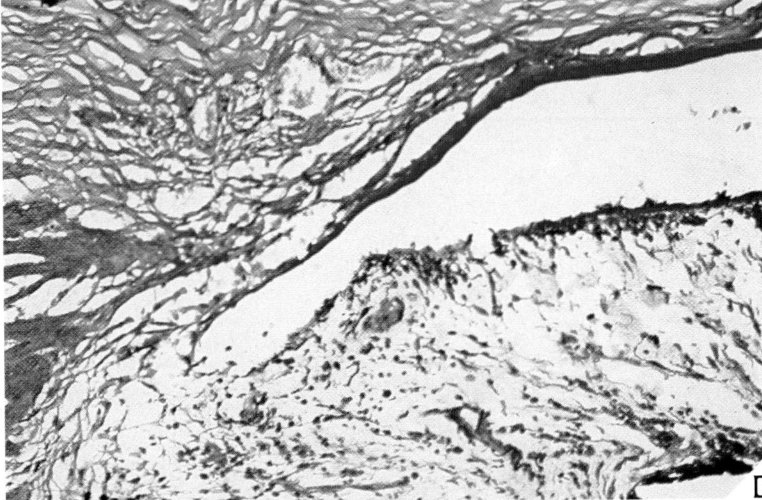

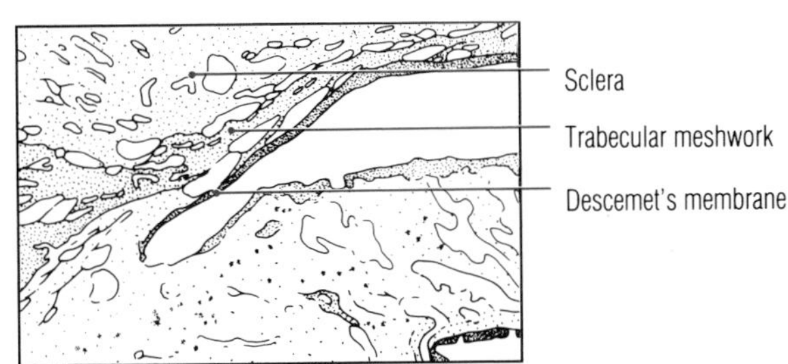

FIGURE 16.15 ICE SYNDROME (ESSENTIAL IRIS ATROPHY VARIANT). **A** Slit-lamp and **B** red-reflex views of the same eye show migration of the iris nasally toward the initial synechia and stretching of the iris temporally, causing a hole clear through the iris. **C** Histologic section of another eye with essential iris atrophy shows a peripheral anterior synechia, various degrees of degeneration and loss of the central iris stroma, and total loss of the central iris pigment epithelium. **D** In an area away from the peripheral anterior synechia, the anterior chamber angle is open but the trabecular meshwork is covered by proliferated corneal endothelium and the Descemet membrane. (**A,B**, courtesy of Dr. HG Scheie; **C,D**, reported in Scheie HG, et al., 1976.)

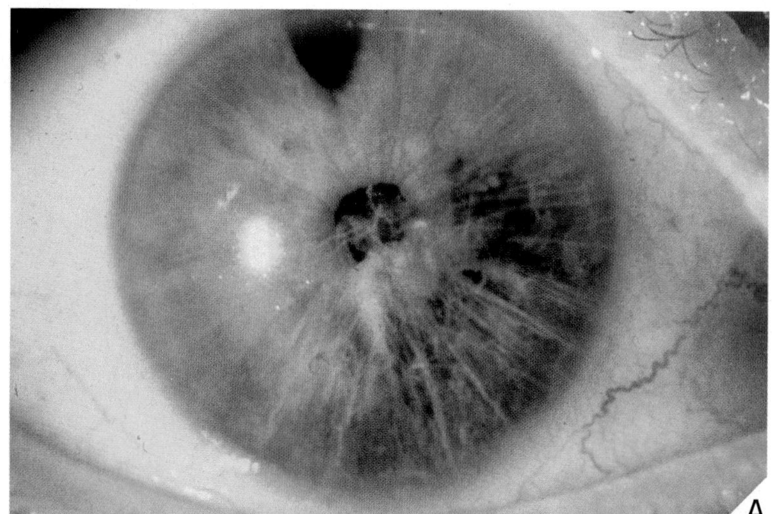

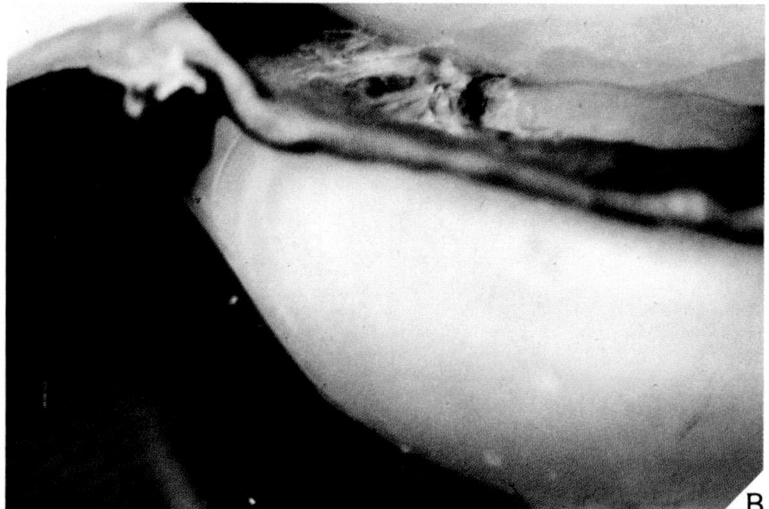

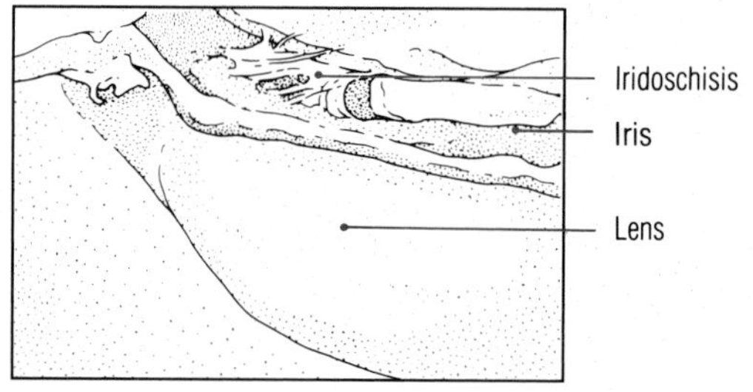

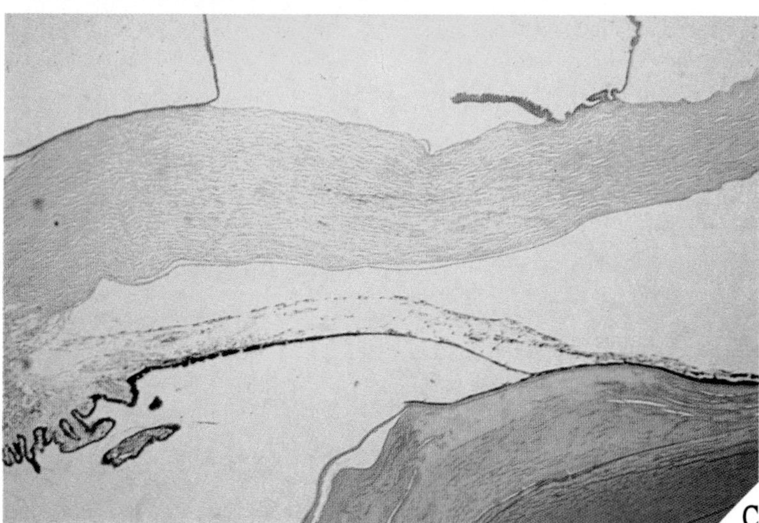

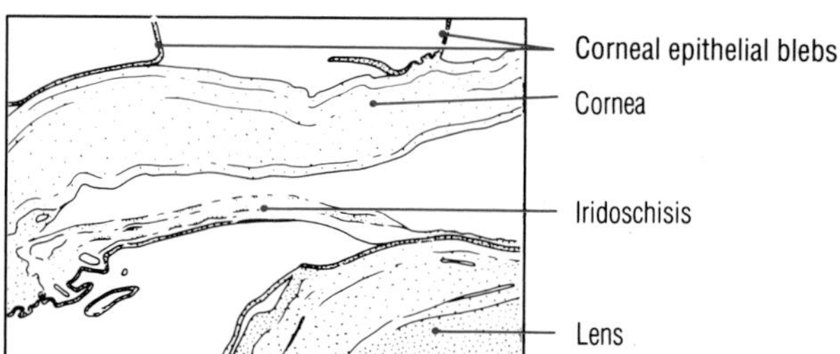

FIGURE 16.16 IRIDOSCHISIS. A The iris is in disarray, with long rolled strips from the 3-o'clock to the 6-o'clock position. **B** The gross specimen from another eye shows separation and breakage of the collagenous columns of the iris stroma. **C** Histologic section of the eye shown in **B** demonstrates epithelial blebs (bullous corneal edema) and separation of the iris stroma into elongated lamellae. (**A**, courtesy of Dr. G. Naumann, from Yanoff M, Fine BS, *Ocular Pathology*, 3rd ed.)

FIGURE 16.17 IRIS NEOVASCULARIZATION. A Large blood vessels growing abnormally over the anterior surface of the iris give it a reddish color, a condition called rubeosis iridis. **B** Histologic section shows vascular channels and fibrous tissue present above the anterior border layer of the iris in the form of iris neovascularization. The membrane has caused a peripheral anterior synechia. Shrinkage of the membrane has produced an ectropion uvea. **C** In a scanning electron microscope (SEM) view, the anterior chamber angle and peripheral iris are covered by a fibrovascular membrane, and the angle is closed by a peripheral anterior synechia. (**B**, PAS stain; **C**, SEM view courtesy of Drs. RC Eagle Jr and JW Sassani.)

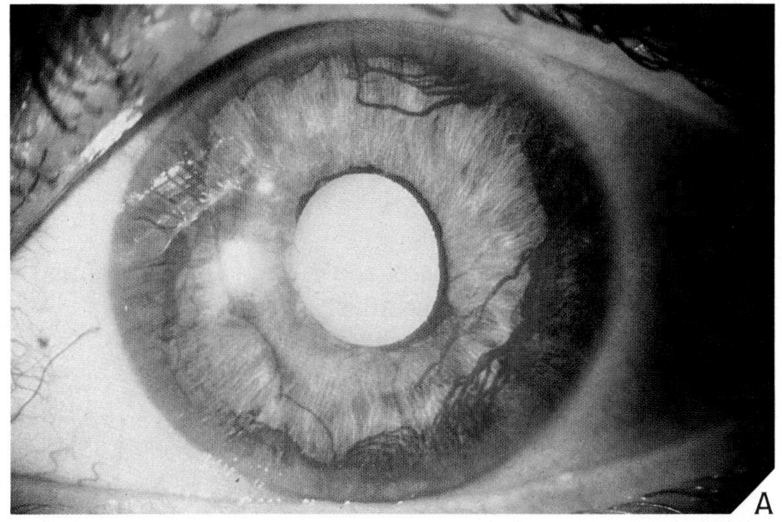

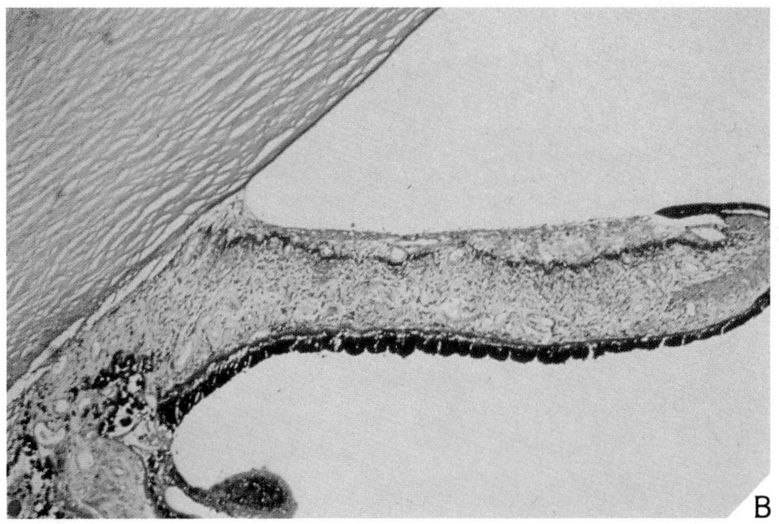

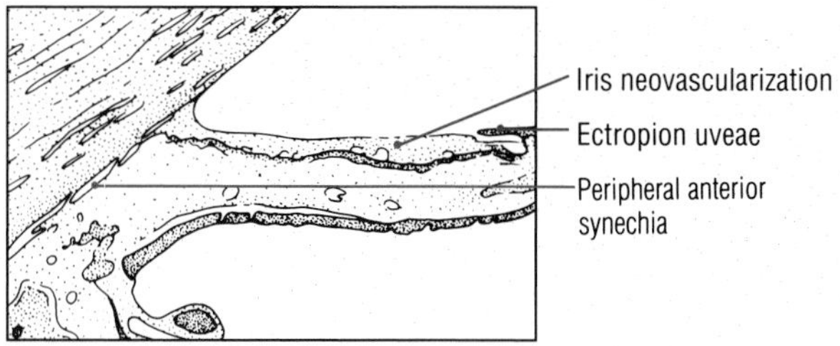

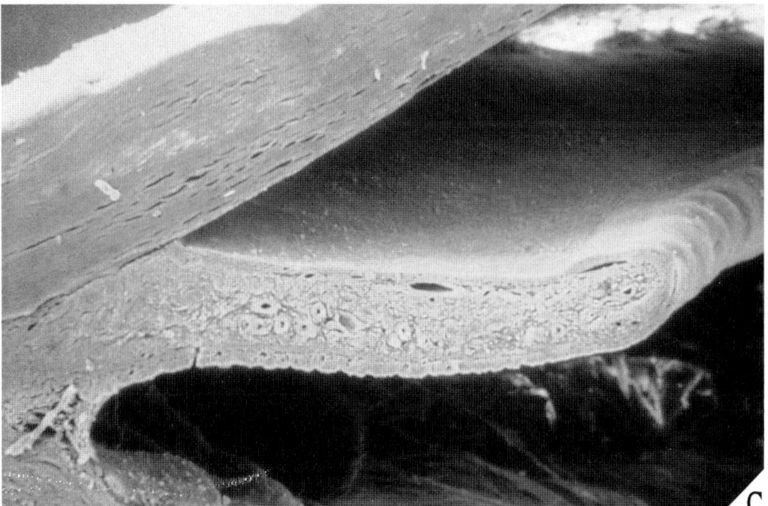

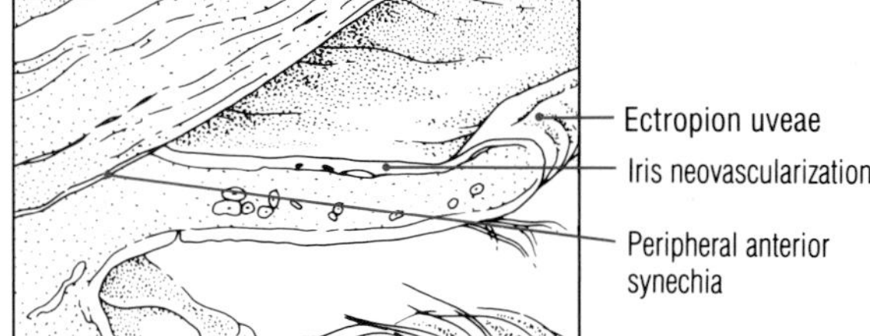

CAUSES OF SECONDARY OPEN-ANGLE GLAUCOMA

Cells or debris in angle
Hyphema
Uveitis
Phacolytic, hemolytic (ghost-cell), and melanomalytic glaucoma
Nondenatured lens material from ruptured lens
Pigment dispersion syndrome
Exfoliation syndrome
Uveal melanoma
Endo- or epithelialization

Damaged outflow channels
Old uveitis
Recurrent attacks of closed-angle glaucoma
Repeated hyphema
Siderosis and hemosiderosis bulbi
Trauma
Cornea guttata
Early iris neovascularization

Unknown mechanisms
Steroids
α-Chymotrypsin

Corneoscleral and extraocular conditions
Interstitial keratitis
Orbital venous thrombosis
Cavernous sinus thrombosis
Carotid-cavernous fistula
Retinal detachment surgery (postsurgical)
Retrobulbar mass
Leukemia
Mediastinal mass

FIGURE 16.18

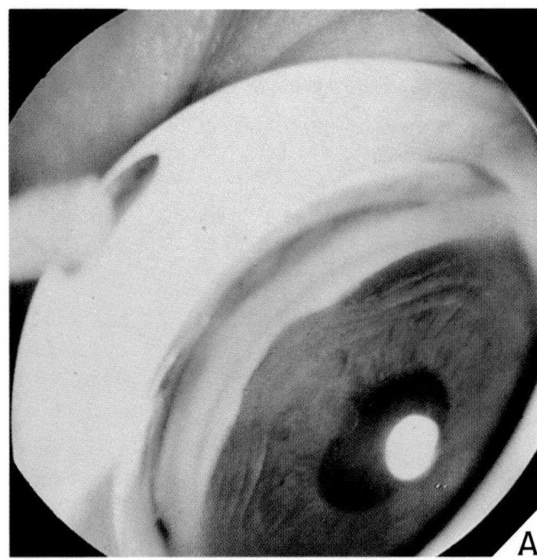
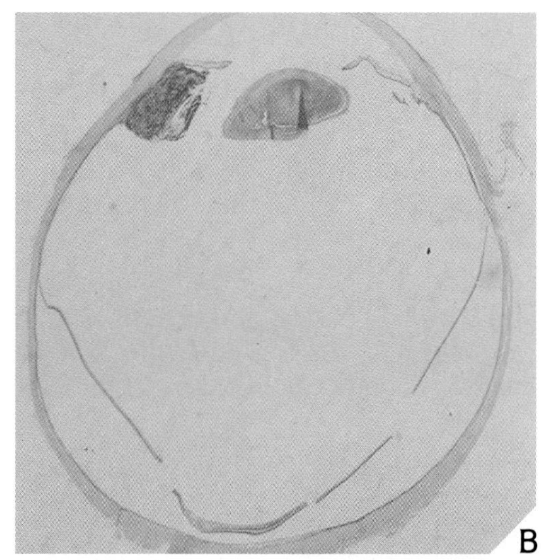
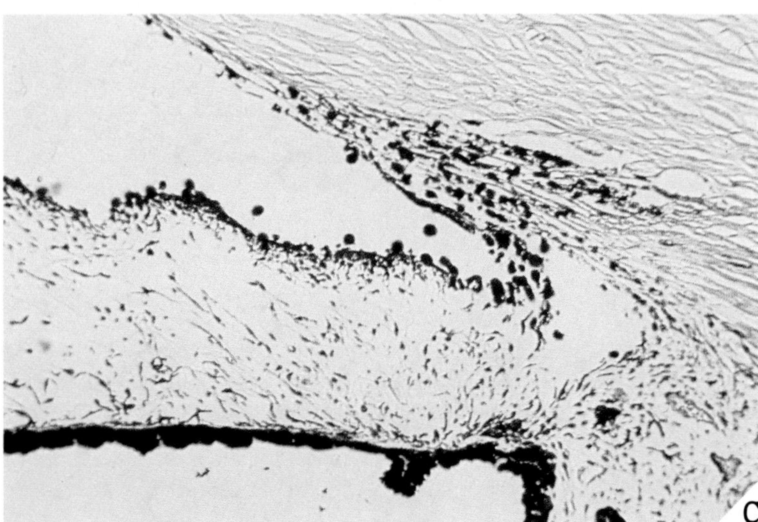

FIGURE 16.19 MELANOMALYTIC GLAUCOMA. A The patient presented with a markedly elevated intraocular pressure, ocular pain, and was seeing halos around lights. The angle, however, was deeply pigmented and wide open, except where it was closed by a pigmented tumor between the 8-o'clock and 9-o'clock positions. **B** The enucleated eye shows a small and completely necrotic ciliary-body melanoma. **C** Pigmented cells are seen over the anterior surface of the iris, the angle recess, and the trabecular meshwork. A bleached section of the pigmented cells showed that they were macrophages filled with pigment. The necrotic cells of the ciliary-body melanoma have lysed and liberated their melanin pigment, which has been phagocytosed by macrophages and carried by the aqueous into the anterior chamber and angle. This is analogous to what happens in phacolytic and hemolytic (ghost-cell) glaucomas. (**A**, courtesy of Dr. HG Scheie; case reported in Yanoff M, Scheie HG, 1970.)

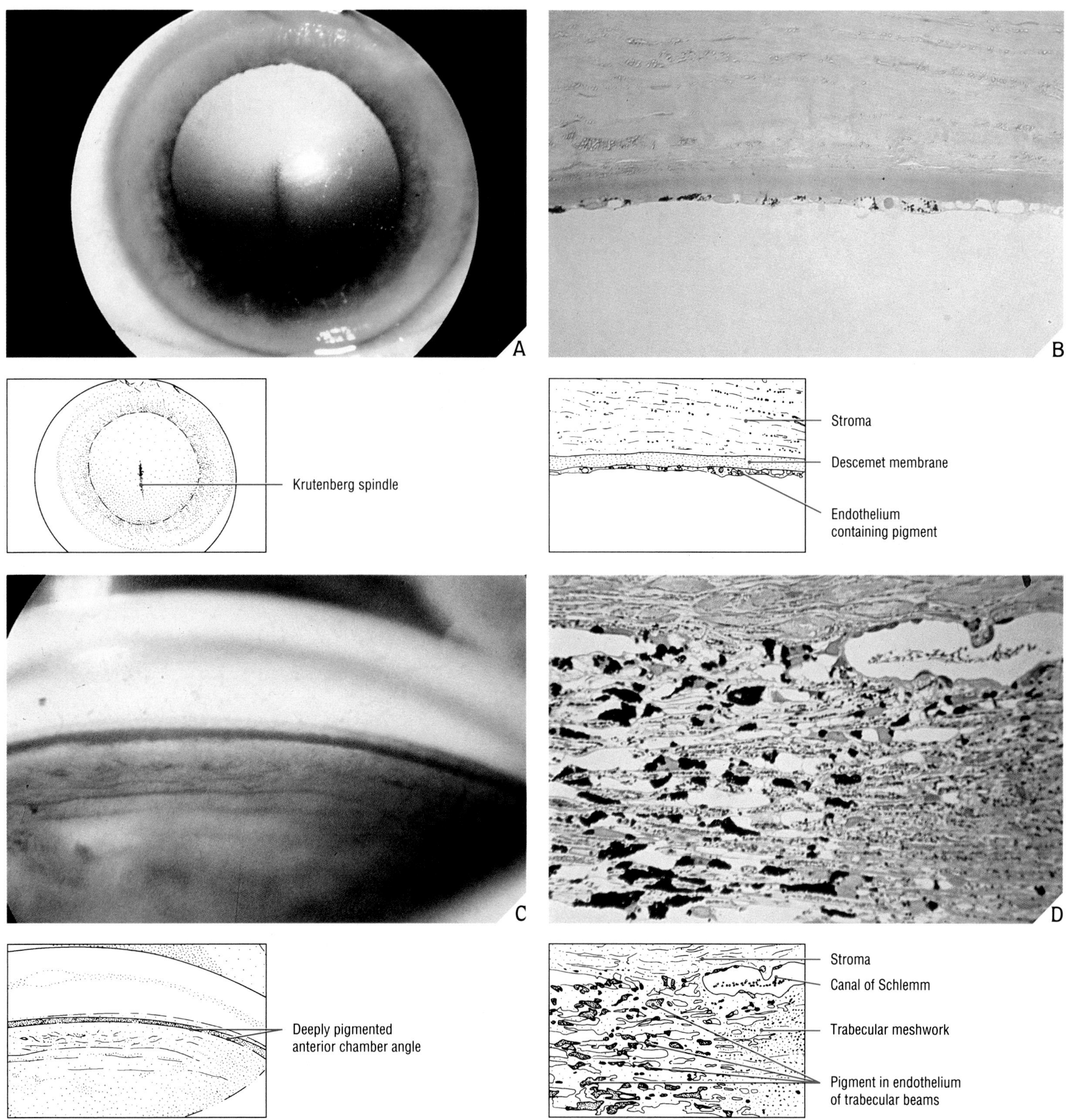

FIGURE 16.20 PIGMENT DISPERSION SYNDROME. A A Krukenberg spindle is seen as a vertical linear deposition of melanin pigment in the central inferior cornea. **B** Granules of melanin pigment are present within corneal endothelial cells. **C** The anterior chamber angle is deeply pigmented. **D** Melanin pigment is present within the endothelial cells lining the beams of the trabecular meshwork.

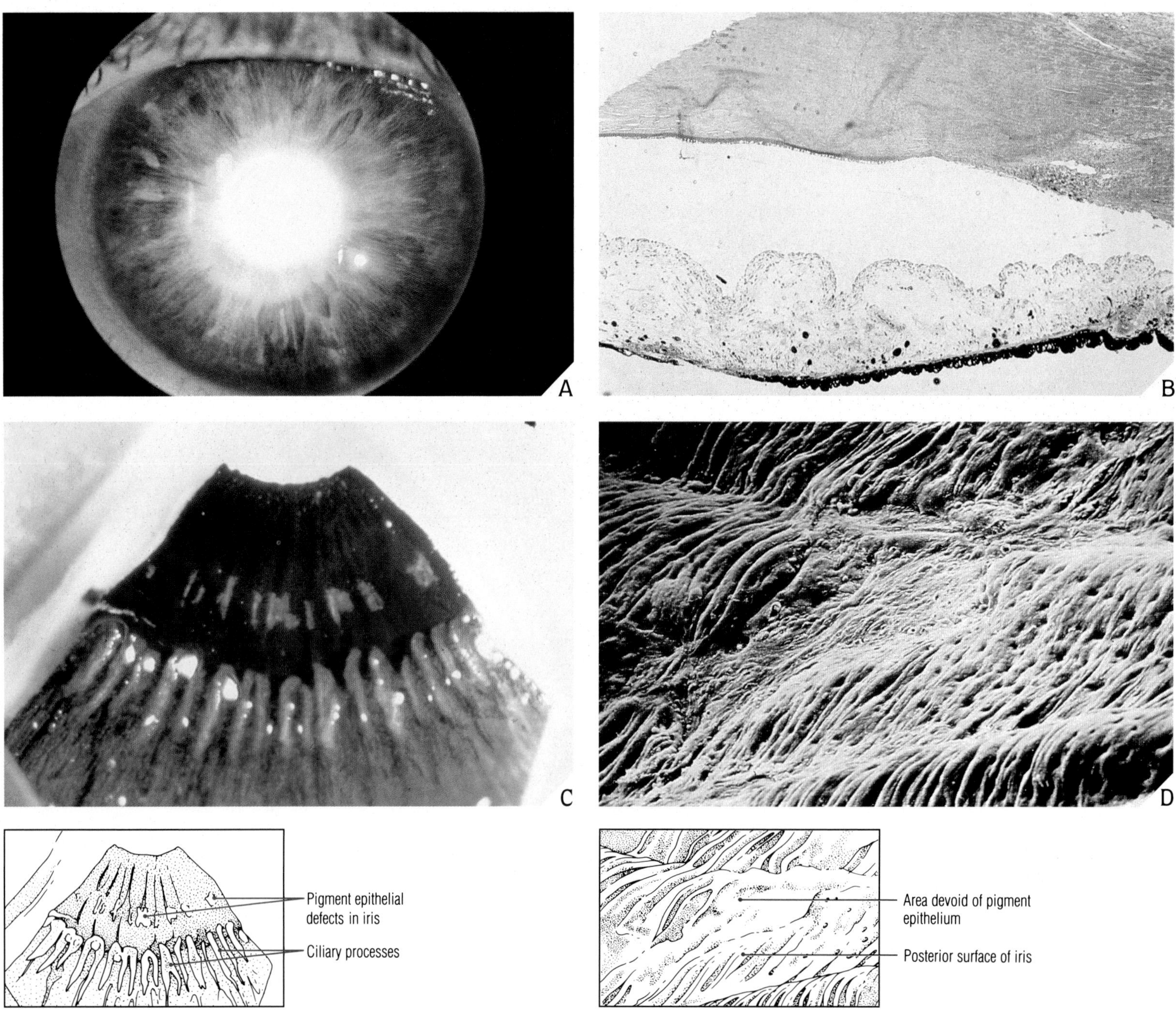

FIGURE 16.21 PIGMENT DISPERSION SYNDROME. A Extensive increased iris transillumination is present, predominantly in the middle third of the iris. **B** The area of increased transillumination corresponds to the area of loss of pigment epithelium from the back of the iris. **C** The gross specimen confirms this, as does **D**, an SEM view of the posterior surface of the iris.

MAJOR TISSUE CHANGES SECONDARY TO GLAUCOMA

Corneal edema	Optic nerve atrophy and cupping
Degeneration of inner retinal layers	Cavernous (Schnabel) optic atrophy

FIGURE 16.22

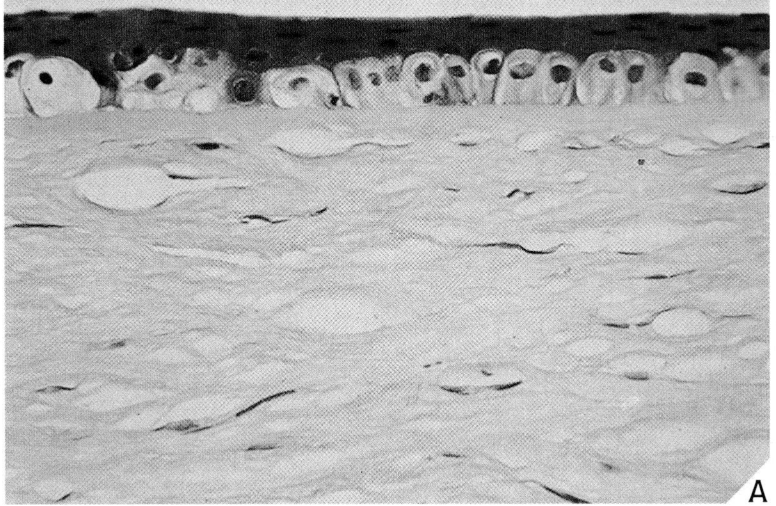

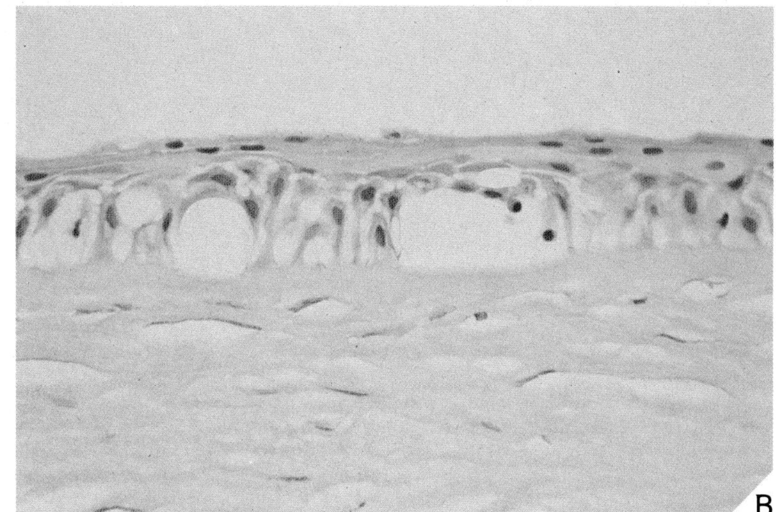

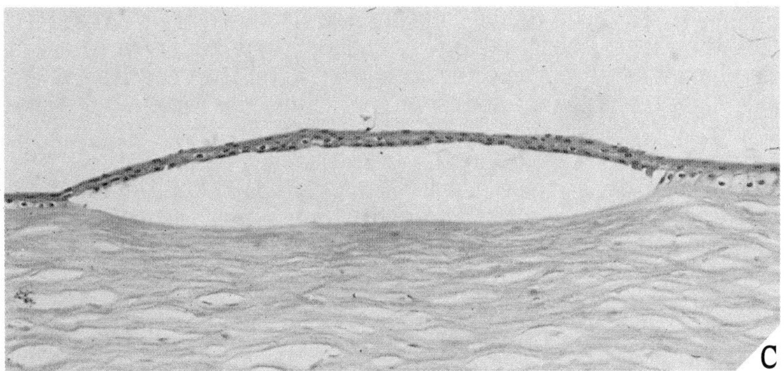

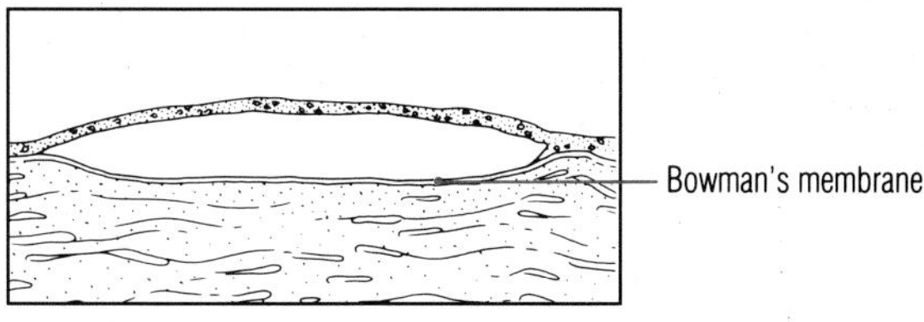

FIGURE 16.23 CORNEAL EDEMA. A Fluid present in the basal layer of the corneal epithelium causes swelling of the cells. Clinically, this would appear as bedewing. **B** The edema has spread both within and between the epithelial cells. **C** Further collection of fluid has caused the entire epithelium to lift off the Bowman membrane, forming a large bleb. The bleb may become ulcerated and even lead to corneal infection and perforation (see Fig. 10.6). (**A**, trichrome.)

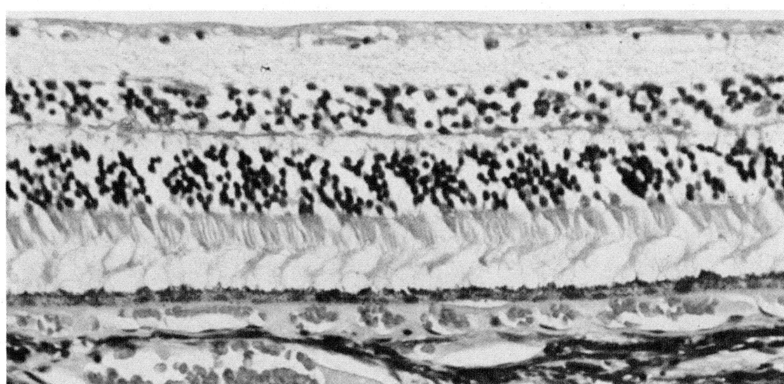

Internal limiting membrane
Atrophic nerve fiber and ganglion cell layers
Rods and cones
Retinal pigment epithelium
Choroid

FIGURE 16.24 GLAUCOMATOUS ATROPHY OF THE RETINA. As a result of glaucoma, marked atrophy of the inner layers of the retina has occurred, especially the nerve fiber layer (which shows thinning) and the ganglion cell layer (which shows only occasional nuclei instead of the normal continuous single layer in this nasal area).

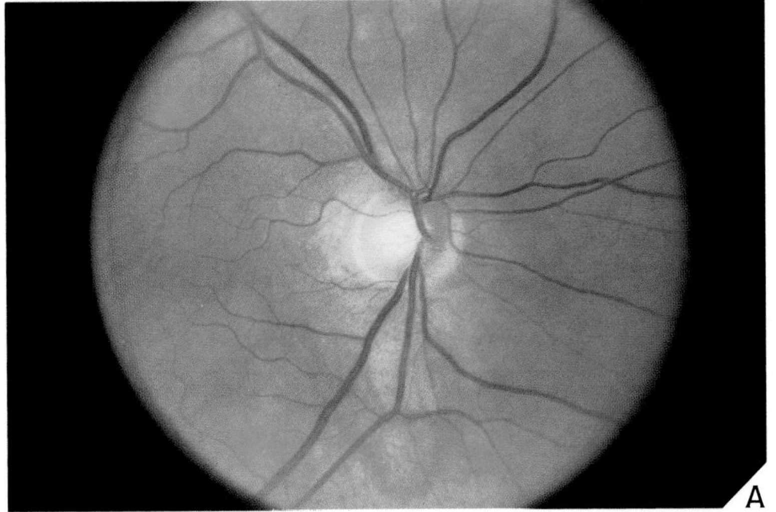

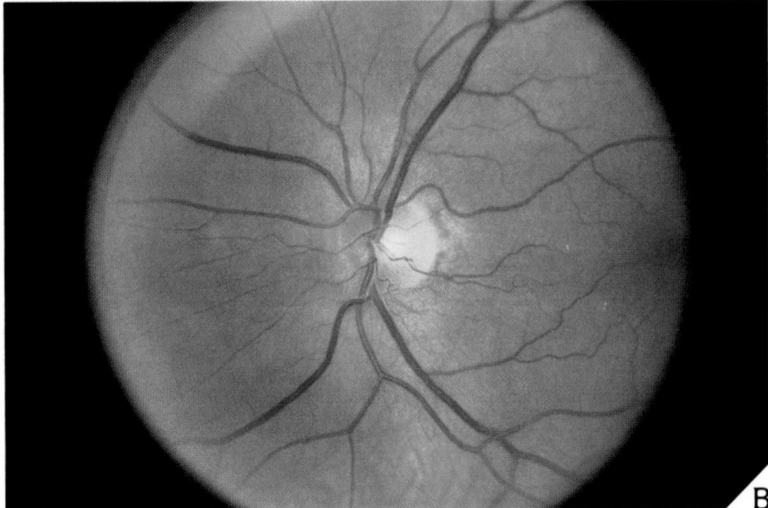

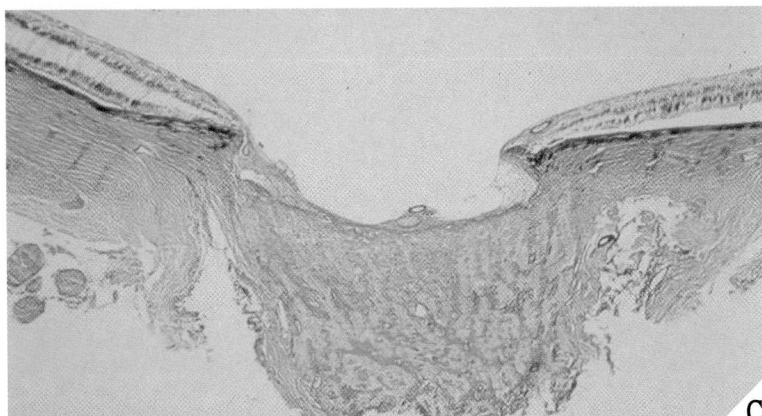

FIGURE 16.25 OPTIC NERVE CUPPING AND ATROPHY. Right **(A)** and left **(B)** eyes of the same patient. The right optic nerve is cupped, secondary to glaucoma. The left optic nerve is less involved (or "less cupped"). **C** The optic nerve head is deeply cupped. Atrophy of the optic nerve is determined by comparing the diameter of the optic nerve at its internal surface and posteriorly where it should double in size. Here it is the same size because of a loss of axons and myelin, which also causes an increase in size of the subarachnoid space and a proliferation of glial cells, resulting in an increased cellularity of the optic nerve.

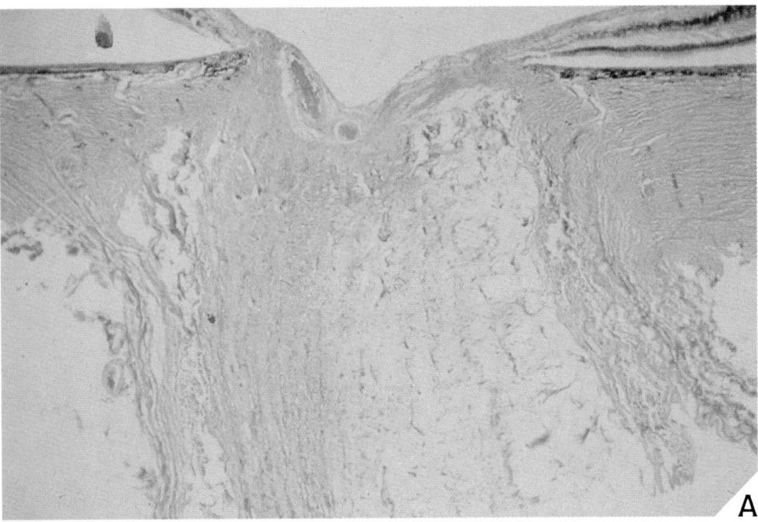

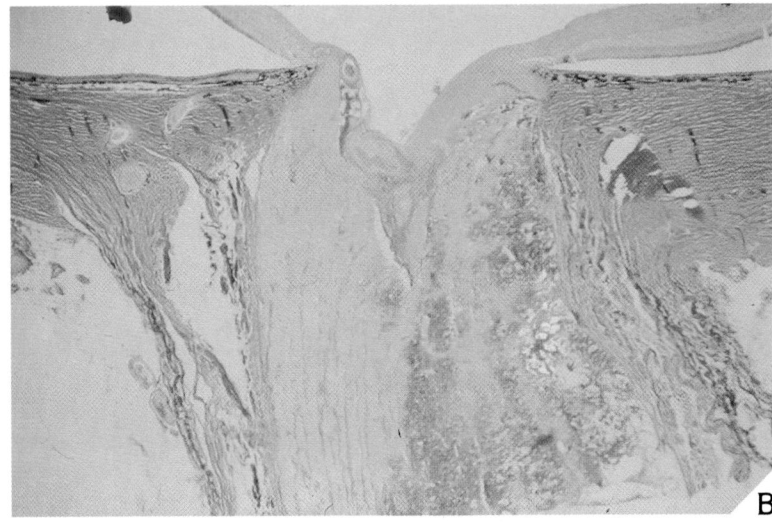

FIGURE 16.26 SCHNABEL CAVERNOUS OPTIC ATROPHY. A The optic nerve head shows cupping of its surface and large cystic spaces in its parenchyma. **B** A special stain to test for the presence of acid mucopolysaccharides (AMP) shows that the cystic spaces are filled with a blue-staining material. Predigestion of the section with hyaluronidase showed empty spaces, demonstrating that they had contained hyaluronic acid. (**A**, from Yanoff M, Fine BS: *Ocular Pathology*, 3rd ed.; **B**, AMP stain.)

Bibliography

Alvarado J, Murphy C, Juster R: Trabecular meshwork cellularity in primary open-angle glaucoma and nonglaucomatous normals. Ophthalmology 91:564, 1984.

Anderson DR: Glaucoma: The damage caused by pressure. Am J Ophthalmol 108:485, 1989.

Bennett SR, Alward LM, Folberg R: An autosomal-dominant form of low-tension glaucoma. Am J Ophthalmol 108:238, 1989.

Caprioli J, et al: Measurements of peripapillary nerve fiber layer contour in glaucoma. Am J Ophthalmol 108:404, 1989.

Eagle RC Jr, et al: Proliferative endotheliopathy with iris abnormalities. The iridocorneal endothelial syndrome. Arch Ophthalmol 97:2014, 1979.

Fine BS, Yanoff M, Stone RA: A clinicopathologic study of four cases of primary open-angle glaucoma compared to normal eyes. Am J Ophthalmol 91:88, 1981.

Hernandez MR, Andrzejewska WM, Neufeld AH: Changes in the extracellular matrix of the human optic nerve head in primary open-angle glaucoma. Am J Ophthalmol 109:180, 1990.

Hoskins HD Jr, Shaffer RN, Hetherington J: Anatomical classification of the developmental glaucomas. Arch Ophthalmol 102:1331, 1984.

Jakobiec FA, et al: Solitary iris nevus with peripheral anterior synechiae and iris endothelialization: a variant of the iris nevus syndrome. Am J Ophthalmol 83:884, 1977.

Jonas JB, Naumann GOH: Parapapillary chorioretinal atrophy in normal and glaucoma eyes. II. Correlations. Invest Ophthalmol Vis Sci 30:919, 1989.

Jonas JB, Naumann GOH: Parapapillary retinal vessel diameter in normal and glaucoma eyes. II. Correlations. Invest Ophthalmol Vis Sci 30:1604, 1989.

Jonas JB, et al: Parapapillary chorioretinal atrophy in normal and glaucoma eyes. I. Morphometric data. Invest Ophthalmol Vis Sci 30:908, 1989.

Jonas JB, et al: Parapapillary retinal vessel diameter in normal and glaucoma eyes. I. Morphometric data. Invest Ophthalmol Vis Sci 30:1599, 1989.

Rodrigues MM, Streeten BW, Spaeth GL: Chandler's syndrome as a variant of essential iris atrophy. A clinicopathologic study. Arch Ophthalmol 96:643, 1978.

Scheie HG, Yanoff M, Kellogg WT: Essential iris atrophy: report of a case. Arch Ophthalmol 94:1315, 1976.

Semple HC, Ball SF: Pigmentary glaucoma in the black population. Am J Ophthalmol 109:518, 1990.

Shin DH, et al: Reversal of glaucomatous optic disc cupping in adult patients. Arch Ophthalmol 107:1599, 1989.

Tsai CS, et al: Antibodies to Epstein-Barr virus in iridocorneal endothelial syndrome. Arch Ophthalmol 108:1572, 1990.

Yanoff M, Fine BS: *Ocular Pathology: A Text and Atlas*, 2nd ed. Philadelphia, JB Lippincott, 1982, and 3rd ed., 1989.

Yanoff M, Scheie HG: Melanomalytic glaucoma: report of patient. Arch Ophthalmol 84:471, 1970.

Ocular Melanotic Tumors

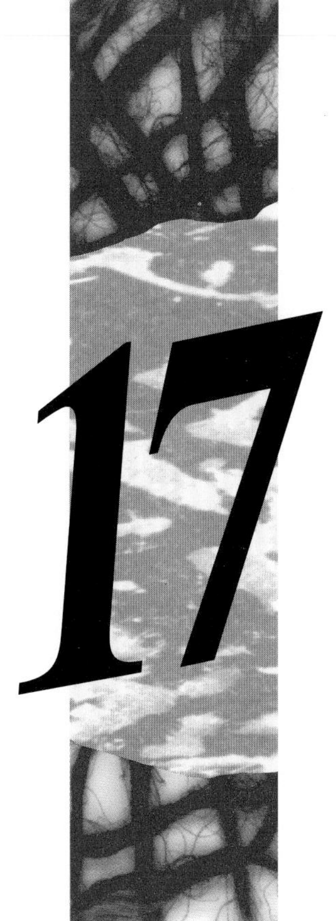

Ocular melanocytes, derived from the neural crest, are present in the eyelids, the conjunctiva, the uvea, and the pigment epithelium. Dermal melanocytes, conjunctival melanocytes, and uveal melanocytes tend to be solitary and dendritic. Pigment epithelial cells, however, form sheets of cuboidal cells which contain large easily visualized pigment granules; this is unlike the fine barely visualized dust-like melanin granules of the uveal melanocytes. While pigment epithelial cells readily undergo reactive proliferation, they rarely become neoplastic. Conversely, dermal, conjunctival, and uveal melanocytes almost never undergo reactive proliferation (except uveal melanocytes in patients who have occult carcinoma), but do give rise to neoplastic processes.

Medulloepitheliomas (previously called diktyomas) most commonly arise from the ciliary epithelium; they also may arise from pigment epithelium elsewhere, and even from the optic nerve. Medulloepitheliomas are tumors composed of elements that closely resemble the primitive medulloepithelium. They may be benign or malignant. The benign and the malignant forms may each contain heteroplastic elements (e.g., cartilage or brain-like tissue); in this case, they are called teratoid medulloepitheliomas.

In general, congenital pigmented ocular lesions fall into three categories: 1) ocular melanocytosis, 2) oculodermal melanocytosis (nevus of Ota), and 3) nevi. All three have a nevus component and may give rise in adulthood to melanomas. In ocular melanocytosis, the melanoma arises in the uveal tract. In oculodermal melanocytosis, the melanoma arises in the uveal tract or skin. Although oculodermal melanocytosis is most common in blacks and orientals, it rarely progresses to a melanoma except in whites. In nevi, the melanoma may arise in the skin, the conjunctiva, or the uvea. A rare congenital nevus involving the optic nerve head is called a melanocytoma or magnocellular nevus. Very rarely, this can give rise to a melanoma. Melanocytomas also may arise in the uveal tract.

Acquired pigmented tumors are unusual in ocular structures. Primary acquired melanosis (PAM) arises in the conjunctiva, generally during the patient's fifth and sixth decades. It may give rise to a melanoma. Adenomas and adenocarcinomas, both incidentally pigmented, may arise from the pigment epithelium of the ciliary body or iris. Fuchs adenoma arises from the nonpigmented ciliary epithelium of the pars plicata and is a reactive lesion rather than a neoplastic one (see Chapter 9). Melanoma of the uveal tract is the most common malignant primary intraocular tumor. Melanomas may arise from pre-existing nevi, as mentioned above, or may appear de novo.

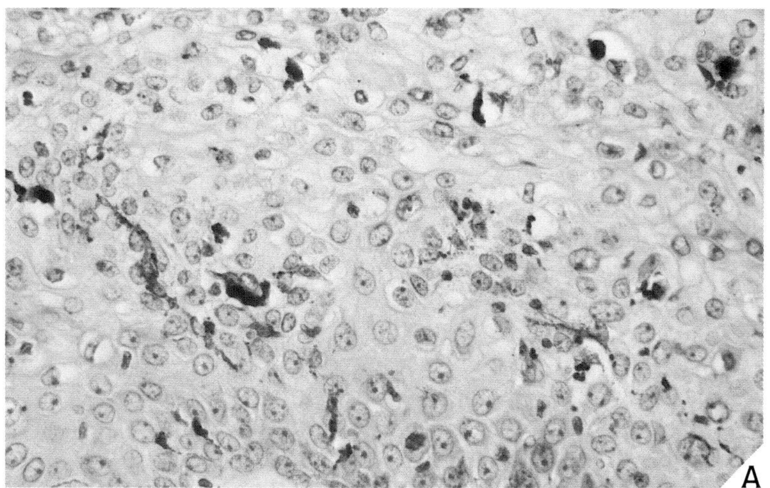

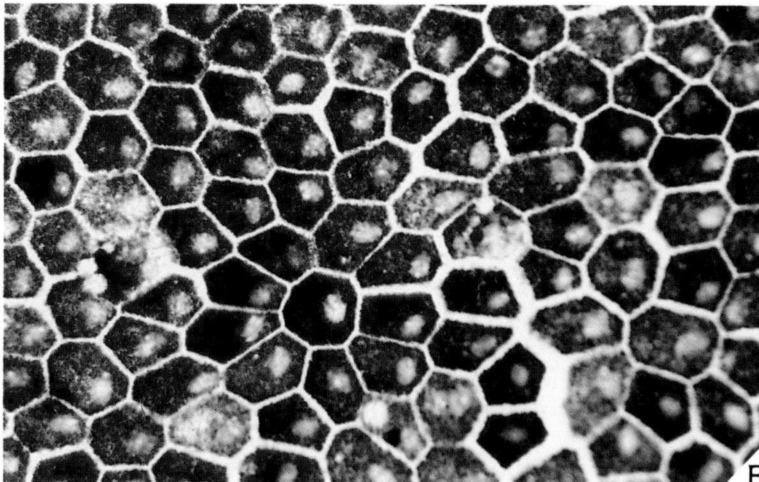

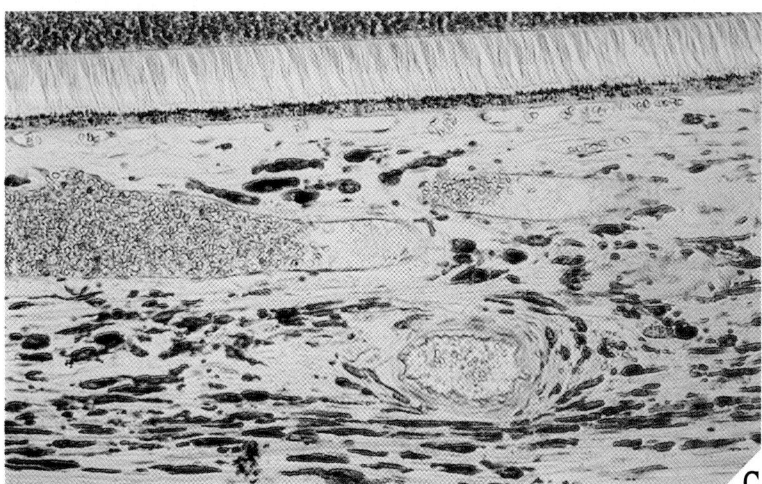

FIGURE 17.1 OCULAR MELANOCYTES. Normally, the epidermal melanocytes appear in hematoxylin and eosin-stained sections as clear cells wedged between basal epithelial cells. Melanin is transferred by the dendritic processes of the melanocytes to the basal keratocytes, where it is stored and later degraded. **A** In this tangential section of "reactive" epidermis, the usually clear melanocytes contain pigment around their nuclei and in their dendritic processes, making them easily visible (See Fig. 1.12C). **B** A flat preparation of retinal pigment epithelium (RPE) of owl monkey shows the epithelial sheet configuration. RPE cells have a basement membrane (inner or cuticular portion of the Bruch membrane) and are attached to one another near their apexes by terminal bars that contain "tight junctions." **C** Cross-section of the retina and choroid compares the epithelial nature of RPE with the nonepithelial individual and solitary choroidal melanocytes. The RPE cells have larger pigment granules than the choroidal melanocytes (see Fig. 9.2C).

CONGENITAL MELANOCYTIC LESIONS

Ocular melanocytosis

Oculodermal melanocytosis (nevus of Ota)

Nevi
Skin
Conjunctiva
Uvea

Medulloepithelioma

Melanocytoma (magnocellular nevus)

FIGURE 17.2

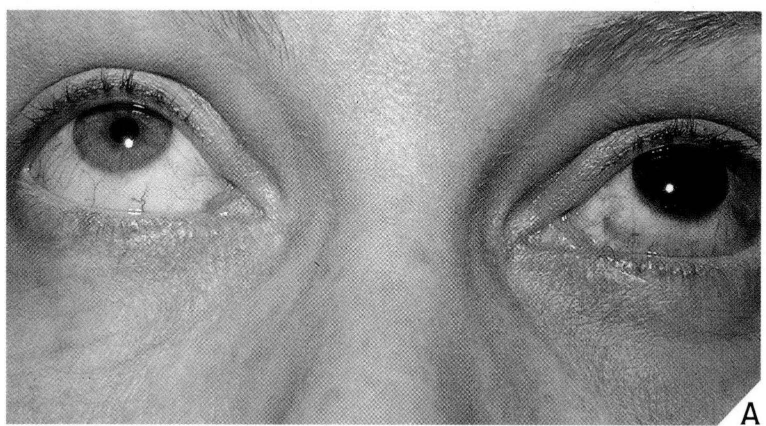

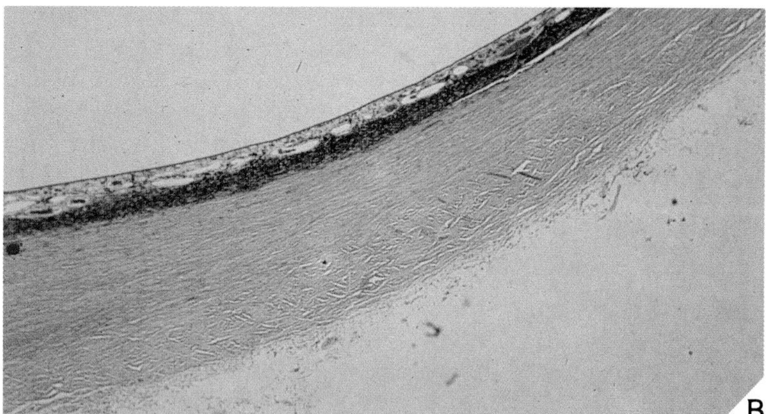

FIGURE 17.3 CONGENITAL OCULODERMAL MELANOCYTOSIS (NEVUS OF OTA). A The patient has heterochromia (the left iris is darker than the right) and increased pigmentation of the left eyelids and sclera. **B** The patient, from whom the eye illustrated here was removed because of secondary closed-angle glaucoma, had congenital ocular melanocytosis; this eye was the involved eye. The histologic section shows hyperpigmentation of the choroid, secondary to a diffuse maximally pigmented choroidal nevus characteristic of the uveal lesion in congenital ocular melanocytosis.

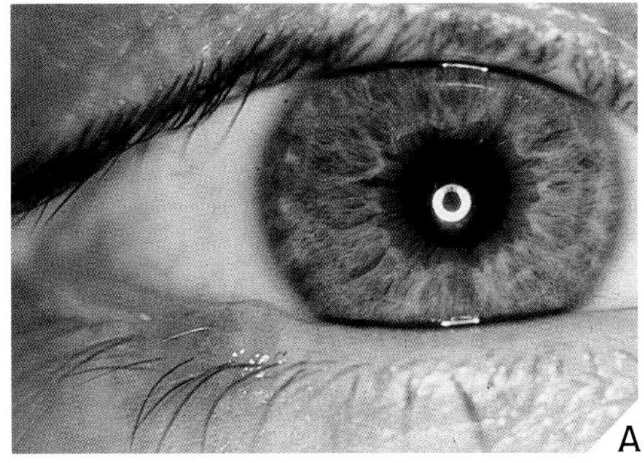

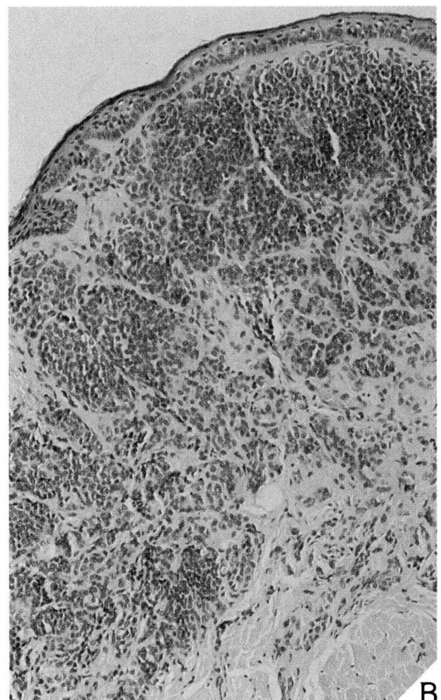

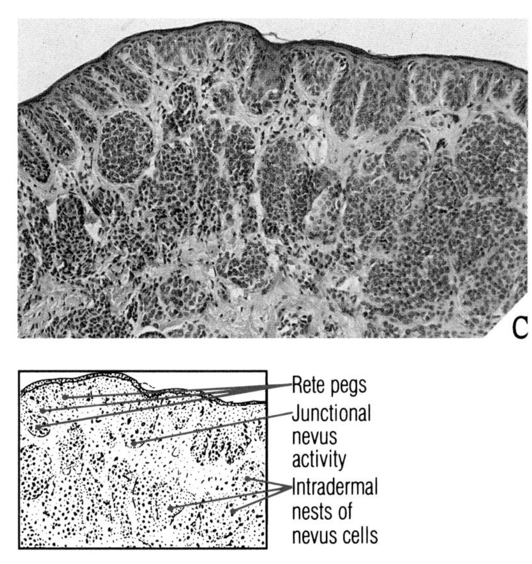

FIGURE 17.4 NEVUS OF SKIN. **A** A lightly pigmented lesion is present at the outer aspect of the right lower lid margin. **B** A histologic section shows that the nests of nevus cells are confined to the dermis, and so the lesion is called an intradermal nevus. The nevus cells have a tendency to become smaller the deeper they appear in the dermis (this is the normal polarity). Multiple lentigines (particularly of the head and neck) and blue nevi may be associated with Carney complex. **C** In another case, nests of nevus cells are present both within the dermis and in the junctional region between epidermis and dermis, thus forming a compound nevus. Rarely, nevus cells may be present only at the junctional region, producing a junctional nevus. Malignant melanomas appear to arise only from the junctional component. (**C**, from Yanoff M, Fine BS: *Ocular Pathology,* 2nd ed.)

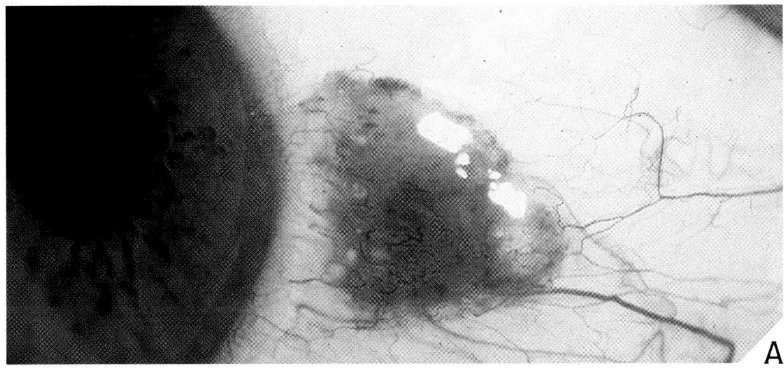

FIGURE 17.5 CONJUNCTIVAL NEVUS. **A** A conjunctival nevus near the limbus shows variable pigmentation and both small and large cystic structures. **B** A histologic section of another case shows nevus cells both in the junctional region between the epithelial and subepithelial tissue (the substantia propria) and in the subepithelial tissue, producing a compound nevus. As in the skin, the nevus cells tend to become smaller the deeper they are in the subepithelial tissue, representing the normal polarity of the nevus. **C** In addition to nevus cells, epithelial-lined cysts are present. These cysts are often found within the nevus and are part of the hamartomatous lesion. The cysts may be noted clinically, as seen in **A**. (**A**, from Yanoff M, Fine BS: *Ocular Pathology,* 2nd ed.)

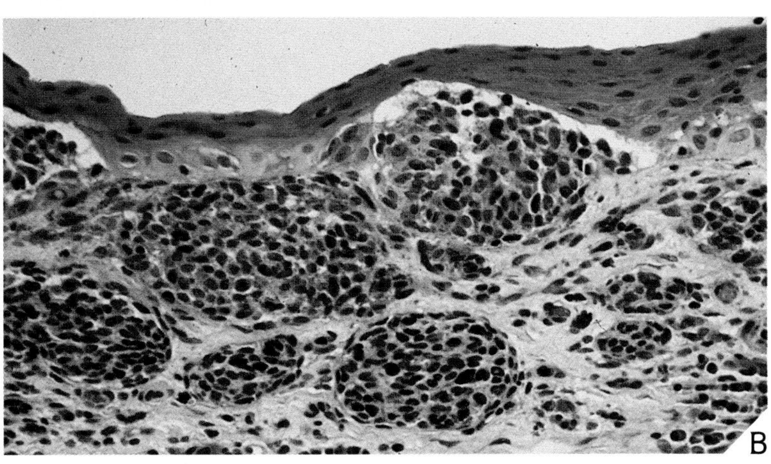

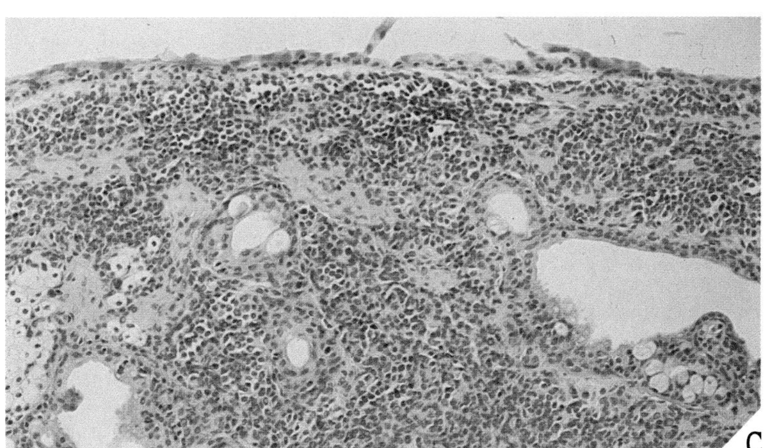

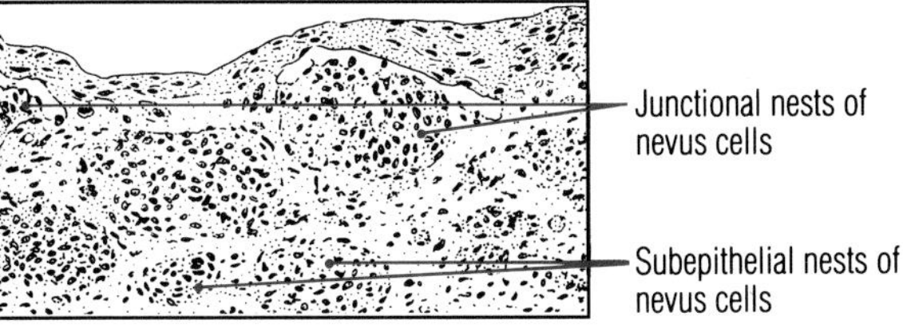

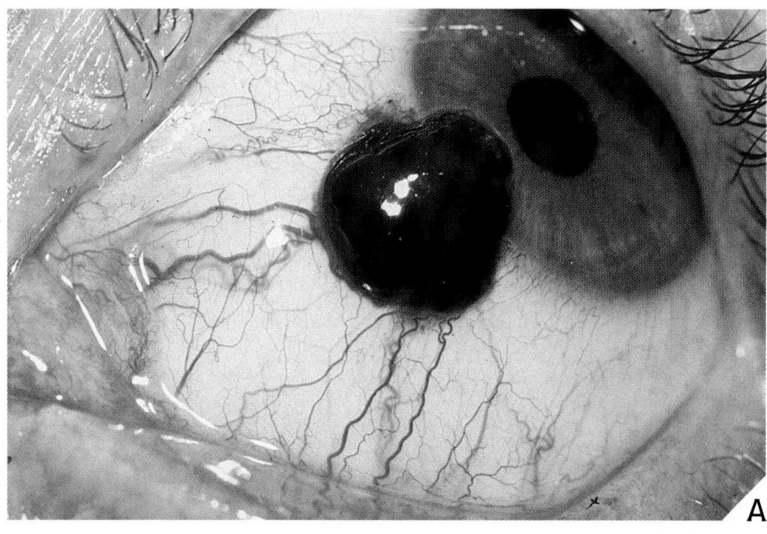

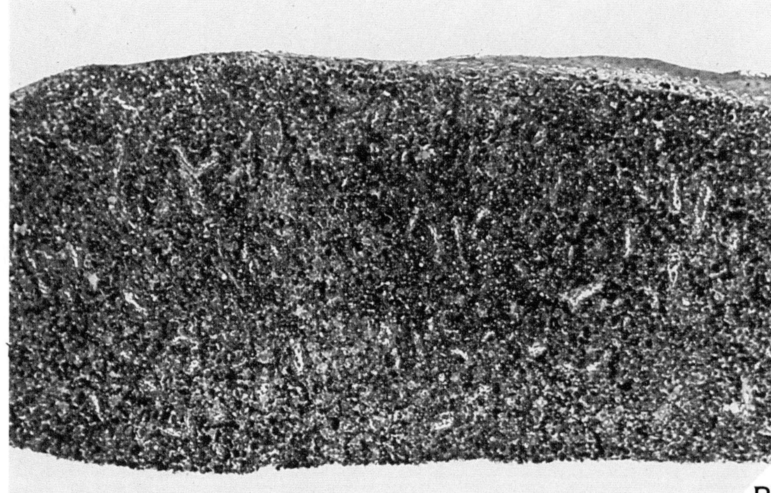

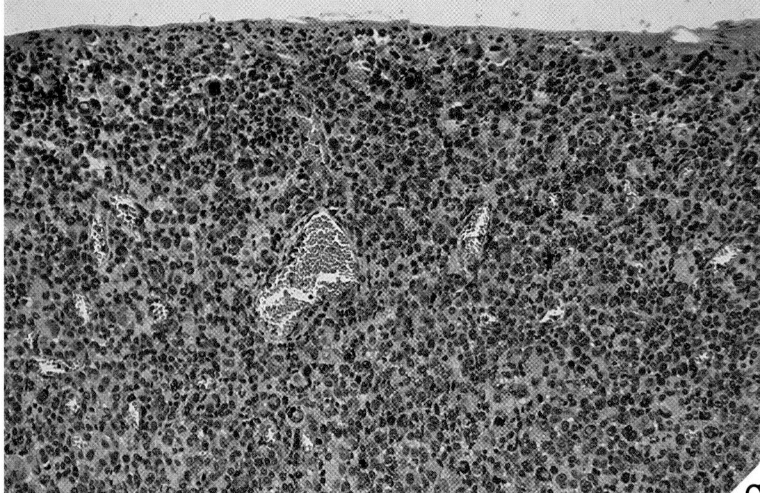

FIGURE 17.6 MALIGNANT MELANOMA. A A pigmented conjunctival lesion near the limbus, present since childhood, had undergone recent rapid growth. **B** A histological section of an incomplete excisional biopsy shows a heavily pigmented tumor. **C** A bleached section shows a loss of normal polarity, i.e., the cells deep in the lesion are of the same size as those nearer the surface instead of being smaller. Generally, conjunctival melanomas not thicker than 1.5 mm have an excellent prognosis, whereas those thicker than that tend to be fatal.

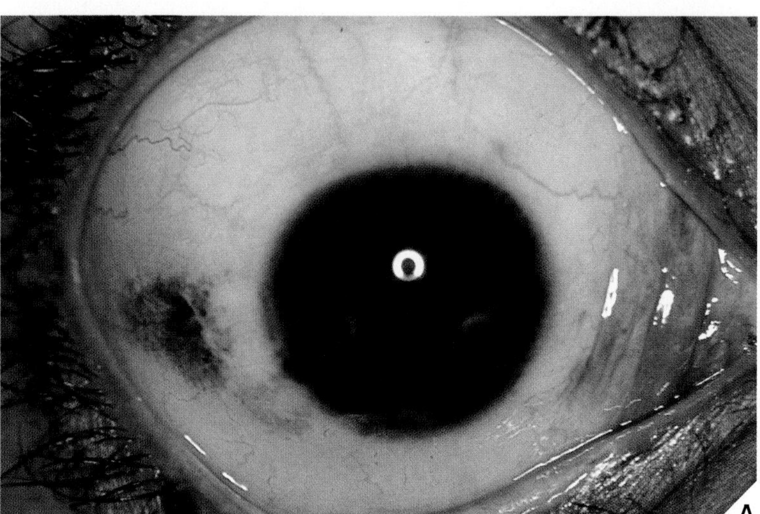

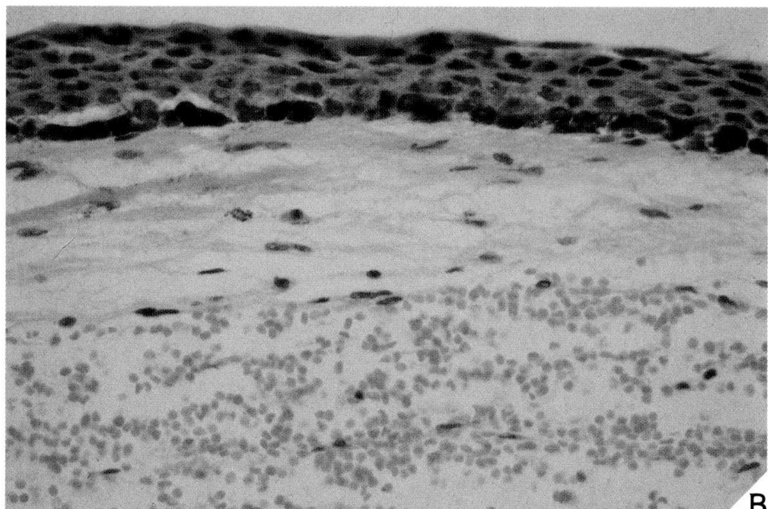

FIGURE 17.7 PRIMARY ACQUIRED MELANOSIS (PAM), BENIGN. A The patient noted pigmentation of the conjunctiva in adulthood. **B** A histological section of a biopsy of the lesion shows increased epithelial pigmentation, most marked in the basal layer but also scattered throughout the epithelial layers. Benign PAM may appear like this or may show benign pigmented nevus cells in the junctional position (see Fig. 17.8C).

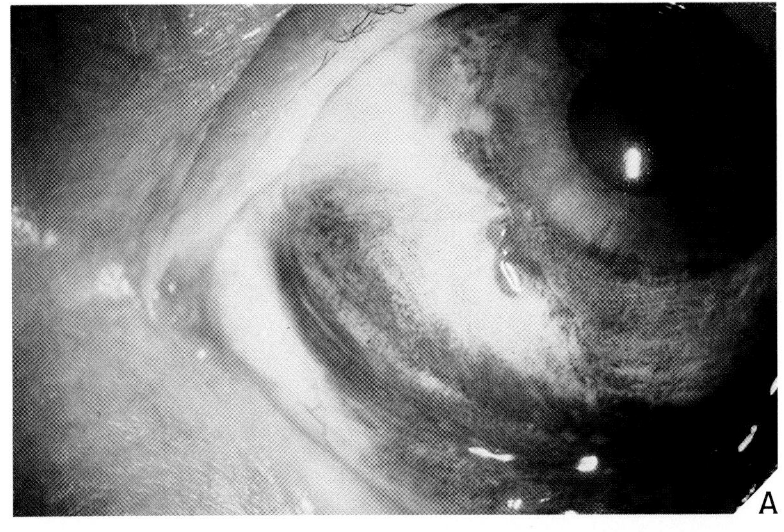

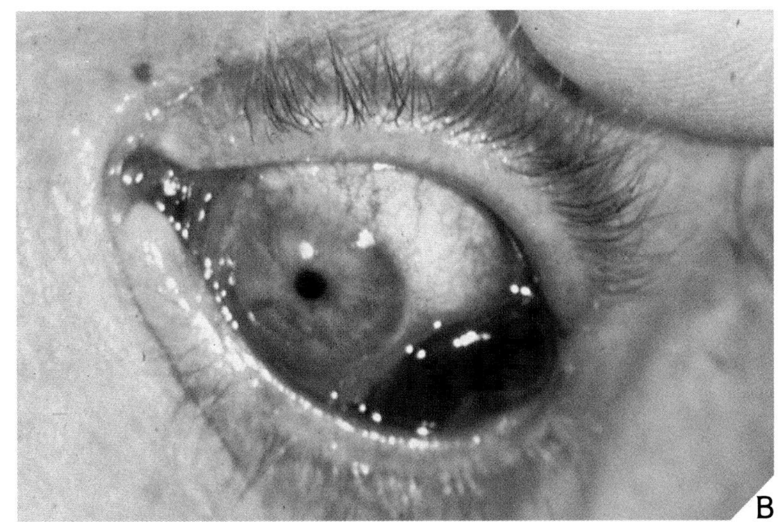

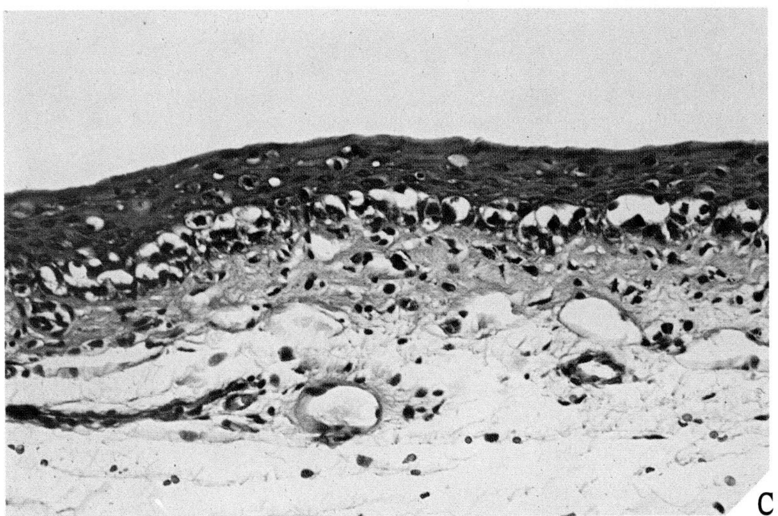

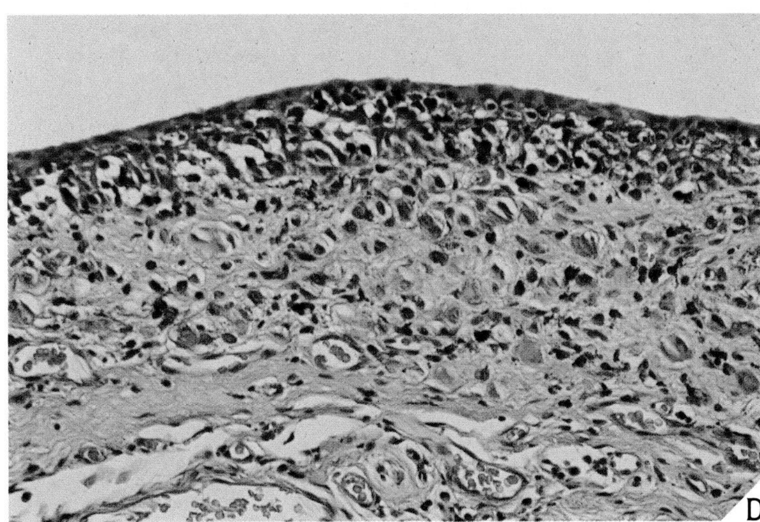

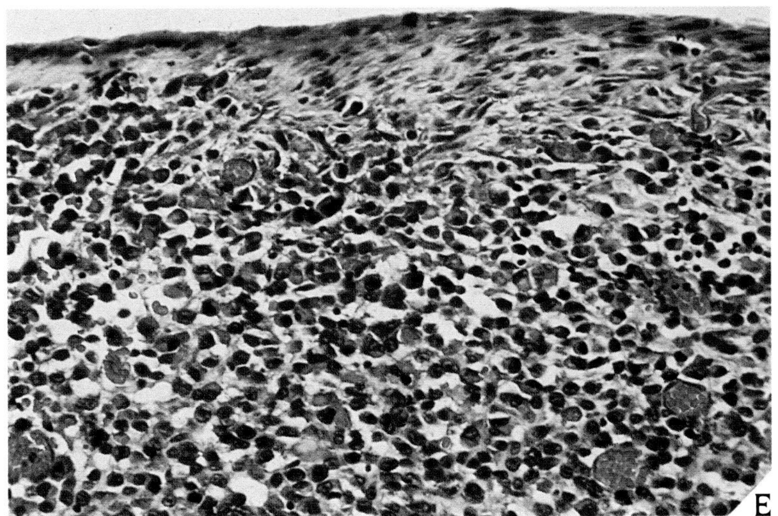

FIGURE 17.8 PRIMARY ACQUIRED MELANOSIS (PAM), CANCEROUS. **A** The patient developed unilateral conjunctival pigmentation in adulthood. The pigmentation was completely flat and also involved the peripheral cornea. As long as the pigmentation is flat, it is unlikely that a melanoma is present. **B** This patient also had adult-onset conjunctival pigmentation. A mass developed and an excisional biopsy was performed. **C** Some areas of the lesion showed benign PAM, as represented here by nests of nevus cells in the junctional position. **D** Other areas showed cancerous PAM (here at an early stage) with invasion of the superficial subepithelial tissue. **E** Still other areas showed frank malignant melanoma characterized by deep invasion of the subepithelial tissue. The cells are large and atypical; they show no tendency for maturation or for following the normal cell-size polarity demonstrated in earlier figures. (**B**, from Yanoff M, Fine BS: *Ocular Pathology,* 2nd ed.)

NONREACTIVE RETINAL PIGMENTAL EPITHELIAL TUMORS

Congenital
Glioneuroma
Medulloepithelioma (diktyoma)
Hypertrophy
Hyperplasia (hamartoma)

Acquired
Adenoma (see Fig. 17.16)
Adenocarcinoma

FIGURE 17.9

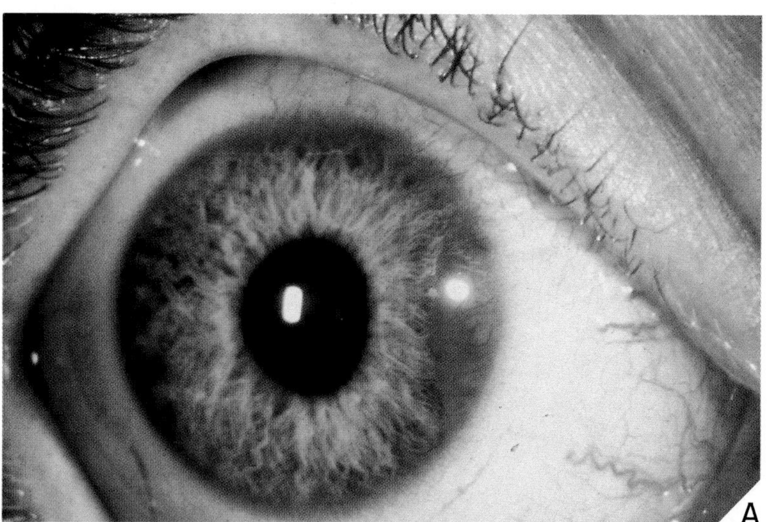

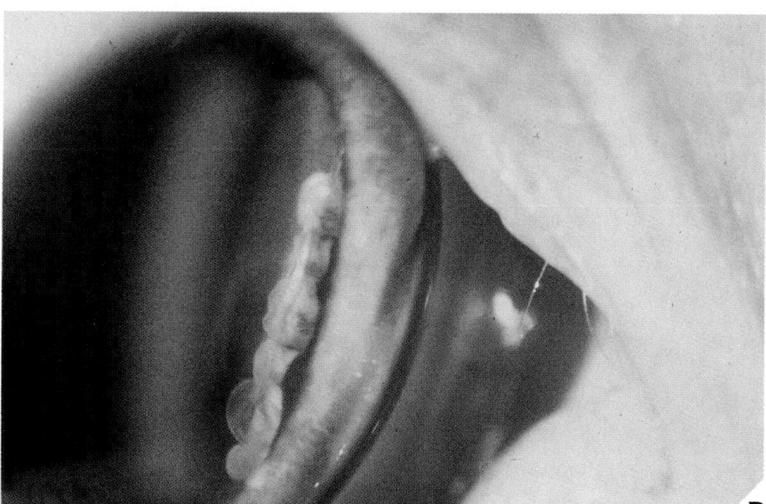

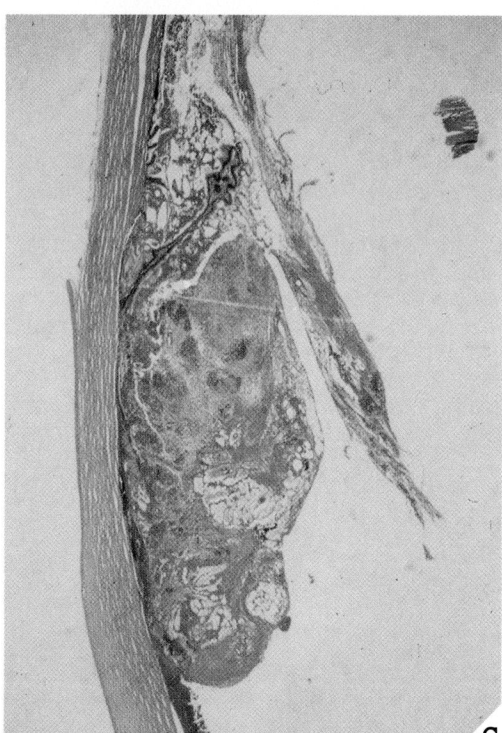

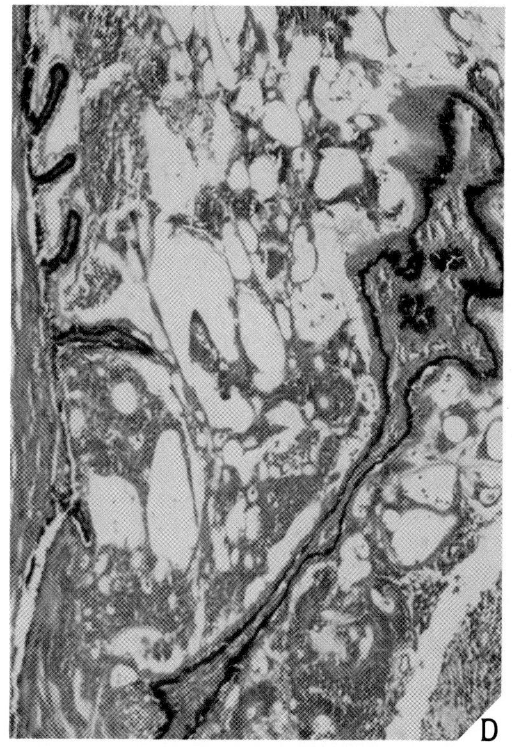

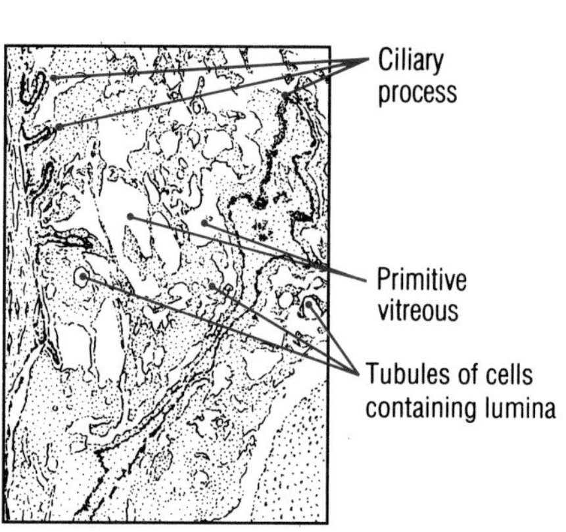

FIGURE 17.10 BENIGN MEDULLOEPITHELIOMA. A The tumor seen in the anterior chamber angle nasally had originated in the ciliary body, best seen in **B** (shown after pupillary dilatation). **C** A histologic section of another case shows structures that resemble primitive medullary epithelium, ciliary epithelium, and retina. The tumor arises from nonpigmented ciliary epithelium. **D** Increased magnification shows the cell tubules. Structures analogous to external limiting membranes of the retina appear on one surface of the tubules (in some areas forming lumina), while the less well defined opposite surface is in contact with a primitive vitreous. (**A, B**, courtesy of Dr. JA Shields; **C, D**, courtesy of Dr. JS McGavic.)

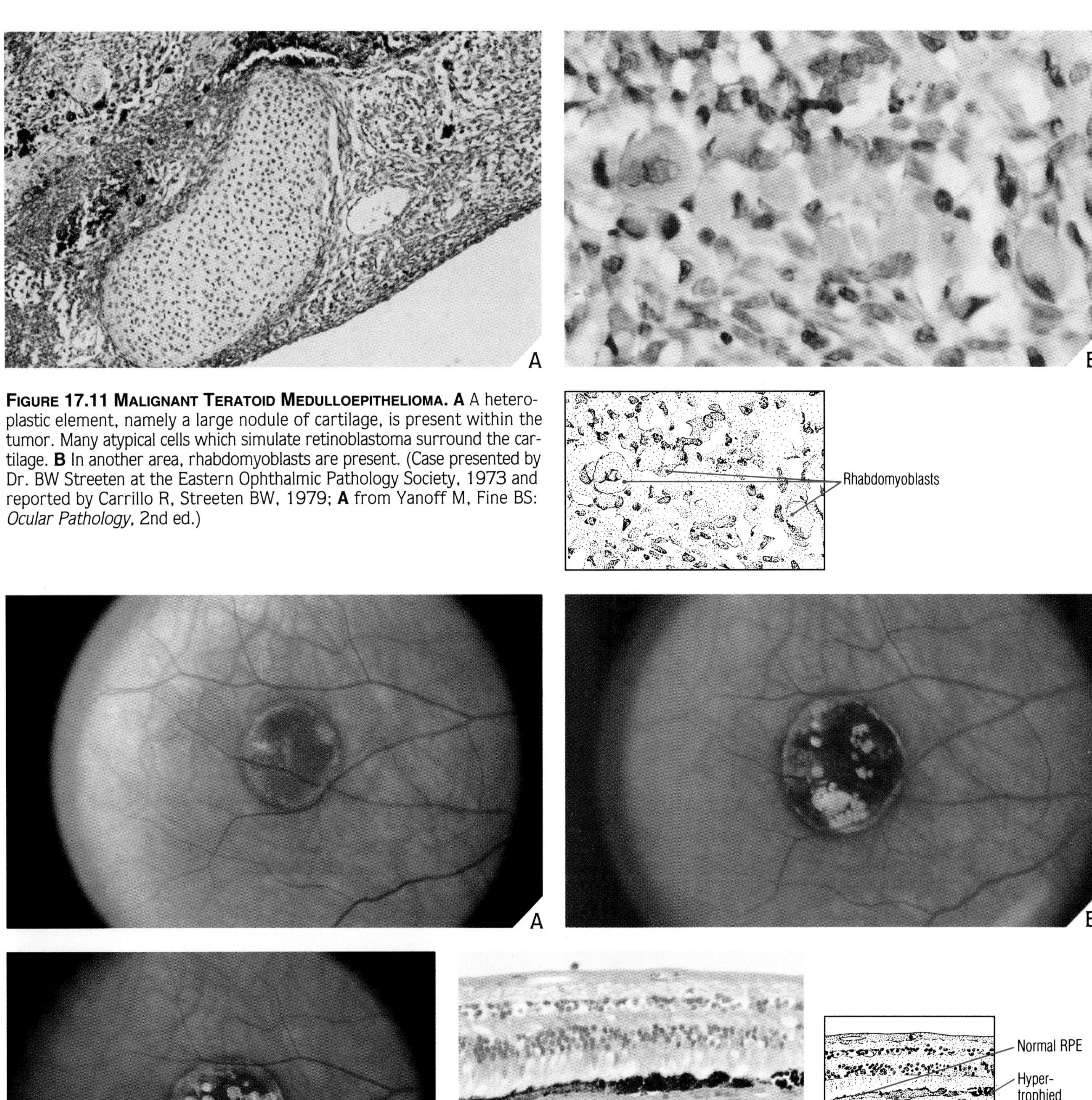

FIGURE 17.11 MALIGNANT TERATOID MEDULLOEPITHELIOMA. A A heteroplastic element, namely a large nodule of cartilage, is present within the tumor. Many atypical cells which simulate retinoblastoma surround the cartilage. **B** In another area, rhabdomyoblasts are present. (Case presented by Dr. BW Streeten at the Eastern Ophthalmic Pathology Society, 1973 and reported by Carrillo R, Streeten BW, 1979; **A** from Yanoff M, Fine BS: *Ocular Pathology,* 2nd ed.)

FIGURE 17.12 RETINAL PIGMENT EPITHELIAL HYPERTROPHY. A The characteristic jet-black lesion, surrounded by a halo, contains yellow patches of irregular size and shape. **B** The same lesion, six years later, has increased in size and changed in appearance. **C** After 12 years, most of the lesion is occupied by large yellow lacunae. **D** A histologic section of another case shows a sudden transition from normal retinal pigment epithelium (RPE) on the left to markedly enlarged cells. The enlarged cells contain enlarged pigment granules (called macromelanosomes). Often, at the edge of such a lesion the RPE cells are depigmented, giving rise to the halo seen clinically around the lesion. Congenital hypertrophy of the RPE may be found in familial adenomatous polyposis (Gardner or Turcot syndromes). (**C**, presented by Dr. WR Lee at the European Ophthalmic Pathology Society, 1982.)

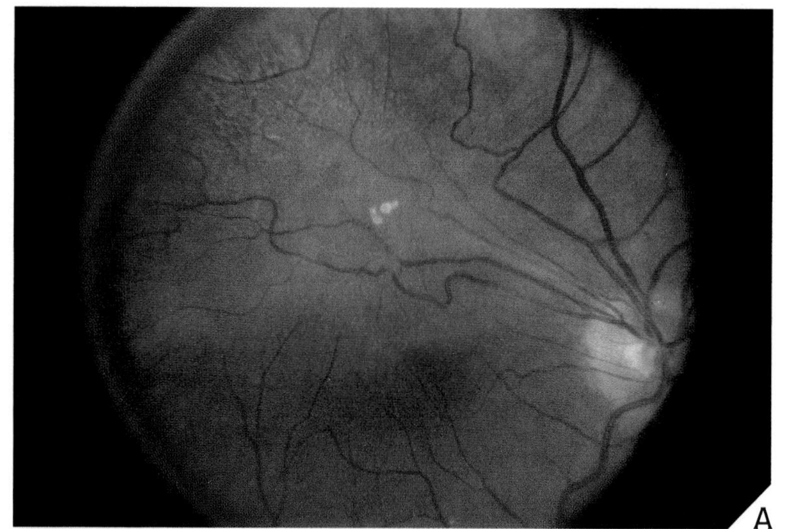

FIGURE 17.13 HAMARTOMA OF THE RETINAL PIGMENT EPITHELIUM. **A** A 23-year-old nurse had esotropia of the right eye since childhood. Examination shows a thickened retina superior to the fovea. A few specks of what appears to be calcium are present in the lesion. **B** Fluorescein angiography shows a highly vascularized lesion which contains abnormal blood vessels. **C** A histologic section of another case shows that the RPE has proliferated into the retina in the juxtapapillary area. Both proliferating pigmented cells and abnormal retinal blood vessels are seen. **D** In another area, an abnormal extension of the outer nuclear layer reaches into the outer plexiform layer, along with abnormally located small blood vessels. (**C, D**, courtesy of Dr. E Howes, reported by Vogel MH, et al., 1969.)

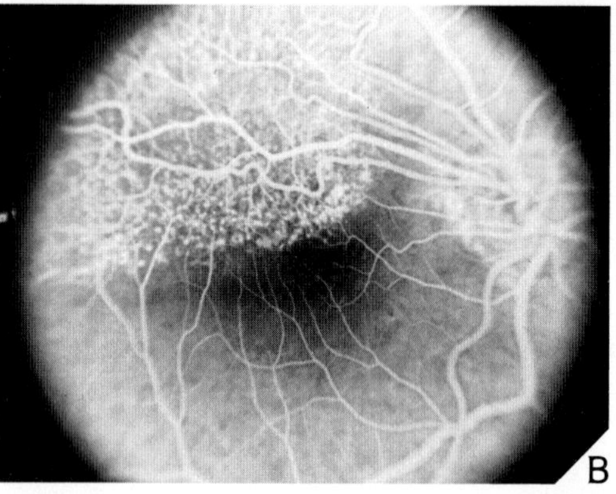

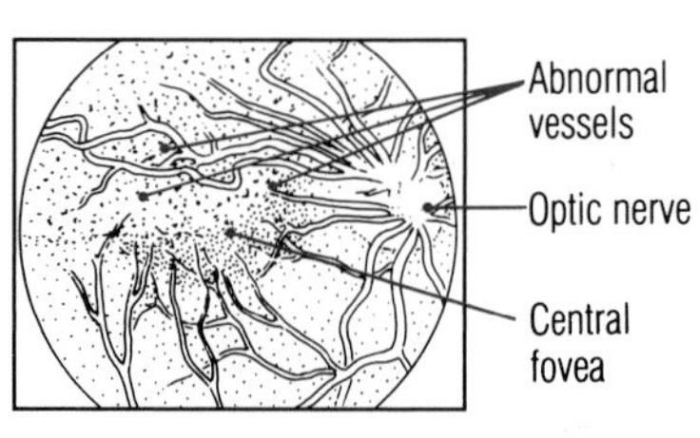

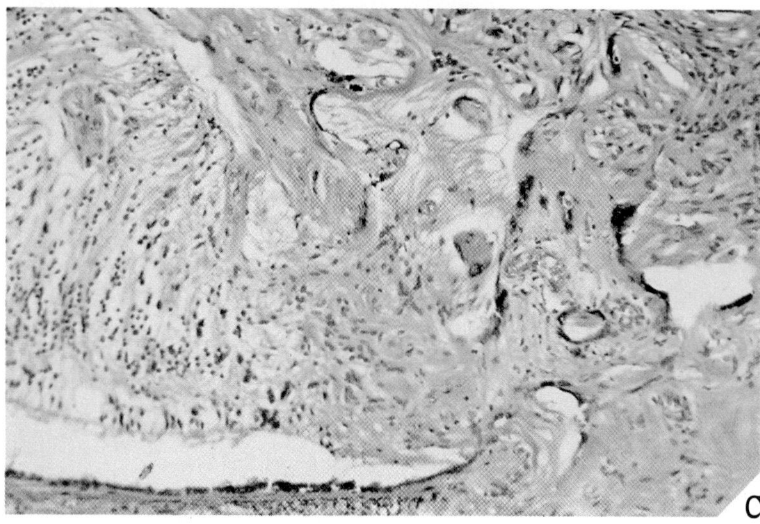

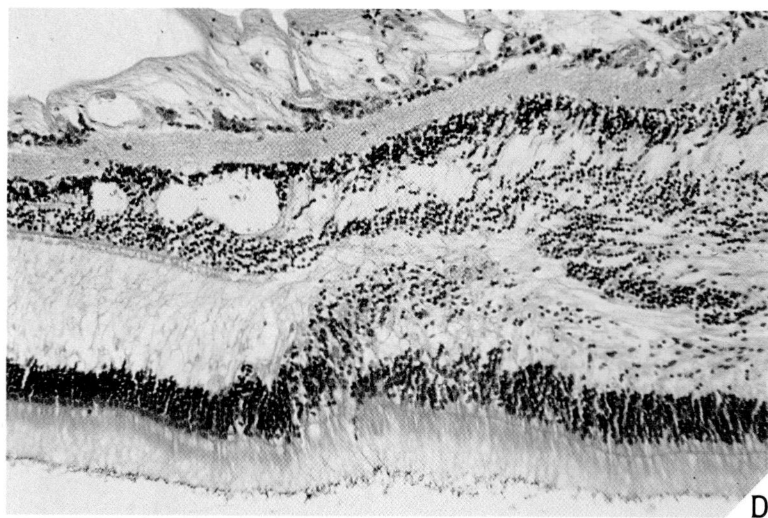

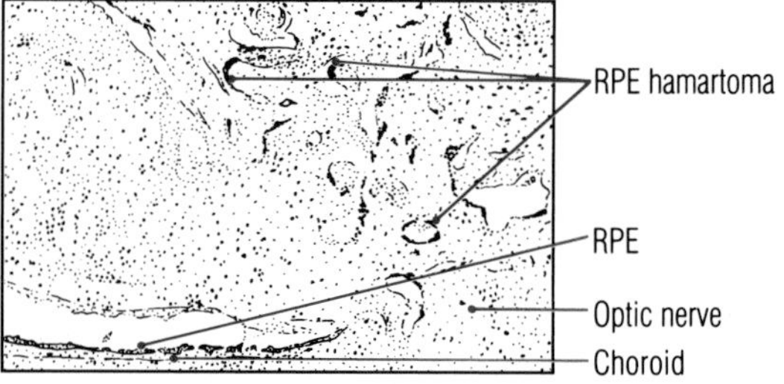

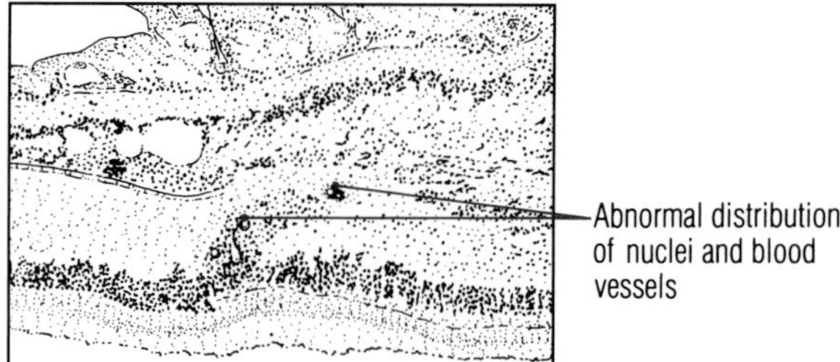

RPE REACTIVE LESIONS

Drusen (see Chapter 11)
Migration (e.g., in retinitis pigmentosa)
Hyperplasia
Metaplasia (fibrous and perhaps osseous)

FIGURE 17.14

UVEAL TUMORS

Congenital ocular (and oculodermal) melanocytosis
Nevus
Melanoma

FIGURE 17.15

FIGURE 17.16 NEVUS AND ADENOMA. A A round pigmented nevus is present in the fundus. The nevus contains scattered drusen on its surface superiorly. Nevi are quite common, being found in the ciliary body and choroid in at least one eye in about 30% of patients. **B** A histologic section from another case shows two benign lesions, an adenoma which arises from the ciliary epithelium, and a nevus of the choroid. **C** Increased magnification of the nevus shows plump polyhedral nevus cells along with slender spindle-like nevus cells. The sparing of the choriocapillaris is characteristic. **D** The adenoma has a papillary appearance. The tumor is composed of chords of predominantly nonpigmented epithelial cells, but some pigmented cells also are present. **E** Alcian-blue stain, for acid mucopolysaccharides, shows a positive reaction. The blue color was not observed when the unstained sections were treated with hyaluronidase prior to alcian-blue staining, signifying that the material is hyaluronic acid ("vitreous").

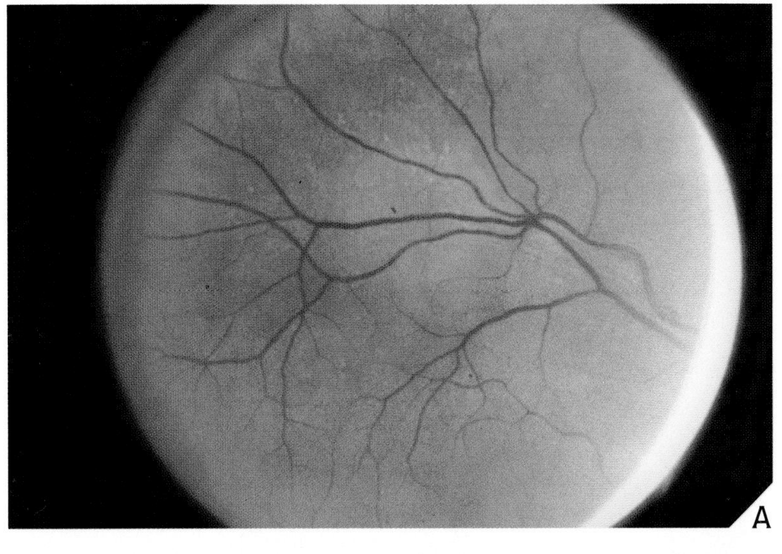

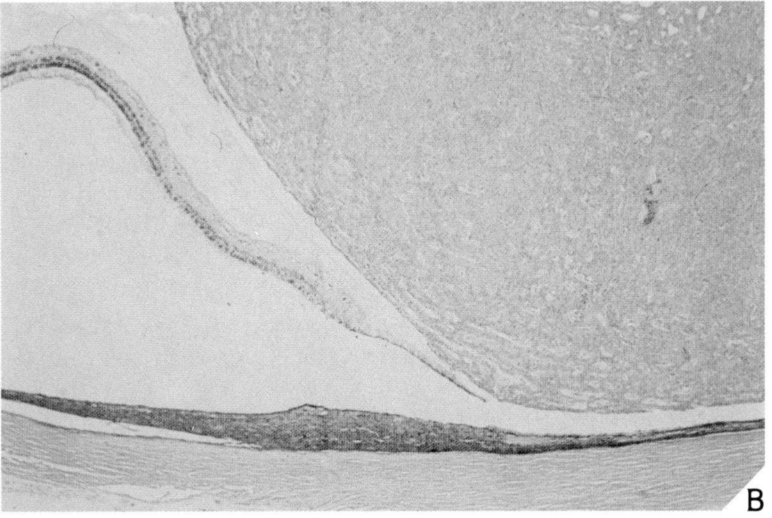

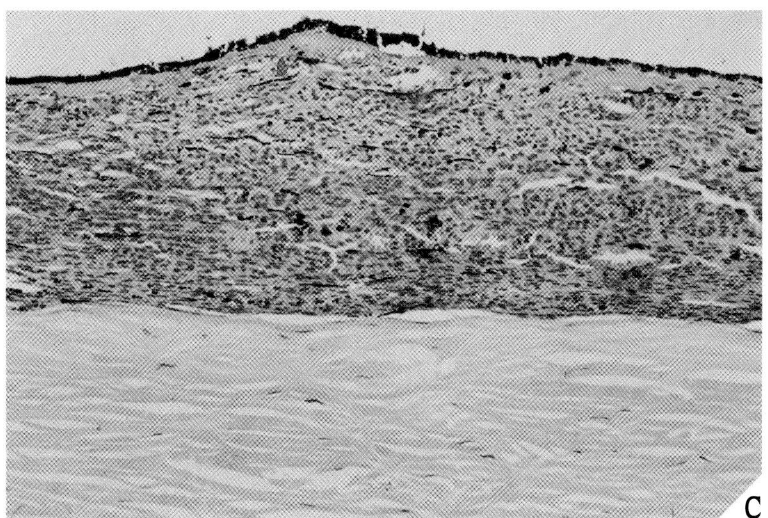

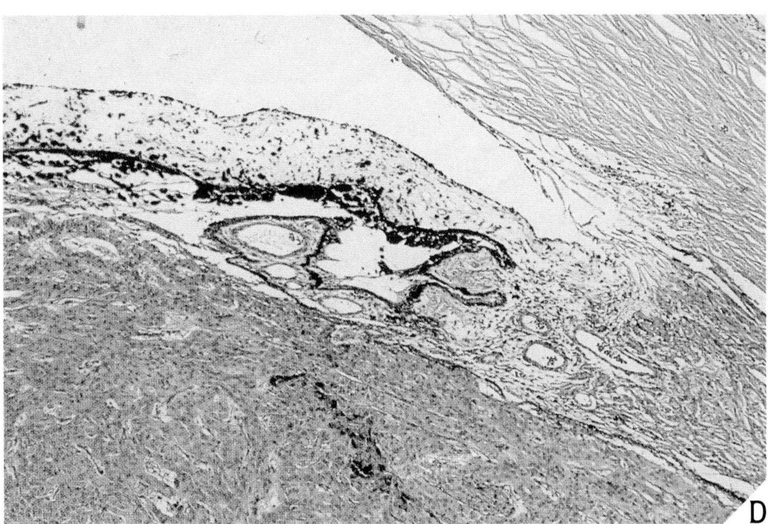

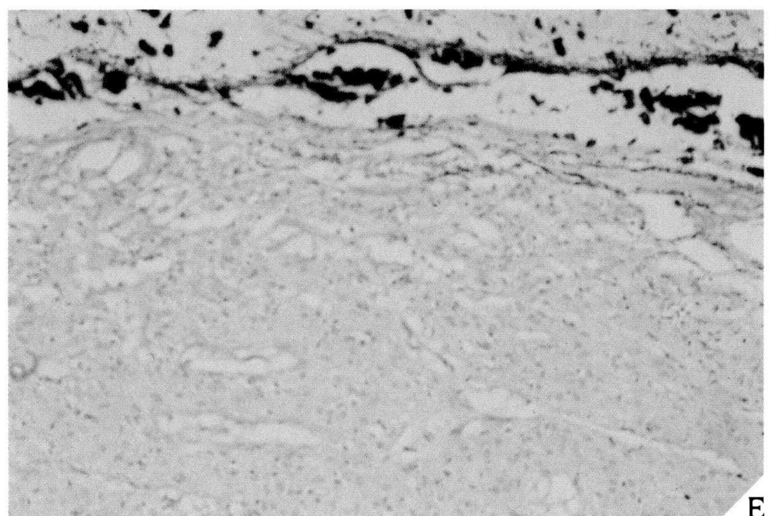

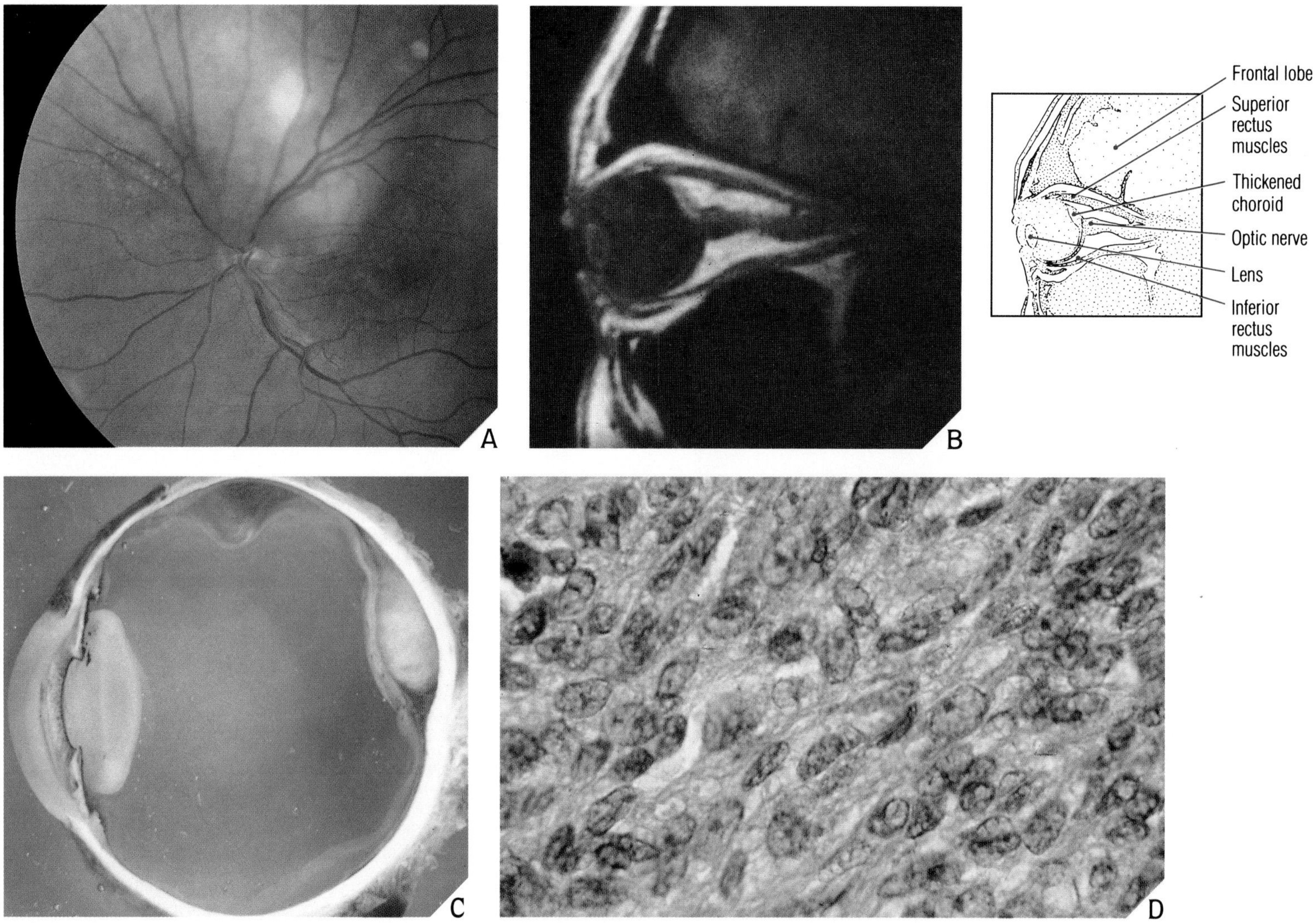

Frontal lobe
Superior rectus muscles
Thickened choroid
Optic nerve
Lens
Inferior rectus muscles

FIGURE 17.17 CHOROIDAL MALIGNANT MELANOMA. A The patient had a slowly enlarging choroidal tumor which was followed for over a 9-year period. **B** Magnetic resonance imaging (mainly T_1) shows the choroidal tumor just above the optic nerve. Mainly T_2-imaging showed that the tumor became less white, characteristic of a malignant melanoma (a hemangioma of the choroid, for example, becomes whiter with T_2-imaging). **C** The enucleated eye shows the gross appearance of the tumor. **D** A histologic section demonstrates a malignant melanoma of the spindle-B type.

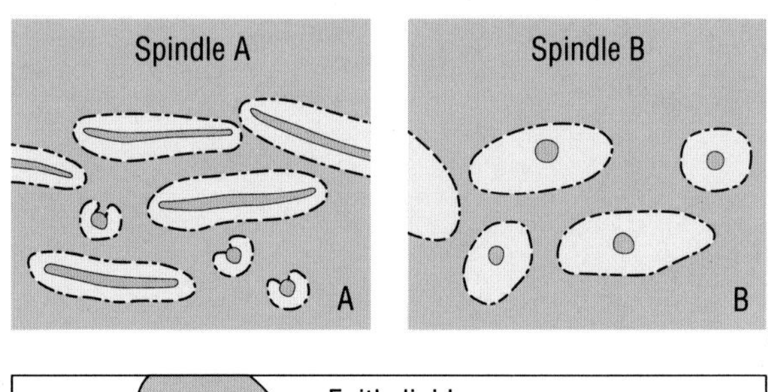

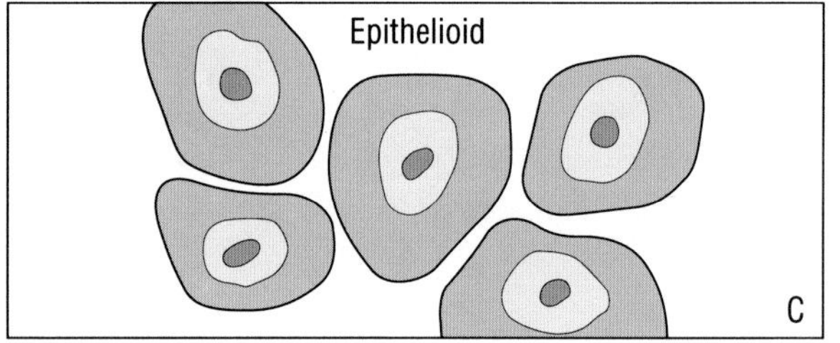

FIGURE 17.18 UVEAL MELANOMA CELL TYPES. A Spindle A cells are shown in longitudinal and transverse cross-sections. The cells are cohesive and have poorly defined cell borders. The nuclei contain nuclear folds that appear as dark stripes parallel to the long axis of the nuclei. The stripe is caused by an infolding of the nucleus, as noted in cross-section. **B** Spindle B nuclei are larger and plumper than spindle A nuclei and contain prominent nucleoli rather than nuclear folds. The cells, similar to spindle A, are cohesive and have poorly defined cell borders. **C** Epithelioid cells are not cohesive, have distinct cell borders, and show large oval nuclei which contain prominent nucleoli. The cells are larger than spindle A and spindle B cells.

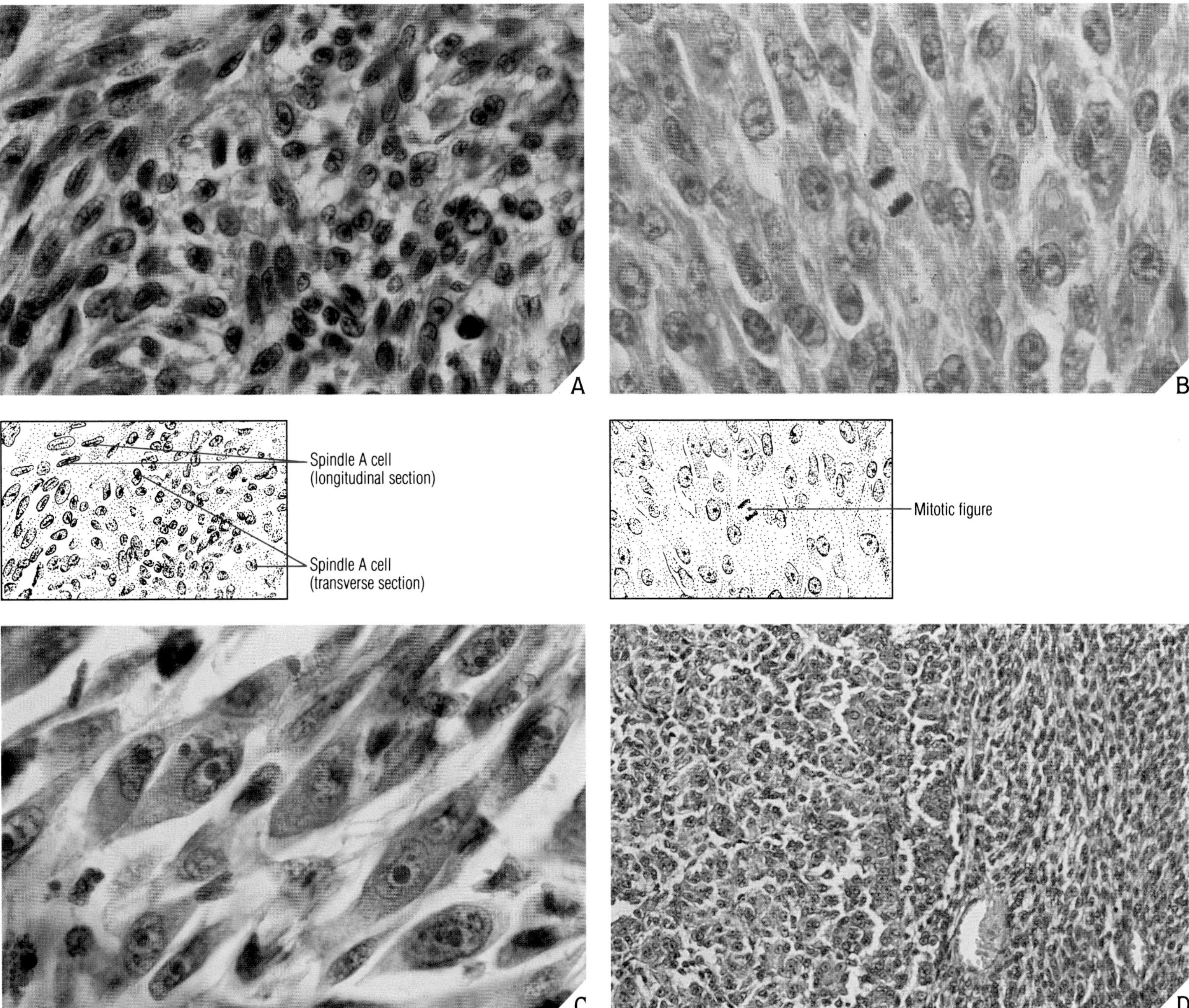

Figure 17.19 Uveal Melanoma Cells. A Spindle-A cells, identified by a dark stripe parallel to the long axis of the nucleus, are seen in longitudinal section. They are identified in transverse cross-section by the infolding of the nuclear membrane that causes the dark stripe. **B** Spindle B cells are identified by their prominent nucleoli. Note the mitotic figure. Both spindle A and spindle B cells tend to be quite cohesive and have poorly defined cell borders. **C** Epithelioid cells are the largest of the melanoma cells, tend not to be cohesive, and have irregular shapes and sizes as well as very prominent nucleoli within the large nuclei. **D** Some melanomas contain a mixture of spindle cells and epithelioid cells. The left half of this figure is occupied by epithelioid cells and the right half by spindle cells (this is called a mixed-cell type melanoma).

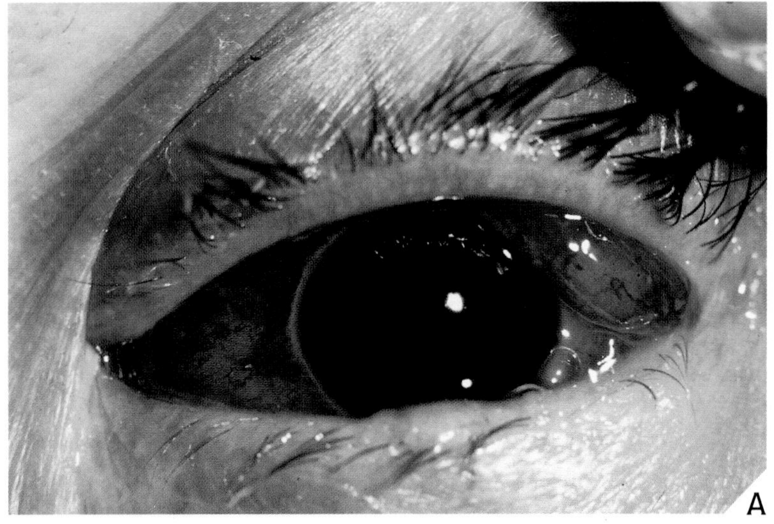
A

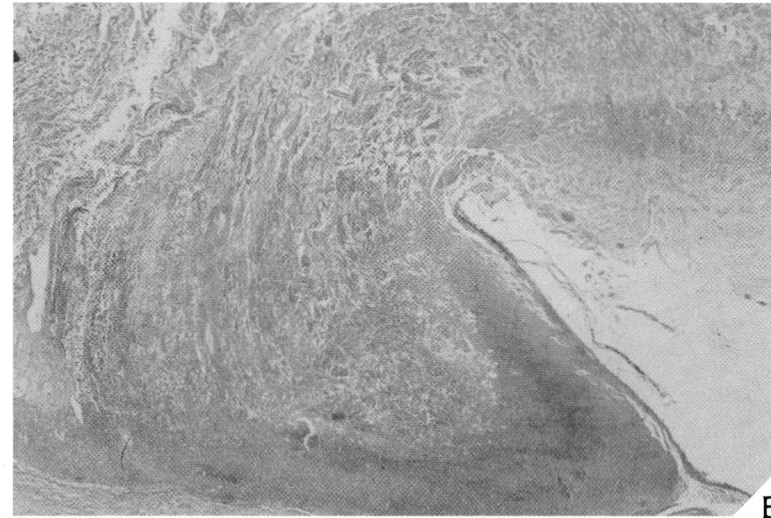
B

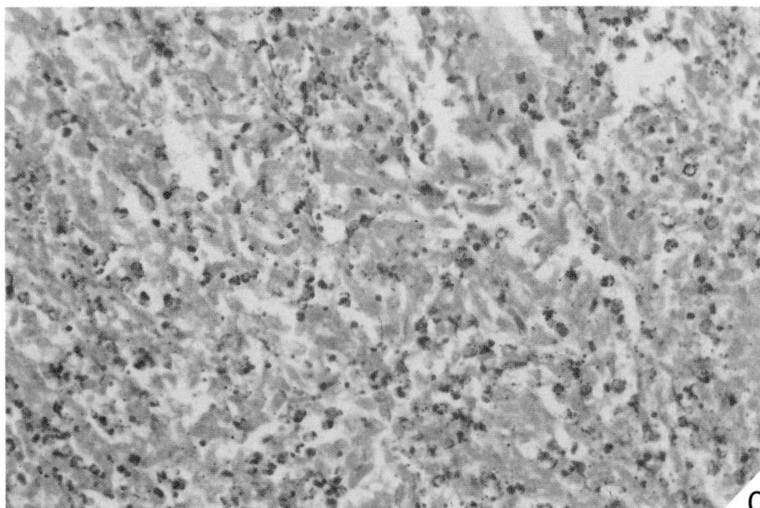
C

FIGURE 17.20 NECROTIC UVEAL MELANOMA. A The patient presented with recent onset of blindness, pain, redness, and chemosis. Examination by ultrasonography showed a solid tumor. The eye was enucleated. **B** A histologic section shows that the typical "mushroom" tumor had undergone spontaneous necrosis, making identification of the melanoma cell type almost impossible. This type, shown with increased magnification in **C**, is therefore called the necrotic-cell type melanoma. Completely necrotic melanomas often present clinically, as this patient's did, with the appearance of inflammation.

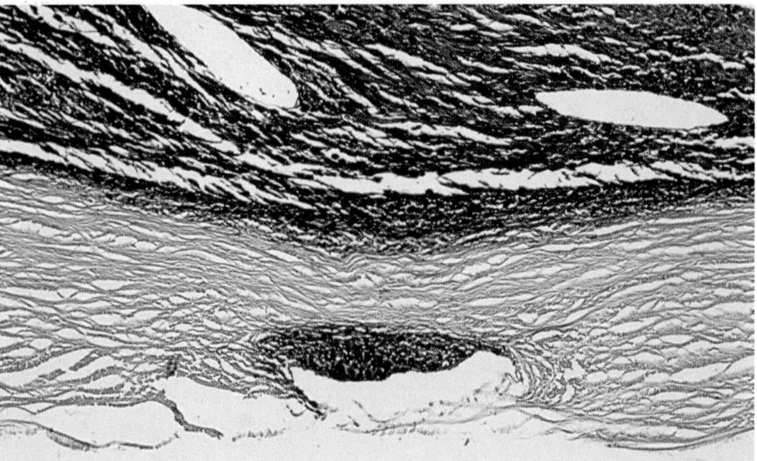

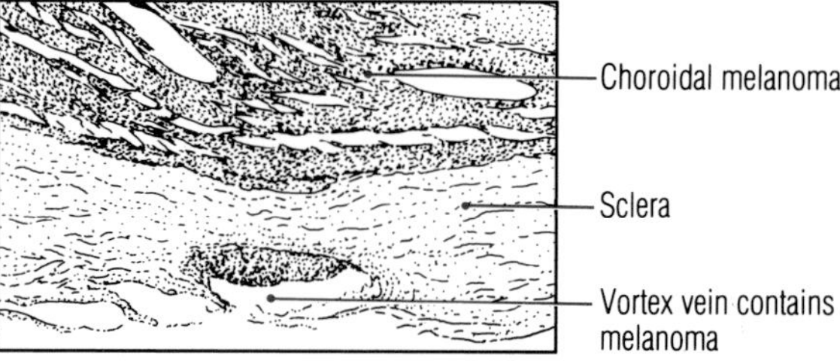

FIGURE 17.21 VORTEX VEIN INVASION. A large pigmented choroidal melanoma is present within the eye and is filling most of an intrascleral vortex vein. Obviously, vortex vein invasion, like extraocular extension into the orbit, carries a life-threatening prognosis. (From Yanoff M, Fine BS: *Ocular Pathology*, 2nd ed.)

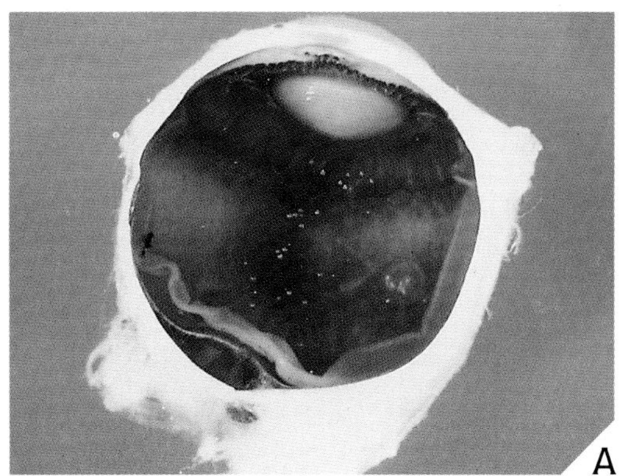

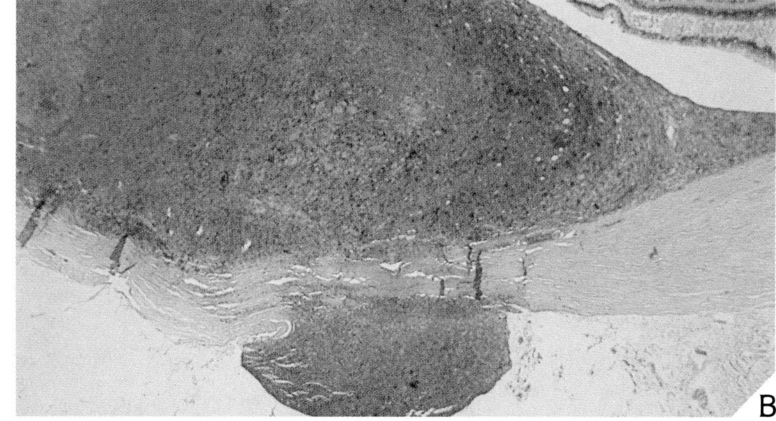

FIGURE 17.22 EXTRAOCULAR EXTENSION. A Note the oval pigmented melanoma of the choroid within the eye and the small pigmented lesion on the surface of the sclera. **B** A histologic section shows the uveal melanoma within the eye and a nodule of extrascleral extension.

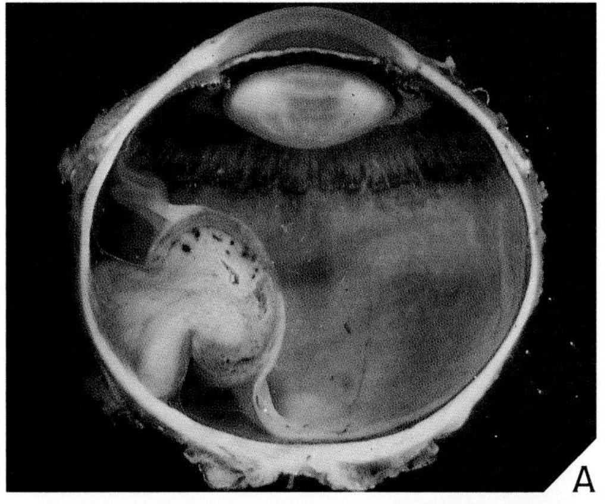

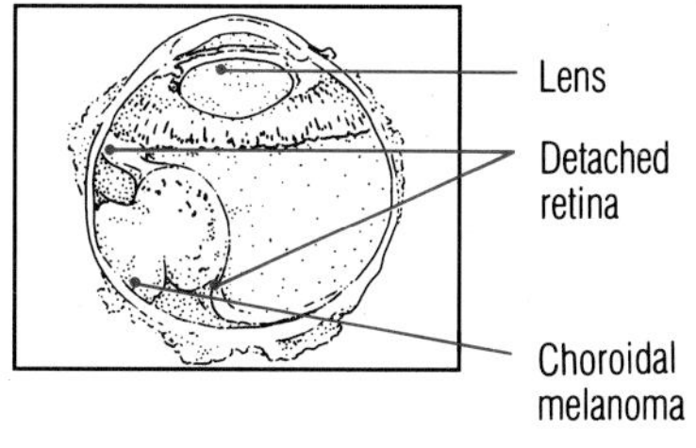

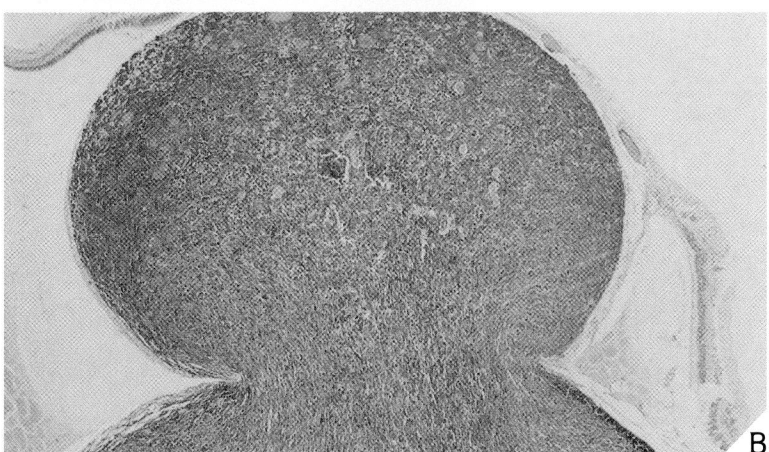

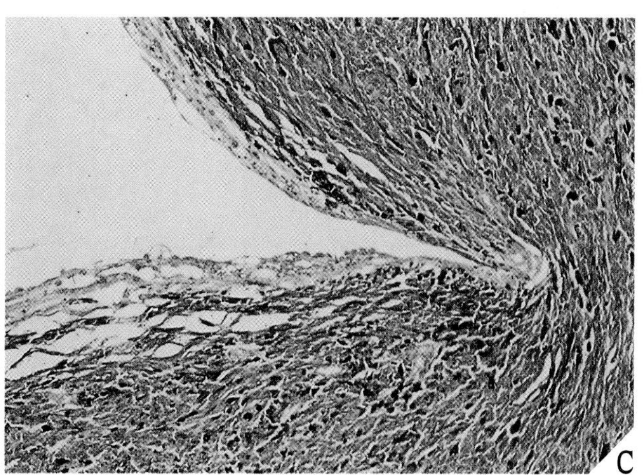

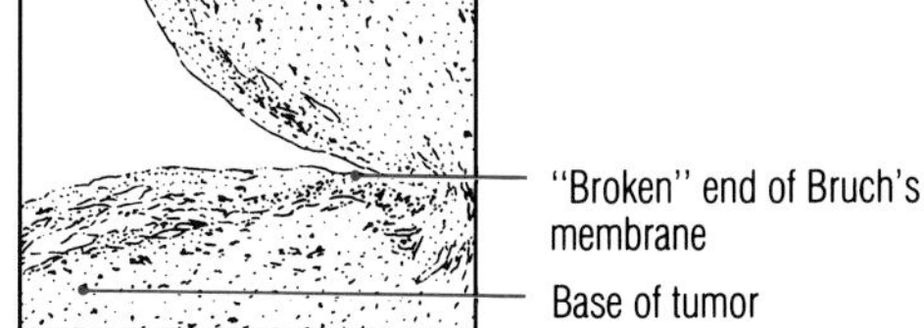

FIGURE 17.23 UVEAL "MUSHROOM" MELANOMA. A The melanoma has ruptured through the Bruch membrane, causing a mushroom configuration. The elastic Bruch membrane remains around the base of the mushroom, acting as a tourniquet. Arteriolar blood gains access to the head of the mushroom, but venous blood has difficulty leaving, giving rise to dilated and engorged blood vessels in the head of the mushroom, as shown here. **B** A histologic section shows the ruptured ends of the Bruch membrane (seen with increased magnification in **C**) and the dilated engorged blood vessels in the head of the tumor. (**A**, courtesy of Dr. RC Eagle Jr.)

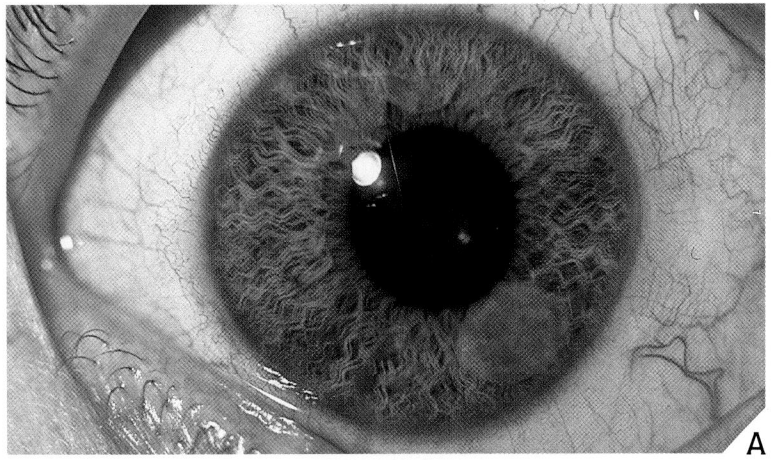

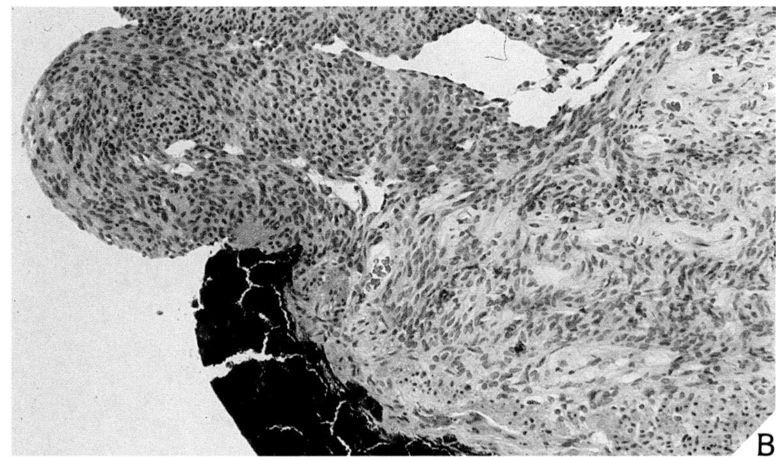

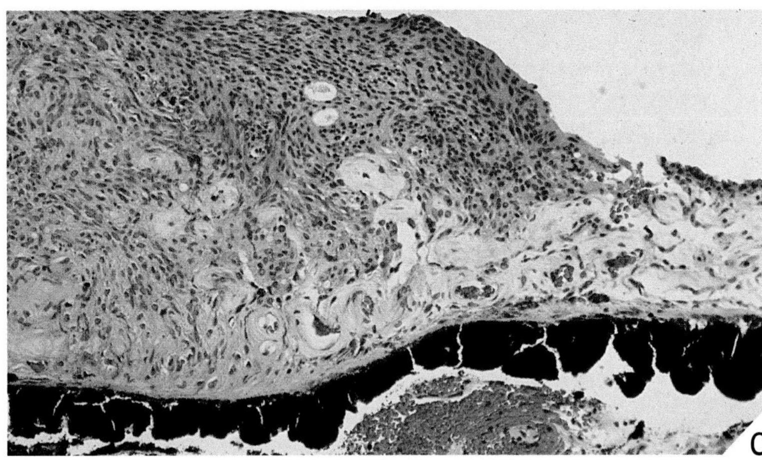

FIGURE 17.24 IRIS MELANOMA. A A lightly pigmented vascularized tumor is present in the iris inferonasally. The tumor has caused some blunting of the pupillary border in that region. **B** A histologic section shows spindle melanoma cells "spilling" over the pupillary border. **C** The cells invade the stroma of the iris. Often, as in this case, the spindle-cells appear different from ciliary body and choroidal spindle-A and -B cells; they seem to be more benign and often are classified as spindle-cell nevae rather than melanoma.

MELANOCYTOMA (MAGNOCELLULAR NEVUS)

FIGURE 17.25

Optic nerve head — Uvea

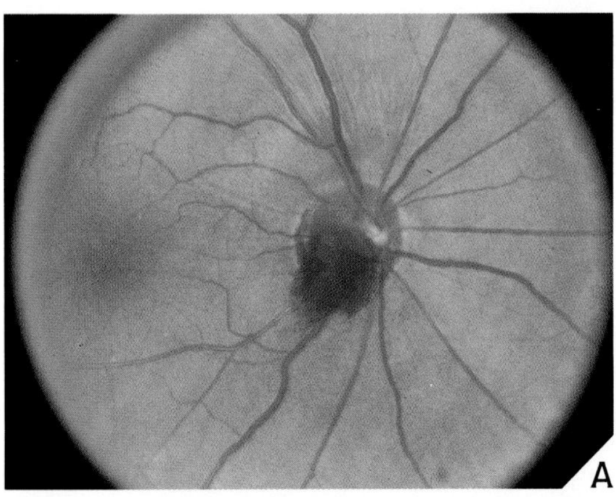

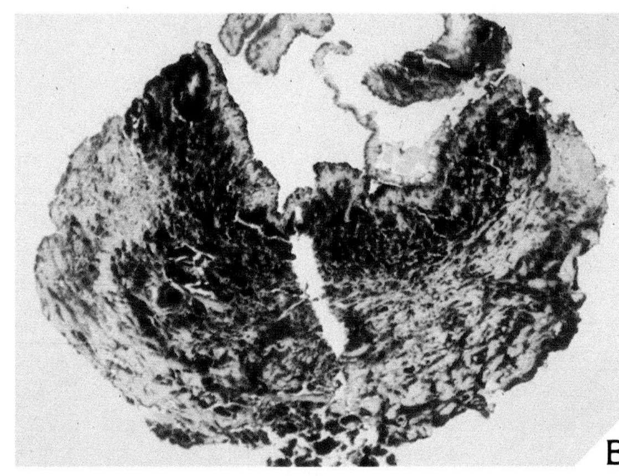

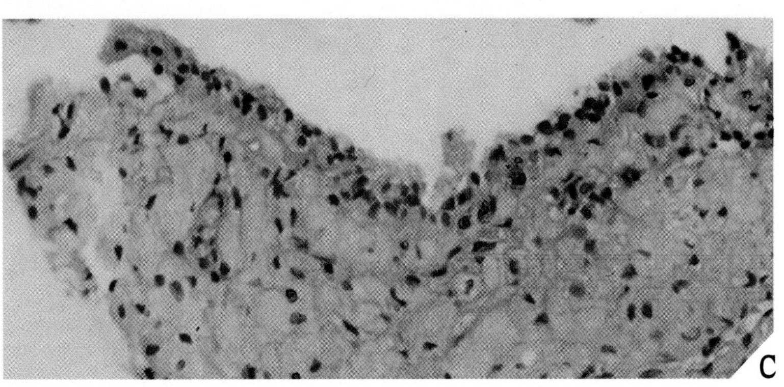

FIGURE 17.26 MELANOCYTOMA. A Melanocytoma of the optic disc characteristically is black in color, has an inferior temporal location, and contains feathered edges. Similar tumors may occur in the choroid and ciliary body. **B** A histologic section of a ciliary body melanocytoma shows that the tumor is composed of maximally pigmented nevus cells. **C** A bleached section shows benign plump polyhedral nevus cells. A melanocytoma is simply a nevus that is composed entirely of maximally pigmented polyhedral nevus cells. (**B, C**, reported by Scheie HG, Yanoff M, 1967.)

Bibliography

Carrillo R, Streeten BW: Malignant teratoid medulloepithelioma in an adult. Arch Ophthalmol 97:695, 1979.

Chang M, Zimmerman LE, McLean I: The persisting pseudomelanoma problem. Arch Ophthalmol 102:726, 1984.

Eagle RC Jr: Iris pigmentation and pigmented lesions: an ultrastructural study. Trans Am Ophthalmol Soc 86:581, 1988.

Folberg R, et al: Comparison of direct and microslide pathology measurements of uveal melanomas. Invest Ophthalmol Vis Sci 86:178, 1985.

Folberg R, McLean IW, Zimmerman LE: Conjunctival melanosis and melanoma. Ophthalmology 91:673, 1984.

Font RL, et al: Combined hamartoma of sensory retina and retinal pigment epithelium. Retina 9:302, 1989.

Gass JDM: Comparison of uveal melanoma growth rates with mitotic index and mortality. Arch Ophthalmol 103:924, 1985.

Gass JDM, et al: Bilateral diffuse uveal melanocytic proliferation in patients with occult carcinoma. Arch Ophthalmol 108:527, 1990.

Grossniklaus HE, Zimmerman LE, Kachmer ML: Pleomorphic adenocarcinoma of ciliary epithelium. Immunohistochemical and electron microscopic features. Ophthalmology 97:753, 1990.

Kivelä T, Tarkkanen A: Recurrent medulloepithelioma of the ciliary body. Immunohistochemical characteristics. Ophthalmology 95:1565, 1988.

Lauritzen K, Augsburger JJ, Timmes J: Vitreous seeding associated with melanocytoma of the optic disc. Retina 10:60, 1990.

Lloyd WC III, et al: Congenital hypertrophy of the retinal pigment epithelium. Electron microscopic and morphometric observations. Ophthalmology 97:1052, 1990.

Lieb WE, et al: Cystic adenoma of the pigmented ciliary epithelium. Clinical, pathologic and immunohistopathologic findings. Ophthalmology 97:1489, 1990.

Martin-Relay DG, Shattuck MC, Guthrie FW: Psammomatous melanotic schwannoma: an additional component of Carney's complex. Report of a case. Am J Clin Pathol 95:484, 1991.

Mooy CM, et al: Ki-67 immunostaining in uveal melanoma. The effect of pre-enucleation radiotherapy. Ophthalmology 97:1275, 1990.

Munden PM, Sobol WM, Weingeist TA: Ocular findings in Turcot syndrome (glioma-polyposis). Ophthalmology 98:111, 1991.

Nakleh RE, et al: Morphologic diversity in malignant melanomas. Am J Clin Pathol 93:731, 1990.

Naumann G, Zimmerman LE, Yanoff M: Histogenesis of malignant melanomas of the uvea. I. Histopathologic characteristics of nevi of the choroid and ciliary body. Arch Ophthalmol 76:784, 1966.

Scheie HG, Yanoff M: Pseudomelanoma of ciliary body, report of a patient. Arch Ophthalmol 77:81, 1967.

Shields JA, et al: Malignant melanoma associated with melanocytoma of the optic disc. Ophthalmology 97:225, 1990.

Teekhasaenee C, Ritch R, Leelawongs N: Ocular findings in oculodermal melanocytosis. Arch Ophthalmol 108:1114, 1990.

Traboulsi EI, et al: A clinicopathologic study of the eyes in familial adenomatous polyposis with extracolonic manifestations (Gardner's syndrome). Am J Ophthalmol 110:550, 1990.

Vogel MH, Zimmerman LE, Gass JDM: Proliferation of the juxtapapillary retinal pigment epithelium simulating malignant melanoma. Doc Ophthalmol 26:461, 1969.

Yanoff M, Fine BS: Ocular Pathology: A Text and Atlas, 2nd ed. Philadelphia, JB Lippincott, 1982.

Yanoff M, Zimmerman LE: Histogenesis of malignant melanoma of the uvea. II. Relationship of uveal nevi to malignant melanomas. Cancer 20:493, 1967.

Zimmerman LE, McLean IW: Do growth and onset of symptoms of uveal melanomas indicate subclinical metastasis? Ophthalmology 91:685, 1984.

Retinoblastoma

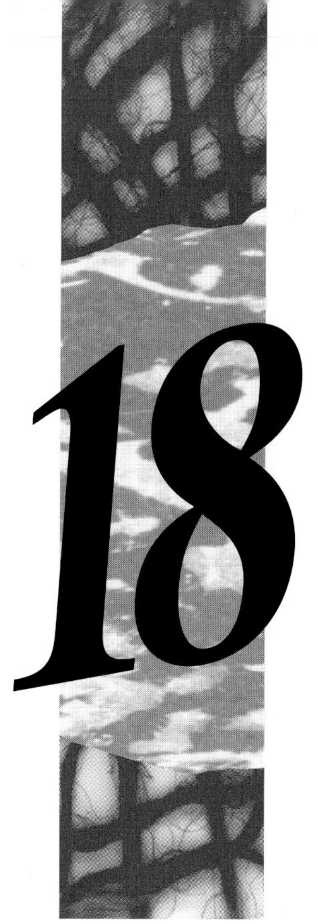

Retinoblastoma is one of the more common childhood malignancies. It is the most common malignant intraocular childhood neoplasm and follows only uveal melanomas and metastatic carcinomas as the most common human intraocular malignancy. The frequency is approximately 1 in 18,000 live births. The average age at the time of initial diagnosis is 13 months; 89% are diagnosed before 3 years of age.

Retinoblastoma in affected families behaves as an autosomal-dominant mendelian trait that has 90% penetrance and variable expressivity. The normal allele at chromosome band 13q14 acts as a mendelian dominant in inhibiting retinoblastoma development. If one of the two alleles normally found at this site is absent, as may occur in the chromosome 13 deletion syndrome, retinoblastoma will still not develop unless a second "hit" occurs that makes the individual homozygous with respect to the absence of the normal allele. Therefore, at the cellular level, retinoblastoma is inherited as an autosomal-recessive. Familial (inherited) cases constitute 10% of the total incidence of retinoblastoma; 90% of the cases are sporadic. Among the sporadic cases, 25% arise as mutations in the germ line and, therefore, will become inheritable. The rest of the cases arise as a result of mutations in the somatic (retinal) cells and cannot be inherited. Bilateral retinoblastoma and multifocal retinoblastoma in one eye generally are caused by inherited retinoblastoma. Retinoblastoma may arise simultaneously and primarily in both eyes and in the pineal gland (trilateral retinoblastoma).

At the cellular level, retinoblastomas are quite primitive and undifferentiated. Structures such as Flexner-Wintersteiner and Homer Wright rosettes, as well as fleurettes, may be found. A patient whose tumor shows abundant Flexner-Wintersteiner rosettes has about a sixfold better prognosis than a patient whose tumor has no rosettes. A tumor composed entirely of fleurettes also indicates an excellent prognosis. The mortality rate is around 25% if the tumor invades the choroid slightly; this rises to 65% when the invasion is massive. When the tumor does not invade the optic nerve, the mortality rate is approximately 8%. If invasion extends to the lamina cribosa, but not beyond, the mortality rate rises to around 15%. When the invasion is posterior to the lamina cribosa, but not in the cut end of the nerve, the mortality rate is about 44%. If the invasion is to the point of surgical transection or to the posterior point of exit of the central retinal vessels from the optic nerve, the mortality rate is about 65%. Unfortunately, even when the retinoblastoma is "cured," a significant proportion of patients will develop a second malignancy, which may prove fatal. The increased incidence of second malignancies, especially with osteosarcoma, is not necessarily related to radiation therapy from treatment of the primary retinoblastoma.

Retinoblastomas often present clinically with a "cat's eye" reflex, called leukokoria. A number of conditions may mimic retinoblastoma and also present with leukokoria; these are called pseudogliomas (the old term for retinoblastoma was glioma, hence the term pseudoglioma). The most common pseudogliomas are persistent hyperplastic primary vitreous, retinal dysplasia (most often associated with 13 trisomy—see Chapter 2), retinopathy of prematurity, toxocara endophthalmitis, and Coats disease. Not only may the pseudogliomas present with leukokoria, they also may present as small localized lesions resembling those of endophytic and exophytic retinoblastomas.

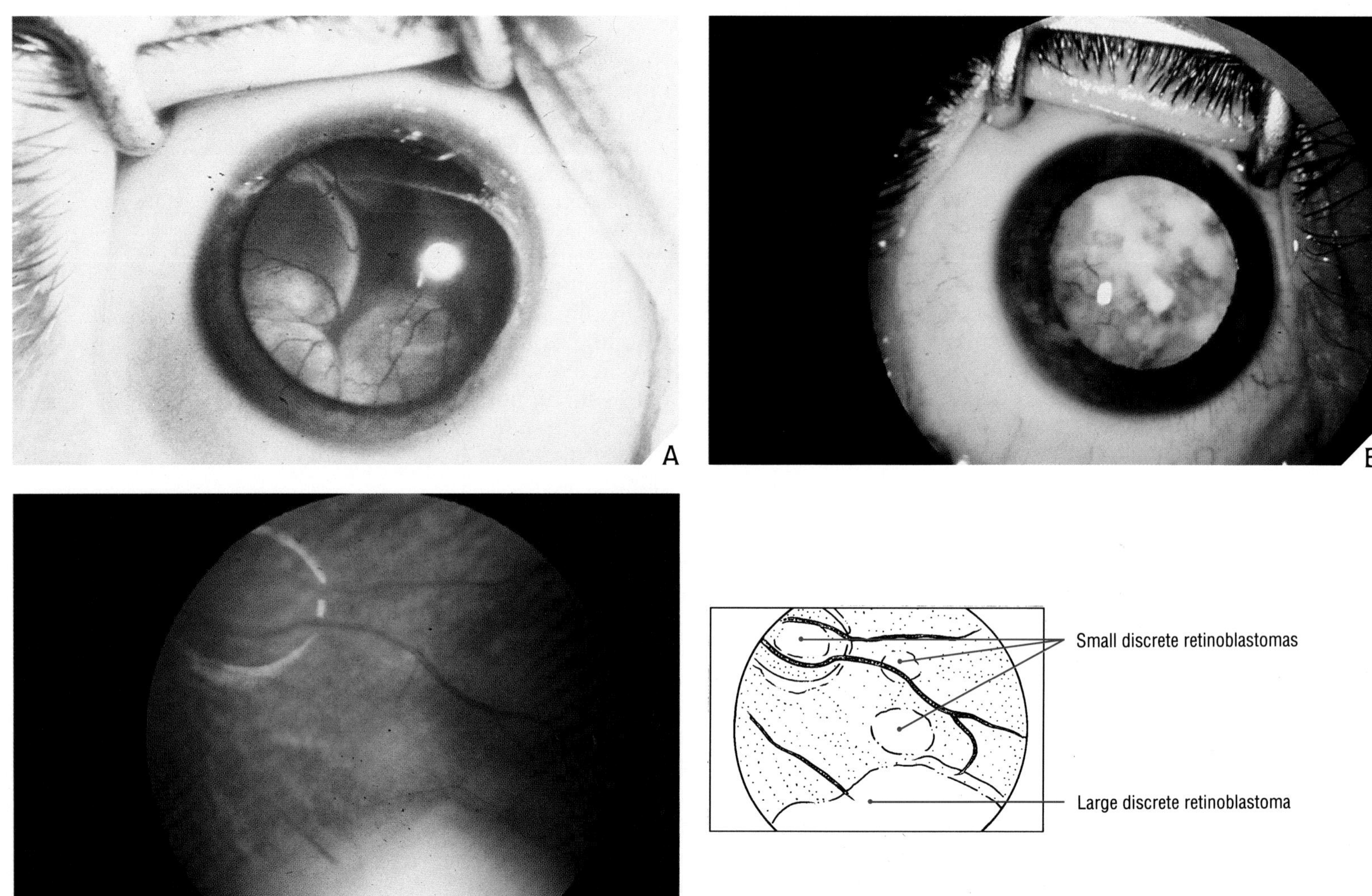

FIGURE 18.1 RETINOBLASTOMA. A Retinoblastomas may arise mainly from the external retinal layers, grow externally (exophytic growth), and cause a retinal detachment. This patient, who presented with leukokoria, had a solid tumor under the retinal detachment. **B** Retinoblastomas may grow predominantly from the inner layers of the retina (endophytic growth) into the vitreous. Their clinical appearance, as here, closely resembles that of brain tissue. Often, the retinoblastoma arises at different levels of the retina and grows both inward and outward. **C** The retinoblastoma may grow as individual discrete retinal tumors. Here we see three small tumors and one large tumor inferiorly.(**A**, **B**, courtesy of Dr. HG Scheie, from Yanoff M, Fine BS, *Ocular Pathology*, 3rd ed. **C**, courtesy of Dr. DB Schaffer.)

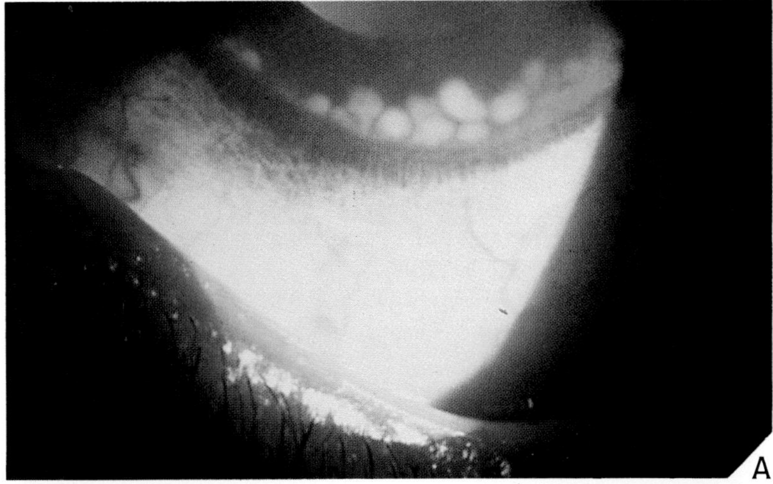

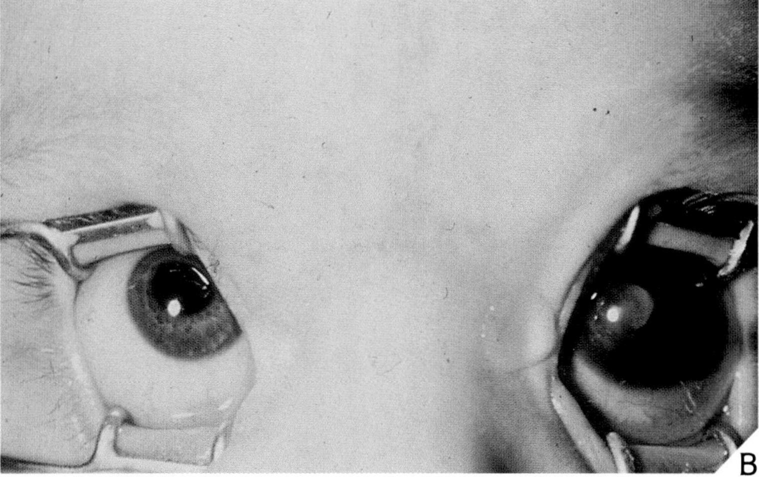

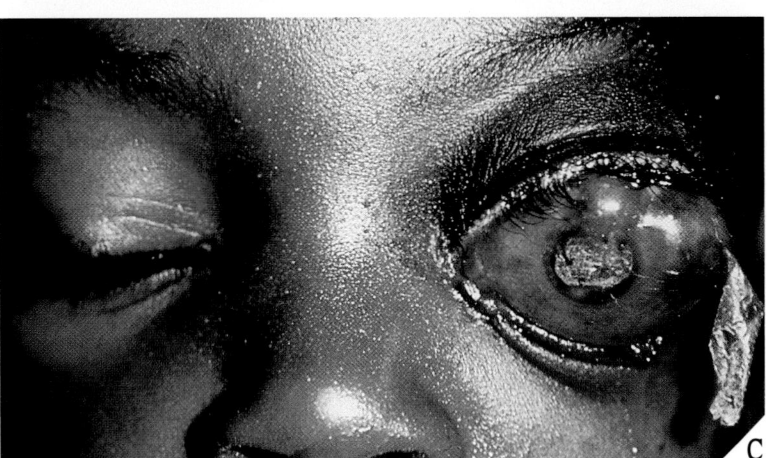

Figure 18.2 Retinoblastoma. A Retinoblastoma cells have formed balls of tumor in the anterior chamber inferiorly, simulating a hypopyon, thus "pseudohypopyon". **B** Iris neovascularization may arise secondary to the retinal process. The iris neovascularization can lead to peripheral anterior synechiae and a secondary closed-angle glaucoma. In infants, this may give rise to buphthalmos (as occurred here). **C** Rarely, an untreated retinoblastoma may invade the orbit and result in proptosis. (**A**, courtesy of Dr. AJ Shields; **B**, courtesy of Dr. HG Scheie, from Yanoff M, Fine BS, *Ocular Pathology*, 3rd ed., **C**, courtesy of Dr. RE Shannon.)

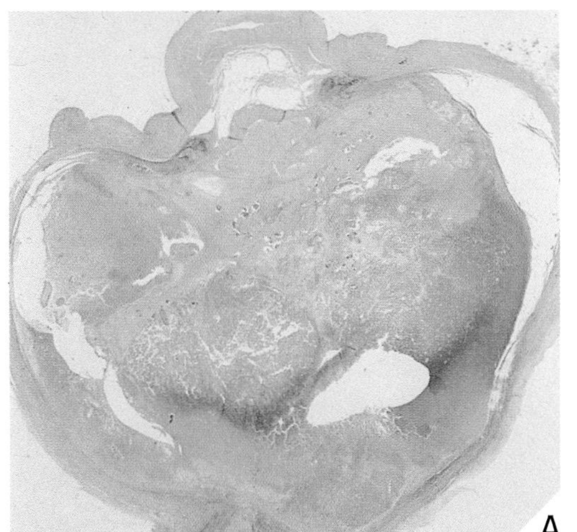

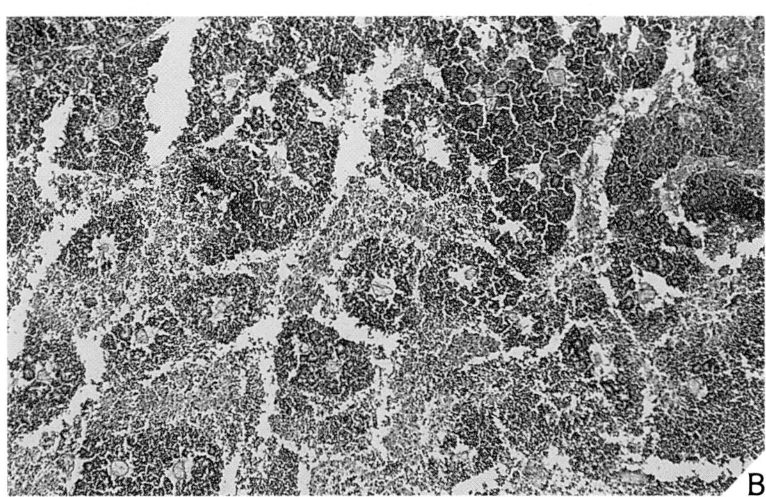

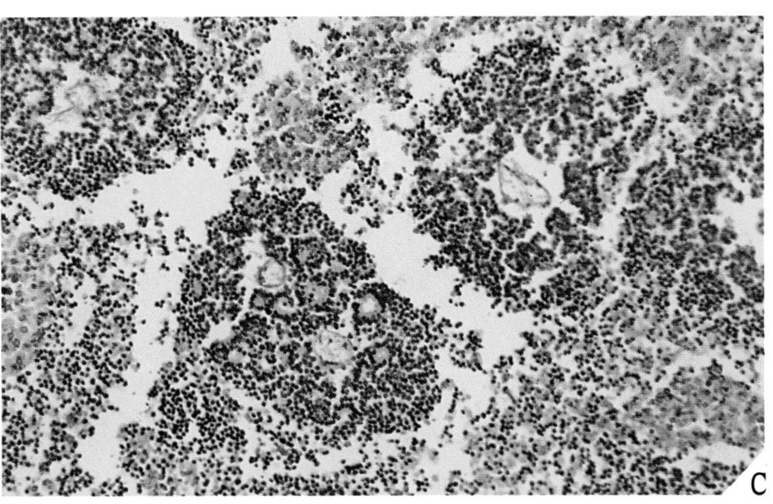

Figure 18.3 Retinoblastoma. A Characteristically, sections of retinoblastoma stained with hematoxylin and eosin and viewed under low magnification show dark blue areas surrounded by light pink areas. The dark areas represent the viable cells and calcium deposition, while the light areas represent tumor necrosis. **B** Increased magnification shows viable (dark blue) tumor cells clustered around central blood vessels and surrounded in turn by a mantle of necrotic (pink) cells. Numerous Flexner-Wintersteiner rosettes are present. **C** Further increased magnification shows the viable tumor cells around blood vessels, the necrotic areas, and the Flexner-Wintersteiner rosettes.

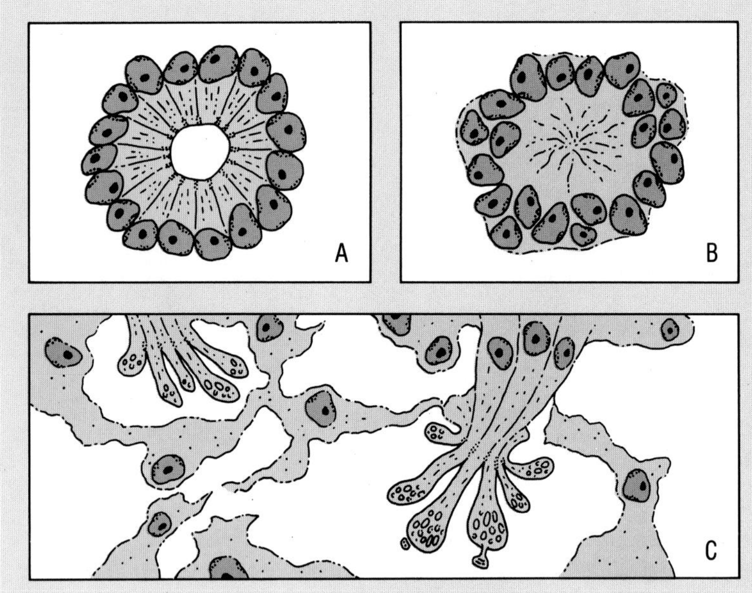

FIGURE 18.4 TYPES OF ROSETTES. A A Flexner-Wintersteiner rosette consists of a central lumen lined by cuboidal tumor cells that contain nuclei positioned basally (away from the lumen). Delicate limiting membranes are seen at the apices of the cells which surround the lumen. **B** Homer Wright rosettes are found more frequently in medulloblastomas and neuroblastomas than in retinoblastomas. In these rosettes, the cells line up around an acellular area which contains cobweb-like material. **C** Fleurettes are flower-like groupings of tumor cells within the retinoblastoma. The cells of fleurettes show clear evidence of differentiation into photoreceptor elements.

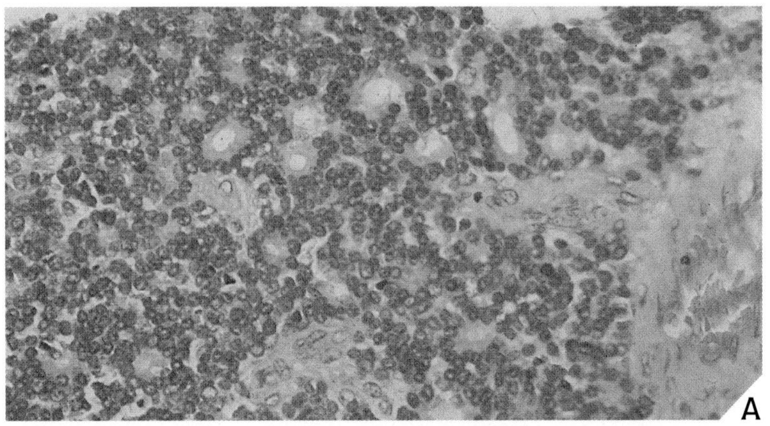

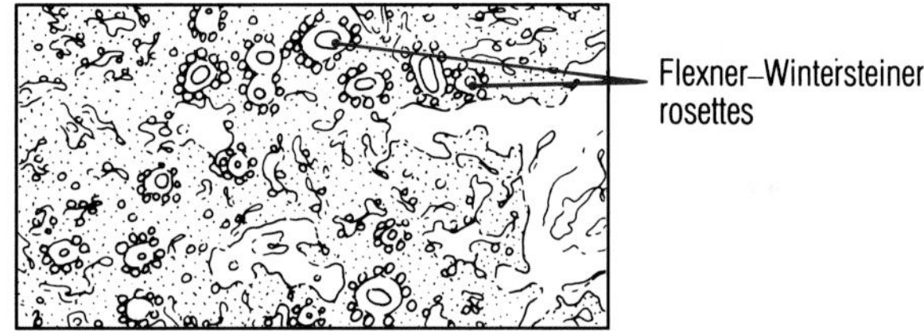

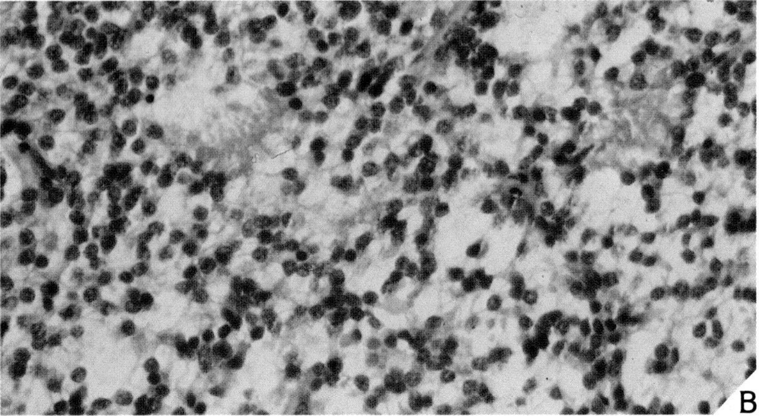

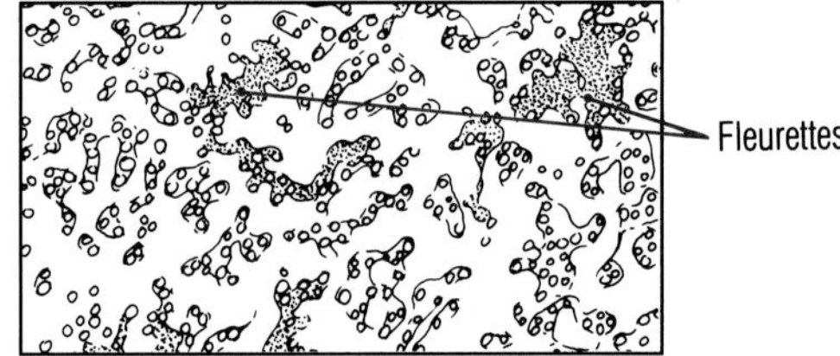

FIGURE 18.5 ROSETTES AND FLEURETTES. A Flexner-Wintersteiner rosettes show clear lumina lined by a delicate limiting membrane and cuboidal retinoblastoma cells that contain basally located nuclei. **B** In this histologic section of a retinoblastoma, almost all of the cells show photoreceptor differentiation, indicated by the pale eosinophilic cellular regions. The differentiated areas are forming fleurettes.

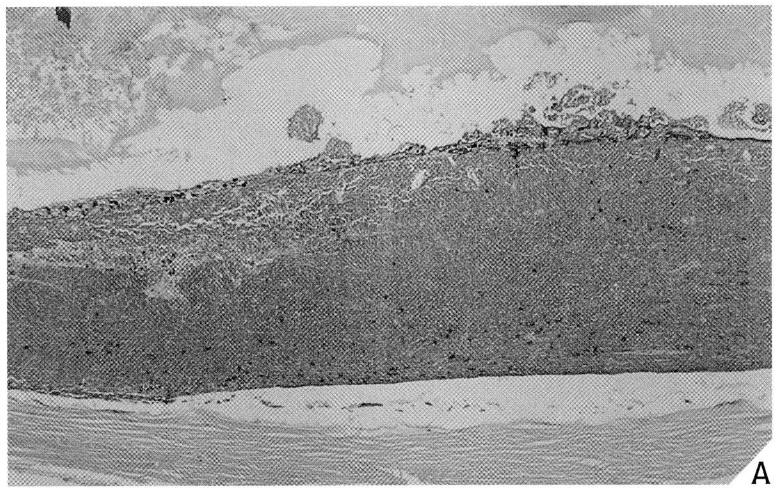

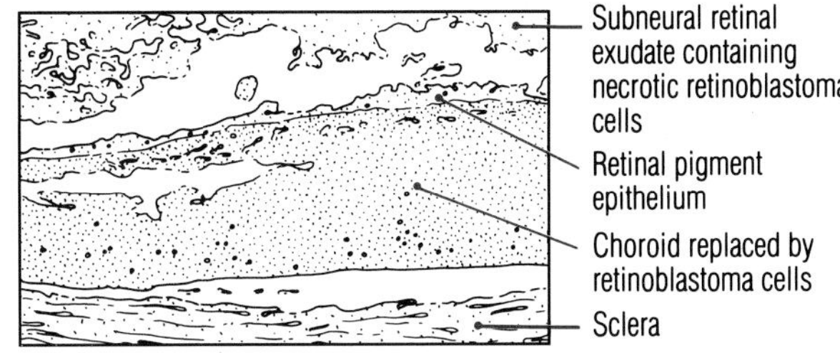

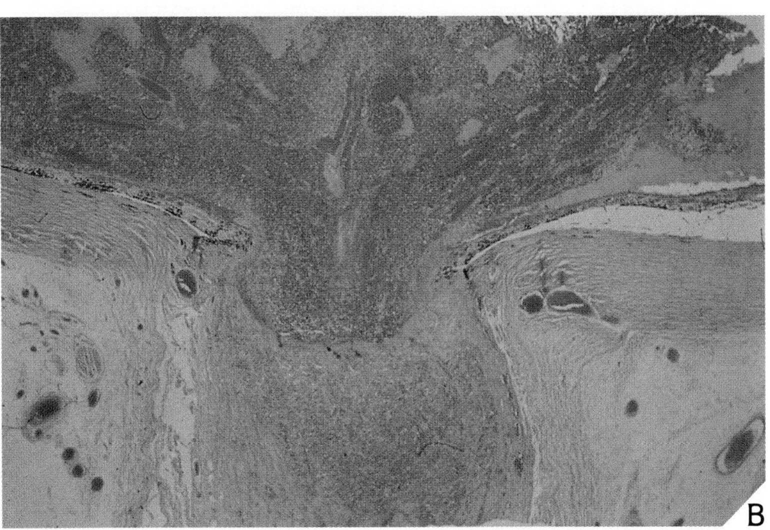

FIGURE 18.6 INVASION BY RETINOBLASTOMA. A The retinoblastoma has invaded through the Bruch membrane, massively replacing the choroid. Among patients with mild invasion of the choroid, there is a 25% mortality rate. Those with massive invasion, as shown here, have a mortality rate of about 65%. **B** The retinoblastoma has invaded the optic nerve up to the cut end. For those patients in whom the substance of the optic nerve has been invaded posterior to the lamina cribosa, the mortality rate is around 44%. If retinoblastoma is present at the cut end of the optic nerve, the mortality rate is approximately 65%.

PSEUDOGLIOMAS—LEUKOKORIA

Persistent hyperplastic primary vitreous (PHPV)
Retinal dysplasia (see Chapter 2)
Retinopathy of prematurity
Toxocara endophthalmitis
Coats disease
Norrie disease
Incontinentia pigmenti
Massive retinal fibrosis
Metastatic retinitis
Congenital nonattachment of the retina
Secondary retinal detachment
Juvenile retinoschisis (see Chapter 11)
Embryonal medulloepithelioma (see Chapter 17)

FIGURE 18.7

PERSISTENT HYPERPLASTIC PRIMARY VITREOUS

Congenital and unilateral
Present at birth
Microphthalmos
Shallow anterior chamber
Long ciliary processes
Persistent hyaloid artery
Posterior lens capsule dehiscence

FIGURE 18.8

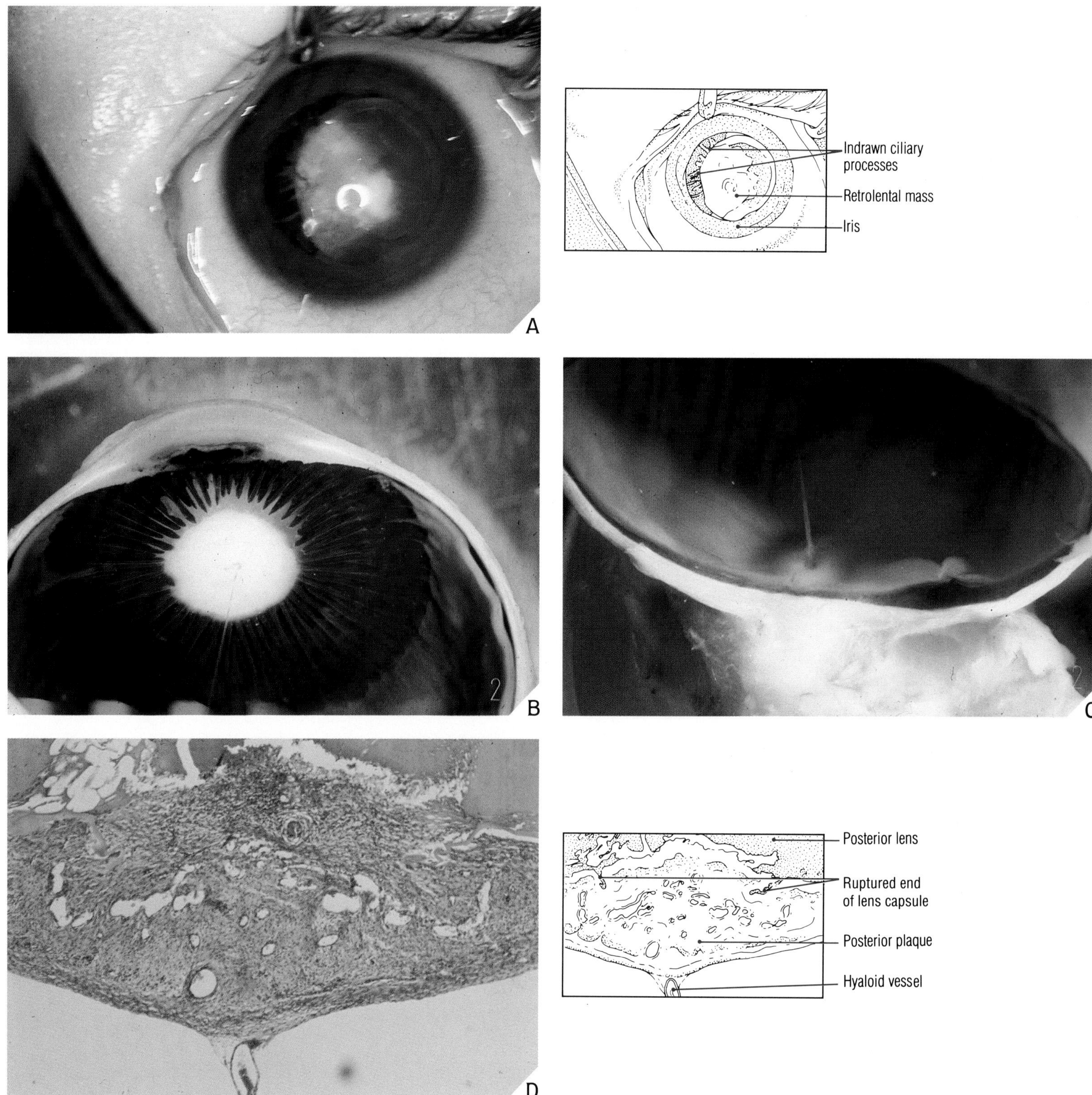

FIGURE 18.9 PERSISTENT HYPERPLASTIC PRIMARY VITREOUS (PHPV). **A** Clinically, the ciliary processes are characteristically drawn inward and a posterior lens opacity is noted. **B, C** Gross specimens of another case show a persistent hyaloid vessel and the ciliary processes stretched inward toward a posterior lens plaque (**B**); in **C** the hyaloid vessel extends to the optic nerve. **D** A histologic section shows abundant mesenchymal fibrovascular tissue just behind and within the posterior lens. Note the ends of the ruptured lens capsule. A persistent hyaloid vessel also is present. (**A**, from Yanoff M, Fine BS, *Ocular Pathology*, 3rd ed., **B, C, D**, courtesy of Dr. BW Streeten and reported in Caudill JW, et al., 1985.)

RETINOPATHY OF PREMATURITY

Not congenital*
Not present at birth
Eyes normal size at birth but may become microphthalmic

*Atypical forms may be present at birth.

Related to prematurity and oxygen administration

FIGURE 18.10

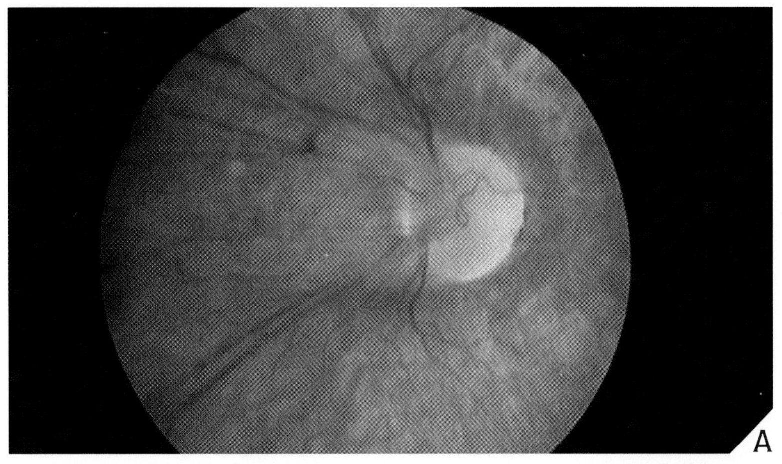

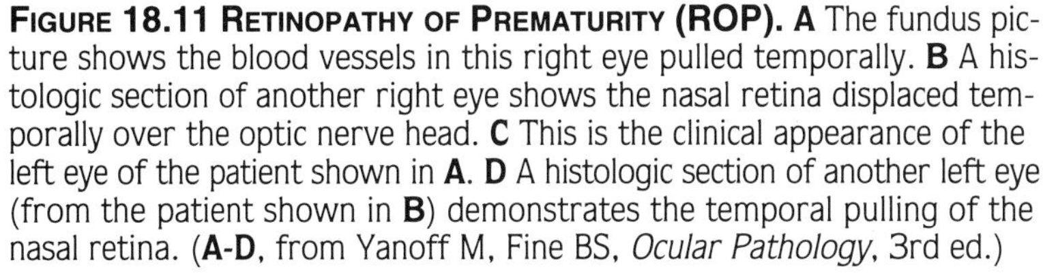

FIGURE 18.11 RETINOPATHY OF PREMATURITY (ROP). A The fundus picture shows the blood vessels in this right eye pulled temporally. **B** A histologic section of another right eye shows the nasal retina displaced temporally over the optic nerve head. **C** This is the clinical appearance of the left eye of the patient shown in **A**. **D** A histologic section of another left eye (from the patient shown in **B**) demonstrates the temporal pulling of the nasal retina. (**A-D**, from Yanoff M, Fine BS, *Ocular Pathology*, 3rd ed.)

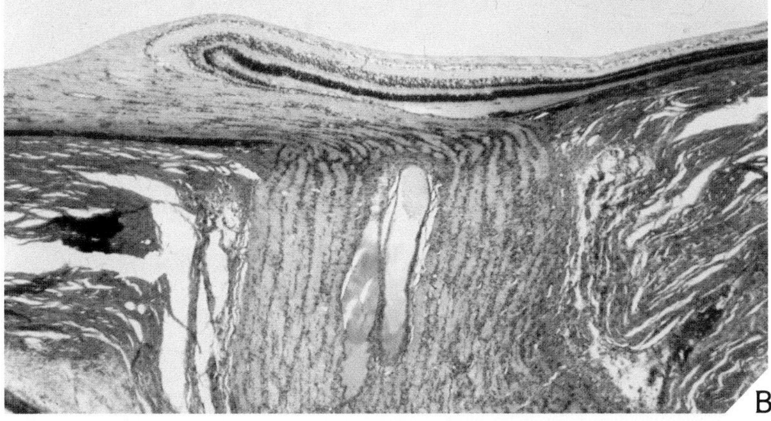

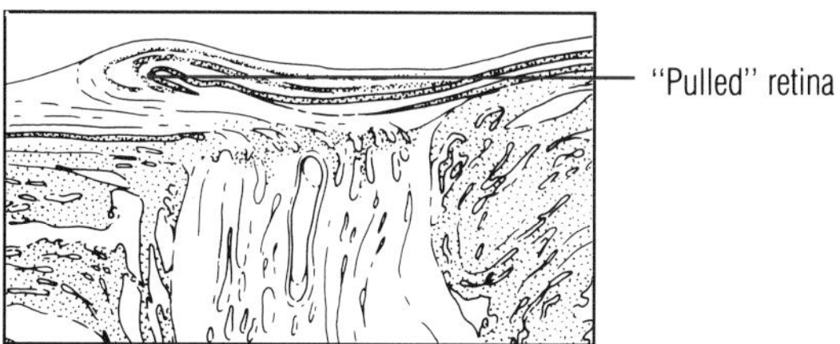

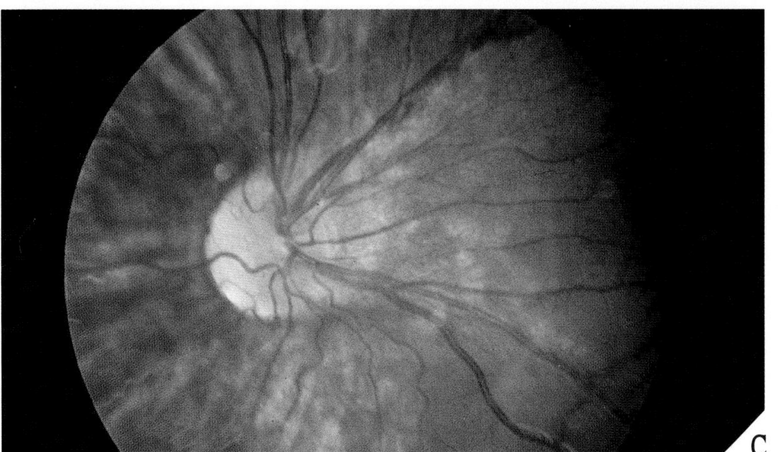

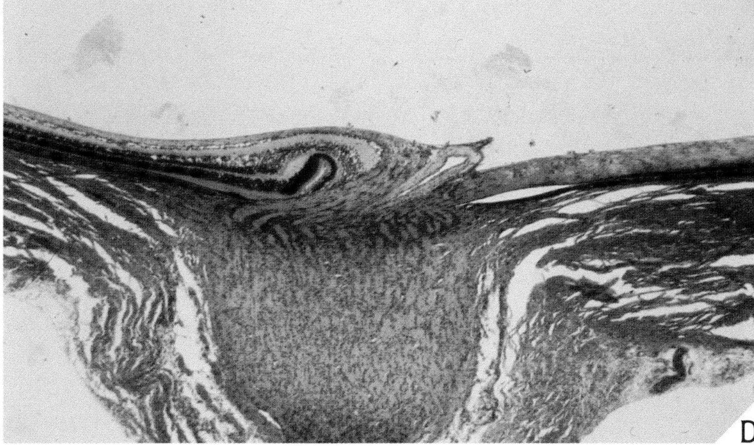

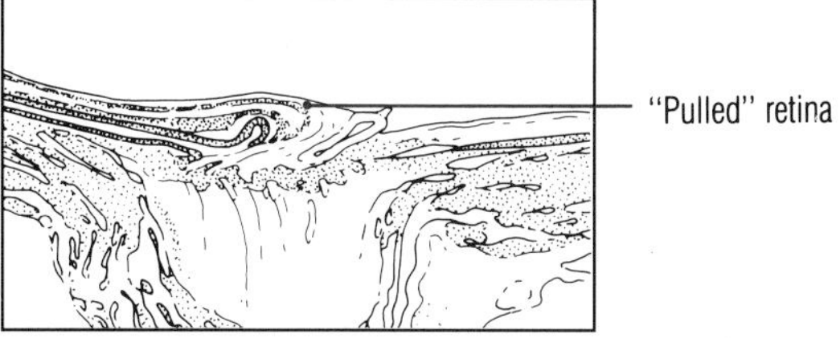

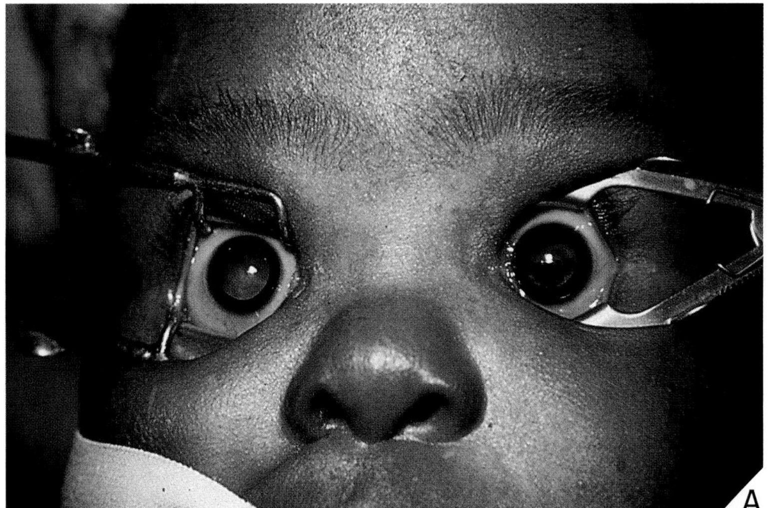

FIGURE 18.12 RETINOPATHY OF PREMATURITY. A A 6-month-old baby shows bilateral leukokoria secondary to ROP. **B** A histologic section of another eye shows the detached retina drawn by fibrovascular tissue into a mass behind the lens (hence the old term retrolental fibroplasia). **C** Neovascularization of the retina has occurred anterior to the equator, forming fibrovascular bands and causing a traction detachment of the retina. (**A**, from Yanoff M, Fine BS, *Ocular Pathology*, 3rd ed.)

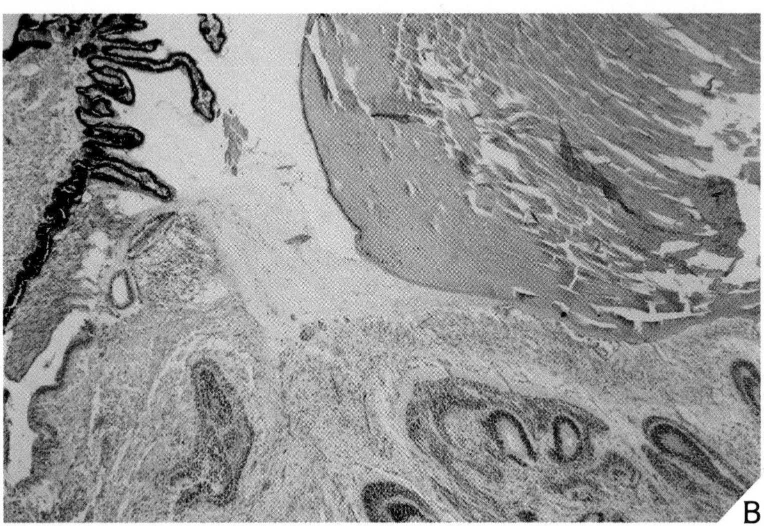

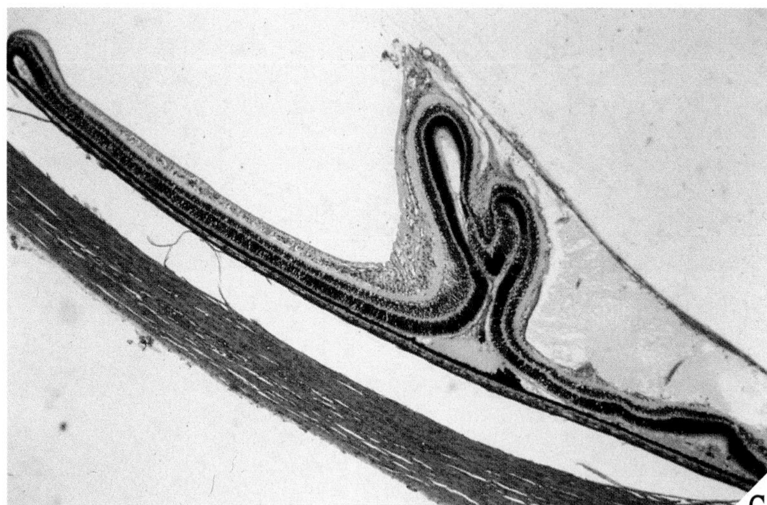

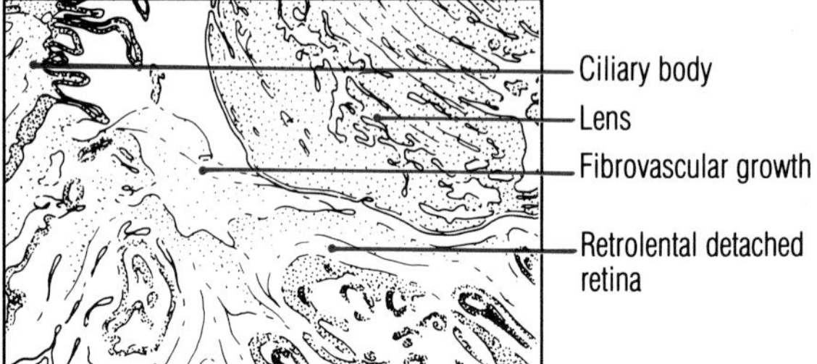

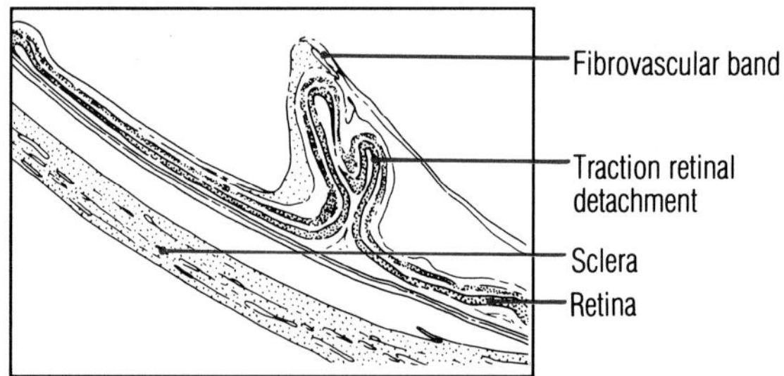

TOXOCARIASIS (*TOXOCARA CANIS*)

Ocular manifestation of visceral larva migrans
Involves children between 6 and 11 years of age
Two forms: leukokoria and discrete lesions
Zonal granulomatous reaction around eosinophilic abscess and worm

FIGURE 18.13

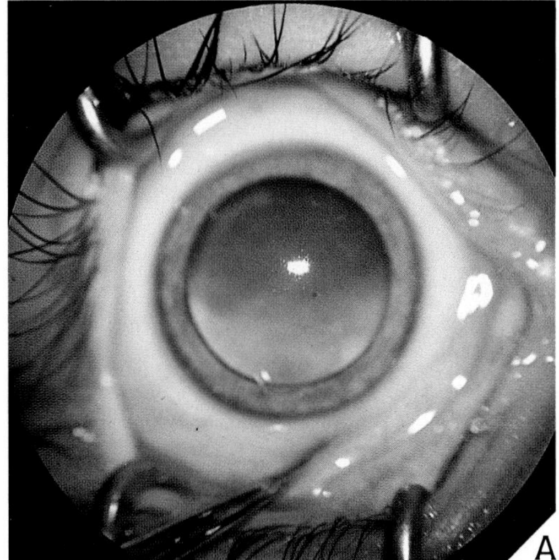
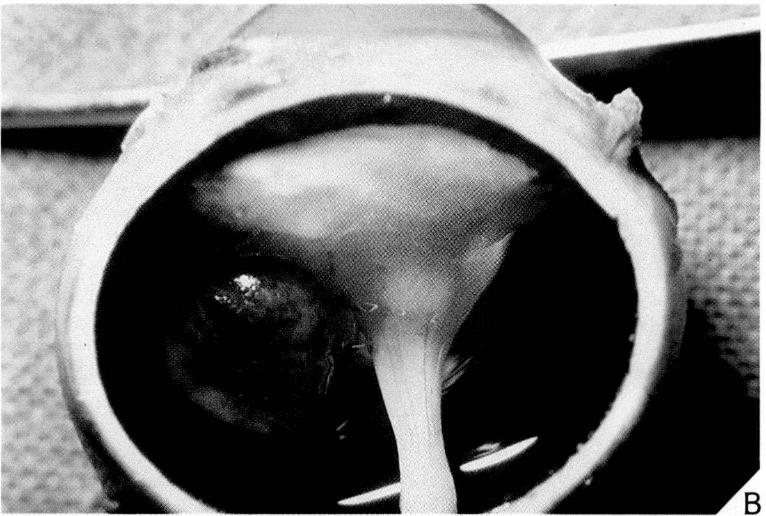
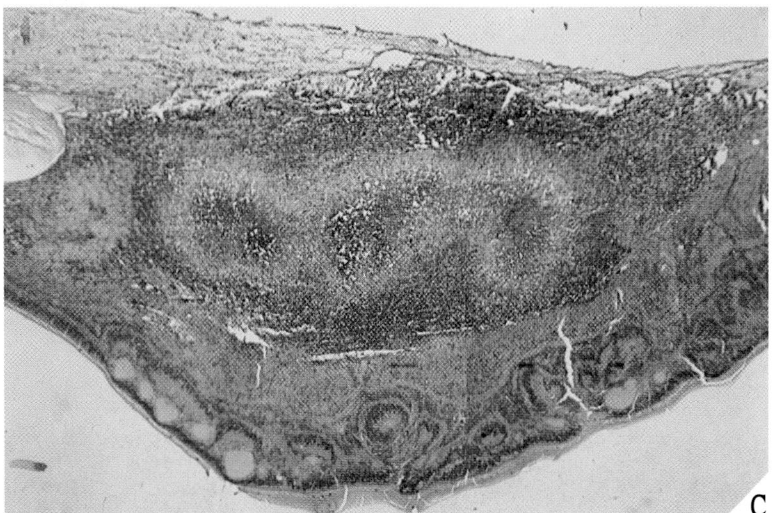
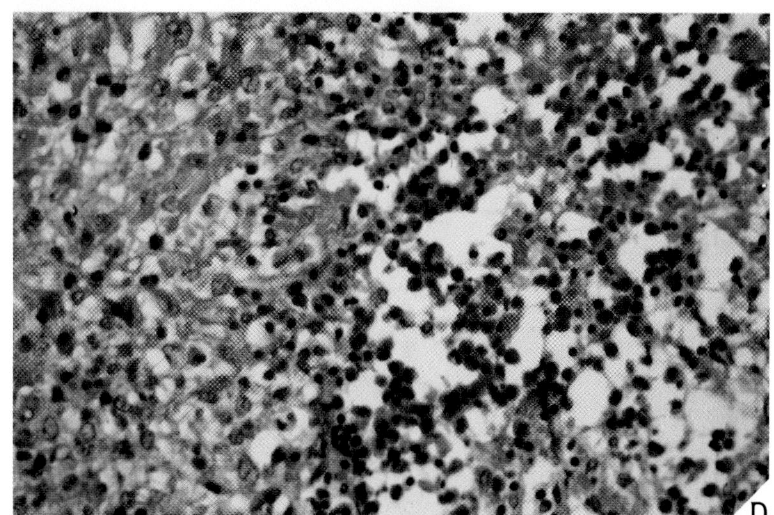

FIGURE 18.14 TOXOCARIASIS. A This 8-year-old boy presented with leukokoria. The eye was white, and other than loss of vision, no additional symptoms were present. **B** Another eye displaying leukokoria was enucleated to rule out retinoblastoma. A total retinal detachment and a peripheral retinal mass are seen. **C** A histologic section shows the peripheral retinal mass which contains an eosinophilic abscess. **D** Increased magnification shows a collection of eosinophils surrounded by a chronic granulomatous inflammatory reaction. Often, the worm itself is not found but the eosinophils are evidence of its presence prior to dissolution. Granulomas (called Splendore-Hoeppli phenomena) may develop in the eyelid, the episclera, or the conjunctiva, and are caused by different agents, including toxocariasis.

COATS DISEASE

Unilateral
Occurs mainly between the ages of 8 months and 18 years
Two-thirds occur in male children
Retinal telangiectasis is the earliest sign
Exudative bullous retinal detachment may be the end result

FIGURE 18.15

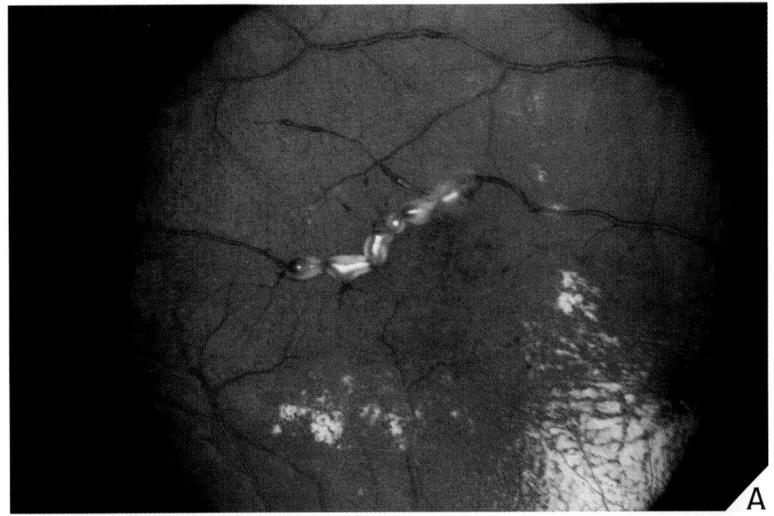

FIGURE 18.16 COATS DISEASE. A Abnormal telangiectatic retinal vessels show the typical "light bulb" appearance. These vessels leak fluid into and under the neural retina. **B** Fluorescein angiography of the same case shows the abnormal telangiectatic vessels. **C** The exudation may increase and result in an exudative retinal detachment, as occurred in this case. Note the telangiectatic vessels on the surface of the retina. **D** A histologic section of another case shows large telangiectatic vessels in the peripheral retina. The vessels have leaked fluid into the outer layers of the retina, causing a spreading and necrosis of the outer retina. **E** Increased magnification shows foamy (lipoidal) histiocytes engulfing the lipid-rich exudate in the outer layers of the retina and in the subretinal space. (**C**, from Yanoff M, Fine BS, *Ocular Pathology*, 3rd ed.)

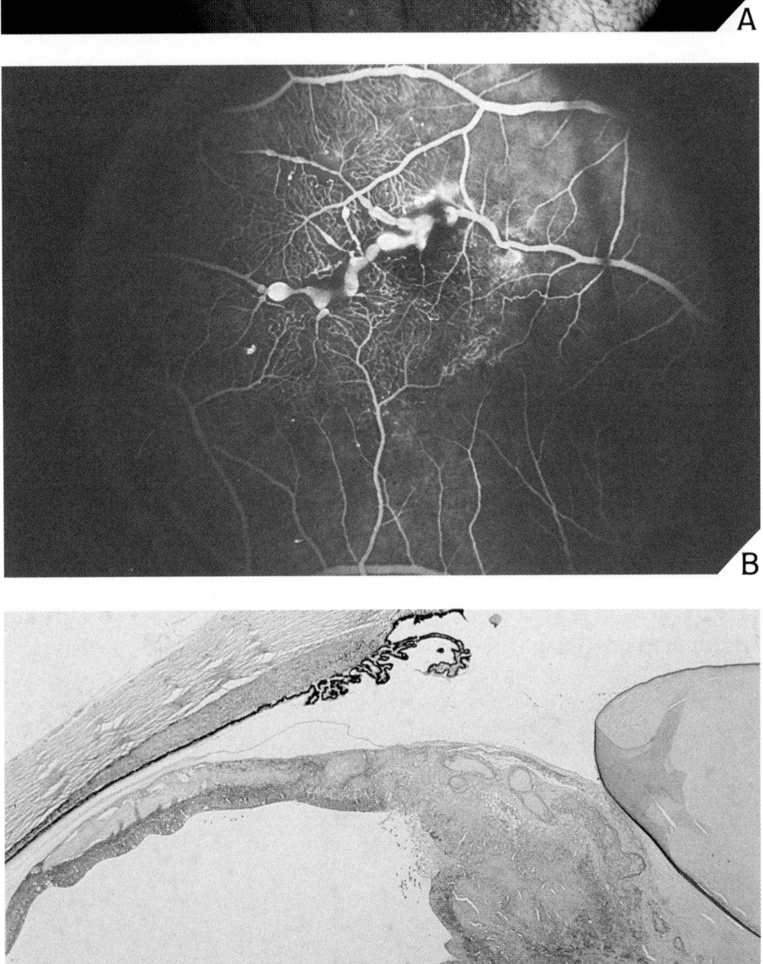

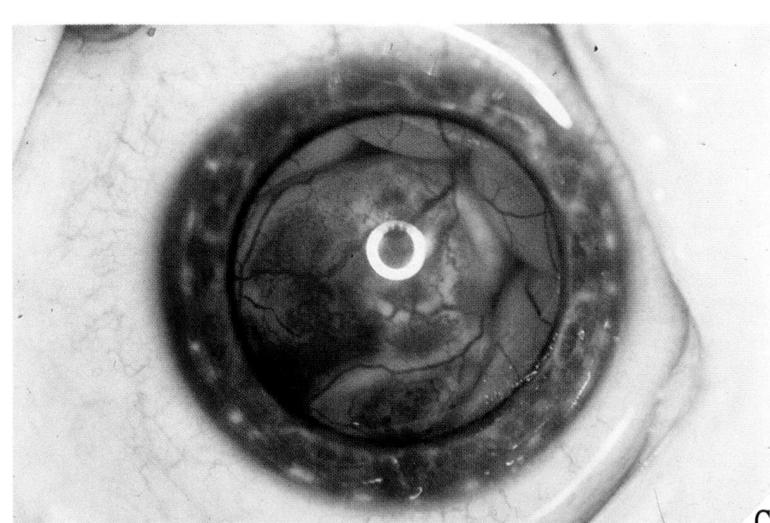

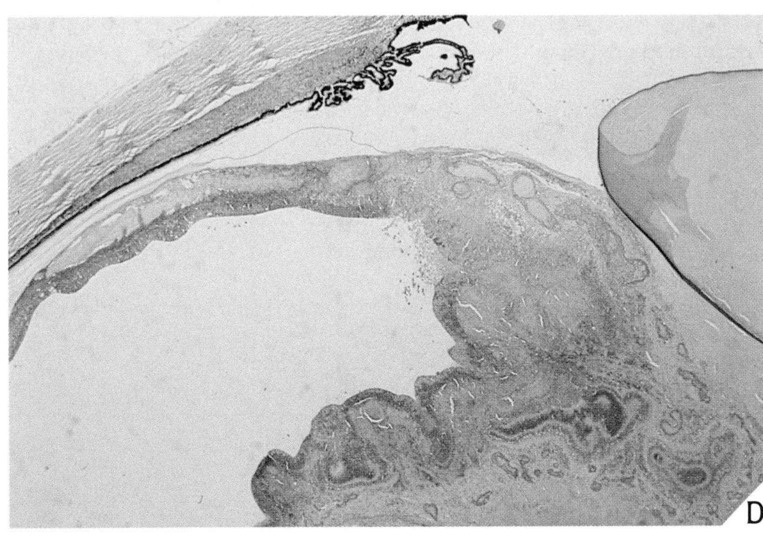

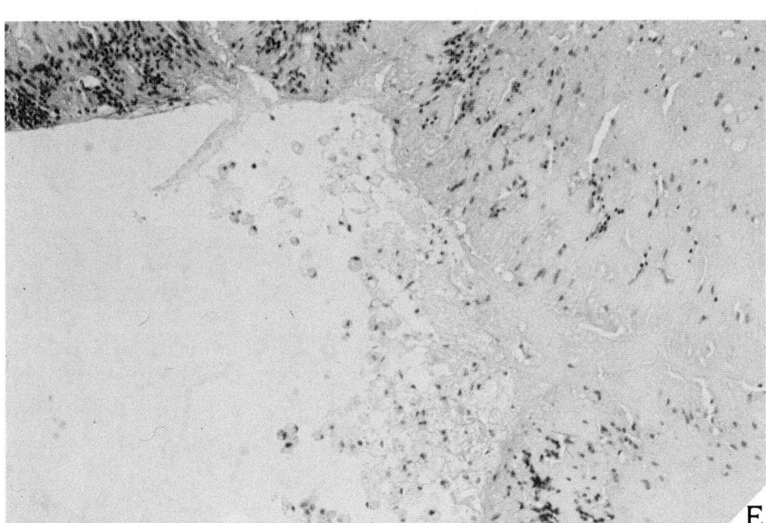

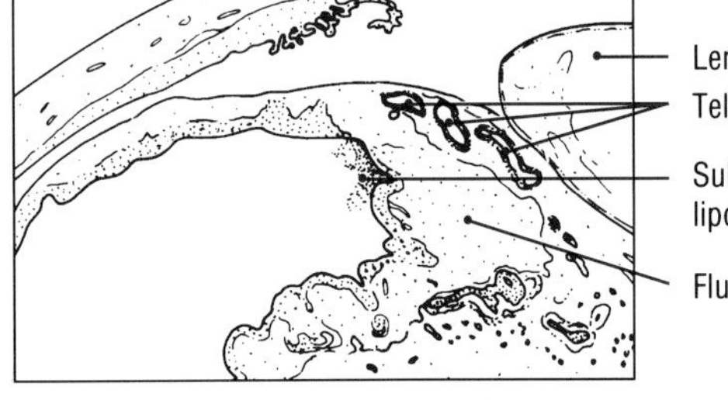

Bibliography

Ben Sira I, Nissenkorn I, Kremer I: Retinopathy of prematurity. Surv Ophthalmol 33:1, 1988.

Bunin GR, et al: Frequency of 13q abnormalities among 203 patients with retinoblastoma. J Natl Cancer Inst 81:370, 1989.

Burnier MN, et al: Retinoblastoma: the relationship of proliferating cells to blood vessels. Invest Ophthalmol Vis Sci 31:2037, 1990.

Catalano RA: Incontinentia pigmenti. Am J Ophthalmol 110:696, 1990.

Caudill JW, Streeten BW, Tso MOM: Phacoanaphylactoid reaction in persistent hyperplastic primary vitreous. Ophthalmology 92:1153, 1985.

Chang M, McLean IW, Merrit JC: Coats' disease—a study of 62 histologically confirmed cases. J Pediatr Ophthalmol Strabismus 21:163, 1984.

Enyedi LB, de Juan E, Gaitan A: Ultrastructural study of Norrie's disease. Am J Ophthalmol 111:439, 1991.

Font RL, Yanoff M, Zimmerman LE: Intraocular adipose tissue and persistent hyperplastic primary vitreous. Arch Ophthalmol 82:43, 1969.

Lawson JMM, Dart JK, McCartney ACE: Conjunctival nodules associated with Splendore-Hoeppli phenomenon. Arch Ophthalmol 109:426, 1991.

Lemieux J, et al: First cytogenic evidence of homozygosity for the retinoblastoma deletion in chromosome 13. Cancer Genet Cytogenet 43:73, 1989.

Lin CCL, Tso MOM: An electron microscopic study of calcification of retinoblastoma. Am J Ophthalmol 96:765, 1983.

Messmer EP, et al: Risk factors for metastases in patients with retinoblastoma. Ophthalmology 98:136, 1991.

Pesin SR, Shields JA: Seven cases of trilateral retinoblastoma. Am J Ophthalmol 107:121, 1989.

Scheffer H, et al: Linkage analysis of families with hereditary retinoblastoma: nonpenetrance of mutation, revealed by combined use of markers within and flanking the RBI gene. Am J Hum Genet 45:252, 1989.

Shields JA: Ocular toxocariasis. A review. Surv Ophthalmol 28:361, 1984.

Shields CL, Shields JA, Shah P: Retinoblastoma in older children. Ophthalmology 98:395, 1991.

Tamboli A, Podgor MJ, Horm JW: The incidence of retinoblastoma in the United States: 1974 through 1985. Arch Ophthalmol 108:128, 1990.

Traboulsi EI, Zimmerman LE, Manz HJ: Cutaneous malignant melanoma in survivors of heritable retinoblastoma. Arch Ophthalmol 106:1059, 1988.

Yanoff M: The rosettes of James Homer Wright (Correspondence). Arch Ophthalmol 108:167, 1990.

Yanoff M, Fine BS: Ocular Pathology: A Text and Atlas, 2nd ed. Philadelphia, JB Lippincott, 1982, and 3rd ed. 1989.

Zhu X, et al: Preferential germline mutation of the paternal allele in retinoblastoma. Nature 340:312, 1989.

INDEX

Note: Numbers in **boldface** refer to figures.